Veterinary Endocrinology
and Reproduction

Veterinary Endocrinology and Reproduction

L. E. McDONALD, D.V.M., Ph.D., Editor

Professor of Physiology and Pharmacology
University of Georgia, Athens, Georgia

M. H. PINEDA, D.V.M., Ph.D., Associate Editor

Professor of Physiology and Pharmacology
Iowa State University, Ames, Iowa

FOURTH EDITION

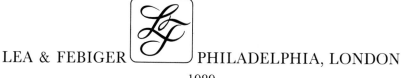

LEA & FEBIGER PHILADELPHIA, LONDON

1989

Lea & Febiger
600 Washington Square
Philadelphia, PA 19106–4198
U.S.A.
(215) 922–1330

1st Edition, 1969
Reprinted March, 1971
Reprinted April, 1974
2nd Edition, 1975
Reprinted August, 1977
Reprinted September, 1979
3rd Edition, 1980
Reprinted July, 1983
4th Edition, 1989

Library of Congress Cataloging-in-Publication Data

Veterinary endocrinology and reproduction/
  L.E. McDonald, editor; N.H. Pineda, associate editor.
  — 4th ed.
      p.   cm.
  Rev. ed. of: Veterinary endocrinology and
  reproduction/L.E. McDonald. 3rd ed. 1980.
  Includes bibliographies and index.
  ISBN 0-8121-1134-6
  1. Veterinary endocrinology.   2. Domestic animals —
Reproduction. I. McDonald, L.E. (Leslie Ernest),
1923–   . II. Pineda, M.H. III. McDonald, L.E. (Leslie
Ernest), 1923–   Veterinary endocrinology and
reproduction.
SF768.3.V48   1988
636.089′64—dc19   88-9015
                                                        CIP

PRINTED IN THE UNITED STATES OF AMERICA

Print Number: 4   3   2   1

To my Father
who had mastered the art of breeding and rearing
animals. Although he lacked an understanding of the
sciences of endocrinology and reproduction, few people
possessed his intuition concerning reproduction of farm
animals.

Preface

THIS book attempts to bring to students of veterinary medicine and animal science a concise and practical consideration of endocrinology and reproduction in domestic animals. Few college students, professional or otherwise, are faced with as much information to comprehend in such a short time as are veterinary medical students. A great deal of information is available in endocrinology and reproduction in domestic animals, but it is scattered through numerous textbooks and other sources of literature. This textbook brings together some of the literature and material available with emphasis on practical considerations and the efficient use of students' time. Often this has meant an arbitrary approach in order to condense the information available in such a form that the student obtains a background for clinical medicine.

This book is designed to serve as a textbook and not a reference book, since it is impossible for one publication to serve as both. Many references are given to guide the students should they wish further study.

We are all students—professors, clinicians, researchers, and students alike. Too often students look at their formal years of training as the culmination of their studies, but in veterinary medicine, as in other sciences, they have only begun their studies. It is hoped that the students using this textbook will be sufficiently motivated to continue their education throughout the rest of their professional life.

A detailed outline is presented at the beginning of each chapter, and the reader is encouraged to spend some time studying this outline before delving into the chapter proper. Only by an orderly cataloging of information are we able to recall and use such material. Consequently, it is felt that the outline will give the student an overview of the material so he can comprehend and tie together the information as it is presented.

Whenever possible, the example used is drawn from domestic animals in order to demonstrate and discuss the principle under consideration. On some occasions the laboratory animal or the primate is a better model. Sometimes the information sought is available only for species other than the domestic animal; consequently, these species must be used. Nonetheless, wherever possible the domestic animal is stressed.

Special attention has been given to the five domestic farm species and the two companion species, the dog and the cat. The veterinarian is called upon to treat many other species, and it is with some reluctance that this book has been limited in its scope. On the other hand, the student must be protected at this stage of his training from becoming confused with the many species differences. At this stage there must be some emphasis on concepts and principles with a moderate application in other species, and it is hoped that a basic understanding will prepare the student for further training if his interest lies in other species.

This edition makes a major change in contributing authorship. New information is accumulating so rapidly that a multiauthored textbook became necessary. Also, specialization in the profession warrants an even more in-depth presentation. Doctors Capen and Martin have undertaken a complete revision of the chapters on the pituitary and the thyroid. Their extensive experience in these areas brings more depth as well as clinical information.

Doctors Hsu and Crump have expanded the presentation on the endocrine pancreas as well as the adrenal cortex. Dr. Pineda has increased our coverage in the female reproduction chapter which is the basis of much of the presentation which follows for the individual species. Doctors Hopkins and Evans have had considerable experience in artificial insemination so their expansion of that chapter is welcomed.

Dr. Hopkins revised the chapter on cattle reproduction. His experience in this area qualified him to update this important chapter. Dr. Pineda expanded the chapter on reproduction of sheep to include goats since goats are becoming more important to the practicing veterinarian. Dr. Evans is well qualified to revise the chapter on swine reproduction. Reproduction of swine is becoming more important to the practitioner because of the rapid changes occurring in swine husbandry.

Dr. Pineda has thoroughly updated the chapters on reproduction in dogs and cats. This is one of the most rapidly advancing areas and the veterinarian needs access to new information and concepts.

Embryo transfer continues as one of the newer areas for application of modern techniques and information. Doctors Bowen and Pineda bring a wealth of first-hand experience in their authorship of this chapter.

It is with pleasure that I welcome Dr. Pineda as a co-editor of this edition. He has helped a great deal in this effort.

L.E. McDonald

Athens, Georgia

Acknowledgments

The authors of Chapters 5–10, 12, 14–17, and 19 are indebted to Ms. Marlene Bauman and Ms. Glenda Burkheimer for typing the revisions for those chapters. Special thanks are extended to Dr. Michael P. Dooley and Mr. Gary C. Althouse for their editorial assistance and valuable comments.

Contributors

R.A. BOWEN, D.V.M., Ph.D.
Assistant Professor of Physiology and Biophysics
College of Veterinary Medicine and Biomedical Sciences
Colorado State University
Fort Collins, Colorado

C.C. CAPEN, D.V.M., M.Sc., Ph.D.
Professor and Chairman, Department of Pathobiology
Professor of Endocrinology
College of Veterinary Medicine
The Ohio State University
Columbus, Ohio

M.H. CRUMP, D.V.M., M.S., Ph.D.
Associate Professor of Physiology
Department of Veterinary Physiology and Pharmacology
College of Veterinary Medicine
Iowa State University
Ames, Iowa

L.E. EVANS, D.V.M., M.S., Ph.D.
Professor of Veterinary Clinical Sciences
Chairman, Department of Veterinary Clinical Sciences
College of Veterinary Medicine
Iowa State University
Ames, Iowa

S.M. HOPKINS, D.V.M.
Associate Professor of Veterinary Clinical Sciences
College of Veterinary Medicine
Iowa State University
Ames, Iowa

W.H. HSU, B.V.M., Ph.D.
Professor of Pharmacology
Department of Veterinary Physiology and Pharmacology
College of Veterinary Medicine
Iowa State University
Ames, Iowa

L.E. McDONALD, D.V.M., Ph.D.
Professor of Physiology and Pharmacology
College of Veterinary Medicine
University of Georgia
Athens, Georgia

S.L. MARTIN, D.V.M., M.Sc.
Professor, Department of Veterinary Clinical Sciences
College of Veterinary Medicine
The Ohio State University
Columbus, Ohio

M.H. PINEDA, D.V.M., M.S., Ph.D.
Professor of Physiology Department of Veterinary Physiology and Pharmacology
College of Veterinary Medicine
Iowa State University
Ames, Iowa

Contents

Introduction

L. E. McDonald and C. C. Capen

1

ENDOCRINOLOGY and reproductive physiology have been rapidly growing areas in the broad field of domestic animal physiology. From the philosophical point of view, the main purposes of the animal industry are to develop an animal which will grow and reproduce at a fast and economical rate. Since the *growth* and the *reproductive processes* are primarily *under endocrine control*, it follows that these areas of physiology are becoming increasingly important. As a part of a larger perspective, one should also look at the development of a sound animal agriculture as contributing a great deal to the health and economic well-being of mankind. It is more than significant that only in countries that have developed a sound animal agriculture does one find a high standard of living for their citizens. To maintain and improve this standard, we must continually seek to improve the efficiency of animal production. This relationship and dependence of man on his domestic animals date back to early historic times when the animal served not only as a source of food and protection, but also as a beast of burden. For the most part the latter role has been assumed by machines, but with an increasing human population, the competition of man for food of animal origin is increasing.

Endocrinology has the important position of being able to correlate anatomy, physiology, genetics and biochemistry and is able to prepare the student to look at the organism in its entirety with emphasis on a special system much as during the clinical years. It is hoped students will be able to correlate several of their previously studied disciplines throughout endocrinology and reproductive physiology.

DEFINITION OF HORMONE

Endocrinology is an outgrowth from the broad field of physiology much as has been the case with biochemistry. It is truly a twentieth century science, since most of the advances have been made this century and this new knowledge has led to the development of an exciting area in medicine. The *endocrine glands are those ductless glands* of the body whose secretion goes directly into the blood stream which is in contrast to the exocrine glands whose secretion is carried away by a duct. One organ of the body, *the pancreas, contains both an endocrine and an exocrine portion* (Table 1-1). The endocrine portion is composed of the islets of Langerhans whose two major secretory products (or hormones) are

1

Table 1-1   Classification of the Pancreas

Organ	Gland Type	Tissue	Secretion
Pancreas	*Endocrine* or ductless or internal secretion	Islets of Langerhans 1. Alpha cells 2. Beta cells	Glucagon (Hyperglycemic hormone) Insulin (Hypoglycemic hormone)
	Exocrine or duct or external secretion	Acinar cells	Digestive enzymes

glucagon and insulin. In addition, the pancreas has an exocrine portion which is made up of the acinar cells which secrete pancreatic juice, including a number of digestive enzymes which are carried to the gut by the pancreatic duct. Those substances secreted by the endocrine gland have been named *hormones* and are concerned with chemical adjustments throughout the body. Endocrinology has been defined as a *science concerned with chemical integration of the body.* Integration is a key word and as the student already knows, this is a function shared with the nervous system. There are important interrelationships between the nervous and endocrine systems which will be dealt with in greater detail.

Hormone is a Greek word meaning "I stir up or stimulate" and was first used by Bayliss and Starling in 1902.[5] *A hormone is a chemical substance produced in one part of the body (restricted area) that diffuses or is transported to another area where it influences activity and tends to integrate component parts of the organism.* It should be pointed out that *hormones regulate* (decrease or increase) the rates of specific processes but do not contribute energy to the process or initiate metabolic reactions. Instead, hormones influence rates of existing reactions which usually involve activity of enzymes. Consequently an excess of hormone may be as detrimental as a deficiency, since an existing reaction could be stimulated to excess. Starling's original definition of a hormone must now be broadened to include other "local hormones" or parahormones. These chemical messengers or regulators which are not hormones in the strictest sense include (1) prostaglandins, present in many tissues, but having important

local effects on reproduction, (2) erythropoietin, released by the anoxic kidney and stimulating bone marrow production of red blood cells, and (3) histamine, produced by injured tissues and acting locally on the surrounding tissue.

HISTORICAL BACKGROUND

The writings of Hippocrates and Aristotle as early as 460 to 322 B.C. contain information that there might be internal control over some of the functions of the body. Aristotle described the effects of castration in birds and man although there was no understanding of the mechanism involved. It was another two thousand years before the records indicate much insight into the actual mechanisms involved. As early as 1775 Bordeu claimed that the testis formed a substance which became bloodborne and affected the animal. In 1849 Berthold began the first experiments involving castration.[6] By *castration* of cockerels and *transplantation of the testis* of others, he was able to identify the testicular graft as being the organ responsible for normal sexual behavior and development of the accessory sex organs. He also demonstrated that the atrophic comb of the capon was due to a lack of the humoral substance from the excised testis. A memorable year in endocrinology was 1899, since it witnessed the report by the French physician Brown-Sequard that he had accomplished self-rejuvenation at the age of 72 by self-injection of aqueous extracts of dog testes. It is now known that this could not have been possible; he more than likely was experiencing psychological rejuvenation by his antics. Nevertheless, this report stimulated additional investigation. In 1889, Von Mering and Minkowski reported the historic finding that a disease, later to be known as *diabetes mellitus*, could be produced in the dog after surgical removal of the pancreas.[23] This important finding led to the recognition of *insulin* and with it the control of diabetes mellitus in man and animals.

Twentieth century endocrinology got off to a good start by the experiments of Bayliss and Starling published in 1902.[5] They found that a hormone, *secretin*, was released by the duodenal mucosa following the emptying of the acid ingesta from the stomach. Secretin was found to be carried by the circulation to the pancreas where it caused a discharge of pancreatic juice into the pancreatic duct. This was one of the first observations that the endocrine system could bring about an *integrative act* without the help of the nervous system. This also led Bayliss and Starling to coin the word *hormone* for their newly discovered substance, secretin.

The first quarter of this century was characterized by findings which showed that a specific endocrine organ influenced a particular reaction and that the mediator was a humoral substance. It was not until the second quarter of this century that identification of these humoral substances began to occur. Their identification was dependent upon development of proper biochemical techniques for their extraction and identification. The identification and synthesis of various hormones during the last 50 years has been an exciting story. Perhaps the pinnacle of this excitement came in 1949 when Hench and co-workers announced that a hormone from the adrenal cortex, *cortisone* or compound E, had relieved some of the clinical symptoms of rheumatoid arthritis.[14] This announcement set off a race in the pharmaceutical industry to attempt to synthesize this hormone in quantities sufficient for medical use. Microorganisms were used to effect enzymatic changes in steroid molecules in order to produce cortisone. The Mexican yam provided a steroid from which progesterone could easily be produced and then the

step from progesterone to cortisone was made with the aid of microbial oxygenation. Not only is cortisone readily available today at reasonable prices, but other steroids, which are unnatural to the animal body, such as prednisolone, have been produced which do an even better job than the natural substances, hydrocortisone (cortisol) or corticosterone.

Another example of the advancements in endocrinology and medicine was the discovery in 1953 by Simpson and Tait that the unidentified steroid present in extracts from the adrenal gland was *aldosterone*. One of the reasons for its late discovery was that it was so potent that only microgram quantities were present and more sophisticated techniques had to be employed in order to recover it. This is the hormone responsible for much of the endocrine regulation of *water and electrolyte metabolism*.

Although Banting and Best isolated potent extracts containing insulin as early as 1921,[4] it was *not until 1926 that Abel prepared insulin in crystalline form* and described its polypeptide nature. The exocrine portion of the pancreas contained a proteolytic enzyme which readily destroyed the endocrine secretion, insulin, thereby complicating isolation. It was not until 1954 that Sanger and his colleagues were able to elucidate the chemical structure of insulin.

In 1955 Staub et al. crystallized a hyperglycemic substance from the *islets of Langerhans* and named it *glucagon*.[20] Its amino acid sequence was determined by Bromer in 1957.[7] This was in addition to the already discovered hypoglycemic substance, *insulin*.

In 1978, insulin was synthesized by a strain of genetically engineered *E. coli*, another milestone in biology. Genetically engineered bacteria can produce bovine somatotropin (growth hormone) which is identical to the natural hormone. Daily injections can increase lactation in the cow as much as 20 to 40%.[6a] Du Vigneaud and his coworkers in 1953 determined the structure of *oxytocin* and *vasopressin* which are polypeptide hormones from the posterior pituitary.[10]

Table 1-2 Hormones of the Hypothalamus and the Pituitary Gland

	Hormone	Site of Action (target organ)	Biologic Activity
Hypothalamus	Gonadotropin releasing hormone (GnRH)	Anterior pituitary (AP)	Release LH and FSH
	Thyrotropin releasing hormone (TRH)	AP	Release TSH
	Corticotropin releasing hormone (CRH)	AP	Release ACTH
	Somatotropin releasing hormone (STH-RH)	AP	Release STH
	Somatotropin release-inhibiting hormone (STH-RIH)	AP	Inhibit STH output
	Prolactin inhibitory hormone (PIH)	AP	Inhibit prolactin output
	Prolactin releasing hormone (PRH)	AP	Release prolactin
Adenohypophysis — Pars distalis (anterior lobe)	Somatotropin (STH, growth hormone)	General soma	Body growth (bone, muscle, organs), protein synthesis, carbohydrate metabolism, regulation of renal functions (GFR) and water metabolism. Increase cell permeability to amino acids. Lactation facilitation
	Adrenocorticotropic hormone (ACTH, corticotropin)	Adrenal cortex	Maintenance of structural integrity of adrenal cortex, regulation of glucocorticoid secretion by zona fasciculata
	Thyrotropic hormone (TSH, thyrotropin)	Thyroid	Maintenance of the normal structure and function of the thyroid gland. Production of thyroxine and analogues
	Prolactin (lactogenic hormone)	Mammary gland	Possibly favoring lactation
	Gonadotropins — Follicle-stimulating hormone (FSH)	Ovary	Growth and maturation of ovarian follicles
		Testis seminiferous tubules	Germ-cell production (spermatogenesis)
	Gonadotropins — Interstitial cell-stimulating or luteinizing hormone (ICSH, LH)	Ovary	Synergistically with FSH causing estrogen secretion, follicle maturation, and ovulation. Corpus luteum development in some species
		Testis Leydig cells	Stimulation of interstitial tissue, androgen secretion
Pars intermedia	Intermedin (melanocyte-stimulating hormone, MSH)	Melanophore cells of amphibia and reptiles	Melanophore-expanding activity with resultant maintenance of skin color (in mammals, of negligible importance)
Neurohypophysis	Antidiuretic hormone (ADH, vasopressin)	Renal tubules (distal convoluted)	Regulation of water excretion by reabsorption of water. Pressor effect only in high doses
	Oxytocic hormone	Mammary myoepithelium	Letdown of milk by contraction of myoepithelium
		Uterine myometrium	Contraction of uterine musculature to aid parturition and sperm transport

Each year we see new information forthcoming on the structure and function of additional or existing hormones. It would appear that the discovery of additional hormones would be coming to an end, but this does not seem to be the case. Certainly the determination of the exact structure of all the hormones and finally their synthesis in the laboratory will serve to clarify many of the difficult spots in endocrinology.

Refer to Tables 1-2 and 1-3 for the classification and actions of the hormones.

Table 1-3 Nonpituitary Hormones

Gland	Hormone	Some Principal Functions and Effects
Thyroid	Thyroxine and Tri-iodothyronine (T_4, T_3)	Increase BMR, O_2 consumption. Growth, maturation, and function of all cells.
	Calcitonin	Lowers blood calcium by slowing bone resorption.
Parathyroid	Parathyroid Hormone (PTH) Parathormone	Calcium and phosphorus metabolism via skeleton and/or kidney.
Islets of Langerhans	Insulin	Lower blood glucose by storage or utilization. Also fat & protein metabolism.
	Glucagon	Elevates blood glucose by favoring liver glycogenolysis.
Adrenal Medulla	Epinephrine	Glycogenolysis to raise blood glucose.
	Norepinephrine	Increase cardiovascular function. Pressor effects mainly.
Adrenal Cortex	Glucocorticoids (cortisol) (cortisone) (corticosterone)	Gluconeogenesis. Decrease peripheral glucose utilization. Anti-inflammatory effect. Anti-allergic effect. Euphoric effect.
	Aldosterone	Electrolyte and water metabolism.
Ovary	Estrogens (estradiol) (estrone) (others)	Development, maintenance, and cyclic changes of female tubular genital tract. Glandular duct development of mammae and uterus. Secondary sex characteristics. Behavior. Accessory sex organs. Calcium and fat metabolism of birds.
	Progesterone	With estrogen develops uterus for implantation and pregnancy maintenance. Mammary and uterine gland development.
	Relaxin	Dissolution of symphysis pubis and relaxes pelvic tissues.
Testis	Testosterone	Development of accessory sex organs and secondary sex characteristics. Behavior. Spermatogenesis. Anabolism.
Placenta	Chorionic Gonadotropin (HCG) (primates)	Mainly LH-like although some FSH-like properties.
	Pregnant Mare Gonadotropin (PMSG) (equine only)	Mainly FSH-like although some LH-like properties.
	Estrogens	Like ovary sources.
	Progesterone	Like ovary source.
	Relaxin	Like ovary source.
Many tissues	Prostaglandins	Many effects such as labor induction, abortion, CL destruction, gastric secretion, bronchial dilation, vasodilation, diuresis, GI motility, sweating.

INTERRELATION OF ENDOCRINE AND NERVOUS SYSTEMS

The nervous system was the first to gain attention and it still remains an important coordinating system, but knowledge of the endocrine system, which depends upon a humoral mediator, has developed sufficiently that it now has taken its place alongside the nervous system as the *coordinating systems* of the body. In fact, it is now evident that these two control systems work closely together within the body. For example, the nervous system may serve as an afferent branch bringing the impulse to the hypothalamus; then the endocrine system (hypophysis) releases humoral substances which act peripherally to complete the reflex. In the nervous system, the signal which travels throughout the body is similar, regardless of the eventual effect, but the choice of pathways determines the end result. In the case of the endocrine system the pathway traveled by the humoral mediator is always the same, namely, the circulatory system, but the humoral mediator changes to bring about the intended effects. This humoral substance travels rather slowly, since it is dependent upon the circulatory system for transportation.

Some have likened the *endocrine system* to a "wireless" communication system of the body and the *nervous system* to a "wire" system. Regardless of the comparison which one makes, it is important to remember that these two communication systems are coordinated and are mutually dependent for the maintenance of homeostasis.

Ovulation in the rabbit is a physiological event which calls on both the nervous and endocrine systems for its culmination (Fig. 1-1). Physical stimulation of the cervix during copulation causes an impulse to travel to the spinal cord (1), and thence to the hypothalamus (2). Here a humoral substance, a releasing hormone (3), is carried by the hypophyseal portal vessels to the anterior pituitary (adenohypophysis) (4) where the release of luteinizing hormone occurs. Luteinizing hormone then travels by the circulatory

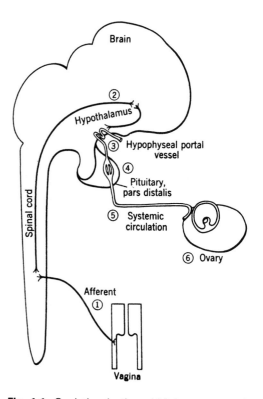

Fig. 1-1. Ovulation in the rabbit is a neuroendocrine reflex arc. (From Gorbman, A., and Bern, H. A.: *Comparative Endocrinology.* New York, John Wiley, Inc. 1962.)

system (5) to the ovary where the ripe ovarian follicle (6) is stimulated to rupture—thus ovulation.

INTERRELATION OF GENETICS AND ENDOCRINOLOGY

The genetic makeup of the individual affects growth and development and especially reproduction. With recent advances in understanding the biochemical mechanism by which heredity is manifested, we know that the phenotypic characteristics of the individual are only manifestations of this biochemical coding in the DNA of the genes. At one time, we considered the meeting of heterologous chromosomes as sufficient explanation for determination of the phenotypic characteristics of the offspring. Now we recognize that these nucleotide molecules constituting the gene are intricate packages of

DNA which are able to program and dictate the detailed development of the offspring. To carry this a bit further, the DNA makeup of these packages is able to dictate the kind of function and the level of function that an endocrine organ carries out. This means that the amount and kind of hormone to be produced have been coded. Consequently, errors or mistakes in coding could result in malfunction of an endocrine organ which could lead to hereditary disease. This could result in an over-production of a hormone, an under-production of a hormone, or the production of an abnormal hormone.

Studies by Baird et al. indicated quite clearly that rate of growth and final size of swine may be selected for and against within a genetic line by retaining as breeding stock either the large animals and breeding therein or the small animals and breeding therein.[2] After many generations a fast growing large line and a slow growing small line were developed. Upon assay of the anterior pituitary glands of these two lines of swine, it was found that the content of somatotropin was high in the large line and low in the small line per unit of tissue. This finding causes one to consider the fact that the selection for body size in domestic animals actually may be selection for the amount of somatotropin that the animal is able to produce. Furthermore, the way genes manifest themselves is by influencing the amount of somatotropin the pituitary is able to produce, which in turn dictates body size.

CHEMICAL CLASSES OF HORMONES

Hormones may be classified into four groups from the chemical point of view. The first group includes the polypeptide hormones which are varied in structure and represent those hormones produced by the hypothalamus, neurohypophysis, adenohypophysis, parathyroid, and islets of Langerhans. Building blocks for these hormones obviously are amino acids, and production of the hormone is dependent upon the proper substrate, presence of an energy supply, and necessary biological stimulation. These hormones must be replaced parenterally, since oral administration would lead to their destruction by the digestive enzymes.

Steroid hormones constitute the second group and include all the gonadal and adrenal cortical hormones. The steroid structure is complex; the building blocks are acetate leading to cholesterol with delicate alterations determining which steroid is finally released. Biogenesis of steroids by the endocrine organs probably involves each steroidogenic organ producing varying amounts of many related steroids. The tropic hormones from the pituitary, such as ACTH, favor a certain pathway thereby causing that target organ (i.e. adrenal cortex) to produce primarily the end steroid intended and desired, cortisol and/or corticosterone. The substrate used may be any of the intermediate substances circulating to the target organ, such as acetate, cholesterol, or even another hormone, such as progesterone, produced elsewhere by the corpus luteum. Furthermore, it can be seen how derangement of steroidogenesis may cause abnormal production of a hormone as when the adrenal cortex produces excessive androgens that cause adrenal virilism.

Attention should be drawn to the structural similarity of several steroid hormones which have widely different physiological-pharmacological effects within the body. For example, the chemical differences between a potent androgen (testosterone) and a life-giving mineralocorticoid (aldosterone) are minor.

The third group includes the catecholamines and iodothyronines. These hormones are tyrosine derivatives. They account for approximately 5% of mammalian hormones and include the catecholamines (epinephrine, norepinephrine) secreted by the adrenal medulla, and the iodothyronines (thyroxine, triiodothyronine) produced by follicular cells of the thyroid gland. Catecholamines share similar mechanisms of action with polypeptide hormones, whereas iodothyronines more closely resemble the characteristics of steroid hormones.

The fourth group consists of several unique fatty acids having hormone-like properties, the prostaglandins.

HORMONE TRANSPORT

After production by a particular gland, the polypeptide hormones are usually stored within that gland until needed. Upon call, they are then secreted into the efferent capillaries. Steroid hormones are not stored in significant quantities; instead they are released as produced. Thyroxine and triiodothyronine are stored in the thyroid follicles until needed.

The steroid hormones do not circulate in the blood as free hormone after release from the endocrine organ. Plasma contains specific carrier proteins for the steroid hormones and thyroxine. These are thyroxine-binding globulin (TBG), corticosteroid-binding globulin (CBG), also called *transcortin*, which binds adrenocorticosteroids and progesterone, and sex-hormone-binding globulin (SHBG), which binds estradiol and testosterone. This binding to plasma proteins restricts diffusion through the tissues, but at the same time prolongs their action, since the binding protects against degradation and elimination. The bound form of a hormone cannot enter the cell and it must be in the free form before it can enter the cell and exert its physiologic function. Pregnancy causes an increase in the protein-bound thyroid hormone or iodine (PBI), but the basal metabolic rate remains essentially the same because the hormone is bound in the blood and only the usual amount gets to the tissues in the free state to stimulate metabolism.

The sex steroids are firmly bound to SHBG thus increasing the solubility of the steroid in the aqueous medium of the blood. The bound steroid is biologically inactive but is in equilibrium with a small amount of the free form which is the form taken up by the target cells.

Thyroxine has a much shorter period of action in the chicken than in mammals, perhaps because the bird has a low ability to bind thyroxine to its plasma proteins. Consequently, thyroxine is lost by metabolism more quickly than from mammals which have a greater ability to bind thyroxine to plasma proteins.

RECEPTOR SITES—TARGET ORGANS—MECHANISM OF HORMONE ACTION

The two chemical classes of hormones, the steroids and the peptides, have different mechanisms of action. Steroid and thyroid hormones are small molecules (ca. MW 300), that diffuse freely into most cells of the body. The plasma membrane is not a barrier. In contrast to the steroid hormones, the peptide hormones are large molecules (MW 10,000 or more), and because of their size do not pass through the plasma membrane. Instead, the peptide hormones exert their action initially on the surface of the target cell.

Although all cells are exposed to hormones, only a few cells can respond; hence these are termed *target cells*. A target cell is able to respond because it has a highly specific *receptor site*. Receptors are on the surface of the cell for peptide hormones, in the nuclear chromatin for thyroid hormones, and in the cytoplasm and nucleus for steroid hormones.

A specific receptor site in a target organ selectively "binds" a particular hormone to the membrane of the cell as the first step in peptide hormone action (see Fig. 1–2 for LH action).

The second step in LH action is the subsequent stimulation of the enzyme, adenyl cyclase, in the cell membrane to convert ATP to cyclic 3, 5 adenosine monophosphate (cAMP). The cAMP (second messenger) conveys the message of the hormone to intracellular sites to initiate the chain of reactions that result in the physiologic effects of the hormone. ACTH, LH, FSH, TSH, and HCG produce their effects by the cAMP second messenger. Depending upon the biochemical and structural uniqueness of a particular target cell the intracellular accumulation of cAMP either modifies enzyme activity, alters membrane permeability, or may stimulate hormone release. Steroid production by the adrenal cortex and gonads also is regulated by cAMP. Since different cells contain recep-

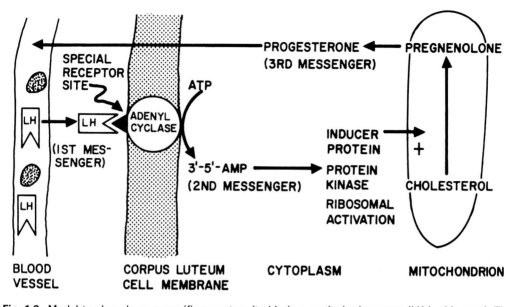

Fig. 1-2. Model to show how a specific receptor site binds a particular hormone (LH in this case). The target organ (corpus luteum cell membrane) contains a *hormone-specific* receptor protein as part of its adenyl cyclase system. Binding of LH results in activation of adenyl cyclase with a resulting increase in the production of cAMP (second messenger). The cAMP then activates the protein kinase in that particular cell which leads to progesterone (third messenger) production by the mitochondrion.

tors for different hormones, cAMP appears to be the common denominator of all peptide hormone action. Each cell would have different enzymes to be affected by cAMP.

Although the foregoing scheme explains the mechanism of action of many peptide hormones, there are other possibilities (for example insulin). A hormone may affect the permeability of, or transport across, the cell membrane or subcellular structures to make substrate more available, such as insulin increasing the uptake of glucose by muscle cells or somatotropin facilitating the entrance of amino acids through the cell membrane.

Steroid and thyroid hormones stimulate their target cells by *intracellular* action on the control of synthesis of specific proteins (Fig. 1-3). Only a target cell has the specific receptor protein to bind the steroid in question. Once the hormone-receptor complex is formed, it can move from the cytoplasm into the nucleus where there is an acceptor site on the chromosome. At this point the gene responds in a programmed way to form a specific messenger RNA which then leaves

the nucleus and directs the synthesis of a particular protein necessary for the function of the particular steroid hormone.

The effector tissues have the ability to "trap or bind" the hormone concerned with their function and hold it firmly at the receptor site. This is especially true in the case of insulin, since we know that tissues which use insulin, namely, muscle, adipose and mammary tissues, take up insulin with such an affinity that it is difficult to wash away. This is not true of brain tissue or red blood cells, since these tissues do not use insulin and consequently do not hold it. Likewise, the gonads appear to bind the gonadotropins and hold them in close association in order that the effector tissue has an opportunity to be acted upon by the hormone. This "trapping" mechanism means that the hormone is attached to the receptor site.

Although most hormones have a target organ that responds to a greater extent than any other tissue, other tissues may have some receptors. For example, the female sex hormone from the ovarian follicle, estradiol, has

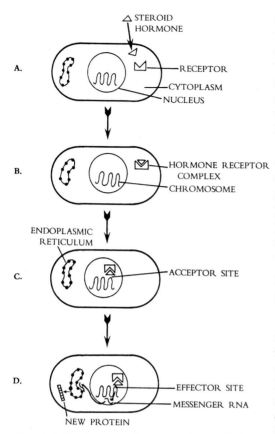

Fig. 1-3. Mechanism of action of steroid hormones. Steroids can enter all cells, but only target cells contain the specific receptors (A) that bind the hormone (B). The receptor-hormone complex passes into the cell nucleus (C) and attaches to an acceptor site on the chromosome which contains the genes (DNA) of the cell. At the effector site the receptor-steroid complex causes synthesis of a messenger RNA depending on the particular gene. Messenger RNA then migrates to the endoplasmic reticulum (D), where it directs synthesis of new protein.

as its target organ the accessory sex organs such as the uterus and vagina. Estradiol exerts a most profound influence in their growth, development, and function. But there are other tissues which also have receptor sites and respond to estrogen such as skin, hair, and bone. Thus it is important to keep in mind that a hormone may have several effects in the body even though its main effect may be on the primary target organ.

Target organs can function at a minimal level even in the absence of the hormone. Thus nature has provided a base level of function which may be sufficient to maintain life in the absence of the hormone. *In vitro* slices of the thyroid, adrenals, or even gonads produce some of their respective hormones in the absence of trophic hormones; likewise all tissues are able to use carbohydrates at a minimal level even in the absence of insulin.

Some physiologic processes need more than one hormone for full function. Development of full lactation potential by the mammary gland requires a sequential effect by estrogen, progesterone, and possibly some adenohypophyseal hormones. In addition, thyroxine and adrenal corticoids are essential. Thus lactation is a response to several hormones.

REGULATION OF HORMONE SECRETION

The endocrine glands are important regulators of many processes in the body; therefore it is obvious that careful regulation of endocrine output is critical. Regulation of hormone secretion depends on several mechanisms. A particular hormone output may depend on more than one control mechanism. Some are fairly well understood, but others are still being studied. With current information we can categorize these (Table 1-4).

Humoral control is the mechanism we usually think of first, and the concentration of a particular blood constituent is one of the simplest control schemes. For example, a rising level of blood glucose signals for a blood sugar lowering hormone, insulin, to be released. Insulin facilitates glucose movement

Table 1-4 Types of Control of Endocrine Secretion

I. Humoral
a. Concentration of a blood constituent
b. Concentration of another hormone
II. Nervous
a. Peripheral nerve connection
b. Hypothalamic connection (pituitary)
III. Genetic

After Gorbman, A., and Bern, H. A.: Comparative Endocrinology, New York, John Wiley & Sons, Inc., 1962.

through the cell membrane where it is either metabolized or stored for later use, usually in the form of glycogen. Either route lowers blood glucose. Should the blood glucose level drop below normal, a blood glucose raising hormone, glucagon, released from the alpha cells of the pancreatic islets acts to stimulate the release of sugar from the glycogen stores of the liver thereby raising the glucose level back to normal.

Regulation of hormone output by *concentration of another hormone* is best depicted via the adenohypophysis, which secretes tropic hormones which regulate other glands. This is a "feedback mechanism" or "servomechanism." The anterior pituitary is in turn inhibited directly or indirectly (via the hypothalamic releasing factors) by hormones produced by the target endocrine organs. Therefore a balance is finally achieved between the stimulating effects of the adenohypophyseal hormone and the resultant inhibitory effects on adenohypophyseal hormone output by the target organ hormone (Fig. 1-4). A *servo-mechanism* as used in endocrinology is an automatic means of correcting the hormone output of a gland to a desired level by a level-sensing feedback of another hormone.

Peripheral nervous control of hormone output is difficult to separate entirely except in the case of the adrenal medulla where a peripheral nerve connection (preganglionic sympathetic fiber) can cause increased output of epinephrine. This impulse could have arisen in the cerebral cortex after the animal recorded a frightful image on the visual cortex.

Another method involves the *hypothalamic connection* as a means of mediating *nervous control*. A good example of this is the way light affects the reproductive cycle of certain animals. In some species increasing day length signals the hypothalamus which in turn increases the output or changes the ratio of adenohypophyseal gonadotropins (FSH and LH). This awakens the gonad causing germ cell and sex hormone production to resume.

Finally we must consider, especially in

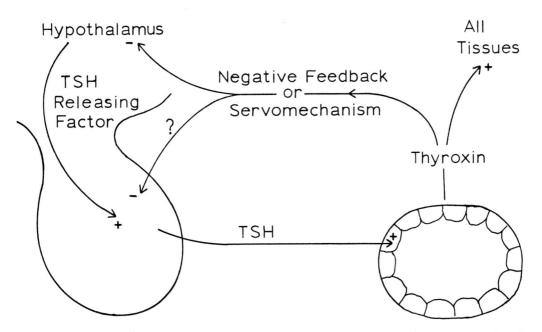

Fig. 1-4. A typical negative feedback or servomechanism type of regulation of hormone output. There is a continuing effort by the hypothalamus to produce TSH releasing hormone. This causes TSH to be released which in turn causes thyroxine output. Thyroxine "feeds" back to inhibit the hypothalamus from producing TSH releasing hormone. If thyroxine levels fall, then the brake is released and TSH production rises.

domestic animals, the influence of the *genetic makeup* of the animal on endocrine secretion. The possible effects of genetic coding on the *level* of hormone output and the effect of hormones on protein synthesis were considered earlier, as was the practical aspect of this in terms of pituitary somatotropin content and output in fast growing swine.

Thus one can see that the endocrine system serves as an important control mechanism, but it in turn is controlled by and is obedient to other forces. There appears to be no central control, and the old reference to the anterior pituitary as being "the master gland" is no longer tenable. There are so many external influences on the function of the adenohypophysis that we cannot look upon it as a control headquarters, but instead we must consider it as an important link in a circuitous control scheme.

PROLIFERATIVE LESIONS IN ENDOCRINE GLANDS

The development of proliferative lesions in adult to aged animals is important clinically and may result in diseases associated with abnormal endocrine function. Neoplasms derived from polypeptide hormone-secreting endocrine cells usually consist of one predominant cell type and may be associated with the hypersecretion of one polypeptide hormone. However, evidence is accumulating from immunocytochemical and electron microscopic investigations to suggest that some endocrine tumors are composed of more than one type of neoplastic cell and are capable of synthesizing multiple hormones.

The histopathologic classification as between nodular hyperplasia, adenoma, or carcinoma often is difficult in endocrine glands since in many (especially thyroid C-cells, secretory cells of the adrenal medulla, and specific tropic hormone-secreting cells of the adenohypophysis) there appears to be a continuous spectrum of proliferative lesions between diffuse or focal hyperplasia and adenomas derived from a specific population of cells. It appears to be a common feature of endocrine glands that prolonged stimulation of a population of secretory cells predisposes to the subsequent development of a higher than expected incidence of tumors. Long-term stimulation may lead to the development of clones of cells within the hyperplastic endocrine gland that grow more rapidly than the rest and are more susceptible to neoplastic transformation when exposed to the right combination of promoting carcinogens.

Many neoplasms derived from endocrine glands are functionally active, secrete an excessive amount of hormone either continuously or episodically, and cause dramatic clinical syndromes of hormone excess. Classical examples include the hypoglycemia of insulin-secreting neoplasms of the pancreatic islets in dogs, hyperthyroidism associated with adenomas and carcinomas derived from thyroid follicular cells in cats and dogs, hypercalcitoninism in bulls and other animal species with thyroid C-cell tumors, and hypercortisolism associated either with ACTH-secreting pituitary ("corticotroph") adenomas or neoplasms derived from the adrenal cortex (zona fasciculata) in dogs. Quantitation of hormone levels in serum or plasma in the basal, suppressed, or stimulated state, and the measurement of hormonal metabolites in the urine over a 24-hour period of excretion are essential to confirm that an endocrine tumor is functional.

PATHOGENETIC MECHANISMS OF ENDOCRINE DISEASE

Disorders of the endocrine system are encountered in many animal species and present challenging diagnostic problems. The following examples are the major pathogenetic mechanisms responsible for disturbances of endocrine function that result in clinically important diseases in animals. For each major category, several specific disease problems have been selected to illustrate the response of a particular endocrine gland to the disruption of function.

Many diseases of the endocrine system are characterized by dramatic functional disturbances and characteristic clinicopathologic alterations affecting one or several body systems. The affected animal may be presented because of changes that primarily involve the skin (hair loss caused by hypothyroidism), nervous system (seizures caused by hyperinsulinism), urinary system (polyuria caused by diabetes mellitus, diabetes insipidus, or hypercortisolism), or skeletal system (fractures induced by hyperparathyroidism). If the underlying endocrine problem is recognized early in the course of the disease, it often is amenable to either surgical removal of the source of excess hormone production or supplementation of the specific hormone secreted in inadequate amounts by the diseased gland.

Primary Hyperfunction of an Endocrine Gland

One of the most important pathologic mechanisms is primary hyperfunction of an endocrine gland. A lesion, often a neoplasm derived from endocrine cells, synthesizes and secretes hormone at an uncontrolled (autonomous) rate in excess of the body's ability to utilize and subsequently degrade the hormone, thereby resulting in functional disturbances of hormone excess. Several examples that occur in different animal species are summarized in Table 1-5. These include hyper-

function of parathyroid chief cells, thyroid C- (parafollicular) cells, beta cells of the pancreatic islets, secretory cells of the adrenal medulla, and follicular cells of the thyroid, amongst others.

The autonomous secretion of parathyroid hormone results in progressive and generalized demineralization of the skeleton, leading to hypercalcemia, which results in soft tissue mineralization and the development of renal calculi. The accelerated osteoclastic resorption of bone results in marked thinning and osteoclastic tunneling of cortical bone, and predisposes bone to the development of pathological fractures.

The autonomous hypersecretion of T_4 and T_3 are being recognized with increasing frequency in cats, and are associated with a spectrum of proliferative lesions of follicular cells. Functional thyroid lesions in cats should be considered to be potentially malignant because a low percentage are adenocarcinomas that may metastasize to regional lymph nodes. The functional disturbances of hyperactivity, weight loss despite increased appetite, hyperthermia, and tachycardia reflect long-term stimulation of multiple populations of target cells by the abnormally elevated blood levels of thyroid hormones.

Table 1-5 *Examples of Primary Hyperfunction of Endocrine Glands*

Disease	Hormone Secreted in Excess	Animal Most Frequently Affected	Principal Lesion or Functional Disturbances
Chief cell adenoma or carcinoma	Parathyroid hormone	Dog	Generalized osteitis fibrosa
Thyroid C-cell adenoma or carcinoma	Calcitonin	Bull	Osteosclerosis
Beta cell adenoma or carcinoma	Insulin	Dog	Hypoglycemia
Sertoli cell tumor (Testis)	Estrogens	Dog	Feminization of the male
Pheochromocytoma (Adrenal medulla)	Norepinephrine, epinephrine	Dog	Hypertension. hyperglycemia
Thyroid follicular cell adenoma or carcinoma	Thyroxine, triiodothyronine	Cat	Increased metabolic rate, weight loss
Adrenal cortical adenoma or carcinoma (Zona fasciculata)	Cortisol	Dog	Cushing's syndrome

Secondary Hyperfunction of an Endocrine Gland

In secondary hyperfunction of an endocrine gland, a lesion in one organ secretes an excess of a tropic hormone that leads to long-term stimulation and hypersecretion of hormone by a target endocrine organ. The classical example of this pathogenetic mechanism in animals is the ACTH-secreting tumor derived from pituitary corticotrophs in dogs. The clinical signs and lesions in the patient primarily are the result of the elevated blood cortisol levels associated with the ACTH-stimulated hypertrophy and hyperplasia of the zonae fasciculata and reticularis of the adrenal cortex. The syndrome of cortisol excess in dogs is characterized by progressive alopecia, hyperpigmentation, and muscle wasting caused by the protein catabolic effects of glucocorticoids. In some dogs, particularly Poodles, having a similar marked adrenocortical enlargement and clinical evidence of cortisol excess, there is no evidence of a tumor in the pituitary gland. These dogs may have a change in their set point to the negative feed-back signal (blood cortisol). This can be caused by an abnormal accumulation of certain neurotransmitter substances (serotonin) near neurons in the hypothalamus that secrete corticotropic hormone-releasing factor. The end result is corticotroph hyperplasia, elevated ACTH levels in the blood, and long-term stimulation of the adrenal cortex, which result in hyperplasia of the zonae fasciculata and reticularis and the clinical syndrome of cortisol excess.

Primary Hypofunction of an Endocrine Gland

In primary hypofunction of an endocrine gland, hormone secretion is subnormal because of extensive destruction of secretory cells by a disease process, the failure of an endocrine gland to develop properly, or the result of a specific biochemical defect in the synthetic pathway of a hormone.

Immune-mediated injury causes hypofunction of several endocrine glands in ani-mals, including the parathyroid, adrenal cortex, and thyroid. Thyroiditis caused by this mechanism is characterized by marked infiltration of lymphocytes and plasmacytes, and deposition of electron-dense immune complexes along the follicular basement membranes with progressive destruction of secretory parenchyma.

Failure of development also results in primary hypofunction of an endocrine gland. The classical example of this mechanism in animals is the failure of oropharyngeal ectoderm to differentiate completely into tropic hormone-secreting cells of the adenohypophysis in dogs, resulting in pituitary dwarfism and a failure to attain somatic maturation. A large, multicompartmented cyst is present on the ventral aspect of the brain in the pituitary region of these dogs. The cyst compresses the normally developed neurohypophysis and results in disturbances of water metabolism.

Another form of primary hypofunction recognized recently is a failure of hormone synthesis caused by a genetically determined defect in a biosynthetic pathway or lack of a specific enzyme. One of the best documented examples of this condition in animals is vitamin D-dependent rickets in pigs. It is caused by the lack of an enzyme in the proximal convoluted tubules of the kidney that is needed to synthesize the hormonal form of vitamin D. Blood calcium and phosphorus levels progressively decrease due to the subnormal ability of the pig to produce the biologically active, hormonal form of vitamin D (1,25-dihydroxy-cholecalciferol) in the kidney. The lowered blood concentrations of calcium and phosphorus lead to failure of mineralization of osteoid, overgrowth of cartilage in the physes, and associated severe skeletal deformities.

Congenital dyshormonogenetic goiter in sheep, goats, and cattle is another example of primary hypofunction caused by failure of hormone synthesis. The low blood T_4 and T_3 levels and clinical evidence of severe hypothyroidism in these animals are due to an inability of follicular cells to synthesize thyroglobulin. The molecular defect has been shown to be due to defective processing of the primary transcripts for thyroglobulin messenger ribonucleic acid (mRNA) and aberrant transport of mRNA from the nucleus to the ribosomes. This results in subnormal amounts of thyroglobulin mRNA in follicular cells, particularly mRNA that is attached to membranes of the endoplasmic reticulum in the cytoplasm.

Secondary Hypofunction of an Endocrine Gland

In secondary hypofunction of an endocrine gland, a destructive lesion in one organ, such as the pituitary, interferes with the secretion of tropic hormone. This results in hypofunction of the target endocrine glands. Large, endocrinologically inactive, pituitary neoplasms in adult dogs, cats, and other species may interfere with the secretion of the multiple pituitary tropic hormones and result in clinically detectable hypofunction of the adrenal cortex, follicular cells of the thyroid, and gonads. The adrenal cortex of animals with a large pituitary neoplasm of this type has marked atrophy and degeneration of the ACTH-dependent inner zones; however, the aldosterone-secreting zona glomerulosa, which is not under direct ACTH control, remains intact. Thyroid function may be subnormal due to a lack of thyrotropin and atrophy of follicular cells, but the calcitonin secreting C-cells function normally since they are not controlled by pituitary tropic hormones.

Endocrine Hyperactivity Secondary to Diseases of Other Organs

The best characterized example of endocrine hyperactivity secondary to diseases of other organs in animals is the hyperparathyroidism that develops secondary to chronic renal failure or nutritional imbalances. In the renal form, the early retention of phosphorus and subsequent progressive destruction of cells in the proximal convoluted tubules interfere with the metabolic activation of vitamin D by an enzyme in the kidney. This rate-limiting step in the metabolic activation of vitamin D is tightly controlled by parathyroid hormone and several other factors. The impaired intestinal absorption of calcium results in the development of progressive hypocalcemia, which leads to long-term parathyroid stimulation and subsequent development of generalized demineralization of the skeleton. Many bones, particularly the cancellous bone of the skull, become weakened and more susceptible to fractures.

Nutritional hyperparathyroidism develops in animals fed abnormal diets that are low in calcium, high in phosphorus, or (for certain nonhuman primates) deficient in cholecalciferol. Unsupplemented all-meat diets fed to carnivores fail to supply the daily requirements for calcium, leading to progressive hypocalcemia that stimulates the parathyroid gland activity. The normal kidneys in these animals respond to the increased parathyroid hormone by increasing phosphorus excretion and lowering the blood phosphorus level. After a carnivore is fed this imbalanced diet for several months, its skeleton becomes severely demineralized and predisposed to fractures.

Hypersecretion of Hormones or Hormone-like Substances by Nonendocrine Tumors

The hypersecretion by nonendocrine tumors of "hormone-like humoral substances" that may be similar chemically or biologically (or both) to the native hormone secreted by the endocrine gland has been recognized recently in animals including man. Most of these substances secreted by nonendocrine tumors are peptides. Steroids and iodothyronines require more complex biosynthetic pathways and do not appear to be secreted by nonendocrine tumors. A classical example of this mechanism is the adenocarcinoma derived from apocrine glands of the anal sac in dogs. This tumor produces a humoral substance that stimulates osteoclasts both *in vivo* and *in vitro*. The resulting accelerated mobilization of calcium from bone leads to the development of persistent hypercalcemia, even though the animal's parathyroid glands are smaller than normal and composed of inactive chief cells and parathyroid hormone levels are subnormal. This neoplasm develops predominantly in elderly female dogs and is composed of solid and glandular areas.

Following surgical removal of the apocrine adenocarcinoma, the serum calcium and phosphorus levels return to normal, immunoreactive parathyroid hormone levels increase rapidly, and the active vitamin D metabolite level in blood decreases. The tumor cells appear to secrete a parathyroid-hormone-like humoral substance that stimulates osteoclastic resorption of bone distant from the tumor and results in the development of persistent hypercalcemia.

Endocrine Dysfunction Due to Failure of Target Cell Response

Such dysfunctions have been more appreciated recently, coincident with our more complete understanding of how hormones convey their biologic message by interacting with target cells. Steroid and iodothyronine hormones penetrate the cell membrane, bind to cytosolic receptors, and are transported to the nucleus where they interact with the genetic information in the cell to increase new protein synthesis. Polypeptide and catecholamine hormones bind to receptors on the surface of target cells and activate a membrane-bound enzyme that generates an intracellular messenger (cAMP) and elicits the physiological response.

Failure of target cells to respond to hormone may be due to a lack of adenylate cyclase in the cell membrane or to an alteration in hormone receptors on the cell surface. Hormone is secreted in normal or increased amounts by cells of the endocrine gland. Certain forms of insulin-resistance associated with obesity result from a decrease in the number of receptors on the surface target cells. This develops in response to the chronic increased insulin secretion stimulated by the hyperglycemia resulting from excessive food intake. Secretory cells in the corresponding endocrine gland (pancreatic islets) undergo

compensatory hypertrophy and hyperplasia in an attempt to secrete additional hormone. The normal pancreatic islets contain predominantly granulated beta cells, whereas the beta cells in the enlarged islets from an obese diabetic animal are markedly hyperplastic and depleted of insulin-containing secretory granules.

Failure of Fetal Endocrine Function

Endocrine disorders also may be due to a failure of fetal endocrine function. Subnormal function of the fetal endocrine system, especially in ruminants, may disrupt normal fetal development and result in prolonged gestation. In some breeds of cattle, a genetically determined failure of the adenohypophysis to develop (although the neurohypophysis develops normally) results in a lack of fetal pituitary tropic hormone secretion during the last trimester and hypoplastic development of target endocrine organs, such as adrenal cortex, gonads, and follicular cells of the thyroid gland. Fetal development is normal up to approximately 7 months, but subsequently ceases, irrespective of how long the viable fetus is retained in the uterus.

Prolongation of gestation in sheep results after maternal ingestion early in gestation of a plant that results in extensive malformations of the CNS and hypothalamus in the lamb. Although the adenohypophysis is present, it lacks the necessary fine control derived from the releasing hormones of the hypothalamus to be able to secrete normal amounts of tropic hormones (eg. adrenocorticotropin).

The concepts that have emerged from the study of these two syndromes are: (1) fetal hormones are necessary for final growth and development *in utero* in certain animals, and (2) normal parturition at term in these species requires an intact fetal hypothalamic-adenohypophyseal-adrenocortical axis working in concert with trophoblasts of the placenta.

Although the presence of absence of functional adenohypophyseal tissue determines whether the fetus continues to grow *in utero*, the pathogenesis of prolongation of the gestation is similar in these two examples. The subnormal development of the fetal adrenal cortex in calves and lambs results in an inadequate secretion of cortisol and a failure of induction of the 17-hydroxylase in the placenta that converts precursor molecules, such as progesterone, to estrogens. As a result, the circulating progesterone levels in the dam remain high and the marked increase in estrogens necessary for parturition, normally seen at term, does not occur. The estrogen surge under normal conditions stimulates the synthesis of prostaglandins in the uterus, which cause smooth muscle contractions and biochemical changes in collagen along the birth canal that normally permit delivery of the fetus.

Endocrine Dysfunction Resulting from Abnormal Degradation of Hormone

With abnormal degradation of hormone, the secretion of hormone by an endocrine gland is normal but blood levels are elevated persistently. A decreased rate of degradation simulates a state of hypersecretion. The syndrome of feminization due to hyperestrogenism, associated with cirrhosis and decreased hepatic degradation of estrogens in men, is a classical example of this pathogenic mechanism.

Chronic renal disease in animals may be associated with subnormal, normal, or elevated blood concentrations of calcium. The hypercalcemia associated with certain forms of renal disease may be related, in part, to diminished degradation of parathyroid hormone along with decreased urinary excretion of calcium by the diseased kidney. Biologically active parathyroid hormone is degraded in the kidney either by peptidases on the surface of tubular cells or by lysosomal enzymes after uptake of the hormone from the glomerular filtrate. In animals with hypercalcemia and renal failure, parathyroid glands often are atrophic and composed of inactive chief cells.

Iatrogenic Syndromes of Hormone Excess

The administration of hormone, either directly or indirectly, influences the activity of target cells and results in clinical disturbances. It is well recognized that daily administration of potent preparations of adrenal corticosteroids at inappropriate doses for prolonged intervals in the symptomatic treatment of various diseases, will reproduce most of the functional disturbances associated with endogenous hypersecretion of cortisol. These disturbances include muscle weakness, marked hair loss, and mineral deposition in the skin. The elevated blood levels of exogenous cortisol result in marked trophic atrophy of the adrenal cortex, particularly the ACTH-dependent zonae fasciculata and reticularis.

It has been reported recently that the administration of certain progestagens will indirectly result in a syndrome of hormone excess. The injection of medroxyprogesterone acetate for the prevention of estrus in dogs stimulates increased secretion of growth hormone by pituitary somatotrophs, resulting in many of the clinical manifestations of acromegaly. The excessive skin folds, expansion of interdental spaces, and abdominal enlargement in dogs with iatrogenic acromegaly are related to the protein anabolic effects of growth hormone on connective tissues.

REFERENCES

1. Ariens, E. J., and Beld, A. J. (1977): The receptor concept in evolution. Biochem. Pharmacol. *26*:913.
2. Baird, D. M., Nalbandov, A. V., and Norton, H. W. (1952): Some physiological causes of genetically different rates of growth in swine. J. Animal Sci. *11*:292.
3. Ballard, P. L. (1977): Glucocorticoid receptors in the lung. Fed. Proc. *36*:2660.
4. Banting, F., and Best, C. H. (1922): The internal secretion of the pancreas. J. Lab. Clin. Med. *7*:251.
5. Bayliss, W. M., and Starling, E. H. (1902): The mechanism of pancreatic secretion. J. Physiol. *28*:325.
6. Berthold, A. A. (1849): Transplantation der hoden. Arch. Anat. Physiol u. wiss. Med. *16*:42.
6a. Bauman, D. E., Eppard, P. J., DeGetter, M. J., and Lanza, G. M. (1985): Responses of high producing dairy cows to long term treatment with pituitary somatotrophin and recombinant somatotrophin. J. Dairy Sci. *68*:1352.
7. Bromer, W. W., Sinn, L. G., and Behrens, O. K. (1957): The amino acid sequence of glucagon. J. Amer. Chem. Soc. *79*:2807.
8. Clark, J. H., and Hardin, J. W. (1977): Steroid hormone receptors and mechanism of action. Res. Repro. *9(6)*:2.
9. Devynck, M. A., and Meyer, P. (1978): Angiotensin receptors. Biochem. Pharmacol. *27*:1.
10. du Vigneaud, V., Ressler, C., and Trippett, S.

(1953): The sequence of amino acids in oxytocin, with a proposal for the structure of oxytocin. J. Biol. Chem. *205*:949.

11. du Vigneaud, V. (1956): Hormones of the posterior pituitary gland: oxytocin and vasopressin. Harvey Lec., New York, Academic Press, Inc.

12. Gorbman, A., and Bern, H. A. (1962): Comparative Endocrinology. New York, John Wiley & Sons, Inc.

13. Hechter, O., and Halkerston, I. D. K. (1965): Effects of steroid hormones on gene regulation and cell metabolism. Ann. Rev. Physiol. *27*:133, 162.

14. Hench, P. S., et al. (1949): The effect of a hormone of the adrenal cortex (17-hydroxy-11-dehydrocorticosterone: compound E) and of pituitary adrenocorticotrophic hormone on rheumatoid arthritis, Preliminary Report, Proc. Staff Meet., Mayo Clin. *24*:181.

15. Jacob, F., and Monod, J. (1961): Genetic regulatory mechanisms in the synthesis of proteins. J. Mol. Biol. *3*:318.

16. Kleinsmith, L. J. (1972): Molecular mechanisms for the regulation of cell function. Bioscience *22*: 343.

17. McEwen, B. S. (1976): Interactions between hormones and nerve tissue. Sci. Am. *235(1)*:48.

18. Mellen, W. J., and Hardy, L. B., Jr. (1957): Blood-bound iodine in the fowl, Endocrinology *60*:547.

19. O'Malley, B. W., and Schrader, W. T. (1976): The receptors of steroid hormones. Sci. Am. *234(2)*:32.

20. Staub, A., Sinn, L. and Behrens, O. K. (1955). Purification and crystallization of glucagon. J. Biol. Chem. *214*:619.

21. Sutherland, E. W. (1972): Studies on the mechanism of hormone action. Science *177*:401.

22. Turner, C. D. (1966): General Endocrinology. Philadelphia, W. B. Saunders Co.

23. Von Mering, J., and Minkowski, O. (1889): Diabetes melitus nach pankreas-extirpation. Arch. Exp. Pathol. Pharmakol. *26*:371.

The Pituitary Gland

C. C. CAPEN and S. L. MARTIN

2

INTRODUCTION

THE pituitary gland has received a great deal of attention, some of which dates back to the time of Galen when his writings mentioned the pituitary as a source of one of the four humors. During the first half of this century the pituitary was looked upon by most endocrinologists as the "center" of endocrinology and was often referred to as "the leader of the orchestra." Its location at the base of the brain was thought to be only coincident to its function of regulating other endocrine glands of the body. Early attempts to remove the gland (hypophysectomy) were usually fatal; consequently the feeling developed that it was essential for life. Early in this century hypophysectomy was accomplished in the dog and then simplified in the rat. Thereafter, it was concluded that the pituitary was not essential to life.

Hypophysectomy permitted various experiments to be carried out so that finally the complexities of the pituitary began to unravel. Only the adrenal cortex can match the complexity of the pituitary in the multiple hormones formed. But the adrenal cortex secretes closely related hormones (i.e. steroids), whereas the pituitary secretes numerous peptide hormones, many of which are quite different in chemical structure and size. These vary from the octapeptides from the pars nervosa, to ACTH (composed of 39 amino acids), to others that are larger and are true proteins.

The last three decades have witnessed many advances which have led to an understanding of the function of the pituitary gland. We now realize that the pituitary gland is located at the base of the brain so it can function as an anatomical and functional extension of the central nervous system. Therefore, the adenohypophysis and the hypothalamus are parts of an integrated and functional information relay system which ties the nervous and the endocrine systems together.

Endocrine glands such as the pituitary are concerned exclusively with endocrine function. They are small in comparison with other body organs and connected with other endocrine glands by the bloodstream. They are richly supplied with blood, and there is a close anatomic relationship between endocrine cells and the capillary network. The peripheral cytoplasmic extensions of the capillary endothelial cells have fenestrae covered by a single membrane in order to facilitate rapid transport of raw materials and secretory products between the bloodstream and endocrine cells. Endocrine cells working in concert with the nervous system integrate and coordinate a wide variety of physiologic activities concerned with maintaining a constant internal environment. Endocrine glands are interposed as sensing or signalling devices to detect changes in a constituent of the extracellular fluid compartment (Fig. 2-1).

Cells concerned with the production of polypeptide hormones, such as the adenohypophysis, have a well-developed endoplasmic reticulum, with many attached ribosomes for assembly of hormone and a prominent Golgi apparatus for packaging of hormone into granules for intracellular storage and transport (Fig. 2-2). Secretory granules are unique to endocrine cells synthesizing polypeptide and catecholamine hormones,

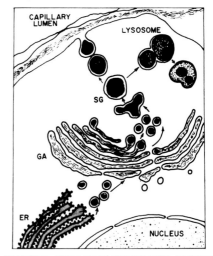

POLYPEPTIDE HORMONE SYNTHESIS, PACKAGING, SECRETION AND DEGRADATION

Fig. 2-2. Synthesis of polypeptide hormones from endocrine glands, e.g., adenohypophysis, begins on ribosomes attached to membranes of the rough endoplasmic reticulum (ER). Precursor hormone molecules accumulate within the cisternae of the ER and are transported to the Golgi apparatus (GA), where they are concentrated and packaged into membrane-limited secretory granules. Secretory granules (SG) are macromolecular aggregations of preformed hormone that are moved to the periphery of the cell by contraction of microfilaments and are released into the perivascular spaces either by exocytosis or emiocytosis. Hormone synthesized in excess of the body's requirement is degraded by fusion of secretory granules with lysosomes, a process termed "crinophagy."

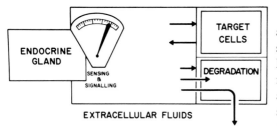

EXTRACELLULAR FLUIDS

Fig. 2-1. Schematic representation of the endocrine system. Endocrine glands are interposed as sensing and signaling devices to detect changes in constituents of the extracellular fluid compartment. Hormones interact with specific target cells in the body to elicit a biologic response. In addition, hormones are degraded by cell surface enzymes, lysosomal enzymes within the cells, or are conjugated with glucuronic acid and sulfate for excretion in the urine or bile. (From Roth, J.: Cell Membrane Receptors for Viruses, Antigens and Antibiotics, Polypeptide Hormones, and Small Molecules. New York, Raven Press).

and provide a mechanism for intracellular storage of substantial amounts of preformed hormone. These membrane-limited granules represent macromolecular aggregations of active hormone, often in association with specific binding proteins. Upon receipt of an appropriate signal for hormone secretion, secretary granules are directed to the periphery of the endocrine cell, probably by the contraction of microfilaments and the limiting membrane of the granule fuses with the plasma membrane of the cell. The hormone-containing granule core is extruded into the extracellular perivascular space by either emiocytosis or exocytosis. Subsequently, the granule core is fragmented and rapidly transported through capillary fenestrae into the circulation. Hormone synthesized in excess of the body's requirement is degraded by fusion of the hormone-containing granules with lysosomes, a process termed crinophagy.

DEVELOPMENTAL ANATOMY

The two distinct parts of the pituitary gland, viz., neurohypophysis and the adenohypophysis, arise from different primordia, although both are ectodermal. The neurohypophysis originates from the infundibulum of the brain and remains attached to the hypothalamus by a neural stalk. By contrast, the adenohypophysis arises from the roof of the mouth in the form of an invagination commonly referred to as craniopharyngeal duct (Rathke's pouch). When this pouch reaches the infundibulum as shown in Figure 2-3, it loses its connection with the oro-

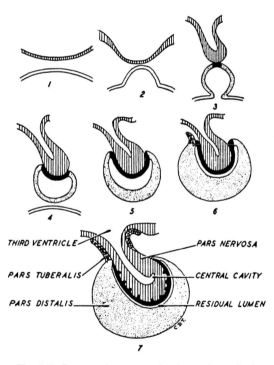

Fig. 2-3. Progressive stages in the embryonic development of the mammalian hypophysis. Cross hatching indicates the neurohypophysis, solid black indicates the pars intermedia, stippling represents the pars distalis, and circles represent the pars tuberalis. Rathke's pouch (craniopharyngeal duct) becomes detached from the oral epithelium. (From Turner, C. D. General Endocrinology. Courtesy W. B. Saunders Co.)

Labels in figure:
THIRD VENTRICLE
PARS TUBERALIS
PARS DISTALIS
PARS NERVOSA
CENTRAL CAVITY
RESIDUAL LUMEN

pharynx. After Rathke's pouch has become separated, it proceeds to encircle the infundibular process to varying degrees and thickens on the ventral side to form the pars distalis, the main secretory part of the anterior pituitary.

The embryologic development is in keeping with the final innervation of these two lobes. The neurohypophysis retains an attachment to the hypothalamus and retains its direct innervation from hypothalamic nuclei. Because the adenohypophysis does not have direct neural connections with the hypothalamus, it follows that it would be dependent upon a humoral connection with the hypothalamus. The pars intermedia normally forms from the craniopharyngeal duct near the point that fuses with the pars nervosa.

STRUCTURE AND FUNCTION OF THE PITUITARY GLAND

The pituitary gland in the adult is completely separated from the oral cavity. It is situated in the sella turcica, a concavity of the sphenoid bone, and enveloped by an extension of dura mater. The pituitary gland (hypophysis) is subdivided anatomically into the adenohypophysis (anterior lobe) and neurohypophysis (posterior lobe).

The adenohypophysis surrounds the pars nervosa of the neurohypophyseal system to varying degrees in a different animal species (Fig. 2-4). The adenohypophysis consists of three portions, viz. the pars distalis, the pars tuberalis, and the pars intermedia. The pars distalis is the largest of the three portions and contains the multiple populations of endocrine cells that secrete the pituitary trophic hormones (Fig. 2-5). The secretory cells are supplied with abundant capillaries that have fenestrae in the cytoplasm and are supported by the cytoplasmic processes of stellate follicular (substentacular) cells (Fig. 2-6). The pars tuberalis consists of dorsal projections of cells along the infundibular stalk. It functions primarily as a scaffold for the capillary network of the hypophyseal portal system during its course from the median eminence to the

COMPARATIVE ANATOMY OF HYPOPHYSIS

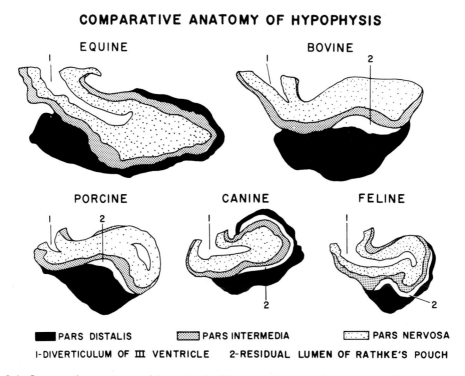

EQUINE   BOVINE

PORCINE   CANINE   FELINE

■ PARS DISTALIS   ▨ PARS INTERMEDIA   ▢ PARS NERVOSA

1-DIVERTICULUM OF III VENTRICLE   2-RESIDUAL LUMEN OF RATHKE'S POUCH

Fig. 2-4. Comparative anatomy of hypophysis. The adenohypophysis surrounds the pars nervosa to varying degrees in different species of animals. The pars intermedia is particularly well developed in the pituitary glands of horses and cattle. There are two cavities in the pituitary: (1) diverticulum of the third ventricle, and (2) residual lumen of Rathke's pouch. (Modified from: Trautman, A. and Febiger, J. (1952). Fundamentals of the Histology of Domestic Animals. Ithaca, NY, Comstock Publishing Associates)

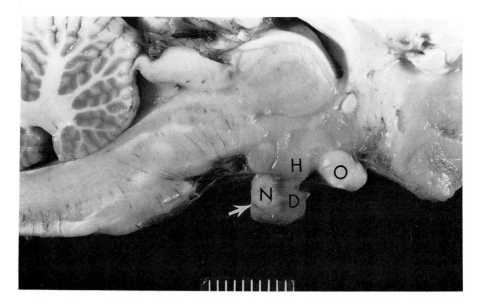

Fig. 2-5. The pituitary region from a dog illustrating the close relationship to the optic chiasm (O), hypothalamus (H), and overlying brain. The pars distalis (D) forms a major part of the adenohypophysis and completely surrounds the pars nervosa (N). The residual lumen of Rathke's pouch (white arrow) separates the pars distalis and pars nervosa, and is lined by the pars intermedia. The scale at the bottom represents 1 cm.

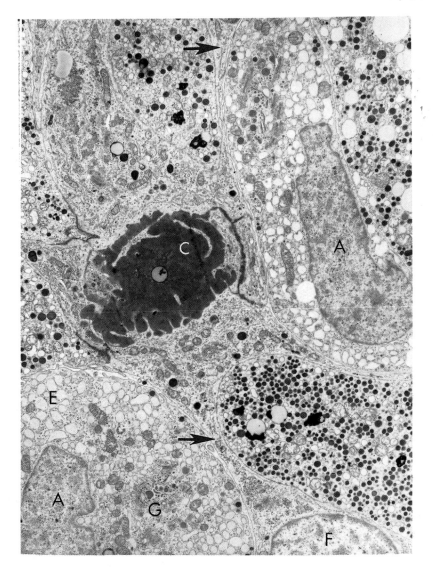

Fig. 2-6. Pars distalis from a dog. Acidophils in the storage (S) phase of the secretory cycle have numerous secretory granules and acidophils in the actively synthesizing (A) phase have an expanded cytoplasmic area with distended cisternae of endoplasmic reticulum (E) and a prominent Golgi apparatus (A). The acidophils are supported by the cytoplasmic processes (arrows) of follicular cells that surround the extracellular accumulations of colloid (C). (From Capen and Koestner, 1967.)

pars distalis. The pars intermedia forms the junction between the pars distalis and pars nervosa.[73] It lines the residual lumen of Rathke's pouch and contains two populations of cells in the dog, one of which synthesizes adrenocorticotrophic hormone (ACTH).[35,62]

A specific population of endocrine cells is present in the pars distalis (and in the pars intermedia for ACTH in the dog) that synthesizes and secretes each of the pituitary trophic hormones.[118] Secretory cells in the adenohypophysis are subdivided into acidophils, basophils, and chromophobes based on interaction of their secretory granules with pH-dependent histochemical stains.

Pituitary cells have a secretory cycle and enter an actively synthesizing phase in response to increased demand for a particular trophic hormone (Fig. 2-7). During this phase the cytoplasm is chromophobic because

SECRETORY CYCLE OF PITUITARY CELLS

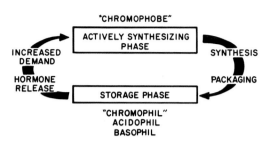

Fig. 2-7. Secretory cycle of cells in the adenohypophysis. During the actively synthesizing phase all pituitary cells are "chromophobic," since their cytoplasm contains abundant endoplasmic reticulum and Golgi apparatus but few secretory granules. When the cell enters the storage phase, the accumulation of hormone-containing secretory granules permits the cells to be subdivided into acidophils, basophils, or chromophobes, based upon their reaction with specific pH-dependent stains.

it contains predominately rough endoplasmic reticulum and Golgi apparatus but few secretory granules. As the batch of recently synthesized hormone is packaged into secretory granules by the Golgi apparatus, the cell enters the storage phase and can be selectively stained by histochemical procedures as either acidophils, basophils, or chromophobes (Fig. 2-6).

Acidophils are further subdivided into somatotrophs and luteotrophs that secrete growth hormone (GH, somatotropin)[150] and luteotrophic hormone (LTH, prolactin),[108] respectively. Basophils include both gonadotrophs that secrete luteinizing hormone (LH) and follicle-stimulating hormone (FSH)[36] and thyrotrophs that secrete thyrotrophic hormone (TTH).[39] Chromophobes are pituitary cells that do not have obvious cytoplasmic secretory granules by light microscopy. They include the endocrine cells concerned with the synthesis of ACTH and melanocyte-stimulating hormone (MSH), nonsecretory follicular cells (Fig. 2-6), and undifferentiated stem cells.

The recent development of radioimmuno-assays for plasma ACTH in the dog has demonstrated a mean concentration of 45.8 pg/ml (range 17 to 98 pg/ml).[47] Assays for

plasma ACTH will be useful in differentiating between pituitary-dependent and other causes of adrenal cortical hyperplasia associated with the syndrome of cortisol-excess. Dogs with functional adrenal cortical neoplasms have plasma ACTH concentrations two standard deviations or more below the mean value for normal dogs.[46] In addition, the development of a homologous radio-immunoassay for canine thyrotropin will facilitate the evaluation of the pituitary-thyroid axis and the diagnosis of certain thyroid diseases. Quinlan and Michaelson[114] reported mean serum thyrotropin levels of 7.0 ± 0.9 ng/ml in euthyroid dogs (9 to 10 years of age, 7 to 14 kg body weight), which increased in response to propylthiouracil administration (334 mg/day intramuscularly) for 1 week. This response was abolished by moderately high doses (1,000 Rad) of X-radiation to the head.

Immunocytochemical staining demonstrated that ACTH- and MSH-staining cells (antisera to porcine ACTH, synthetic ACTH $\beta(1-24)$ and ACTH $\beta(17-39)$, and bovine β-MSH) are polyhedral to round, sparsely granuled, and most numerous in the ventro-central and cranial portions of the pars distalis in dogs where they occur in large groups.[35] They are less numerous in the dorsal and caudal regions of the pars distalis and throughout the pars tuberalis. In the pars intermedia of dogs most cells have immunoreactivity to either pACTH, α-MSH, or β-MSH. Thyrotrophs in the dog are large polyhedral cells situated singly or in small groups ventrocentrally in the para-median plane of the pars distalis.[39] Gonadotrophs (cells reacting with antisera to human FSHβ and/or bovine LHβ) are oval to polyhedral and distributed singly in the pars distalis, particularly in the dorsal-cranial region and in caudal extensions along the pars intermedia.[36] Immunoreactive prolactin cells occur in small groups of large polygonal cells with prominent granules in the ventro-central and cranial portion of the canine pars distalis.[37] A diffuse increase in this population of cells occurs in female dogs near parturition.[42] Growth hormone-secreting cells are present singly along capillaries in the dorsal region of the pars distalis near the pars intermedia.[37] They are small, round to oval, and have fine cytoplasmic granules. Somatotrophs frequently undergo diffuse hyperplasia and hypertrophy in old dogs, especially females with mammary dysplasia or neoplasia.[42]

Endocrine cells in the adenohypophysis are under the control of a corresponding releasing hormone (factor) from the hypothalamus (Fig. 2-8). These releasing hormones are small peptides synthesized by neurosecretion in neurons of the hypothalamus.[129] They are transported by axonal processes to the median eminence, where they are released into capillaries and conveyed by the hypophyseal portal system to specific endocrine cells in the adenohypophysis; there they stimulate the rapid release of preformed trophic hormones (Fig. 2-8).

There appear to be separate hypothalamic releasing hormones that regulate the rate of secretion of each trophic hormone secreted by the adenohypophysis. For most pituitary trophic hormones, negative feedback control is accomplished by the blood concentration of the hormone produced by the target endocrine gland (e.g., thyroid gland, adrenal cortex, ovary, and testis) (Fig. 2-9). The hormone produced by the endocrine glands exerts negative feedback control on the neurosecretory neurons in the hypothalamus that synthesize the corresponding releasing hormone and, to a lesser extent, on the adenohypophysis. Growth hormone, prolactin, and MSH do not act on target endocrine organs to stimulate secretion of a hormone. For example, negative feedback control of growth hormone is effected by production of a corresponding release-inhibiting hormone by neurons in the hypothalamus. The relative local concentrations of the specific releasing hormone and release-inhibiting hormone appear to govern the rate of release of GH from the adenohypophysis. The feedback mechanism of homeostatic control of adrenal cortical secretion is functional in the dog at birth. The newborn dog responds to the administration of ACTH (two

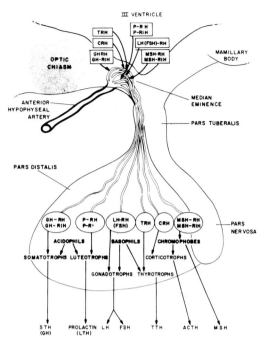

Fig. 2-8. Control of trophic hormone secretion from the adenohypophysis by hypothalamic releasing hormones (RH) and release-inhibiting hormones (R-IH). The releasing and release-inhibiting hormones are synthesized by neurones in the hypothalamus, transported by axonal processes, and released into capillary plexus in the median eminence. They are transported to the adenohypophysis by the hypothalamic-hypophyseal portal system where they interact with specific populations of trophic hormone-secreting cells to govern the rate of release of preformed hormones, such as somatotropin (GH, STH), prolactin (LTH), lutenizing hormone (LH), follicle-stimulating hormone (FSH), thyrotropic hormone (TTH), adrenocorticotropic hormone (ACTH), and melanocyte-stimulating hormone (MSH).

units) or dexamethasone (0.01 to 0.02 mg/kg body weight) with the expected increase or decrease in plasma cortisol concentrations.[99]

HYPOPHYSECTOMY

A classic way of studying the function of an endocrine organ involves surgical removal of the organ and observations to see the effects of its removal. Although this seems to be a simplified approach to studying the endocrine organ it is of tremendous importance to the clinician, since spontaneous failure of the gland will bring about, in varying degrees, the same group of clinical signs as

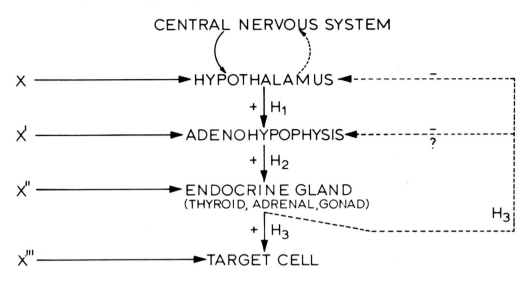

Fig. 2-9. Endocrine control by pituitary gland involving interrelationship with the central nervous system. Receptors in the nervous system detect changes in the internal or external environment and convey this information through neural impulses to neurosecretory neurons in the hypothalamus. Releasing hormones (H1) produced in response to the neural input stimulate the rapid release of corresponding trophic hormone (H2) from the adenohypophysis. Trophic hormones influence the rates of existing reactions in the corresponding endocrine gland (thyroid, adrenal cortex, gonad) and increase the secretion of their hormone (H3), which is carried by the bloodstream to specific target cells to elicit a biologic response. Negative feedback control is affected by the blood concentration of the final endocrine product (H3), on cells in the hypothalamus and the adenohypophysis. Local autoregulatory mechanisms (X) influence the functional activity of each component of the endocrine control system.

does surgical removal. A ventral or transphenoidal approach to the pituitary gland was employed as early as 1910 in the dog by Cushing and others and by Smith in the rat about 1926. Smith's approach was referred to as parapharyngeal. The technique in the rat has become simplified, and technicians can be trained to do hypophysectomies on an assembly line basis. Likewise in the chicken the approach is ventral with a dental drill being used to pierce the sphenoid bone and removal of the hypophysis effected by applying negative pressure through a pipet.

The operation in the domestic animal is more complicated. In swine the approach is anterior in order to avoid the vascular bed (rete mirabile) on the ventral aspect of the hypophysis. French workers have developed a technique of hypophysectomy in the pig by approaching the pituitary from the frontal region through the orbit after having enucleated one eye and elevated the brain. With

surgical forceps the pituitary can be lifted out of the sella turcica.

The effects of removal of the adenohypophysis or of total hypophysectomy are varied since the adenohypophysis regulates the function of so many other organs (Table 2-1). Age has considerable effect on the manifestations of hypophysectomy, since the prepubertal animal would show primarily a deficiency in the rate of growth with an accompanying decrease in the activity of the thyroid and adrenal glands. Since the gonads have not reached a peak of function, gonadal insufficiency would be less recognizable. If hypophysectomy occurs after puberty, then growth would not be affected because the animal would have reached adult body size, but deficiencies in thyroid and adrenal functions would appear, as well as a failure of reproduction and cessation of lactation. In general, the clinical picture would be one of a maintenance level of bodily activities which are

Table 2-1   Some Effects of Hypophysectomy

Clinical Sign	Hormone Deficiency
Low basal metabolic rate	TSH, then thyroxine
Lack of libido in male Anestrus in female Ovulation failure in female Failure to develop ova Lack of secondary sex characteristics Failure of function of accessory sex organs	Gonadotropins (FSH and LH); then gonadal hormones (testosterone or estrogens)
Degeneration of seminiferous tubules of cockerel similar to end of breeding season of wild birds	Gonadotropins; then testosterone.
Atrophy of adrenal cortex	ACTH
Cessation of growth	Somatotropin (STH) plus others (TSH, ACTH)
General depression of metabolism of fat, carbohydrate, and protein	Adrenal steroids, STH, TSH, ACTH, gonadotropins
Cessation of lactation	Prolactin and STH; others like ACTH and TSH to lesser degree

influenced by the adenohypophysis. It is important to note that the pituitary gland is not essential for life and that the essential organs such as the adrenal cortex are capable of continued function to the extent that the basic life processes are preserved. Functions above the maintenance level of the body, such as growth, reproduction, and lactation, are most drastically affected.

There are some species differences in growth when immature animals are hypophysectomized. Hypophysectomy of the immature pig, guinea pig, goat, or calf leads to a reduced growth rate but not complete cessation. However, the puppy or young monkey has a cessation of skeletal growth after hypophysectomy. This suggests a species difference in dependency on somatotropin for growth.

RELEASING HORMONES

The hypothalamic releasing and release-inhibiting hormones are substances that either stimulate or inhibit the release of adenohypophyseal hormones. These factors, which are formed in the hypothalamus, pass via the hypophyseal portal system to influence the release of hormones of the adenohypophysis. Because of the portal system and the proximity of the hypothalamus to the anterior pituitary, only a small amount of RH is needed locally to stimulate the release of pituitary hormones.

Corticotropin-releasing hormone (CRH) was the first releasing hormone to be discovered. LH- and FSH-releasing hormones are probably identical. This RH is referred to as GnRH, or gonadotropin-releasing hormone. Thyrotropin-releasing hormone (TRH) and growth hormone-releasing hormone stimulate the secretion of TSH and STH, respectively. An inhibitory hormone negatively influences STH release. This inhibitory hormone is called growth hormone release-inhibiting hormone or somatostatin.

The identity of most releasing hormones and the finding that they are small peptides led to their chemical identification and synthesis. The chemical structure is known for CRH, TRH (Fig. 2-10), and GnRH (Fig. 2-11). The availability of these releasing hormones and inhibitory hormones permits control of several vital physiologic processes in domestic animals.

The mechanism of action of the releasing hormones appears to be similar to other peptide hormones, i.e. binding to a specific receptor or on the surface of trophic hormone-secreting cells, activation of adenylate cyclase, and generation of an intracellular

TRH

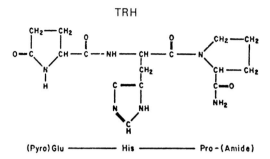

(Pyro) Glu ———————— His ———————— Pro - (Amide)

Fig. 2-10. Amino acid sequence of thyrotropin releasing hormone (TRH).

messenger (cyclic AMP). The cAMP makes the cell more permeable to calcium ion, thereby increasing the intracellular concentration. The increased cytosolic calcium causes the contraction of microfilaments which direct the movement of hormone-containing granules to the periphery of the cell where they are released into capillaries of the portal system.

After the administration of a hypothalamic releasing hormone, there is a pituitary response in a matter of minutes. The circulating half-life of the releasing hormone is short, only a few minutes.

The control of production and release of the releasing hormones by the hypothalamus is modified by a hormone feedback system from the target glands of the tropic hormones. In addition to the feedback control, stimuli from the external environment also influence hypothalamic releasing hormone output, thereby regulating anterior pituitary hormone release. In seasonal breeding animals such as the ewe, bitch, or mare the photoperiod strongly influences the hypothalamic output of releasing hormones. Many other external stimuli such as pain, emotional disturbance, restraint, anesthetics, sexual excitation, or milking influence the output of various releasing hormones.[26]

HORMONES OF THE ADENOHYPOPHYSIS

The hormones of the adenohypophysis can be divided into two main groups according to

GnRH

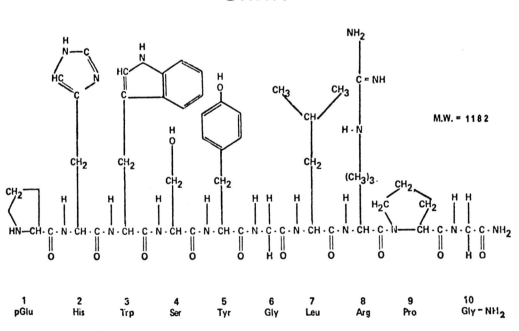

1	2	3	4	5	6	7	8	9	10
pGlu	His	Trp	Ser	Tyr	Gly	Leu	Arg	Pro	Gly - NH$_2$

Fig. 2-11. Amino acid sequence of gonadotropin releasing hormone (GnRH).

their mode of action. In the first group are those hormones which act *directly* on the body tissues. In the second group are those hormones which act *indirectly by first stimulating a target endocrine organ* to release a hormone to bring about another effect. In the first group, acting directly on the general body tissues are somatotropin (growth hormone) and prolactin, which act specifically on the mammary glands and affect milk secretion. Another role for prolactin is as luteotropin in rats which would place it in the second group. In the second group are the thyrotropic, adrenocorticotropic, and gonadotropic hormones which act on their respective target endocrine organs. The various hormones from the pituitary, their source, site of action, and activity within the body are summarized in Table 1-2.

Another hormone of the adenohypophysis is the melanocyte-stimulating hormone (MSH). Although MSH is present in mammals and in the pars distalis of birds, its functional significance is less clear than in amphibia and reptiles where it regulates the pigmentation of the skin. It is a peptide that shares 24 of the 39 amino acids of ACTH. Because the first 13 amino acids in both hormones are identical, there is some possible "overlapping" of effects of these hormones in some species. The predominant control of MSH output is inhibitory from the hypothalamus.

Somatotropin (STH)

Somatotropin or growth hormone (GH) is a complex protein which has been studied by many groups for several decades. There are species differences, but they appear to be more similar than once thought and the molecular weight is approximately 22,000 for most species. The structure of human STH, which has been elucidated by Li and co-workers, has 188 amino acids with two disulfide bridges (Fig. 2-12). There is considerable species specificity for STH and most investigators attempt to use homologous hormone for experimental studies. Refractoriness develops with heterologous hormone, as well as other adverse effects from the injection of a foreign substance. The rat responds to most STH except fish STH. The human responds only to human or monkey STH. Most domestic animals respond best to homologous STH and least to heterologous STH.

The complete protein molecule is not necessary for STH activity. Some peptide sequences may be deleted without altering the biological potency. In fact, fragments of 38 to 40 amino acids have been found to be active.

Control of STH Output

The control of STH output is achieved by a balance between the growth hormone-releasing hormone (GH-RH) and growth-

Table 2-2 *Comparative Pituitary Content of Gonadotropic Hormones*

Species	Pituitary LH Content	Pituitary FSH Content	Occurrence of "Silent Estrus"	Relative Length of Estrus
Cattle	highest	lowest	frequent	short, 14 to 18 hours (ovulation failure seldom a cause of infertility)
Sheep, pigs	high	intermediate	sheep—often pig—rarely	intermediate, 24 to 35 hours for sheep, 2 to 3 days for pigs
Rabbits, rats	intermediate	high		
Horses	lowest	highest	rare	long, 5 to 10 days (LH-like hormone often administered to terminate estrus and cause ovulation, since ovulation failure often a cause of infertility)

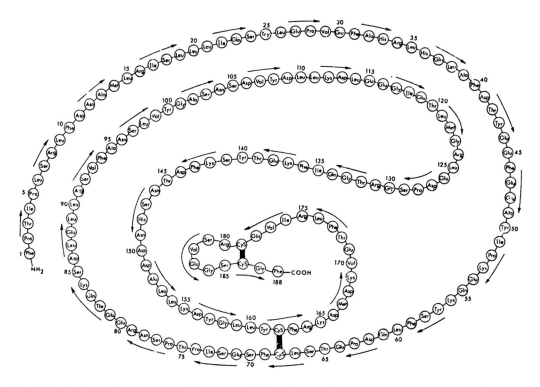

Fig. 2-12. Amino acid sequence of the human STH molecule. (From Li, C. H.: Recent studies on the chemistry of human growth hormone, *In* La spécificité zoologique des hormones hypophysaires et de leurs activités, edited by M. Fontaine, Paris, Centre National de la Recherche Scientifique, 1969.)

hormone release-inhibiting hormone (GH-RIH or somatostatin). Low blood glucose is believed to be the primary cause of GH-RH release which in turn causes STH secretion. In addition, stress, exercise, fasting, high protein food intake, and sleep increase the levels of plasma STH. The amino acid arginine, vasopressin, and alpha-adrenergic agents have a STH-releasing effect, although their mechanism is not understood. Acromegaly follows prolonged elevated STH output (Fig. 2-13), whereas dwarfism results from an early onset deficiency of STH output. Insulin, by lowering the blood glucose level, causes an increased secretion of STH, whereas high doses of glucocorticoids elevate blood glucose and thereby decrease the circulating levels of STH. Fatty acids, hyperglycemia, and beta-adrenergic agents inhibit STH output.

STH appears to be released at a rather similar rate throughout the life of the animal. Although skeletal growth ceases after puberty, STH has a biologic role throughout life as an anabolic agent as well as a synergistic role by enhancing the action of ACTH, TSH, LH, and FSH on their target organs.

Normal Effects in the Body

Somatotropin increases both the soft and osseous tissues of the body and has an effect on lactation. Growth of the long bones continues so long as the epiphyseal lines do not close and in species such as the rat, where the epiphyseal lines do not close, "giants" can be created by prolonged administration of the hormone (Fig. 2-14). In domestic animals, closure of epiphyseal lines soon after puberty results in cessation of skeletal growth under normal conditions.

Protein metabolism is markedly influenced by STH. One of the most important ways that it affects protein metabolism is to increase the retention of nitrogen by the body. The loss of nitrogen into the urine as urea or other

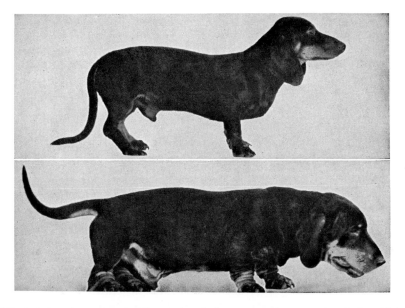

Fig. 2-13. Effect of chronic treatment with anterior pituitary extract in young dog. *Lower,* Male dachshund given daily intraperitoneal injections of pituitary extract containing growth hormone from 6th to 32nd week of life. *Upper,* Littermate male: untreated. (From Evans *et al., Growth and Gonadstimulating Hormone of the Anterior Hypophysis.* Berkeley, University of California Press, 1933.)

nitrogenous waste products is diminished, indicating retention within the body. In addition, another and possibly more *important effect* of STH is to increase cell permeability to amino acids thereby favoring a buildup of the muscle mass of the body. Evidence suggests that STH favors protein synthesis by gene activation, mRNA synthesis, and ribosomal RNA and transfer RNA production by liver cells. The liver cells produce smaller polypeptides called *somatomedins* which act on target cells.

The effect of STH on carbohydrate metabolism is indirect, although it is known that it markedly influences carbohydrate metabolism. For example, the administration of STH to dogs, swine, and several other species will eventually induce a permanent hypergly-

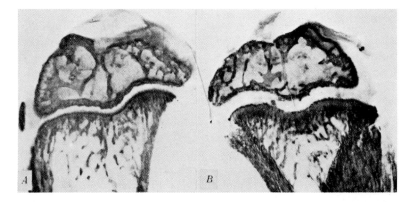

Fig. 2-14. Effect of growth hormone on proximal tibial epiphysis of rat (tibia split longitudinally and stained with silver nitrate). A. Tibia from untreated hypophysectomized rat. *B,* Tibia from hypophysectomized rat treated with growth hormone for 4 days. (Both animals 34 days of age, 16 days postoperative.) Note increase in width of cartilage (unstained band). From Evans *et al., Endocrinology: 32*:14, 1943.)

cemia. The mode of action may involve the elevation of blood sugar through extrapancreatic mechanisms. The high blood sugar level then stimulates the pancreatic beta cells to produce insulin until they are eventually exhausted and undergo degeneration.

It has long been known that diabetes mellitus in the depancreatized dog can be ameliorated by hypophysectomy. The way in which the "Houssay dog" is able to deal with the insulin deficiency most likely is by removing the hyperglycemic effect of STH. STH reduces lipid synthesis, increases fatty acid oxidation, and mobilizes adipose tissue.

In summary, it can be seen that STH favors economical use of proteins and carbohydrates, encouraging the body to retain these building blocks for tissue growth and development or for energy. The metabolism of these substances is complicated with many other hormones and factors being involved in the process. However, STH is one of the important regulating factors of metabolism of carbohydrates, proteins, and fats.

Somatotropin is expensive, is species-specific, and has some adverse side effects. Studies in swine,[31] dogs, and cats indicate that injection of STH frequently leads to the induction of persistent hyperglycemia. Cells of the islet of Langerhans are often damaged. The use of STH produced by recombinant DNA techniques in dairy cows appears to be effective in increasing milk production.

Thyrotropic Hormone (TSH)

Thyroid stimulating hormone (TSH) or thyrotropic hormone is discussed in more detail in the chapter concerned with the thyroid gland. Thyrotropic hormone is a glycoprotein with a molecular weight estimated to be 30,000. There is considerable species specificity to the hormone. TSH has morphological and functional effects on the thyroid. Functionally, the effect of TSH is to increase the synthetic and secretory activity of the follicular cells of the thyroid gland. This activity involves three stages: (1) the uptake of iodide, (2) the production and release of thyroxine and triiodothyronine, and (3) the proteolysis

of thyroglobulin. TSH causes hypertrophy of the follicular cells as well as hyperplasia in the thyroid gland.

The functional level of the thyroid is dependent upon stimulation by TSH. In the hypophysectomized animal the thyroid functions at a low level; consequently, the basal metabolic rate drops to minimal levels. TSH secretion from the adenohypophysis and the thyroxine level from the thyroid gland exist in a state of mutual inhibition and stimulation (Fig. 1-4). A decrease in the level of circulating thyroid hormone results in the release of additional TSH. Conversely, an elevation of thyroid hormone causes inhibition of the output of TSH. This is the previously described "feedback or servomechanism" control. The site of inhibition of thyroxine and triiodothyronine is at the adenohypophysis and to a lesser extent the hypothalamus. In addition to this negative feedback mechanism, there is an effect manifested as a result of environmental temperature. This too is probably mediated through the hypothalamus. In any event, a lower environmental temperature or chilling of the animal either peripherally or centrally causes release of TRH and then TSH which leads to thyroxine secretion, elevation of basal metabolic rate, and heat production to elevate body temperature.

Adrenocorticotropic Hormone (ACTH)

Adrenocorticotropin (ACTH) is a polypeptide which in the sheep, pig, cow, and man contains 39 amino acids in a straight chain. These four species have an identical sequence in the first 24 and last 7 amino acids but show minor differences in amino acid positions 25 through 32. It is in the first 24 amino acids that biological activity resides. The first 13 amino acids are similar to those of MSH which accounts for some overlapping of activity (Fig. 2-15). A polypeptide has been synthesized containing one chain of 17 and one of 19 amino acids which has properties similar to the naturally occurring 39 amino acid chain of the sheep. Schwayzer and Sieber synthesized ACTH which is identical to porcine ACTH in many ways.[135]

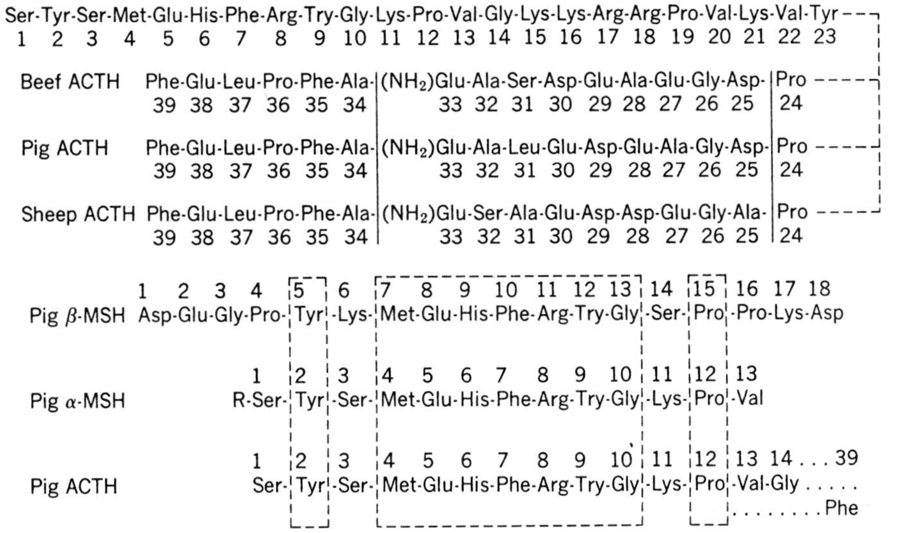

Ser-Tyr-Ser-Met-Glu-His-Phe-Arg-Try-Gly-Lys-Pro-Val-Gly-Lys-Lys-Arg-Arg-Pro-Val-Lys-Val-Tyr ---¬
 1 2 3 4 5 6 7 8 9 10 11 12 13 14 15 16 17 18 19 20 21 22 23   ¦

Beef ACTH   Phe-Glu-Leu-Pro-Phe-Ala-|(NH₂)Glu-Ala-Ser-Asp-Glu-Ala-Glu-Gly-Asp-|Pro ----¬
          39 38 37 36 35 34 | 33 32 31 30 29 28 27 26 25 | 24   ¦

Pig ACTH   Phe-Glu-Leu-Pro-Phe-Ala-|(NH₂)Glu-Ala-Leu-Glu-Asp-Glu-Ala-Gly-Asp-|Pro ----┘
          39 38 37 36 35 34 | 33 32 31 30 29 28 27 26 25 | 24   ¦

Sheep ACTH   Phe-Glu-Leu-Pro-Phe-Ala-|(NH₂)Glu-Ser-Ala-Glu-Asp-Asp-Glu-Gly-Ala-|Pro ----┘
          39 38 37 36 35 34 | 33 32 31 30 29 28 27 26 25 | 24

         1 2 3 4 [5] 6 [7 8 9 10 11 12 13] 14 [15] 16 17 18
Pig β-MSH   Asp-Glu-Gly-Pro-|Tyr|-Lys-|Met-Glu-His-Phe-Arg-Try-Gly|-Ser-|Pro|-Pro-Lys-Asp

            1 [2] 3 [4 5 6 7 8 9 10] 11 [12] 13
Pig α-MSH   R-Ser-|Tyr|-Ser-|Met-Glu-His-Phe-Arg-Try-Gly|-Lys-|Pro|-Val

            1 [2] 3 [4 5 6 7 8 9 10] 11 [12] 13 14 ... 39
Pig ACTH   Ser-|Tyr|-Ser-|Met-Glu-His-Phe-Arg-Try-Gly|-Lys-|Pro|-Val-Gly .....
                                                     .... Phe

Fig. 2-15. Comparative structure of ACTH and MSH.

The regulation of the output of ACTH appears to be intimately associated with the hypothalamus and a feedback control *mechanism* exists similar in principle to the mechanism involved in thyroid function. The adrenal steroids act on the hypothalamus to influence the amount of "corticotropin releasing hormone" (CRH) discharged. In addition, some stressful stimuli such as hemorrhage, temperature, toxins, and emotional status influence the release of ACTH by affecting the release of CRH. The hypophysectomized animal secretes enough corticoids to survive in a protected environment. The third "regulator" of ACTH output is the diurnal influence seen by a morning rise in some, but not all, species.

The primary physiological function of ACTH is to stimulate secretion by the inner two zones (zonae fasciculata and reticularis) of the adrenal cortex, especially of cortisol and/or corticosterone. The adrenal cortex responds to ACTH morphologically by hypertrophy of cells in the zonae fasciculata and reticularis and functionally by an increased production of the glucocorticoids. The specific action of ACTH in the adrenal gland appears to be the stimulation of corticoid biogenesis. The half-life of ACTH is only 6 minutes (in

the rat it may be only 1 minute). See Chapter 8 for further discussion of ACTH.

Prolactin (Lactogenic Hormone)

Prolactin, also called lactogenic hormone, consists of 198 amino acids in the sheep with a MW of 23,300 and a 15-minute half-life. Hypophysectomy of a lactating animal will cause cessation of lactation. This and other data led early workers to believe that prolactin was of considerable importance in lactation. Prolactin increases in the peripheral blood of the cow during milking. Prolactin stimulates the pigeon crop gland to hypertrophy and secrete a caseous "crop milk" which is used as a method of bioassay.

Prolactin also appears to have a corpus luteum-stimulating effect in some species, hence the name "luteotropin," at least in the mouse and rat and possibly the ferret, but not in the ewe, cow, guinea pig, human being, or rabbit.

Pituitary Gonadotropins

Two hormones from the adenohypophysis affect the gonads: follicle-stimulating hormone and luteinizing hormone (interstitial cell-stimulating hormone). Their pituitary content is summarized in Table 2-2.

Follicle-stimulating Hormone (FSH)

FSH is a glycoprotein with MW of approximately 29,000 in the pig but 32,000 in the sheep and a 2- to 4-hour half-life. The pituitary output of FSH is under hypothalamic control including a *feedback* mechanism involving the gonadal hormones. Rising estrogen levels from the follicle feed back to depress GnRH and then FSH output. In addition, environmental conditions such as changing seasons and daylight length must be mediated from some exteroceptors to the hypothalamus to influence GnRH output. The physiologic effect of FSH in the female hypophysectomized animal is to cause multiple follicle growth in the ovaries without estrogen production or ovulation. In the male the effect on the seminiferous tubules is a subtle one leading to spermatogenesis if the Leydig cells have produced androgen. FSH does not stimulate Leydig cell production of androgen. Interstitial cell-stimulating hormone (ICSH) is the hormone that causes steroid synthesis by the Leydig cells.

Luteinizing (LH) or Interstitial Cell-stimulating Hormone (ICSH)

Interstitial cell-stimulating hormone (ICSH) and luteinizing hormone (LH) are the same hormone. The nomenclature reflects the sex of the animal concerned. LH is a glycoprotein which has a MW of 30,000 in sheep and cattle, contains 216 amino acids, and has a half-life of 30 minutes. The pituitary content of LH is highest in cattle, sheep, and cats and lowest in horses and man.

The regulation of LH output from the pituitary gland is dependent upon the hypothalamic control (GnRH), which in part is a feedback control mechanism involving the gonadal hormones. The normal effects of LH in the female are to stimulate the developing follicle toward maturation, estrogen production, and finally ovulation provided FSH has already acted. Its role in corpus luteum function will be considered in Chapter 9 on female reproduction. In the male, ICSH acts directly on the Leydig cells of the testis, causing testos-

terone production which in turn acts throughout the body as well as on the seminiferous tubules.

STRUCTURE AND FUNCTION OF NEUROHYPOPHYSIS

The neurohypophysis consists of three anatomic subdivisions. The pars nervosa (posterior lobe) represents the distal component of the neurohypophyseal system. It is composed of numerous capillaries that are supported by modified glial cells (pituicytes). The capillaries in the pars nervosa are termination sites for the nonmyelinated axonal processes of neurosecretory neurons in the hypothalamus. Secretion granules that contain the neurohypophyseal hormones, i.e., oxytocin and antidiuretic hormone, are synthesized in hypothalamic neurons, but are released into the bloodstream in the pars nervosa. The infundibular stalk joins the pars nervosa to the overlying hypothalamus and is composed of axonal processes from neurosecretory neurons.

Neurosecretory neurons in the hypothalamus receive neural input from higher centers and translate this into endocrine output in the form of hormonal secretion (Fig. 2-16). In addition to the usual structural features of neurons they contain prominent arrays of rough endoplasmic reticulum, large Golgi apparatuses, and numerous membrane-limited secretory granules in the cell body and axonal process (Fig. 2-16). The neurosecretory neurons concerned with hormone synthesis are segregated into anatomically defined regions called nuclei in the hypothalamus. The supraoptic nucleus is concerned primarily with the synthesis of antidiuretic hormone, whereas oxytocin is produced predominately by neurons in the paraventricular nucleus.

The neurohypophysis in most animals is supplied directly by the posterior (inferior) hypophyseal arteries that branch from the internal carotid arteries (Fig. 2-17). Branches of the anterior (superior) hypophyseal arteries originate from the internal carotid arteries and

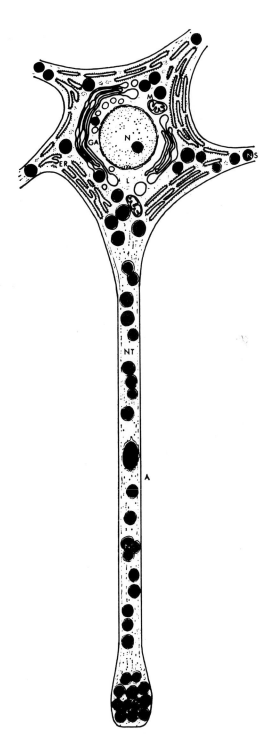

from the posterior communicating arteries of the circle of Willis. Arteriolar branches penetrate the pars tuberalis (infundibularis), lose their muscular coat, and form a capillary plexus near the median eminence. These vessels subsequently drain into hypophyseal portal veins that supply the pars distalis. There also may be a small direct arterial supply to the adenohypophysis of minor physiologic importance that arises from the posterior hypophyseal arteries (Fig. 2-17).

Antidiuretic hormone (ADH; vasopressin) is an octapeptide synthesized by neurons situated primarily in the supraoptic nucleus of the hypothalamus. The hormone is packaged into membrane-limited granules with a corresponding binding protein (neurophysin) and transported to the pituitary gland by axonal processes of the neurosecretory neurons (Fig. 2-16). These axons terminate on fenestrated capillaries in the pars nervosa and release ADH into the circulation.

ADH is transported by the bloodstream to the kidney, where it binds to specific isoreceptors in the distal part of the nephron and collecting ducts. The overall effect of ADH on the kidney is to increase the active renal tubular reabsorption of water from the glomerular filtrate. The hormone (ADH)-receptor complex activates the membrane-bound enzyme, adenylate cyclase, resulting in the intracellular formation of cyclic adenosine monophosphate (cAMP) from ATP (17) (Fig. 2-18). The accumulation of cAMP appears to activate protein kinases involved in the phosphorylation of proteins in the luminal membrane that increase the permeability of the cell to water.

Fig. 2-16. Structural characteristics of a neurosecretory neurone in the hypothalamus. The nerve cell body (N, nucleus) has dendritic and axonal (A) processes with arrays of rough endoplasmic reticulum, a prominent Golgi apparatus, and neurotubules (NT). Hormone-containing, membrane-limited neurosecretory granules (NS) are formed in the Golgi apparatus and transported along the axon to the site of release at the termination on capillaries. Neurosecretory neurones synthesize the releasing and release-inhibiting hormones of the adenohypophysis and the hormones of the neurohypophysis (oxytocin, antidiuretic hormone).

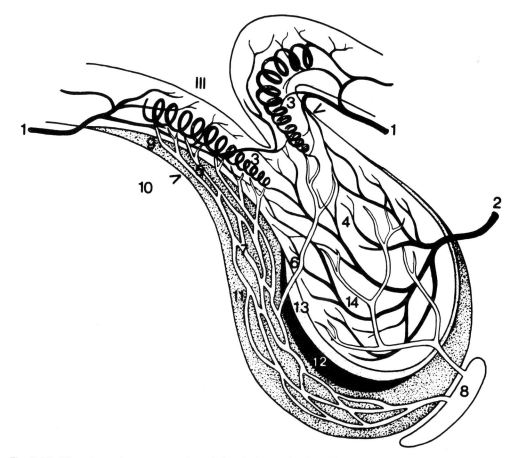

Fig. 2-17. Diagrammatic representation of the pituitary gland and its vascular supply. 1, superior hypophyseal artery; 2, inferior hypophyseal artery; 3, primary plexus of the infundibular stem; 4, primary plexus of the infundibular process; 5, long portal vessels; 6, short portal vessels; 7, secondary plexus in the adenohypophysis; 8, collecting vein; 9, pars tuberalis (infundibularis) of the adenohypophysis; 10, pituitary stalk; 11, pars distalis; 12, residual hypophyseal lumen (intraglandular cleft); 13, pars intermedia; 14, infundibular process of the neurohypophysis; III, infundibular recess of the third ventricle. (From Meijer, J. C.: An investigation of the pathogenesis of pituitary-dependent hyperadrenocorticism in the dog. Thesis, The University of Utrecht, The Netherlands, 1980.)

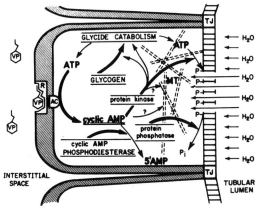

Fig. 2-18. Subcellular mechanism of action of anti-diuretic hormone (vasopressin) in the kidney. The hormone (VP) binds to isoreceptors on target cells of collecting ducts and activates adenylate cyclase (AC) in the plasma membrane on the basilar aspect of the cell. The intracellular accumulation of cyclic adenosine monophosphate (cAMP) may activate certain protein kinases that phosphorylate proteins in the luminal plasma membrane that increase the permeability to water. (From Dousa, T. P.: Cellular action of anti-diuretic hormone in nephrogenic diabetes insipidus, Mayo Clin. Proc. *49*:188, 1974.)

Six of the 8 amino acids are identical in the two hormones produced by hypothalamic nuclei and released in the pars nervosa. Antidiuretic hormone (ADH or vasopressin) has a dual action, affecting the water reabsorption mechanism of the kidney and causing pressor effects on the vascular system when given in high doses. Oxytocin has its primary action upon the smooth muscle of the mammary gland and the uterus. Antidiuretic hormone (ADH) is a peptide containing 8 amino acids (2 molecules of cysteine are S-S bonded to form a single cystine molecule which causes the hormone to contain only 8 *different* amino acids). There are species differences in ADH composition since cattle, man, and most mammals contain arginine and swine ADH contains lysine (Fig. 2-19).

The output of ADH is directly related to the degree of hydration of the body. In fact, the osmoreceptors may be located in the supraoptic and paraventricular nuclei. Hydration of the body or injection of water into the blood going to the hypothalamus inhibits release of ADH, which in turn causes less water resorption from glomerular filtrate thereby removing excess water from the body. Dehydration of the body or injection of hypertonic electrolyte solutions into the hypothalamic artery favors release of ADH, which in turn

causes increased water resorption from the glomerular filtrate. The body water is increased and electrolytes are diluted. Consequently, less urine is formed. Concentrated body fluids cause ADH release, and dilute body fluids hinder ADH release. Other factors such as barbiturates, ether, chloroform, morphine, acetylcholine, nicotine, and pain increase ADH release leading to less urine formation. Ethyl alcohol inhibits ADH release leading to diuresis.

The pressor effect of ADH is less prominent than the antidiuretic effect. At a dosage several hundred times larger than the antidiuretic dosage, ADH has a pronounced pressor effect which may also lead to serious coronary constriction. The contractile mechanism of the capillaries, as well as gastrointestinal and uterine muscle, is stimulated and a rather prolonged elevation of blood pressure follows.

The half-life of ADH is only a few minutes, but ADH is available in forms that slowly release small amounts. The most frequently used preparation is Pitressin Tannate in oil (Parke Davis). The subcutaneous or IM dose for the dog is one to three units each 36 to 48 hours. A higher dose, three to five units, can be used as a diagnostic test for diabetes insipidus. This higher dose would decrease

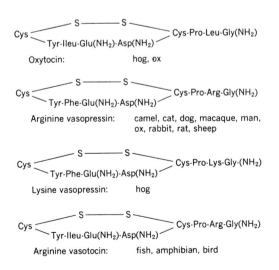

Fig. 2-19. A comparison of amino acid sequences of oxytocin and several vasopressins of various species.

urine formation and differentiate diabetes insipidus from other disturbances of water metabolism.

Oxytocin is similar to ADH insofar as its origin and chemistry (Fig. 2-19). Oxytocin does not possess pharmacological activities similar to those of ADH; instead it has specific effects on the smooth muscle of the uterus and the myoepithelial cells of the mammary gland. An exception is its ability to lower blood pressure of birds—an effect sometimes used for bioassay purposes. Its activity will be further discussed in Chapters 18 and 20 on parturition and lactation. *Oxytocic* is Greek meaning "rapid birth." Oxytocin has no physiological function in the male, although there are suggestions that oxytocin may affect sperm transport through the male tract.[1]

DISORDERS OF PITUITARY FUNCTION

Juvenile Panhypopituitarism ("Pituitary Dwarfism")

Juvenile panhypopituitarism occurs most frequently in German shepherd dogs, but is has also been reported in other breeds, such as the spitz, toy pinscher, and Carelian bear dogs from Denmark.[3,8,9,14,75,87,96,151] Pituitary dwarfism in German shepherd dogs usually is associated with a failure of the oropharyngeal ectoderm of Rathke's pouch to differentiate into trophic hormone-secreting cells of the pars distalis (Fig. 2-20). This results in progressively enlarging, multiloculated cysts in the sella turcica and an absence of the adenohypophysis (Fig. 2-21). The

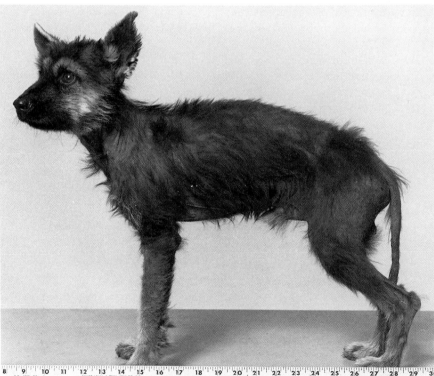

Fig. 2-20. Panhypopituitarism due to a failure of oropharyngeal ectoderm to differentiate into trophic hormone-secreting cells of the adenohypophysis resulting in "pituitary dwarfism" in a German shepherd. Note the failure of somatic maturation (at 1 year of age), large areas of alopecia, and coyote- (or fox-) like facial features.

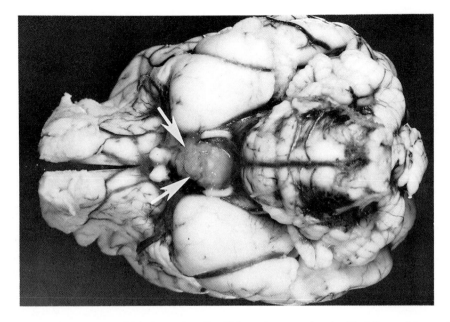

Fig. 2-21. Panhypopituitarism ("pituitary dwarfism") in a dog associated with failure of the embryonic oropharyngeal epithelium of Rathke's pouch to differentiate into secretory cells of the adenohypophysis. Ventral view of the brain and pituitary region and brain to illustrate the large multiloculated cyst (arrows). The pars nervosa was formed normally but was compressed by the mucin-filled cyst.

cyst(s) are lined by pseudostratified, often ciliated, columnar epithelium with interspersed mucin-secreting goblet cells. The mucin-filled cysts eventually occupy the entire pituitary area in the sella turcica and severely compress the pars nervosa and infundibular stalk (Fig. 2-21). Few differentiated, trophic hormone-secreting pituitary cells are present in the pituitary region of dwarf pups that immunocytochemically stain for the specific trophic hormones. An occasional small nest or rosette of poorly differentiated epithelial cells is interspersed between the multiloculated cysts, but their cytoplasm usually is devoid of hormone-containing secretory granules.

The dwarf pups appear normal or are indistinguishable from littermates at birth and up to about 2 months of age. Subsequently, the slower growth rate than the littermates, retention of puppy hair coat, and lack of primary guard hairs gradually become evident in dwarf pups (Fig. 2-22). German shepherd dogs with pituitary dwarfism appear coyote- or fox-like owing to their diminutive size and soft woolly hair coat (Fig. 2-21).[100,101] A bilaterally symmetric alopecia develops gradually and often progresses to complete alopecia except for the head and tufts of hair on the legs. There is progressive hyperpigmentation of the skin until it is uniformly brown-black over most of the body. Adult German shepherd dogs with panhypopituitarism vary in size from as tiny as 4 pounds up to nearly half the normal size, apparently depending upon whether the failure of formation of the adenohypophysis is complete or only partial.

Permanent dentition is delayed or completely absent. Closure of epiphyses is delayed as long as 4 years depending on the severity of hormonal insufficiency. There are few trabeculae in the primary and secondary spongiosa of the metaphysis of long bones, and osteoblasts are decreased in dwarf pups, as compared with normal littermates. The external genitalia usually remain infantile. The testes and penis are small, calcification of the os penis is delayed or incomplete, and the penile sheath is flaccid. In females the

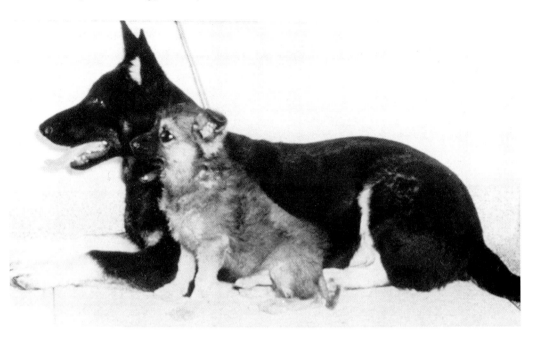

Fig. 2-22. Panhypopituitarism ("pituitary dwarfism") in a 5-month-old German shepherd. An unaffected littermate weighed 60 pounds and the dwarf, 8.8 pounds. Note the retention of the puppy hair coat on the dwarf. (Courtesy of Dr. J. Alexander and the Canadian Veterinary Journal, 1962.)

ovarian cortex is hypoplastic and estrus irregular or absent. The shortened lifespan in these dogs results not only from the panhypopituitarism, but also from the resulting secondary endocrine dysfunction, such as hypothyroidism and hypoadrenocorticism. The increase in blood thyroxine and cortisol levels in response to challenge by exogenous thyrotropin and adrenocorticotropin are subnormal, owing to the hypoplasia of the thyroid gland and cortisol-secreting zone of the adrenal cortex.[136] The variation in severity and onset of the lesions in pituitary dwarfism appears to be related to the degree that the oropharyngeal epithelium fails to differentiate and the rapidity with which the mucin-filled cysts enlarge and exert pressure on adjacent structures.[4]

Other useful diagnostic aids include comparison of height with littermates (Fig. 2-22), radiographs of open epiphyseal lines, thyroid function tests, and skin biopsy. Cutaneous lesions include hyperkeratosis, follicular keratosis, hyperpigmentation, adnexal atrophy and a loss of elastin fibers, and the loose network of collagen fibers in the dermis. Hair shafts are absent and hair follicles are primarily in the telogen (resting) phase of the growth cycle.[4,19,77,101]

Panhypopituitarism in German shepherd dogs often occurs in littermates and related litters, suggesting a simple autosomal recessive mode of inheritance.[7-9,93,104,151] The activity of somatomedin (a cartilage growth-promoting peptide whose production in the liver and plasma activity is controlled by somatotropin) is low in dwarf dogs.[93] Intermediate somatomedin activity is present in the phenotypically normal ancestors suspected to be heterozygous carriers. Assays for somatomedin (a non-species-specific, somatotropin-dependent peptide) provide an indirect measurement of circulating growth hormone activity in dogs suspected to be heterozygous carriers.[147,151] Basal levels of circulating canine growth hormone are reported to be detectable but low (normal range: 1.75 ± 0.17 ng/ml)[63] in pituitary dwarfs and fail to increase following a provocative test for growth hormone secretion provided by clonidine injection (30 μg/kg, intravenously) as in normal dogs.[75] Insulin hypersensitivity has been demonstrated in pituitary dwarf dogs, probably due to a change in insulin receptor numbers or affinity of binding in response to the low growth hormone levels.[136] Dwarf dogs develop hypoglycemia of greater magnitude in response to an insulin injection (0.025 U/kg) than that in normal dogs but similar to that in experimentally hypophysectomized dogs.

In affected Carelian bear dogs there is low somatomedin activity. A simple autosomal recessive pattern of inheritance appears likely in these dogs which were heavily crossbred with Greman shepherd dogs and apparently acquired the gene for dwarfism.[7,8]

The interesting dwarf German shepherd dog reported by Müller-Peddinghaus et al.[102] with a cystic pituitary had surprisingly high (4.1 ng/ml) serum growth hormone levels (normal range 1.8 to 3.8 ng/ml) but an abnormally low (0.13 unit/ml) serum somatomedin level (normal for dog more than 0.50 unit/ml, as determined by ^{35}S incorporation into piglet rib cartilage). These changes in growth hormone and somatomedin levels resemble those found in Laron's syndrome of dwarfism in human infants in which there is a peripheral resistance to the action of somatotropin. In this dog the adenohypophysis apparently had developed but subsequently underwent pressure atrophy from the multiple cysts in the pituitary gland derived from the craniopharyngeal duct. Only remnants of the adenohypophysis remained with compressed, immunocytochemically stained, trophic hormone-secreting cells.

Roth et al.[125] investigated the pathogenesis of retarded growth in an inbred colony of Weimaraner dogs. Affected pups developed a wasting disease characterized by unthriftiness, emaciation, chronic anemia, stunted growth, and persistent infections. The thymus was small owing to a markedly diminished cortex. In pups that developed the wasting syndrome there was a lack of lymphocytes in paracortical areas of lymph nodes and around periarteriolar lymphoid sheaths of splenic white pulp. One pup that survived the wasting syndrome had a depressed lymphocyte blastogenic response to phytohemagglutinin compared with that of its surviving littermates. Pups with this syndrome also lacked the increase in plasma growth hormone concentration that occurs in normal dogs after injection of clonidine hydrochloride.

Acromegaly

Acromegaly is a disease characterized by an overgrowth of connective tissue, increased appositional growth of bone, coarsening of facial features, and enlargement of viscera due to a chronic excessive secretion of growth hormone (somatotropin). Under experimental conditions, acromegalic characteristics have been induced in dogs by the long-term injection of anterior pituitary extracts.[44,113] Harris and Heaney[67] increased skeletal mass of adult dogs of both sexes by the exogenous administration of bovine growth hormone (0.5 mg/kg/day) without inducing acromegaly or diabetes. Although growth hormone-secreting acidophils are one of the major cell types in the adenohypophysis of dogs, the development of adenomas and primary hyperplasia derived from this population of acidophils is of infrequent occurrence in dogs. Lucksch[92] reported an acidophil adenoma in a dog with thickened cranial bones. An acidophil tumor reported by King et al.[83] was accompanied by metahypophyseal diabetes with fewer pancreatic islets than present in normal dogs.

Rijnberk et al.[122] detected the development of acromegalic features in a 6-year-old female Belgian shepherd that had been frequently administered large doses of a progestational drug to prevent estrus. Initial clinical signs included polyphagia, exercise intolerance, intolerance to warmth (frequent panting, preference for cool places to sleep), exaggerated growth of the hair coat, slight exophthalmos, increase in abdominal size, mucometra, and inspiratory stridor. Subsequently, the body weight increased and there was a disproportionate increase in the size of the head and limbs. The interdental spaces between incisors was considerably widened owing to the proliferation of connective tissue (Fig. 2-23). The hair coat was thick and curly and large skin folds were present on the ventral surface of the trunk and neck. Radiographically, there was spondylosis of the lumbar vertebrae and widening of the metaphalangeal bones, with a slight periosteal reaction.

Plasma growth hormone levels, determined by radioimmunoassay, were initially high (over 45 ng/ml) compared with 1.75 ng/ml ± 0.17 for clinically normal dogs[63] but progressively decreased toward normal over a period of about 1 year. The dog did not receive additional injections of medroxyprogesterone acetate during the interval of declining growth hormone levels. An oral glucose load resulted in a prolonged elevation of the blood glucose concentration, exaggerated insulin response with a prolonged elevation of plasma insulin levels, and a lack of suppression

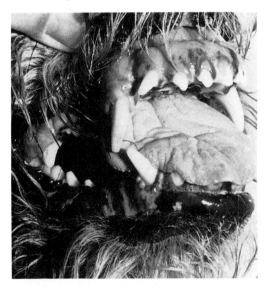

Fig. 2-23. Iatrogenic acromegaly in a dog illustrating widening of the interdental spaces between the incisors due to the proliferation of connective tissue. The increased growth hormone secretion was stimulated by the administration of medroxyprogesterone acetate. (From Rijnberk et al. Small Animal Clinic, Faculty of Veterinary Medicine, State University of Utrecht, The Netherlands.)

of the high immunoreactive growth hormone levels in the blood.[122] During the interval of declining growth hormone levels, signs of respiratory distress and exercise intolerance progressively disappeared. The increased connective tissue mass appeared to regress, but the skeletal abnormalities remained unchanged. The glucose tolerance curve, insulin response to a glucose load, and growth hormone levels returned to normal over the 3-year-period of observation.

A stimulation of growth hormone-secreting acidophils in the adenohypophysis by progestational agents also has been reported under experimental conditions in the dog.[38,40,41] El Etreby and Fath El Bab[36] observed increased numbers of somatotrophs after the administration of progesterone and cyproterone acetate. Diabetes mellitus has been reported in experimental dogs following the administration of medroxyprogesterone acetate[64] and megestrol acetate.[148] The stimulation of growth hormone release in dogs by progestogens differs from the situation in human beings in whom high prolactin levels result from treatment with these drugs.

Concannon et al.[24] evaluated changes in plasma growth hormone, prolactin, cortisol, and progesterone levels in beagles following intramuscular injection of medroxyprogesterone acetate (6α-methyl-17-acetoxyprogesterone) (75 mg/kg) every 3 months for 17 months. Circulating hormone levels were correlated with the development of acromegalic features (Fig. 2-24) and mammary nodules. The extent of acromegalic-like appearance was scored from 0 to 4 according to the following criteria: 0-normal; 1-coarse hair with slightly thickened and folded skin on the face, shoulders, back, and flank; 2-in addition to 1, enlargement of the feet, thickening and folding of the skin on the forelegs; 3-in addition to 1 and 2, prominent folds of thick skin on and about the face; 4-in addition to all of the foregoing, more prominent facial changes and folds of thick skin extending over the body to the hind legs (Fig. 2-25).

Medroxyprogesterone acetate increased mean growth hormone levels, incidence of

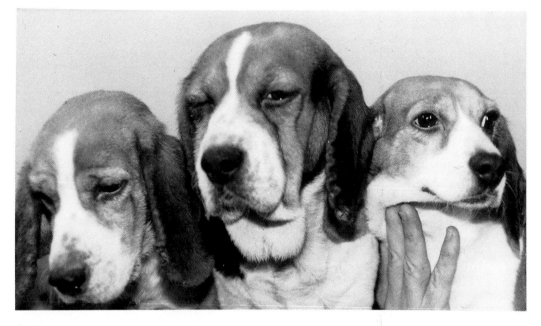

Fig. 2-24. Acromegaly in a beagle (center) compared to unaffected littermates (left and right). Note the coarseness of facial features and marked thickening and folding of the skin of the face. (Courtesy of Dr. P. Concannon, Department of Physical Biology, New York State College of Veterinary Medicine, Cornell University.)

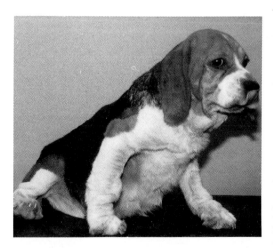

Fig. 2-25. Acromegaly in a beagle caused by chronic stimulation of growth hormone secretion following the administration of medroxyprogesterone acetate (75 mg/kg every 3 months for 17 months). The skin of the face, trunk, and forelegs is coarsely thickened and folded. (Courtesy of Dr. P. Concannon, Department of Physical Biology, New York State College of Veterinary Medicine, Cornell University.)

acromegaly-like changes, and frequency of palpable mammary nodules in beagles under controlled conditions (Table 2-3). Growth hormone levels were elevated (2.5 ng/ml and above) in all female beagles with acromegalic features (mean 12.8 ng/ml) compared with placebo controls and dogs receiving crystalline progesterone implants. All dogs with elevated growth hormone levels had multiple mammary nodules that averaged 9.5 ± 2.2 mm in diameter. The elevation in growth hormone levels and development of acromegalic features was greater in older (mean: 65.4 ± 6.9 months) than in younger (mean: 42.0 ± 1.7 months) dogs. Preliminary studies indicated that initial elevations of growth hormone occurred after 8 months of medroxyprogesterone acetate treatment. Serum prolactin levels were not changed by either medroxyprogesterone acetate or crystalline progesterone implants, but serum cortisol levels were suppressed significantly compared with those in controls (Table 2-3). The latter probably was the result of medroxyprogesterone-induced suppression of pituitary adreno-

Table 2-3 Effects of Medroxyprogesterone Acetate (MPA) (75 mg/kg Every 3 Months for 17 Months) and Progesterone on Beagle Dogs.

	Placebo Controls	MPA (75 mg/kg × 3 mo)	Progesterone Implants[a]
Serum Growth Hormone (ng/ml)	0.4 ± 0.1	9.5 ± 2.8[†**]	0.6 ± 0.2
Serum Prolactin (ng/ml)	12.6 ± 1.2	13.7 ± 2.8	13.6 ± 2.1
Serum Cortisol (ng/ml)	13.7 ± 1.4	1.7 ± 0.2[†**]	14.9 ± 1.2
Serum Progesterone (ng/ml)	5.3 ± 3.1	0.2 ± 0.02[†**]	13.8 ± 2.1[*]
Mammary Nodules: Numbers	2	35	8
Mean (mm) Diameter (range)	2.0 ± 0.0	7.9 ± (2–75)	3.7 (206)
Acromegaly Score	0 ± 0.0	1.3 ± 0.4[**]	0.3 ± 0.3

Different from placebo controls:
* (P < 0.05)
† (P < 0.01)
Different from progesterone implants:
** (P < 0.05–0.01)
[a] Subcutaneous implants crystalline progesterone.

From Concannon, P., et al., Growth hormone, prolactin, and cortisol in dogs developing mammary nodules and an acromegaly-like appearance during treatment with medroxyprogesterone acetate. Endocrinology *106*:1173, 1980.

corticotropin secretion and corresponding decrease in cortisol synthesis by the adrenal cortex.[24,34,38,41] Growth hormone levels also have been reported to be elevated in dogs with spontaneous mammary tumors, and somatotrophs have cytologic evidence of increased secretory activity.[27]

Acth-Secreting Pituitary Tumors Associated with Hypercortisolism

Functional tumors arising in the pituitary gland of dogs often are derived from corticotroph (ACTH-secreting) cells either in the pars distalis or in the pars intermedia. They cause a clinical syndrome of cortisol excess (Cushing's-like disease) (Fig. 2-26). These neoplasms are encountered most frequently in dogs and infrequently in other animal species. They develop in adult to aged dogs and have been reported in a number of breeds.[18a,21,22,65,120,121,149] Boxers, Boston terriers, and dachschunds appear to have a higher incidence of functional (ACTH-secreting) pituitary tumors than other breeds of dogs. The spectrum of dramatic clinical manifestations and lesions that develop is primarily the result of long-term overproduction of cortisol by hyperplastic adrenal cortices

(Fig. 2-27). These changes are the result of the combined gluconeogenic, lipolytic, protein catabolic, and anti-inflammatory action of glucocorticoid hormones on many organ systems of the body.

A number of distinctive clinical and functional alterations develop in dogs with corticotroph (ACTH-secreting) adenomas, resulting in the syndrome of cortisol-excess.[18,18a,91,139] Centripetal redistribution of adipose tissue leads to prominent fat pads on the dorsal midline of the neck giving the neck and shoulders a thick appearance. Appetite and intake of food may be increased or ravenous, either as a direct stimulation of the appetite center by the cortisol-excess or as a result of destruction of the "satiety center" in the ventral-medial nucleus of the hypothalamus by the dorsally expanding adenoma. Muscles of the extremities and abdomen are weakened and atrophied. The loss of tone of abdominal muscles and muscles of the abaxial skeleton results in gradual abdominal enlargement ("pot belly") (Fig. 2-26), lordosis, muscle trembling, and a straight-legged skeletal-braced posture to support the body weight. Profound atrophy of the temporal muscles may result in obvious concave indentations and readily palpable

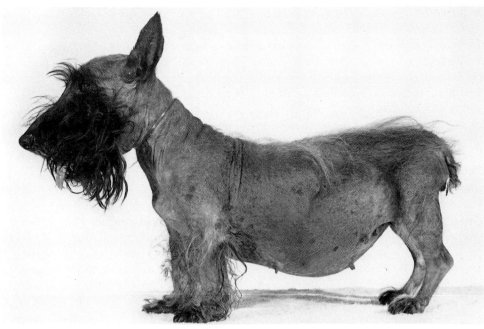

Fig. 2-26. ACTH-secreting pituitary tumor resulting in hypercortisolism in a Scottish terrier. The long-term secretion of excessive cortisol resulted in alopecia that extends over most of the body. Due to the gluconeogenic action of excess cortisol the skin is thin, wrinkled, and hyperpigmented. Muscle asthenia is evident from the pendulous abdomen and swayed back.

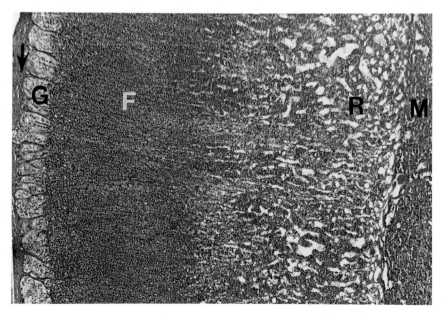

Fig. 2-27. Diffuse hyperplasia of the adrenal cortex in a dog with a ACTH-secreting adenoma of the pituitary. The zonae fasciculata (F) and reticularis (R) are markedly hyperplastic in response to the long-term overproduction of ACTH, whereas the outer zona glomerulosa (G) is compressed immediately beneath the adrenal capsule (arrow). M = cortical-medullary junction.

prominences of the underlying skull bones. Hepatomegaly due in part to increased fat and glycogen deposition and vacuolation of liver cells may contribute to the development of the distended, often pendulous, abdomen.

The pituitary gland consistently is enlarged in dogs with corticotroph adenomas (Fig. 2-28). Neither the occurrence nor the severity of functional disturbances appears to be directly related to the size of the neoplasm. Small adenomas are as likely to be endocrinologically active as are larger neoplasms. The larger adenomas often are firmly attached to the base of the sella turcica without evidence of erosion of the sphenoid bone. Growth of the pituitary tumor along the basilar aspects of the brain may result in incorporation of the second, third, and fourth cranial nerves leading to functional disturbances from a disruption of their function.

There is bilateral enlargement of the adrenal glands in dogs with functional corticotroph adenomas (Fig. 2-28). This enlargement often is striking and is due entirely to increased cortical parenchyma, primarily in the zonae fasciculata and reticularis (Fig. 2-27). Nodules of yellow-orange cortical tissue often are found outside the capsule in the periadrenal fat as well as extending down into the adrenal medulla. The cortico-medullary junction is irregular and the medulla is compressed. The secretion of excess cortisol in these dogs can be diminished by the administration of the adrenocytotoxic drug, ortho, para'-DDD.[68,133]

Pituitary corticotroph adenomas are composed of well-differentiated secretory cells supported by fine connective tissue septa. They are composed of either large or small chromophobic cells. The cytoplasm of the tumor cells is devoid of secretory granules

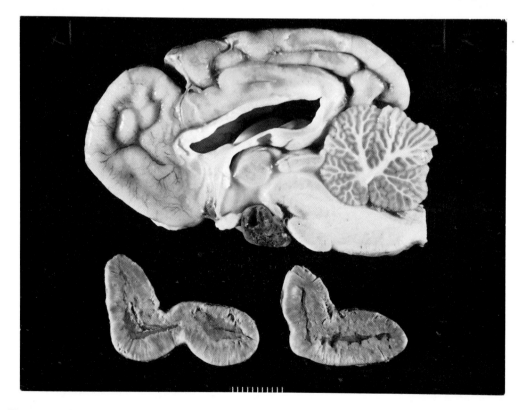

Fig. 2-28. ACTH-secreting adenoma in the pituitary gland from a dog with bilateral enlargement of the adrenal glands. The long-term secretion of ACTH results in hypertrophy and hyperplasia of secretory cells of the zonae fasciculata and reticularis in the adrenal gland and an excessive secretion of cortisol. The scale at the bottom represents 1 cm.

detectable by specific histochemical procedures used for pituitary cytology. However, pituitary adenomas arising in both the pars distalis and the pars intermedia associated with the syndrome of cortisol excess in dogs are composed of polyhedral cells that immunocytochemically stain selectively for ACTH and MSH (26). Nodules of focal hyperplasia and microadenomas, composed of similar ACTH/MSH cells, are also present in both lobes of the adenohypophysis.

Although remnants of the pars distalis can be identified near the periphery of the adenomas, the demarcation is not distinct between the neoplasm and pars distalis. The pars distalis either is partly replaced by the neoplasm or is severely compressed. The pars nervosa and infundibular stalk either are infiltrated and disrupted by tumor cells or are completely incorporated within the larger neoplasms.

Cells comprising functional corticotroph adenomas in dogs have definite ultrastructural evidence of secretory activity.[17] Organelles concerned with protein synthesis (endoplasmic reticulum) and packaging of secretory products (Golgi apparatus) are well developed in tumor cells. Hormone-containing secretory granules can be demonstrated by electron microscopy in cells comprising functional corticotroph adenomas. The granules vary in number from cell to cell, are roughly spherical, and are surrounded by a delicate limiting membrane. They are small (mean diameter of 170 μm), electron-dense, and have a prominent submembranous space.

Adenomas derived from corticotroph cells of the pars intermedia develop more often in nonbrachycephalic breeds of dogs than in brachycephalic breeds.[18a] Adenomas of the pars intermedia in dogs may be associated with the secretion of excessive adrenocorticotropin (ACTH), leading to bilateral adrenocortical hyperplasia and the syndrome of cortisol excess. The clinical signs in dogs with functional corticotroph adenomas arising in the pars intermedia are similar to those arising in the pars distalis, and the neoplastic cells stain immunocytochemically for ACTH and MSH.[42]

Pituitary tumors arising in the pars intermedia of dogs appear to arise from the lining epithelium of the residual hypophyseal lumen covering the infundibular process. They are relatively small, more strictly localized than chromophobe adenomas arising in the pars distalis, and extend across the residual hypophyseal lumen to compress the pars distalis. The neoplastic cells compress and frequently invade the pars nervosa and infundibular stalk, resulting in disturbances of water metabolism early in the course of development of the tumor.[17]

Hypopituitarism Associated with Endocrinologically Inactive Pituitary Tumors

Nonfunctional pituitary tumors occur frequently in dogs, cats, and horses but are uncommon in other species.[16] There does not appear to be any breed or sex predisposition. Although chromophobe adenomas appear to be endocrinologically inactive, they may result in significant functional disturbances and clinical signs by virtue of compression atrophy of adjacent portions of the pituitary gland and dorsal extension into the overlying brain.

Dogs and cats with nonfunctional pituitary adenomas develop clinical disturbances related to lack of secretion of pituitary trophic hormones and diminished target organ function or dysfunction of the central nervous system.[16,45,49] An affected dog often is depressed and has incoordination and other disturbances of balance, weakness, collapse with exercise, and occasionally a change in personality. The animal may become unresponsive to people and develop a tendency to hide at the slightest provocation. In long-standing cases there may be evidence of blindness with dilated and fixed pupils due to compression and disruption of optic nerves by dorsal extension of the pituitary tumor. Affected dogs often have a progressive loss of weight ("pituitary cachexia") with muscle atrophy due to a lack of protein anabolic effects of growth hormone (Fig. 2-29). Compression of the cells that

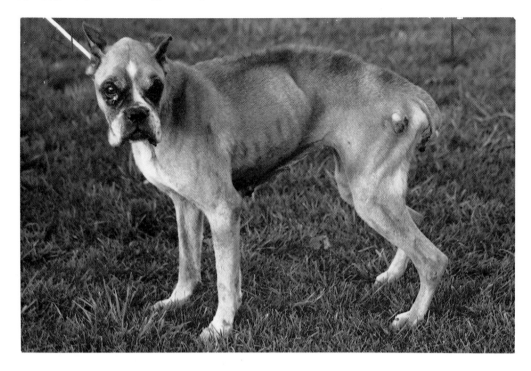

Fig. 2-29. Pituitary cachexia in a dog with a large endocrinologically inactive pituitary adenoma resulting in adult-onset panhypopituitarism.

secrete gonadotrophic hormones or the corresponding hypothalamic releasing hormone results in atrophy of the gonads. They appear to be dehydrated, as evidenced by a lusterless dry hair coat, and the owner may have noticed increased consumption of water.

A consistent finding in dogs and cats with large nonfunctional pituitary tumors is excretion of large volumes of dilute urine with a low specific gravity (approximately 1.007 or lower). Water intake is increased correspondingly and the owner complains that the dog, previously housebroken, urinates frequently in the house. Disturbances of water balance are the result of interference with the synthesis of antidiuretic hormone in the supraoptic nucleus or release of the hormone into capillaries of the pars nervosa.[17] The posterior lobe, infundibular stalk, and hypothalamus are compressed or disrupted by neoplastic cells. This interrupts the non-myelinated axons that transport antidiuretic hormone from its site of production, primarily in the supraoptic nucleus of the hypothalamus, to the site of release in the capillary plexus of the pars nervosa. Compression of neurosecretory neurons in the supraoptic nucleus of the hypothalamus by the dorsally expanding neoplasm also may result in decreased antidiuretic hormone synthesis.

Clinical signs in dogs and cats with nonfunctional pituitary adenomas and hypopituitarism are not highly specific and could be confused with other disorders of the central nervous system such as brain tumors and encephalitis or chronic renal disease. Hypopituitarism caused by pituitary tumors should be included in the differential diagnosis of diseases characterized by incoordination, depression, polyuria, blindness, and a sudden change in personality in adult or old animals. Because the blindness is central in origin, ophthalmoscopic examination usually fails to reveal significant lesions. There is no effect on body stature associated with compression of the pars distalis and interference with growth hormone secretion, because these neoplasms usually arise in adult dogs that have already completed their growth. The atrophy of the skin and loss of muscle mass may be related to a lack of protein anabolic effects of growth hormone in an adult dog or cat (Fig. 2-29). Interference in the secretion of pituitary trophic hormones often results in gonadal atrophy resulting in either decreased libido or anestrus, reduced basal metabolic rate due to diminished thyrotropin secretion, and hypoglycemia from trophic atrophy of the adrenal cortex.

Endocrinologically inactive pituitary adenomas often reach considerable size before they cause obvious signs or kill the animal (Fig. 2-30). The proliferating tumor cells incorporate the remaining structures of the adenohypophysis and infundibular stalk. The entire hypothalamus may be compressed and replaced by the tumor.

The adrenal glands of animals with large nonfunctional pituitary adenomas are small and consist primarily of medullary tissue surrounded by a narrow zone of cortex (Fig. 2-30). The adrenal cortex is a thin yellow-brown rim composed of a moderately thickened capsule and secretory cells of the outer zona glomerulosa, which are not predominately under the control of adrenocortocotropin (ACTH). The zonae fasciculata and reticularis are severely atrophied compared with these zones in normal adrenal glands due to an interference in ACTH secretion. Thyroid glands in dogs and cats with large pituitary adenomas often are smaller than normal, though to a much lesser degree than the adrenal cortex (Fig. 2-30). The majority of the atrophic thyroid follicles are large, lined by a flattened cuboidal epithelium, and have few endocytotic vacuoles near the interface between the colloid and luminal aspect of the follicular cells. The

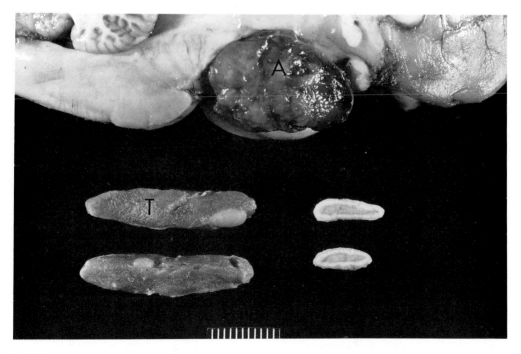

Fig. 2-30. Large, endocrinologically inactive, pituitary adenoma from a dog with extension into the hypothalamus. There is severe trophic atrophy and reduction in size of the adrenal glands (right) due to loss of cells in the zonae fasciculata and reticularis from the subnormal secretion of ACTH. The thyroid glands (left) are approximately normal size due to the distension of follicles with colloid in the absence of thyrotropin secretion. The scale at the bottom represents 1 cm.

thyroid lesion is due to lack of thyrotrophic hormone (TTH)-induced endocytosis of colloid. Seminiferous tubules of the testes are small and have little evidence of active spermatogenesis.

The histogenesis of nonfunctional pituitary adenomas in dogs is uncertain, but they appear to be derived from pituitary cells that are unable to either store or secrete an excess of a specific hypophyseal trophic hormone.

CRANIOPHARYNGIOMA is a benign tumor derived from epithelial remnants of the oropharyngeal ectoderm of the craniopharyngeal duct (Rathke's pouch). Compared with all other types of pituitary neoplasms, craniopharyngiomas occur in younger dogs, and they are present in either a suprasellar or infrasellar location. They cause panhypopituitarism and dwarfism in young dogs through subnormal secretion of somatotropin and other trophic hormones beginning at an early age, prior to closure of the growth plates. Craniopharyngiomas have alternating solid and cystic areas.[16,149] The solid areas are composed of nests of epithelial cells with focal areas of mineralization. The cystic spaces either are lined by columnar or squamous cells and contain keratin debris and colloid.

Craniopharyngiomas in young dogs often are large and grow along the ventral aspect of the brain where they can incorporate several cranial nerves. In addition, they extend dorsally into the hypothalamus and thalamus. The disturbances in function resulting from this type of pituitary tumor often are a combination of: (1) lack of secretion of pituitary trophic hormones resulting in atrophy and subnormal function of the adrenal cortex, thyroid, and gonads plus failure to attain somatic maturation owing to a lack of growth hormone; (2) disturbances in water metabolism (polyuria, polydipsia, and low urine specific gravity and osmolality) from an interference in the release and synthesis of antidiuretic hormone by the large tumor;[127] (3) deficits in cranial nerve function; and (4) central nervous system dysfunction due to extension of the tumor into the overlying brain.

Pituitary Tumors in Horses with Hirsutism

Adenomas derived from cells of the pars intermedia are the most common type of pituitary tumor in horses. They develop in older horses with females affected more frequently than males. The clinical syndrome associated with tumors of the pars intermedia in horses is characterized by polyuria, polydipsia, ravenous appetite, muscle weakness, somnolence, intermittent hyperpyrexia, and generalized hyperhidrosis.[13,90] The affected horses often develop a striking hirsutism (excess growth of hair) because of a failure of the cyclic seasonal shedding of hair. The hair over most of the trunk and extremities is long (up to 4 or 5 inches), abnormally thick, wavy, and often matted together (Fig. 2-31).

Plasma cortisol and immunoreactive adrenocorticotropin (iACTH, molecular weight 4,500) levels are only modestly elevated in horses with adenomas of the pars intermedia. However, the cortisol levels lack the normal diurnal rhythm and are not suppressed by either high or low doses of dexamethasone.[152] Tumor tissue and plasma from horses with

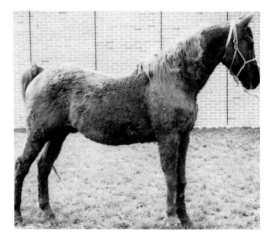

Fig. 2-31. Pituitary tumor in a horse resulting in hirsutism from a failure of cyclic shedding of hair. A large adenoma of pars intermedia had extended out of the pituitary region and into the overlying hypothalamus.

adenomas of the pars intermedia contain high concentrations of immunoreactive peptides (corticotropin-like intermediate lobe peptide [CLIP], alpha and beta melanocyte-stimulating hormones [α and β-MSH]), and beta endorphin [β-END] derived from pro-opiolipomelanocortin [pro-OLMC] and processed in the pars intermedia). This biosynthetic precursor of ACTH and other pituitary peptides is a high molecular weight (31,000 to 37,000 daltons) glycoprotein that undergoes different post-translational processing in the pars distalis and pars intermedia (Fig. 2-32). The modest elevation of plasma iACTH appears to be due to the different processing of pro-OLMC in horses with tumors derived from cells of the pars intermedia. This may explain the normal or slightly elevated blood cortisol levels and normal or mildly hyperplastic adrenal cortices observed in some horses with adenomas of the pars intermedia. Electron microscopy of the cells comprising adenomas of the pars intermedia in horses reveals that the rough endoplasmic reticulum and Golgi apparatus are particularly well developed, suggesting they are synthesizing and packaging considerable amounts of protein (e.g., pro-opiolipomelanocortin for secretion).

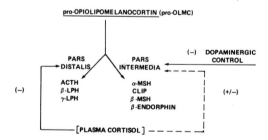

Fig. 2-32. The precursor molecule of ACTH and related peptides, pro-opiolipomelanocortin (pro-OLMC), is processed differently in the pars distalis and pars intermedia. Plasma cortisol exerts primary negative feedback control on the pars distalis whereas the pars intermedia is predominantly under dopaminergic control. Pro-OLMC undergoes post-translational processing in the pars intermedia to α-MSH, corticotrophin-like intermediate lobe peptide (CLIP), β-MSH and β-endorphin.

Horses with larger pituitary tumors often have hyperglycemia (insulin-resistant) and glycosuria, probably the result of a down-regulation of insulin receptors on target cells induced by the chronic excessive intake of food and hyperinsulinemia. The disturbances in carbohydrate metabolism, ravenous appetite, hirsutism (hypertrichosis) and hyperhidrosis are considered to be primarily a reflection of deranged hypothalamic function caused by the large pituitary tumors.[90] Adenomas of the pars intermedia in horses often extend out of the sella turcica and expand dorsally because of the incomplete diaphragm sella and severely compress the overlying hypothalamus. The hypothalamus is known to be the primary center for homeostatic regulation of body temperature, appetite, and cyclic shedding of hair.

Diabetes Insipidus

Diabetes insipidus is a disorder in which inadequate antidiuretic hormone (ADH) is produced or target cells in the kidney lack the biochemical systems necessary to respond to the secretion of normal or elevated circulating levels of hormone. The hypophyseal form of diabetes insipidus develops as a result of compression and destruction of the pars nervosa, infundibular stalk, or supraoptic nucleus in the hypothalamus. The lesions responsible for this disruption of ADH synthesis or secretion include large pituitary neoplasms,[17] a dorsally expanding cyst or inflammatory granuloma, and traumatic injury to the skull with hemorrhage and glial proliferation in the neurohypophyseal system.[68] Axons in the compressed pars nervosa of dogs with hypophyseal diabetes insipidus associated with pituitary neoplasms are depleted of ADH-containing dense secretory granules (Fig. 2-33), compared with normal dogs (Fig. 2-34).

Sporadic cases of hypophyseal diabetes insipidus may be the result of an inherited biochemical defect in the synthesis of ADH and its corresponding binding protein (neurophysin I), as has been well characterized in the Brattleboro strain of rats.[79,144] In the nephrogenic form of diabetes insipidus blood

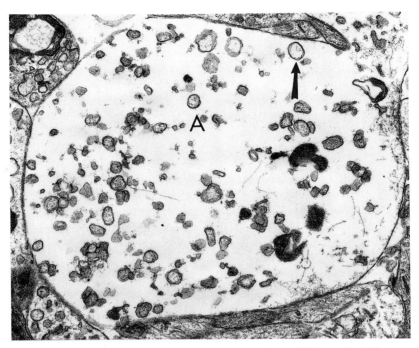

Fig. 2-33. Axonal process in pars nervosa from a dog with hypophyseal diabetes insipidus associated with a large pituitary adenoma. The axonal swelling contains few secretory granules with dense cores but occasional irregularly shaped, empty vesicles. X 19,800. From Koestner, A. and Capen, C. C.: Ultrastructural evaluation of the canine hypothalamic-neurohypophyseal system in diabetes insipidus associated with pituitary neoplasms. (Pathol. Vet. *4*:513,1967.)

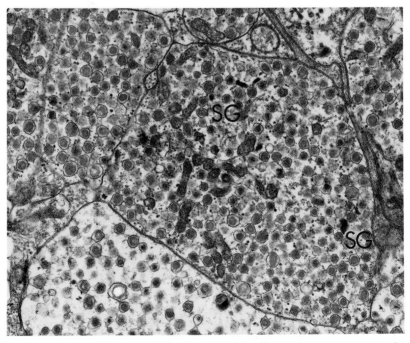

Fig. 2-34. Axonal processes in pars nervosa from a normal dog illustrating numerous membrane-bound, ADH-containing secretory granules (SG). X 17,000. (From Koestner, A. and Capen, C. C.: Ultrastructural evaluation of the canine hypothalamic-neurohypophyseal system in diabetes insipidus associated with pituitary neoplasms. Pathol. Vet. *4*:513,1967.)

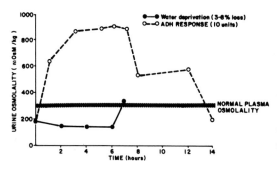

Fig. 2-35. Hypophyseal diabetes insipidus in a Great Dane illustrating the decrease in urine osmolality below that of plasma and rapid increase of urine osmolality above normal plasma osmolality in response to exogenous ADH. (Redrawn from Richards, 1970.)

levels of ADH are normal or elevated, but target cells in the distal nephron and collecting ducts are unable to respond owing to a lack of adenylate cyclase in the plasma membrane.

Animals with diabetes insipidus excrete large volumes of hypotonic urine, which in turn obligates the intake of equally large amounts of water to prevent hyperosmolality of body fluids and dehydration.[17,56] Urine osmolality is decreased below normal plasma osmolality (approximately 300 mOsM/kg) in both hypophyseal (Fig. 2-35) and nephrogenic (Fig. 2-36) forms of diabetes insipidus. In response to water deprivation, urine os-

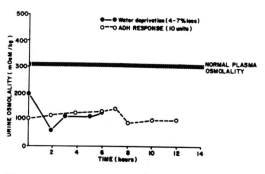

Fig. 2-36. Nephrogenic diabetes in a poodle illustrating the decrease in urine osmolality below plasma and lack of response both to hyperosmotic stimuli provided by water deprivation and to the administration of exogenous ADH. (Redrawn from Richards, 1970.)

molality remains below that of plasma in both forms of diabetes insipidus in contrast to that observed in normal animals. The elevation of urine osmolality above that of plasma in response to exogenous ADH in the hypophyseal form (Fig. 2-35), but not in nephrogenic diabetes insipidus (Fig. 2-36), is useful in the clinical separation of these two forms of the disease.[88,119]

REFERENCES

1. Agmo, A., Anderson, R., and Johansson, C. (1978): Effect of oxytocin on sperm numbers in spontaneous rat ejaculates. Biol. Reprod. *18:*346.
2. Akbar, A. M., Reichert, L. E., Jr., Dunn, T. G., et al. (1973): Bovine FSH in serum measured by radioimmunoassay. J. Animal Sci. *37:*299.
3. Alexander, J. E. (1962): Anomaly of craniopharyngeal duct and hypophysis. Can. Vet. J. *3:*83.
4. Allan, G. S., Huxtable, C. R. R., Howlett, C. R., et al. (1978): Pituitary dwarfism in German shepherd dogs. Small Anim. Pract. *19:*711.
5. Althen, T. G., and Gerrits, R. J. (1973): Pituitary growth hormone levels in selected lines of swine. J. Animal Sci. *37:*299.
6. Anderson, R. R., Hindery, G. A., Parkash, V., et al. (1968): Effectiveness of subcutaneously administered oxytocin hormone upon removal of residual milk cow. J. Dairy Sci. *51:*601.
7. Andresen, E., and Willeberg, P. (1976): Pituitary dwarfism in Carelian bear-dogs: Evidence of simple, autosomal recessive inheritance. Hereditas *384:*232.
8. Andresen, E., and Willeberg, P. (1976): Pituitary dwarfism in German shepherd dogs. Additional evidence of simple, autosomal recessive inheritance. Nord. Vet. Med. *28:*481.
9. Andresen, E., Willeberg, P., and Rasmussen, P. G. (1974): Pituitary dwarfism in German shepherd dogs. Nord. Vet. Med. *26:*692.
10. Archbald, L. F., Schultz, R. H., Fahning, M. L., et al. (1973): Sequential morphologic study of the ovaries of heifers injected with exogenous gonadotropins, Am. J. Vet. Res. *34:*21.
11. Arendarcik, J. (1972): Some recent findings on the structure, synthesis and effect of the hypothalamic LH and FSH releasing hormones and the pituitary gonadotropins (FSH, LH). Folia Vet. *16:*85.
12. Arendarcik, J., and Halagan, J. (1971): Serum gonadotropin (PMSG) of crossbred pony mares—biological and immunological properties. Veterinarni Med. *16:*563.
13. Backstrom, G. (1963): Nagot on hirsuitism i samband med hypofystumorer hos hast. Nord Vet. Med. *15:*778.
14. Baker, E. (1955): Congenital hypoplasia of the pituitary and pancreas glands in the dog. J. Am. Vet. Med. Assoc. *126:*468.
15. Berthelon, M., and Rampin, D. (1972): Serum gonadotropins in the mare. Rev. Med. Vet. *123:*1437.
16. Capen, C. C. (1978): Tumors of the endocrine

glands. *In* Tumors in Domestic Animals, edited by J. E. Moulton. Berkeley and Los Angeles. University of California Press.

17. Capen, C. C. and Koestner, A. (1967): Functional chromophobe adenomas of the canine adenohypophysis. An ultrastructural evaluation of a neoplasm of pituitary corticotrophs. Pathol. Vet. *4:*326.

18. Capen, C. C. and Martin, S. L. (1975): Hyperadrenocorticism in dogs. An animal model for Cushing's syndrome in man. Am. J. Pathol. *81:*459.

18a. Capen, C. C., Martin, L. L., and Koestner, A. (1967): Neoplasms in the adenohypophysis of dogs. Vet. Pathol. *4:*301.

19. Cassel, S. E. (1978): Ovarian imbalance in a German shepherd dwarf. V.M.S.A.C. *73*(2):162.

20. Chakracorty, P. K. and Reeves, J. J. (1973): Pituitary responsiveness to infusion with LH-RH/FSH-RH. J. Animal Sci. *37:*304.

21. Clarkson, T. B., Netsky, M. G. and de la Torre, E. (1959): Chromophobe adenoma in a dog. Angiographic and anatomic study. J. Neuropathol. Exp. Neurol. *18:*559.

22. Coffin, D. I., and Munson, T. O. (1953): Endocrine diseases of the dog associated with hair loss. J. Am. Vet. Med. Assoc. *123:*402.

23. Cohrs, P., and Nieberle, K. (1967): Textbook of Special Pathological Anatomy of Domestic Animals. New York. 1st English ed. Pergamon Press.

24. Concannon, P., Altszuler, N., Hampshire, J., et al. (1980): Growth hormone, prolactin, and cortisol in dogs developing mammary nodules and an acromegaly-like appearance during treatment with medroxyprogesterone acetate. Endocrinology *106:*1173.

25. Cotes, P. M., Crichton, J. A., Folley, S. J., et al. (1949): Galactopoietic activity of purified anterior pituitary growth hormone. Nature *164:*992.

26. Convey, E. M. (1973): Neuroendocrine relationships in farm animals: a review. J. Anim. Sci. *37:*745.

27. Crighton, D. B. (1973): Review of releasing hormones in domestic animals. Vet. Rec. *93:*254.

28. Dobson, H., Hopkinson, C. R. N., and Ward, W. R. (1973): Progesterone, 17-beta-oestradiol and LH in relation to ovulation. Vet. Rec. *93:*76.

29. Dockhorn, W., and Schutzler, H. (1973): Gonadotropin content of pregnant mares serum with reference to the production of PMS gonadotropin. Mht. Veterinarmed. *28:*220.

30. Dousa, T. P. (1974): Cellular action of antidiuretic hormone in nephrogenic diabetes insipidus. Mayo Clin. Proc. *49:*188.

31. Doyle, L. P., Turman, E. J., and Andrews, F. N. (1956): Some pathological effects of anterior pituitary growth hormone preparation on swine. Am. J. Vet. Res. *17:*174.

32. du Vigneaud, V., Lawler, H. C., and Popenoe, E. A. (1953): Enzymatic cleavage of glycinamide from vasopressin and a proposed structure for this pressor-antidiuretic hormone of the posterior pituitary. J. Am. Chem. Soc. *75:*4,880.

33. Dubois, M. P. (1971): Glycoprotein hormone-producing cells of the anterior pituitary: separation by immunofluorescence of the thyrotropic and gonadotropic cells in bovine, ovine and porcine pituitaries,

Ann. Rech. Vet. *2:*197.

34. El Etreby, M. F. (1979): Effect of cyproterone acetate, levonorgestrel and progesterone on adrenal glands and reproductive organs in the beagle bitch. Cell Tissue Res. *200:*229.

35. El Etreby, M. F., and Dubois, M. P. (1980): The utility of antisera to different synthetic adrenocorticotrophins (ACTH) and melanotrophins (MSH) for immunocytochemical staining of the dog pituitary gland. Histochemistry *66:*245.

36. El Etreby, M. F., and Fath El Bab, M. R. (1978): Effect of cyproterone acetate, d-norgestrel and progesterone on cells of the pars distalis of the adenohypophysis in the beagle bitch. Cell Tissue Res. *191:*205.

37. El Etreby, M. F., and Fath El Bab, M. R. (1977): The utility of antisera to canine growth hormone and canine prolactin for immunocytochemical staining of the dog pituitary gland. Histochemistry *53:*1.

38. El Etreby, M. F., and Fath El Bab, M. R. (1978a): Effect of 17β-estradiol on cells stained for FSHβ and/or LHβ in the dog pituitary gland. Cell Tissue Res. *193:*211.

39. El Etreby, M. F., and Fath El Bab, M. R. (1978b): Localization of thyrotropin (TSH) in the dog pituitary gland. A study using immunoenzyme histochemistry and chemical staining. Cell Tissue Res. *186:*399.

40. El Etreby, M. F., Friedreich, E., Hasan, S. H., et al. (1979): Role of the pituitary gland in experimental hormonal induction and prevention of benign prostatic hyperplasia in the dog. Cell Tissue Res. *204:*367.

41. El Etreby, M. F., Gräf, K. J., Günzel, P., et al. (1979a): Evaluation of effects of sexual steroids on the hypothalamic-pituitary system of animals and man. Arch. Toxicol. Suppl. *2:*11.

42. El Etreby, M. F., Müller-Peddinghaus, R., Bhargava, A. S., et al. (1980): Functional morphology of spontaneous hyperplastic and neoplastic lesions in the canine pituitary gland. Vet. Pathol. *17:*109.

43. El Etreby, M. F., Müller-Peddinghaus, R., Bhargava, A. S., et al. (1980a): The role of the pituitary gland in spontaneous canine mammary tumorogenesis. Vet. Pathol. *17:*2.

44. Evans, H. M., Meijer, K., and Simpson, J. E. (1933): The growth- and gonad-stimulating hormone of the anterior hypophysis. *In* Memoirs of The University of California. Berkeley. University of California Press.

45. Farrow, B. R. H. (1969): Chromophobe adenoma of the pituitary in a dog. Vet. Rec. *84:*609.

46. Feldman, E. C. (1981): Effect of functional adrenocortical tumors on plasma cortisol and corticotropin concentrations in dogs. J. Am. Vet. Med. Assoc. *178:*823.

47. Feldman, E. C., Bohannon, N. V., and Tyrrell, J. B. (1977): Plasma adrenocorticotropin levels in normal dogs. Am J. Vet. Res. *38*(10):1643.

48. Francis, K. C., and Mulligan, R. M. (1949): The weight of the pituitary gland of the male dog in relation to body weight and age, with a differential cell count of the anterior lobe. J. Morphol. *85:*141.

49. Gilbert, G. J., and Willey, E. N. (1969): Pituitary chromophobe adenoma in the bulldog. J. Am. Vet.

Med. Assoc. *154:*1071.

50. Ginther, O. J., and Wentworth, B. C. (1974): Effect of a synthetic gonadotropin-releasing hormone on plasma concentrations of luteinizing hormone in ponies. Am. J. Vet. Res. *35:*79.

51. Glawischnig, E. (1970): Agalactia in the sow: treatment and prevention with desamino-oxytocin (synthetic oxytocin). Wien. Tierarztl. Mschr. *57:*102.

52. Golter, T. D., Reeves, J. J., and O'Mary, C. C. (1973): Serum LH levels in bulls treated with synthetic luteinizing hormone-releasing hormone/follicle stimulating hormone-releasing hormone. J. Anim. Sci. *37:*123.

53. Gorbman, A., and Bern, H. A. (1962): A Textbook of Comparative Endocrinology. New York, John Wiley & Sons.

54. Graves, W. E., Lauderdale, J. W., Hauser, E. R., et al. (1968): Relation of post partum interval to pituitary gonadotropins ovarian follicular development and fertility in beef cows. Wis. Agr. Exp. Sta. Res. Bul. *270:*23.

55. Green, J. D., and Maxwell, D. S. (1959): Comparative anatomy of the hypophysis and observations on the mechanism of neurosecretion. *In* Comparative Endocrinology, edited by A. Gorbman. New York, John Wiley & Sons.

56. Green, R. A., and Farrow, C. S. (1974): Diabetes insipidus in a cat. J. Am. Vet. Med. Assoc. *164:*524.

57. Greig, W. A. (1963): Diabetes insipidus in the dog and cat. Proc. 17th World Vet. Cong., Hannover *2:*1,117.

58. Grunert, E., and Pohlmeyer, K. (1973): Effect of exogenous oxytocin on first insemination results in cattle. Prakt. Tierarzt. *54:*239.

59. Hackett, A. J., Turner, E. M., Bonavita, N. J., et al. (1973): Luteinizing hormone in dairy cattle from parturition to first estrus and ovulation. J. Dairy Sci. *56:*641.

60. Hackett, A. J., and Hafs, H. D. (1969): Pituitary and hypothalamic endocrine changes during the bovine estrous cycle. J. Anim. Sci. *28:*531.

61. Hall, Peter (1968): Personal communication.

62. Halmi, N. S., Peterson, M. E., Colurso, G. J., et al. (1981): Pituitary intermediate lobe in dog: Two cell types and high bioactive adrenocorticotropin content. Science *211:*72.

63. Hampshire, J., Altszuler, N., Steele, R., et al. (1975): Radioimmunoassay of canine growth hormone: Enzymatic radioiodination. Endocrinology *96:*822.

64. Hansel, W., Concannon, P. W., and McEntee, K. (1977): Plasma hormone profiles and pathological observations in medroxy-progesterone acetate treated beagle bitches. In Pharmacology of Steroid Contraceptive Drugs, edited by S. Garattini, and H. W. Berendes. New York, Raven Press.

65. Hare, T. (1935): Chromophobe cell adenoma of the pituitary gland associated with dystrophia adiposogenitalis in a maiden bitch. Proc. Roy. Soc. Med. *25:*1493.

66. Harris, G. W., and Donovan, B. T. (1966): The Pituitary Gland, Vol. I, II, III. Berkeley. The University of California Press.

67. Harris, W. H., and Heaney, R. P. (1969): Effect of growth hormone on skeletal mass in adult dogs.

Nature *223:*403.

68. Hart, M. M., Reagan, R. L., and Adamson, R. H. (1973): The effect of isomers of DDD on the ACTH-induced steroid output, histology and ultrastructure of the dog adrenal cortex. Toxicol. Appl. Pharm. *24:*101.

69. Head, H. H., and Wilcox, C. J. (1969): Short-term effects of bovine growth hormone on plasma glucose, insulin, nonesterified fatty acids and amino nitrogen. J. Dairy Sci. *52:*561.

70. Henry, W. B., Jr., and Sieber, S. E. (1965): Traumatic diabetes insipidus in a dog. J. Am. Vet. Med. Assoc. *146:*1,317.

71. Hewitt, W. F., Jr. (1950): Age and sex differences in weight of pituitary gland in dogs. Proc. Soc. Exptl. Biol. Med. *74:*781.

72. Hill, J. R., Jr., Dickey, J. F., and Hendricks, D. M. (1973): Estrus and ovulation in PGF$_2$/PMS treated heifers. J. Anim. Sci. *37:*315.

73. Howe, A. (1973): The mammalian pars intermedia: A review of its structure and function. J. Endocrinol. *59:*385.

74. Jeffcott, L. B., Atherton, J. G., and Mingay, J. (1969): Equine pregnancy diagnosis—a comparison of 2 methods for the detection of gonadotrophin in serum. Vet. Rec. *84:*80.

75. Jensen, E. C. (1959): Hypopituitarism associated with cystic Rathke's cleft in a dog. J. Am. Vet. Med. Assoc. *135:*572.

76. Johnson, K. G. (1972): The effect of vasopressin on urinary excretion of Bos taurus and Bos indicus—crossbred cows. Res. Vet. Sci. *13:*431.

77. Jones, S. R. (1979): Panhypopituitary dwarfism. In Spontaneous Animal Models of Human Disease, edited by E. J. Andrews, B. C. Ward, and N. H. Altman. New York, Academic Press.

78. Jubb, K. V., and McEntee, K. (1955): Observations on the bovine pituitary glands. Cornell Vet. *45:*576.

79. Kalimo, H., and Rinne, U. K. (1972): Ultrastructural studies on the hypothalamic neurosecretory neurons of the rat. II. The hypothalamo-neurohypophysial system in rats with hereditary hypothalamic diabetes insipidus. Z. Zellforsch. Mikrosk. Anat. *134:*205.

80. Kaltenbach, C. C., Dunn, T. G., Kiser, T. E., et al. (1974): Release of FSH and LH in beef heifers by synthetic gonadotrophin releasing hormone. J. Anim. Sci. *38:*357.

81. Karg, H., Hoffmann, B., and Schams, D. (1969): Content of progesterone, LH and prolactin in blood of a cow during the estrus cycle. Zuchthygiene *4:*149.

82. Keenan, T. W., Saacke, R. G., and Patton, S. (1970): Prolactin, the Golgi apparatus, and milk secretion: brief interpretive review. J. Dairy Sci. *53:*1349.

83. King, J. M., Kavanaugh, J. F., and Bentinck-Smith, J. (1962): Diabetes mellitus with pituitary neoplasms in a horse and a dog. Cornell Vet. *52:*133.

84. Koestner, A., and Capen, C. C. (1967): Ultrastructural evaluation of the canine hypothalamic-neurohypophyseal system in diabetes insipidus associated with pituitary neoplasms. Pathol. Vet. *4:*513.

85. Koprowski, J. A., Tucker, H. A., and Convey, E. M. (1970): Prolactin and growth hormone circadian

periodicity. J. Anim. Sci. *31:*224.

86. Kraeling, R. R., and Gerrits, R. J. (1971): Effects of PMS, HCG and cortisone on the ovary of the immature hypophysectomized pig. J. Anim. Sci. *33:* 1159.

87. Krook, L. (1969): Metabolic bone diseases of endocrine origin: Hypopituitarism. In Handbook of the Special Pathological Anatomy of Domestic Animals, edited by J. Dobberstein, G. Pallaske, and H. Stunzi. Berlin, Paul Parcy Verlag.

88. Lage, A. L. (1973): Nephrogenic diabetes insipidus in a dog. J. Am. Vet. Med. Assoc. *163:*251.

89. Lauderdale, J. W., Graves, W. E., Hauser, E. R., et al. (1968): Relation of post partum interval to corpus luteum development, pituitary prolactin activity and uterine involution in beef cows. Wis. Agr. Exp. Sta. Res. Bull. 270.

90. Loeb, W. F., Capen, C. C., and Johnson, L. E. (1966): Adenomas of the pars intermedia associated with hyperglycemia and glycosuria in two horses. Cornell Vet. *56:*623.

91. Lubberink, A. A. M. E., Rijnberk, A., der Kinderen, P. J., et al. (1971): Hyperfunction of the adrenal cortex. A review. Aust. Vet. J. *47:*504.

92. Lucksch, F. (1923): Uber hypophysentumoren beim hunde. Tierarztl. Arch. *3:*1.

93. Lund-Larsen, T. R., and Grondalen, J. (1976): Ateliotic dwarfism in the German shepherd dog: Low somatomedin activity associated with apparently normal pituitary function (2 cases) and with panadenopituitary dysfunction (1 case). Acta Vet. Scand. *17:*293.

94. McGrath, P. (1974): The pharyngeal hypophysis in some laboratory animals. J. Anat. *117:*95.

95. McKenzie, B. E., and Kenney, R. M. (1973): Histologic features of ovarian follicles of gonadotropin-injected heifers. Am. J. Vet. Res. *34:*1033.

96. Moch, R., and Haase, G. (1953): Hypofunction der adenohypophyse eins hundes. Tierarztl. Umsch. *8:* 242.

97. Momongan, V. G., and Schmidt, G. H. (1970): Oxytocin levels in the plasma of Holstein-Friesian cows during milking with and without a premilking stimulus. J. Dairy Sci. *53:*747.

98. Morag, M. (1968): The effect of regular intravenous injections of oxytocin at milking time on the proportion of the yield obtained as residual milk in the ewe. J. Dairy Res. *35:*377.

99. Muelheims, G. H., Kinsella, R. A., Jr., and Francis, F. E. (1973): Maturity of the pituitary-adrenal axis in the newborn dog. Proc. Soc. Exp. Biol. Med. *143:* 1197.

100. Muller, G. H. (1979): Pituitary dwarfism: Cutaneous manifestations of an endocrine disorder. Vet. Clin. North Am. *9:*41.

101. Muller, G. H., and Jones, S. R. (1973): Pituitary dwarfism and alopecia in a German shepherd with a cystic Rathke's cleft. J. Am. Anim. Hosp. Assoc. *9:*567.

102. Müller-Peddinghaus, R., El Etreby, M. F., Siebert, J., et al. (1980): Hypophysärer Zwergwuchs beim Deutschen Schäferhund. Vet. Pathol. *17:*406.

103. Muzikant, J., and Pedany, J. (1972): Effect of oxytocin injection on the volume and quality of boar semen. Veterinaria, Sofia *14:*293.

104. Nicholas, F. (1978): Pituitary dwarfism in German shepherd dogs: A genetic analysis of some Australian data. Small Anim. Pract. *19:*167.

105. Ono, K., Kraeling, R. R., Woods, D. R., et al. (1973): Hypophysectomy and glycolysis in the hog. J. Anim. Sci. *37:*268.

106. Osborne, C. A., Low, D. G., and Finco, D.R. (1972): Canine and Feline Urology. Philadelphia, W. B. Saunders Co.

107. Paatsama, S., Rokkanen, P., Jussila, J., et al. (1971): Somatotropin, thyrotropin and corticotropin hormone-induced changes in the cartilages and bones of the shoulder and knee joint in young dogs. An experimental study using histological oxytetracycline bone labeling and microradiographic methods. J. Small Anim. Pract. *12:*595.

108. Papkoff, H. (1976): Canine pituitary prolactin: Isolation and partial characterization. Proc. Soc. Exp. Biol. Med. *153:*498.

109. Parkash, V., and Anderson, R. R. (1972): Pituitary and blood plasma oxytocic activity and oxytocin disappearance rates in cattle. J. Dairy Sci. *55:*75.

110. Payne, F. (1943): The cytology of the anterior pituitary of broody fowls, Anat, Rec. *86:*1.

111. Pineda, M. H., Garcia, M. C., and Ginther, O. J. (1973): Effect of antiserum against an equine pituitary fraction in corpus luteum and follicles in mares during diestrus. Am. J. Vet. Res. *34:*181.

112. Pineda, M. H., Ginther, O. J., and McShan, W. H. (1972): Regression of corpus luteum in mares treated with an anti-serum against an equine pituitary fraction. Am. J. Vet. Res. *33:*1767.

113. Putnam, T. J., Benedict, F. B., and Teel, H. M. (1929): Studies in acromegaly, VIII. Experimental canine acromegaly produced by injection of anterior lobe pituitary extract. Arch. Surg. *18:*1708.

114. Quinlan, W. J., and Michaelson, S. (1981): Homologous radioimmunoassay for canine thyrotropin: Response of normal and X-irradiated dogs to propylthiouracil. Endocrinology *108:*937.

115. Rao, R. R., and Bhat, N. G. (1971): Incidence of cysts in pars distalis of mongrel dogs. Indian Vet. J. *48:*128.

116. Reeves, J. J., Tarnavsky, G. K., and Chakraborty, P. K. (1973): Serum LH in ewes treated with LH-RH/FSH-RH at three states of anestrus. J. Anim. Sci. *37:*326.

117. Reeves, J. J., Tarnavsky, G. K., and Chakraborty, P. K. (1974): Serum LH in ewes treated with synthetic luteinizing hormone-releasing hormone/follicle stimulating hormone-releasing hormone (LH-RH/FSH-RH) at three periods of anestrus. J. Anim. Sci. *38:*369.

118. Ricci, V., and Russolo, M. (1973): Immunocytological observations on the localization of ACTH in the hypophysis of the dog. Acta Anat. *84:*10.

119. Richards, M. A. (1970): Polydipsia in the dog. The differential diagnosis of polyuric syndromes in the dog. J. Small Anim. Pract. *10:*651.

120. Rijnberk, A., der Kinderen, P. J., and Thijssen, J. H. H. (1967): "Cushing's syndrome (spontaneous hyperadrenocorticism) in the dog." J. Endocrinol. *37:*Proceedings ii.

121. Rijnberk, A., der Kinderen, P. J., and Thijssen, J. H. H. (1969): Canine Cushing's syndrome. Zen-

tralbl. Vet. Med. *16:*13.

122. Rijnberk, A., Eigenmann, J. E., Belshaw, B. E., Hampshire, J., et al. (1980): Acromegaly associated with transient overproduction of growth hormone in a dog. J. Am. Vet. Med. Assoc. *177:*534.

123. Rogers, W. G., Valdez, H., Anderson, B. C., et al. (1977): Partial deficiency of antidiuretic hormone in a cat. J. Am. Vet. Med. Assoc. *170:*545.

124. Roth, J. (1976): Introduction to session. In Cell Membrane Receptors for Viruses, Antigens and Antibiotics, Polypeptide Hormones, and Small Molecules, edited by R. F. Beers, Jr., and E. G. Bassett. New York, Raven Press.

125. Roth, J. A., Lomax, L. G., Altszuler, N., et al. (1980): Thymic abnormalities and growth hormone deficiency in dogs. Am. J. Vet. Res. *41:*1256.

126. Sandholm, M., Vasenius, H., and Kivisto, A. K. (1975): Pathogenesis of canine pyometra. J. Am. Vet. Med. Assoc. *167:*1006.

127. Saunders, L. Z. and Rickard, C. G. (1952): Cranio-pharyngioma in a dog with apparent adiposogenital syndrome and diabetes insipidus. Cornell Vet. *42:*490.

128. Schally, A. V. (1973): Hypothalamic regulatory hormones. Science *179:*341.

129. Schally, A. V. (1978): Aspects of hypothalamic regulation of the pituitary gland. Its implications for the control of reproductive processes. Science *202:*18.

130. Schally, A. V., Arimura, A., Kastin, A. J., et al. (1971): Gonadotropin-releasing hormone: one polypeptide regulates secretion of luteinizing and follicle-stimulating hormones. Science *173:*1036.

131. Schams, D., Reinhardt, V., and Karg, H. (1973): Specific manipulation of prolactin secretion in cattle and its influence on lactation. Milchwissenschaft *28:*409.

132. Schams, D., and Bohm, S. (1972): Effect of the stimulus of milking, udder manipulations, genital stimulation and exogenous oxytocin stimulation on the prolactin content of bovine blood. Milchwissenschaft *27:*300.

133. Schechter, R. D., Stabenfeldt, G. H., Gribble, D. H., et al. (1973): Treatment of Cushing's syndrome in the dog with an adrenocorticolytic agent (o,p'DDD). J. Am. Vet. Med. Assoc. *162:*629.

134. Schiefer, B., and Hänichen, T. (1967): Zur Kenntnis und möglichen Bedeutung von Hypophysencysten beim Hund. Acta Neuropath *7:*232.

135. Schwayzer, R., and Sieber, P. (1963): Total synthesis of adrenocorticotrophic hormone. Nature *199:* 172.

136. Scott, D. W., Kirk, R. W., Hampshire, J., and Altszuler, N.: Clinicopathological findings in a German shepherd with pituitary dwarfism. J.A.A.H.A. *14:* 183.

137. Seguin, B. E., Oxender, W. D., and Hafs, H. D. (1972): Androgens after pituitary hormones in bulls.

138. Siegel, E. T. (1968): Assessment of the pituitary-adrenal gland function in the dog. Am. J. Vet. Res. *29:*173.

139. Siegel, E. T., Kelly, D. F., and Berg, P. (1970): Cushing's syndrome in the dog. J. Am. Vet. Med. Assoc. *157:*2081.

140. Siers, D. G., and Trenkle, A. H. (1973): Plasma levels of insulin, glucose, growth hormone, free fatty acids and amino acids in resting swine. J. Anim. Sci. *37:*1180.

141. Siers, D. G., and Swiger, L. A. (1971): Influence of live weight, age, and sex on circulating growth hormone levels in swine. J. Anim. Sci. *32:*1229.

142. Simmons, K. R., Cochrane, D. E., and Pomerantz, D. K. (1970): Bovine pituitary cytology: source of LH. J. Anim. Sci. *30:*73.

143. Slatter, D. H., Schirmer, R. G., and Krehbiel, J. D. (1976): Surgical correction of cystic Rathke's cleft in a dog. J. Am. Anim. Hosp. Assn. *12:*641.

144. Sokol, H. W., and Vatlin, H. (1965): Morphology of the neurosecretory system in rats homozygous and heterozygous for hypothalamic diabetes insipidus (Brattleboro strain). Endocrinology *77:*692.

145. Talanti, S. (1959): Observations on pyometra of dogs with reference to hypothalamic hypophyseal neurosecretory system. Am. J. Vet. Res. *20:*41.

146. Trautmann, A., and Fiebiger, J. (1952): Fundamentals of the Histology of Domestic Animals, 9th Ed. Ithaca, Comstock Publishing Associates.

147. Van Wyk, J. J., Underwood, L. E., Hintz, R. L., et al. (1974): The somatomedins: A family of insulin-like hormones under growth hormone control. *In* Recent Progress in Hormone Research. New York, Academic Press *30:*259.

148. Weikel, J. H., and Nelson, L. W. (1977): Problems in evaluating chronic toxicity of contraceptive steroids in dogs. J. Toxicol. Environ. Health *3:*167.

149. White, E. G. (1938): A suprasellar tumor in a dog. J. Pathol. Bact. *47:*323.

150. Wilhelmi, A. E. (1968): Canine growth hormone. Yale J. Biol. Med. *41:*199.

151. Willeberg, P., Kastrup, K. W., and Andresen, E. (1975): Pituitary dwarfism in German shepherd dogs: Studies on somatomedin activity. Nord. Vet. Med. *27:*448.

152. Wilson, M. G., Nicholson, W. E., Holscher, M. A., et al. (1982): Proopiolipomelanocortin peptides in normal pituitary, pituitary tumor and plasma of normal and Cushing's horses. Endocrinology *110:* 941.

153. Yamanchi, M. (1970): Antihormone against gonadotrophin in cattle. Natl. Inst. Anim. Health Q. *10*(Suppl):149.

154. Yousef, M. K., Takahashi, Y., Robertson, W. D., et al. (1969): Estimation of growth hormone secretion rate in cattle. J. Anim. Sci. *29:*341.

The Thyroid Gland

C. C. CAPEN and S. L. MARTIN

3

deficient animal has long served as a classic example of how an organ hypertrophies in order to compensate for a deficiency of a nutrient until a balance has been again achieved. This compensatory hypertrophy and hyperplasia has been recognized for many centuries even back to the time of the Ebers Papyrus (at least 1500 B.C.). Through the centuries man learned to compensate for an iodine deficiency by eating iodine-rich foods such as seaweed. Thyroid hormones have many functions in the body and, in general, regulate growth, differentiation, and the metabolism of lipids, proteins, and carbohydrates. The advent of radioactive iodine stimulated a voluminous amount of research into thyroid function. Since that time the amount of work on the thyroid gland has equaled or exceeded that on any other endocrine gland of the body. The affinity of the thyroid gland for elemental iodine and its isotopes has permitted more definitive studies on the distribution, synthesis, and metabolism of thyroid hormones.

ORGANOGENESIS

The thyroid gland originates as a thickened plate of epithelium in the floor of the pharynx. It is intimately related to the aortic sac in its development and this association leads to the frequent occurrence of accessory thyroid parenchyma in the mediastinum. This accessory thyroid tissue may undergo neoplastic transformation in the adult dog.[21,34,57,111] Branched cell cords develop from the pharyngeal plate

INTRODUCTION

The thyroid gland is unique in that it is the only tissue of the body which is able to accumulate iodine in large quantities and incorporate it into hormones. The metabolism of iodine is so closely related to thyroid function that the two must be considered together. The enlargement of the thyroid in the iodine-

and migrate dorsolaterally, but remain attached to the pharyngeal area by the narrow thyroglossal duct (Fig. 4-3). The cell cords expand laterally and upward, and these extensions form the anteromedial two-thirds of the adult lobes. The more medial portion remains close to the aortic sac and forms a transitory isthmus. The ultimobranchial bodies fuse with the lateral extensions and deliver C-cells (neural crest origin) to each thyroid lobe. A portion of the thyroglossal duct may persist postnatally and form a cyst due to accumulation of proteinic material secreted by the lining epithelium. Thyroglossal duct cysts are present in the ventral aspect of the anterior cervical region in dogs. Their lining epithelium may undergo neoplastic transformation and give rise to papillary carcinomas.

Accessory thyroid tissue is common in the dog and may be located anywhere from the larynx to the diaphragm. About 50% of adult dogs have accessory thyroids embedded in the fat on the intrapericardial aorta. These nodules are usually 1 to 2 mm in greatest dimension and may number from 1 to 5. They are completely lacking in C-(parafollicular) cells, which secrete calcitonin, but their follicular structure and function are the same as that of the main thyroid glands.[57] The existence of accessory thyroids in the dog was recognized early, but many investigators appear to have been unaware of their frequent occurrence.[34] Attempts to induce hypothyroidism in the dog by a surgical thyroidectomy are not consistently successful because the accessory thyroids readily respond to the prompt increase in endogenous thyroid stimulating hormone (TSH, thyrotropin) secretion and can undergo sufficient hyperplasia to sustain adequate thyroid hormone production.

STRUCTURE AND FUNCTION OF THYROID GLAND

Anatomy

The two thyroid lobes in most animal species are located on the lateral surfaces of the trachea. In pigs the main lobe of the thyroid is on the midline in the ventral cervical region with dorso-lateral projections from each side. In the dog the right lobe of the thyroid is situated slightly cranial to the left lobe and almost touches the caudal aspect of the larynx. The lobes are situated on the lateral surfaces of the trachea. Each lobe is about 2 cm by 1 cm by 0.5 cm in the average size adult dog and the combined weight of the two lobes is about 1 g. Because these lobes are relatively small and are deep to the sternocephalicus muscle, they are not readily palpable except when enlarged. The major blood supply is via the cranial thyroid artery, a branch of the common carotid, and the principal venous drainage is via the caudal thyroid vein, which enters the internal jugular vein.

Lymph drainage from the cranial pole of the thyroid lobes is to the retropharyngeal lymph nodes in dogs. Lymph flow from the caudal aspects of each thyroid lobe is more variable but it often bypasses any lymph nodes before entering the brachiocephalic trunk.[20,106,115] Efferent lymphatics usually enter directly into the cervical lymphatic trunk or internal jugular vein. This explains the frequent occurrence of pulmonary metastases from a thyroid carcinoma in dogs prior to development of secondary foci in regional lymph nodes.[67] Small efferent lymphatics may pass through the caudal cervical lymph nodes along the ventral surface of the trachea before entering the cranial mediastinum.

The vascular supply to the thyroid fluctuates considerably depending upon the activity of the gland. Considering its size, it receives one of the richest supplies of blood of any organ of the body. The thyroid has a rich supply of sympathetic nerves which enter the gland in association with the blood vessels at the hilus on the medial aspect of each lobe. These nerves are thought to regulate only the blood supply to the organ, since transplantation does not affect the function of the thyroid. Only the thyrotrophin (thyroid stimulating hormone, TSH) and the availability of iodine affect the rate of formation of the thyroid hormone.

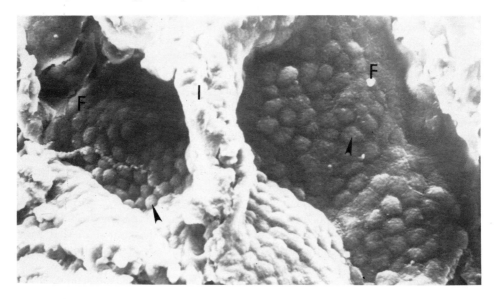

Fig. 3-1. Scanning electron micrograph of thyroid gland of a dog with 2 opened follicles (F). The luminal aspect of individual follicular cells has numerous microvillar projections (arrowheads). I = interfollicular space with connective tissue and capillaries.

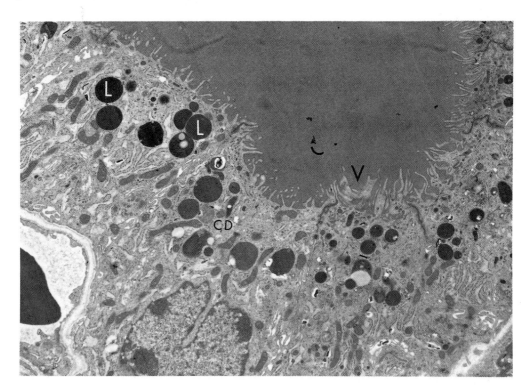

Fig. 3-2. Electron micrograph of normal thyroid follicular cells with long microvilli (V) extending into the luminal colloid (C). Pseudopods from the apical membrane engulf a portion of the colloid to form a colloid droplet (CD). Numerous lysosomes (L) in the apical cytoplasm contribute proteolytic enzymes that hydrolyze the thyroglobulin and release the thyroid hormones, which enter intrafollicular capillaries (left) at base of follicular cells.

Thyroid Histology

The thyroid gland is the largest of the endocrine organs that function exclusively as an endocrine gland. The basic structure of the thyroid is unique for endocrine glands, consisting of follicles of varying size (20 to 250μ) that contain colloid produced by the follicular cells (Fig. 3-1). The follicular cells are cuboidal to columnar and their secretory polarity is directed toward the lumen of the follicles (Fig. 3-2). An extensive network of inter- and intrafollicular capillaries provides the follicular cells with an abundant blood supply. Follicular cells have long profiles of rough endoplasmic reticulum and a large Golgi apparatus in their cytoplasm for synthesis and packaging of substantial amounts of protein that are then transported into the follicular lumen. The interface between the luminal side of follicular cells and the colloid is modified by numerous microvillar projections (Fig. 3-2).

Thyroid Hormone Synthesis

The biosynthesis of thyroid hormones is also unique among endocrine glands because the final assembly of hormones occurs extracellularly within the follicular lumen. Essential raw materials, such as iodide, are trapped efficiently by follicular cells from plasma, transported rapidly against a concentration gradient to the lumen and oxidized by a peroxidase in microvillar membranes to iodine (I_2) (Fig. 3-3). The assembly of thyroid hormones within the follicular lumen is made possible by a unique protein (thyroglobulin) synthesized by follicular cells.

Thyroglobulin is a high molecular weight (600,000 to 750,000) glycoprotein synthesized in successive subunits on the ribosomes of the endoplasmic reticulum in follicular cells. The constituent amino acids (tyrosine and others) and carbohydrates (*i.e.*, mannose, fructose, galactose) come from the circulation. Recently synthesized thyroglobulin (17S) leaving the Golgi apparatus is packaged into apical vesicles and extruded into the follicular lumen.[30,82] The amino acid tyrosine, an essential component of thyroid hormones, is incorporated within the molecular structure of thyroglobulin. Iodine is bound to tyrosyl residues in thyroglobulin at the apical surface of follicular cells to form successively monoiodotyrosine (MIT) and diiodotyrosine (DIT) (Fig. 3-4).[30] The resulting MIT and DIT combine to form the two biologically active iodothyronines (thyroxine-T_4, triiodothyronine-T_3) secreted by the thyroid gland (Fig. 3-5).

Iodine Metabolism

Iodine metabolism and thyroid function should be viewed as an integrated system composed of metabolic subsystems for iodide, the thyroid gland, triiodothyronine (T_3), and thyroxine (T_4). The system is controlled by the feedback mechanism involving the hypothalamus and pituitary gland, and also by the intake of iodine. The function of the system is to provide a carefully regulated supply of T_3 and T_4, which in turn influences the rates of many metabolic processes. There is sufficient flexibility in the system to accommodate day-to-day variations in iodine intake and to sustain a normal metabolic rate even with severe iodine deficiency.

The daily maintenance iodine requirement is about 140 μg for a 10- to 15-kg adult dog.[11] *Ad libitum* consumption of most commercially manufactured dry dog foods provides the average dog with a daily iodine intake of at least 500 μg, and some foods provide as much as 1,500 μg per day. Most iodine in the diet is reduced to iodide in the gastrointestinal tract, and absorption of iodide begins immediately and is essentially complete within 2 hours. In addition to the thyroid gland iodide is cleared from the plasma by the parotid salivary gland and by the gastric mucosa. However, a small amount of iodide is normally lost in the feces (about 20 to 25 μg per day at the usual levels of intake), possibly via secretion in the colon.

The principal features of iodide metabolism in the dog for a daily iodine intake slightly in excess of the normal requirement are shown in Figure 3-6.[9,11] The dietary in-

FOLLICULAR   LUMEN

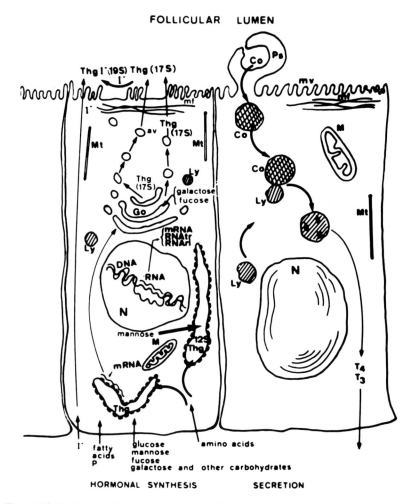

Fig. 3-3. Thyroid follicular cells illustrating two-way traffic of materials from capillaries into the follicular lumen. Raw materials, such as iodine, are concentrated by follicular cells and rapidly transported into the lumen (left side of drawing). Amino acids (tyrosine and others) and sugars are assembled by follicular cells into thyroglobulin (Thg), packaged into apical vesicles (av) and released into the lumen. The iodination of tyrosyl residues occurs within the thyroglobulin molecule to form thyroid hormones in the follicular lumen. Elongation of microvilli and endocytosis of colloid by follicular cells occurs in response to TSH stimulation (right side of drawing). The intracellular colloid droplets (Co) fuse with lysosomal bodies (Ly) and active thyroid hormone is enzymatically cleaved from thyroglobulin and free T_4 and T_3 are released into circulation. (Courtesy of Bastenie et al.[8])

take of 160 μg is augmented by 65 μg of recycled iodide (approximately 50 μg of iodide released by the thyroid and approximately 15 μg derived from peripheral degradation of T_3 and T_4). About two-thirds of this combined input of 225 μg is excreted, chiefly in the urine. The thyroid clears about one-third of the input, to achieve a net daily uptake of about 75 μg.

At the usual levels of iodine intake, the concentration of inorganic iodide in the plasma is about 5 to 10 μg per 100 ml in the dog. In man, plasma iodide concentration is usually about 0.5 μg/100 ml. The principal reasons for the higher level of iodide concentration in the dog are higher intake relative to body weight, proportionately greater recycling of iodide from the thyroid and from peripheral

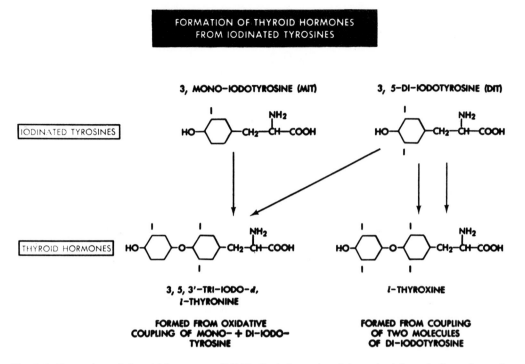

Fig. 3-4. Formation of thyroid hormones (3,5,3'-triiodothyronine, l-thyroxine) from iodinated tyrosines (MIT and DIT) within the follicular lumen of the thyroid gland.

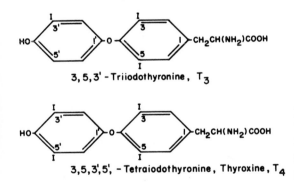

Fig. 3-5. Triiodothyronine (T_3) and tetraiodothyronine (T_4) are the two biologically active iodothyronines secreted by the thyroid gland. They have similar biologic actions and differ by the presence of an additional molecule of iodine on the outer phenolic ring of thyroxine.

degradation of thyroid hormones, and lower fractional clearance by the kidney. Another pertinent difference between canine and human iodide metabolism is that in addition to free iodide and the iodine incorporated in circulating thyroid hormone, canine plasma contains a significant amount of nonhormonal iodine that is bound to plasma proteins (Fig. 3-7). This iodine, usually present in a concentration of 1 μg or more per 100 ml, appears to be incorporated during the synthesis of plasma protein, probably albumin. The total iodine content of the normal canine thyroid is about 1,000 μg. Two-thirds of the iodine is in the form of MIT and DIT, and about one-fourth is in T_3 and T_4, all of which are incorporated in thyroglobulin molecules in the follicular colloid.

Thyroid Hormone Secretion

The secretion of thyroid hormones from stores within luminal colloid is initiated by elongation of microvilli on follicular cells and formation of pseudopods. These elongated cytoplasmic projections are increased by pituitary TSH (Fig. 3-8) and extend into the follicular lumen to indiscriminatingly phagocytize a portion of adjacent colloid. Colloid

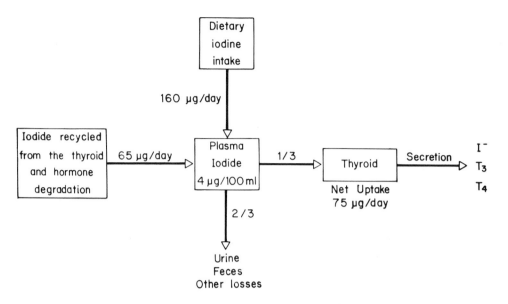

Fig. 3-6. Iodide metabolism in the adult dog at an iodine intake slightly above the normal daily requirement. (Courtesy Dr. Bruce Belshaw.[19])

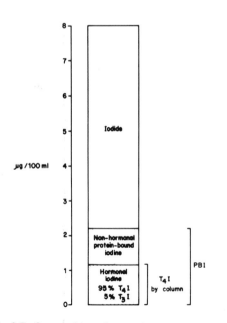

Fig. 3-7. Composition of serum iodine in the normal adult dog at an iodine intake of about 300 μg per day. (Courtesy of Dr. Bruce Belshaw.[19])

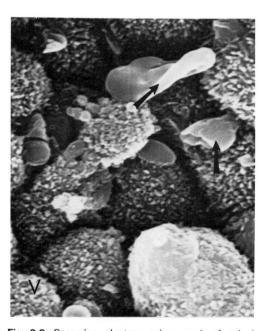

Fig. 3-8. Scanning electron micrograph of apical surface of hypertrophied thyroid follicular cell 4 hours post-TSH stimulation. Numerous elongated microvilli (V) and cytoplasmic projections (arrows) extend into the follicular lumen to engulf colloid as part of the initial stages of thyroid hormone secretion in response to TSH.

droplets within follicular cells fuse with numerous lysosomal bodies that contain proteolytic enzymes (Fig. 3-3). Triiodothyronine and thyroxine are released from the thyroglobulin molecule and secreted into adjacent capillaries. The iodinated tyrosines (MIT and DIT) released from the colloid droplets are deiodinated enzymatically and the iodide generated under normal conditions is either recycled to the lumen to iodinate new tyrosyl residues or released into the circulation. The unique structural and functional characteristics of the phylogenetically oldest endocrine gland suggest that the thyroid may have evolved toward a more "ideal" structure to perform its vital metabolic functions.

Negative feedback control of thyroid hormone secretion is accomplished by the co-ordinated response of the adenohypophysis and certain hypothalamic nuclei to circulating levels of T_4 and T_3. A decrease in thyroid hormone concentration in plasma is sensed by groups of neurosecretory neurones in the hypothalamus that synthesize and secrete a small peptide (molecular weight—361) into the hypophyseal portal circulation.[42] Thyrotrophin-releasing hormone (TRH) binds to isoreceptors on the plasma membrane of thyrotrophic basophils in the adenohypophysis and activates adenylate cyclase, resulting in the formation of 3′,5′ cyclic adenosine monophosphate (cyclic AMP). The intracellular accumulation of cyclic AMP in thyrotrophic basophils results in contraction of microfilaments and peripheral movement and discharge of TSH-containing secretion granules into pituitary capillaries. Thyroid stimulating hormone (TSH) or thyrotrophin is conveyed to thyroid follicular cells where it binds to the basilar aspect of the cell, activates adenylate cyclase, and increases the rate of the biochemical reactions concerned with the synthesis and secretion of thyroid hormones.

One of the initial responses by follicular cells to TSH is the formation of numerous cytoplasmic pseudopodia, resulting in increased endocytosis of colloid and release of preformed hormone stored within the follicular lumen (Fig. 3-8). If the secretion of

TSH is sustained (hours or days), thyroid follicular cells become more columnar and follicular lumens become smaller due to increased endocytosis of colloid (Fig. 3-9). Numerous PAS-positive colloid droplets are present in the luminal aspect of the hypertrophied follicular cells. The converse of what has been just described occurs in response to an increase in circulating thyroid hormone (T_4 and T_3) and a corresponding decrease in circulating pituitary TSH. Thyroid follicles become enlarged and distended with colloid due to decreased TSH-mediated endocytosis of colloid (Fig. 3-10). Follicular cells lining the involuted follicles are low cuboidal and there are few endocytotic vacuoles at the interface between the colloid and follicular cells.

There are marked differences in thyroid morphology and function between canine breeds of European origin and the Basenji, which originated in Africa. At the same level

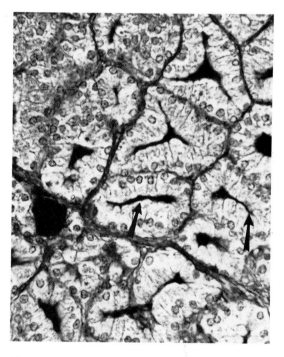

Fig. 3-9. Response of thyroid follicular cells 8 hours post-TSH stimulation. The follicular cells are columnar and many follicles are nearly depleted of colloid and partially collapsed (arrow).

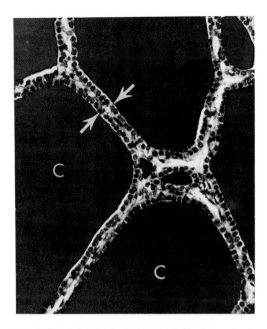

Fig. 3-10. Response of thyroid follicular cells to long-term administration of exogenous thyroxine. The follicular cells (arrows) are cuboidal in response to decreased TSH secretion and thyroid follicles are distended with dense colloid.

of iodine intake, thyroidal turnover of iodine in the Basenji is 2 to 3 times faster than in European breeds.[77] The corresponding differences in thyroid morphology in the Basenji include smaller follicles with more widespread and uniform vacuolation of the colloid, taller follicular epithelium, and ultrastructural features of follicular cells that more closely resemble those of a TSH-stimulated gland in European breeds, such as the Beagle.[78] In addition, younger, rapidly growing dogs have a greater uptake of ^{131}I/g of thyroid and also a faster rate of ^{131}I release.[14]

Metabolism

This discussion on thyroid hormone metabolism will utilize data primarily from the dog since more is known about this species and clinically significant disorders of thyroid function are common in canine patients. In plasma, T_4 is bound to albumin and three globulin fractions, whereas T_3 is bound to albumin and one globulin fraction in dogs.[90] The overall binding affinity of the plasma proteins for T_4 is lower in the dog than in man. Most importantly, the affinity of the canine inter-α globulin fraction for T_4 is much less than that of the thyroxine-binding globulin (TBG) in man. Partly as a result of this weaker binding, total T_4 concentration is lower, the unbound or free fraction of circulating T_4 is higher, and hormone turnover is more rapid in the dog than in man.

About 40% of the extrathyroidal T_4 is in the plasma. Most of the remaining 60% is taken up by the liver and equilibrates rapidly with the plasma. The total plasma-equivalent space of distribution of T_4 is about 12% of body weight. By comparison, T_3 enters peripheral cells more readily than T_4 (partly because it is less firmly bound to plasma proteins), and it reaches a total distribution volume equal to 65% of body weight. Largely owing to the great difference in their respective volumes of distribution, the ratio of T_4 to T_3 in canine plasma is about 20:1, even though they are produced in a ratio of about 2:1 in the thyroid gland. The average plasma T_4 concentration is about 1.8 μg per 100 ml, and the average plasma T_3 level is 84 ng per 100 ml in the dog.[19] These values represent measurements made between 11 AM and noon. The time of measurement is important because there appear to be diurnal oscillations in plasma T_3 and T_4. Peak concentration usually occurs at about midday and the minimum at about midnight.

The equivalent of 115% of total extrathyroidal T_4 and 205% of extrathyroidal T_3 is metabolized and must be replaced each day in dogs. About 45% of the turnover of T_4 is via deiodination and 55% is via fecal excretion; whereas for T_3, 70% is via deiodination and 30% is via fecal excretion.[19] Both the overall rates of turnover and the loss of hormone in the feces are much higher in the dog than in man. Fecal wastage substantially reduces the efficiency of hormone utilization, but it also explains in part the remarkable tolerance of the dog to excess thyroid hormone.[19]

The radiothyroidectomized hypothyroid dog converts a substantial amount of administered T_4 to T_3. The mechanism for production of T_3 may be important because the ratio of T_4 to T_3 in the thyroglobulin is approximately $3.6:1$, while the ratio of the daily production rates (based on plasma concentration and turnover of the two hormones) is $2:1$.

Biologic Action

Thyroxine and triiodothyronine once released into the circulation act on many different target cells in the body. The overall functions of thyroxine and triiodothyronine are similar, though much of the biologic activity is the result of monodeiodination to 3,5,3'-triiodothyronine prior to interacting with target cells[79] (Fig. 3-11). Under certain conditions (protein starvation, neonatal animals, liver and kidney disease, febrile illness, etc.) thyroxine is preferentially monodeiodinated by a 5'-deiodinase to 3, 3',5'-triiodothyronine ("reverse T_3")[66] (Fig. 3-11). Since this form of T_3 formed by target cells is biologically inactive, monodeiodination to form reverse T_3 provides a mechanism to attenuate the metabolic effects of thyroid hormones.

Thyroxine stimulates oxygen utilization and heat production by every cell of the body. It causes increased utilization of carbohydrates, increased protein catabolism as indicated by greater excretion of nitrogen, and greater oxidation of fats as indicated by loss in body weight. The administration of thyroxine will increase the heart rate by a direct effect on heart muscle cells.

Normal function of the central nervous system is dependent upon the normal output of thyroxine. During periods when thyroxine levels are deficient, the central nervous system fails to function in the normal fashion and the animal is lethargic, dull, and mentally deficient. Myelin in the fiber tracts is decreased, cortical neurons are smaller and fewer, and vascularity of the CNS is reduced. The neurons are permanently damaged in the young growing animal by thyroxine deficiency. The neuronal dysfunction caused by thyroxine deficiency is reversible in the adult animal. On the other hand, an excess of thyroxine stimulates CNS activity to the extent that the animal is nervous, jumpy, irritable, and hyperactive.

The subcellular mechanism of action of thyroid hormones appears to resemble steroid hormones in that free hormone enters into target cells and binds to a cytosol-binding protein[80] (Fig. 3-12). Free triiodothyronine (T_3) either binds to receptors on the inner mitochondrial membrane to activate mitochondrial energy metabolism or binds to a nuclear receptor and increases transcription of the genetic message to facilitate new protein synthesis.[42] The overall effects of thyroid hor-

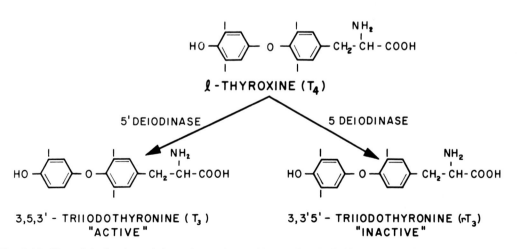

ℓ-THYROXINE (T_4)

5'DEIODINASE　　　　　　　5 DEIODINASE

3,5,3' - TRIIODOTHYRONINE (T_3)
"ACTIVE"

3,3'5' - TRIIODOTHYRONINE (rT_3)
"INACTIVE"

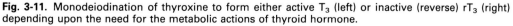

Fig. 3-11. Monodeiodination of thyroxine to form either active T_3 (left) or inactive (reverse) rT_3 (right) depending upon the need for the metabolic actions of thyroid hormone.

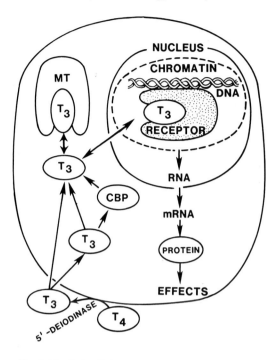

Fig. 3-12. Subcellular mechanism of action of thyroid hormones in target cells. Free triiodothyronine (T_3) primarily enters target cells since most thyroxine (T_4) undergoes monodeiodination in the liver or elsewhere in the periphery to form T_3. Free T_3 in the cell binds either to cytosolic binding proteins (CBP), to high affinity receptors on the inner mitochondrial (MT) membrane and activates oxidative phosphorylation, or to nuclear receptors in target cells. In the nucleus T_3 increases transcription of mRNA which returns to the cytoplasm to direct the synthesis of new proteins. The increased synthesis of new proteins (structural or enzyme) carries out the multiple biologic effects of the thyroid hormones.

mones are to: (1) increase the basal metabolic rate; (2) make more glucose available to meet the elevated metabolic demands by increasing glycolysis, gluconeogenesis, and glucose absorption from the intestine; (3) stimulate new protein synthesis; (4) increase lipid metabolism and conversion of cholesterol into bile acids and other substances, activation of lipoprotein lipase, and increase sensitivity of adipose tissue to lipolysis by other hormones; (5) stimulate the heart rate, cardiac output, and blood flow; and (6) increase neural transmission, cerebration, and neuronal development in young animals.

DISORDERS OF THYROID FUNCTION

Hypothyroidism

Hypothyroidism is a well-recognized clinical entity in dogs.[19,91] Although the disease may occur in many purebred and mixed breed dogs, certain breeds (Doberman Pinschers, Golden Retrievers, Beagles) appear to be more commonly affected.

Clinical hypothyroidism usually is the result of primary diseases of the thyroid gland, especially idiopathic follicular atrophy ("follicular collapse") (Fig. 3-13) and lymphocytic thyroiditis.[36] In "follicular collapse" there is a progressive loss of follicular epithelium and replacement by adipose connective tissue with a minimal inflammatory response. The remaining follicles are small, lined by columnar follicular cells, and contain small amounts of irregularly clumped colloid. The occasional remaining follicular cells have small microfollicles with colloid in their cytoplasm. Nests of unaffected thyroid C-cells are present in the thyroid gland, especially near the hilus. Although the etiology of follicular collapse is uncertain, it is not the result of a pituitary lesion interfering with secretion of thyrotrophic hormone (TSH). Hypertrophy and hyperplasia of thyrotrophic basophils occur in the pars distalis of dogs with follicular collapse and hypothyroidism.

Lymphocytic thyroiditis in dogs closely resembles Hashimoto's disease in humans and appears to be genetically conditioned, at least in certain breeds.[35] Though the exact mechanism in the dog is not well-established, evidence suggests a polygenic pattern of inheritance similar to that observed in the human disease. The immunologic basis for the development of chronic lymphocytic thyroiditis in both man and dog appears to be through production of autoantibodies directed against thyroglobulin, a microsomal antigen, and a second colloid antigen.[37–39,74] Histopathologic alterations in the thyroid glands consist of either a diffuse or nodular infiltration of lymphocytes, plasma cells, and macrophages (Fig. 3-14). Many of the remaining thyroid follicles are small and lined by tall columnar

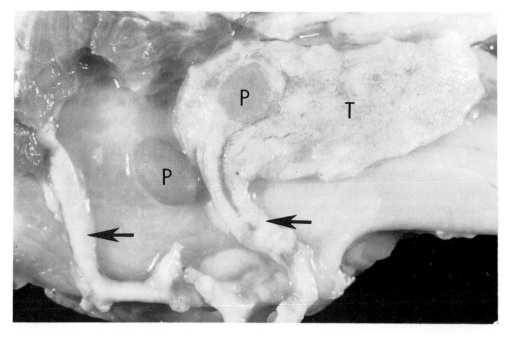

Fig. 3-13. Follicular collapse in a dog with hypothyroidism. The thyroid gland (T) is reduced in size compared to the adjacent parathyroid glands (P) and is lighter in color due to the replacement by adipose connective tissue. Branches of the cranial thyroid artery (arrows) are prominent due to atherosclerosis resulting from severe hyperlipidemia.

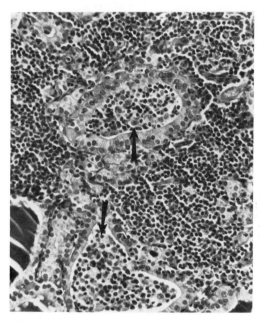

Fig. 3-14. Lymphocytic thyroiditis in a dog with hypothyroidism. Large focal accumulations of lymphocytes and plasma cells are present between the few remaining small thyroid follicles. Numerous lymphocytes and macrophages (arrow) are present within the lumina of thyroid follicles.

follicular cells, reflecting the long-standing stimulation by TSH in an attempt to compensate for the low blood levels of thyroid hormones. Ultrastructurally, numerous lymphocytes and macrophages are observed within the follicular basement membrane extending between follicular cells into the lumens of follicles (Fig. 3-15).

Less common causes of hypothyroidism in dogs are bilateral nonfunctional thyroid tumors or severe iodine-deficient goiter. Hypothyroidism secondary to long-standing pituitary or hypothalamic lesions that prevent the release of either thyrotrophic hormone (TSH) or thyrotrophin-releasing hormone (TRH) is encountered infrequently in the dog. The thyroid gland is moderately reduced in size and composed of colloid-distended follicles lined by flattened follicular cells, owing to a lack of TSH-induced endocytosis of colloid and secretion of thyroid hormones (Fig. 3-16).

Clinical disturbances associated with hypothyroidism vary among affected animals

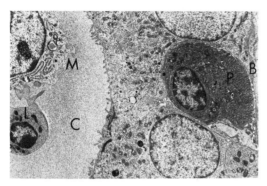

Fig. 3-15. Immune-mediated lymphocytic thyroiditis in a dog with hypothyroidism. A plasma cell is migrating between follicular cells from the basement membrane (B) of the follicle into the colloid (C) in the follicular lumen. Lymphocytes (L) and macrophages (M) are present in the colloid. Continuous release of antigens from the colloid into the interstitial tissues in an animal with defective immune surveillance results in progressive destruction of thyroid follicles, subnormal circulating levels of thyroid hormones, and the clinical syndrome of hypothyroidism.

and not every sign is seen in each patient. Many clinical signs associated with hypothyroidism are due to a reduction in basal metabolic rate. A gain in body weight without an associated change in appetite occurs frequently. The weight gain may vary from slight to striking obesity. The animal usually is less active and the owner may observe a reluctance to play or take walks. The inactivity also contributes to the weight gain.

Dogs with hypothyroidism may have difficulty in maintaining normal body temperature and are often "heat seekers." They will lie on or near sources of heat, such as registers, radiators, and electric blankets, and be reluctant to venture outdoors in cold weather. Excessive shivering may be observed and the skin frequently feels cool.

Changes in the skin and haircoat occur in the majority of affected dogs.[70] Because thy-

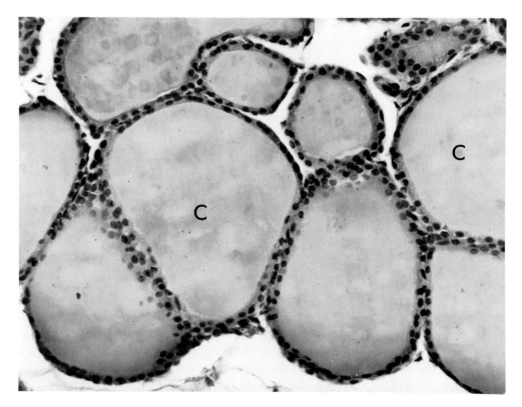

Fig. 3-16. Histologic appearance of the canine thyroid in TSH deficiency caused by a large nonfunctional pituitary tumor. Thyroid follicles are distended by the continued accumulation of colloid (C), and the follicular epithelium is flattened. Note the complete absence of endocytotic vacuoles about the periphery of the colloid.

roxine stimulates the anagen or active phase of hair growth, the reduction in blood levels of thyroid hormones favors the telogen or resting phase. Telogen hairs are more easily dislodged from the hair follicles, resulting in thinning of the haircoat and bilaterally symmetrical alopecia in many dogs. Areas affected by hair loss initially are those receiving frictional wear such as the tail and neck area. The tail may become almost completely bare in dogs with long-standing hypothyroidism. The remaining hairs are often coarse or wiry and dull.

As with other endocrine skin diseases, pruritus (itching) is absent with hypothyroidism. Increased thickness (hyperkeratosis) of the outer skin layer (stratum corneum) is a consistent finding and results in the increased scaliness that is observed clinically. It may become severe and occur in circular patches.

Microscopic examination of skin biopsies from dogs with hypothyroidism consistently reveals marked hyperkeratosis. Most hair follicles are in the telogen phase with hyperkeratosis of the external root sheath. The excessive keratin formation and accumulation within hair follicles often results in follicular keratosis that may cause a grossly observable distention of follicles (Fig. 3-17).

Increased pigmentation occurs in the skin of animals with hypothyroidism, especially in localized areas of alopecia (hair loss) as on the dorsal aspect of the nose and distal portion of the tail. Increased numbers of melanocytes are present in the basal layer of the epidermis. Changes in the thickness of the epidermis are variable in dogs with hypothyroidism. Epidermal atrophy was evident in 48% of a group of hypothyroid dogs studied in our clinic.[95] Normal thickness was observed in 22% and

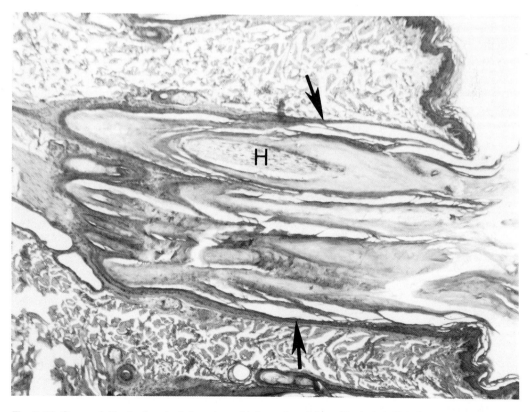

Fig. 3-17. Severe follicular keratosis in a dog with hypothyroidism. The hair follicle (arrows) is in the telogen phase with marked distention by keratin and disruption of attachment at base of hair shaft (H). The stratum corneum is moderately thickened due to the accumulation of multiple layers of keratin.

mild to moderate epidermal thickening due to a prominent stratum granulosum with an atrophic stratum spinosum was present in the remaining 30% of hypothyroid dogs.

The cardiovascular system may be affected by the reduced level of thyroid hormones, resulting in slowing of heart rate. The moderate bradycardia may be difficult to detect unless a normal resting heart rate had been measured previously. A mild, nonregenerative anemia also occurs in dogs with hypothyroidism.

In long-standing and severe hypothyroidism myxedema may develop and produce a characteristic appearance (Fig. 3-18). There is accumulation of mucin (neutral and acid mucopolysaccharides combined with protein) in the dermis and subcutis. This material binds considerable amounts of water and produces marked thickening of the skin. Myxedema is obvious around the face and head where accentuation of the normal skin folds causes a sad or "tragic" appearance (Fig. 3-18). The skin folds of the face are accentuated and the eyelids appear thick and drooping, thus contributing to the facial expression. The skin feels thick and doughy on palpation but the characteristic pitting observed with other types of edema does not occur with myxedema. Histologically, mucin appears as a blue-purple, granular or fibrillar material that disrupts the normal collagen and elastin fibers in the skin.

Another cutaneous manifestation of hypothyroidism is failure of hair regrowth after clipping for either cosmetic or therapeutic purposes. Hair in the clipped area may not regrow for months to years if the hypothyroidism is not recognized clinically and treated appropriately. Diminished circulating levels of thyroid hormones also result in atrophy of accessory skin structures, especially the sebaceous glands. This results in a dry and smooth skin surface in areas of hair loss.

Abnormalities in reproduction are common when a breeding animal develops hypothyroidism. Lack of libido and reduction in sperm count may occur in males, whereas abnormal or absent estrus cycles with reduced conception rates may result in females. Obesity and changes in behavior resulting from hypothyroidism often have detrimental effects on reproduction.

Constipation with passage of scanty, dry, hard feces usually is present in animals with hypothyroidism. Impaired joint function with clinical evidence of pain and joint effusion can result from severe or prolonged hypothyroidism, owing to an accumulation of acid mucopolysaccharides in joint capsules and ligamentous attachments. A change in attitude often is observed by the owner. The affected animal appears dull and less aggressive.

The diagnosis of hypothyroidism is based on the history, clinical signs, and demonstration of lowered levels of circulating thyroid hormones. The condition in dogs is accompanied by low protein-bound iodine levels and decreased ^{131}I uptake by the thyroid gland.[15,91] At present, the most accessible and sensitive method for measurement of blood thyroxine (T_4) and triiodothyronine (T_3) levels is radio-immunoassay (RIA).[10] The normal blood level of thyroxine in the dog is between 1.5 to 3.4 μg/dl and for triiodothyronine between 48 and 154 ng/dl.[10] In dogs with hypothyroidism the thyroxine level usually is below 0.8 μg/dl and triiodothyronine is below 50 ng/dl. When the levels are

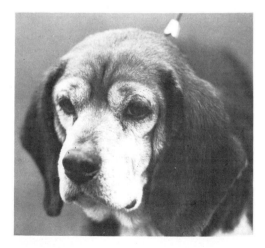

Fig. 3-18. Myxedema in a dog with long-standing and severe hypothyroidism. The thickening of skin folds of the face and eyelids results in a "tragic" facial expression.

borderline, clearer separation of dogs with hypothyroidism from normal dogs can be made by injection of thyrotrophic hormone (TSH).[49]

The serum cholesterol is elevated significantly (400 to 900 mg/dl and above) in many hypothyroid dogs, but diet and other diseases, such as hyperadrenocorticism, diabetes mellitus, and obstructive liver disorders, can result in elevation of cholesterol. The decreased rate of lipid metabolism with diminished intestinal excretion of cholesterol and conversion of lipids into bile acids and other compounds frequently results in hypercholesterolemia. Atherosclerosis of coronary and cerebral vessels may occur in animals with severe hypothyroidism and long-standing hyperlipidemia (Fig. 3-19). This occasionally results in hemorrhage and ischemic necrosis of the myocardium due to impingement of vessel lumina by numerous lipid-laden macrophages in the tunica media and adventitia. In hypo-

thyroid animals with markedly elevated plasma lipids, renal glomeruli may become plugged with lipid, resulting in progressive renal failure (Fig. 3-20). The accumulation of excessive lipid in the liver often results in varying degrees of hepatomegaly with abdominal distention in dogs with long-term hypothyroidism. Corneal lipidosis is observed occasionally in hypothyroid animals with hypercholesterolemia.[25] This lesion is often unilateral because the lipid is deposited in corneas that have been previously injured and have a network of "ghost" vessels from which the lipid diffuses into the connective tissue stroma. It has been reported that hypothyroid dogs have either increased intensity of the alpha$_2$-lipoprotein bands or hypertriglyceridemia with prominent beta-, pre-beta and alpha$_2$-lipoprotein bands in addition to the hypercholesterolemia.[94] High lipid concentrations and altered lipoprotein electrophoretic patterns return to near normal values

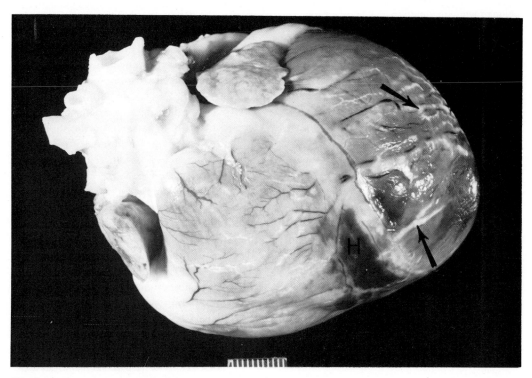

Fig. 3-19. Coronary atherosclerosis (arrows) with areas of ischemic necrosis and hemorrhage of myocardium (H) in a dog with marked hyperlipidemia associated with severe hypothyroidism.

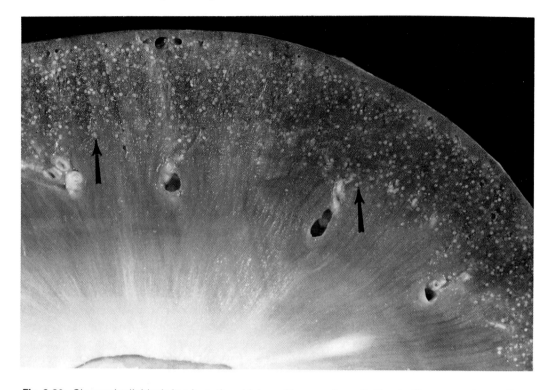

Fig. 3-20. Glomerular lipidosis in a hypothyroid dog with severe hyperlipidemia. Numerous glomeruli are plugged with lipid and are visible macroscopically as small white dots (arrows) in the kidney cortex.

after sodium levothyroxine administration.

The treatment of hypothyroidism involves replacement with either thyroxine or triiodothyronine. By supplying adequate amounts of thyroxine orally, the animal's condition will improve within 2 to 4 weeks. Because of its stability and long shelf life, sodium levothyroxine (a synthetic form of thyroxine) is preferred over desiccated thyroid and triiodothyronine.

Hyperthyroidism

Disturbances of growth in the thyroid-secreting excess thyroid hormones are most common in adult cats. Follicular cell adenomas, often developing in a thyroid with multinodular hyperplasia, are encountered more commonly than malignant thyroid tumors. Most proliferative lesions encountered in the feline thyroid gland until recently were found incidentally at necropsy and were not recognized as being associated with obvious clinical

disturbances. A syndrome of hyperthyroidism is being recognized with greater frequency in aged cats either associated with multinodular hyperplasia, adenomas or adenocarcinomas derived from follicular cells of the thyroid.[50] Large adenomas and carcinomas are detected by palpation or as a swelling in the cranioventral cervical region.

Thyroid adenomas associated with hyperthyroidism in cats usually appear as solitary, soft nodules that enlarge and distort the contour of the affected lobe (Fig. 3-21). A thin, fibrous connective tissue capsule separates the adenoma from the adjacent, often compressed, thyroid parenchyma. Adenomas are composed of hyperactive follicular cells arranged into follicles with variable amounts of colloid. Long microvillar processes extend from the luminal surfaces to phagocytize colloid (Fig. 3-22). As a result of the marked endocytotic activity numerous colloid droplets are present in the cytoplasm of follicular cells in close

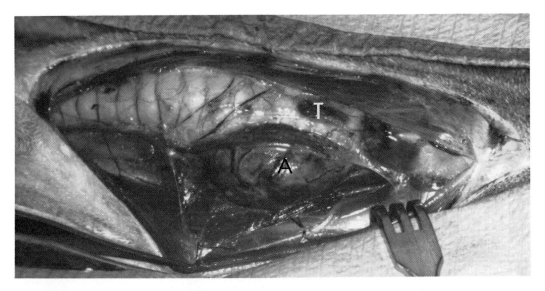

Fig. 3-21. Functional adenoma derived from thyroid follicular cells associated with hyperthyroidism. Surgical exploration of the ventral cervical region revealed a large unilateral adenoma (A) and a small opposite thyroid (T) lobe.

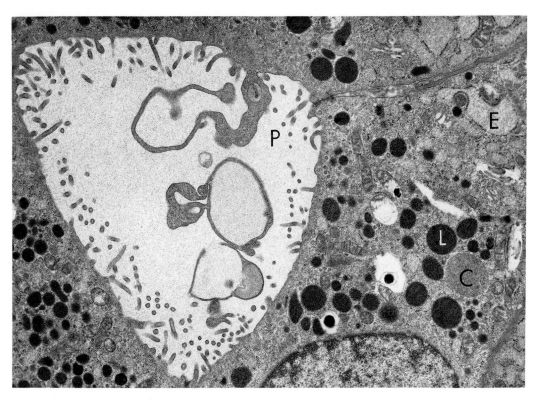

Fig. 3-22. Follicular cell adenoma in a cat associated with hyperthyroidism. Numerous long cytoplasmic processes (P) extend from the luminal surfaces of follicular cells to engulf colloid. Many lysosomal bodies (L), colloid droplets (C), and dilated profiles of rough endoplasmic reticulum (E) are present in follicular cells.

proximity to lysosomal bodies. The neoplastic cells release both T_4 and T_3 at an uncontrolled rate resulting in markedly elevated blood levels of both hormones. Functional thyroid adenomas are partially or completely separated from remnants of the adjacent "normal" thyroid by a fine connective tissue capsule. Follicles in the rim of thyroid around a functional adenoma are markedly enlarged and distended by the accumulation of colloid. The follicular cells are low cuboidal and atrophied with little evidence of endocytotic activity in response to the elevated levels of thyroid hormones. The opposite thyroid lobe should be carefully evaluated in cats with solitary adenomas for evidence of nodular hyperplasia or "microadenomas." These small areas of multinodular hyperplasia of follicular cells may cause recurrence of hyperthyroidism several months to a year or more after surgical removal of the functional adenoma.

Cats with hyperthyroidism usually have markedly elevated serum thyroxine and triiodothyronine levels.[83] Normal serum levels of T_4 in cats by radioimmunoassay are approximately 1.5 to 5.0 μg/dl and serum T_3 levels are 60 to 200 ng/dl. The serum T_4 levels in cats with hyperthyroidism range from 5.0 to over 50 μg/dl and serum T_3 levels range from 100 to 1,000 ng/dl (Fig. 3-23).

The most common disturbance of function in hyperthyroidism is weight loss in spite of a normal or increased appetite (Fig. 3-24). Polydipsia and polyuria occur in some cats with hyperthyroidism. Increased frequency of defecation and increased volume of stools are observed in about half of affected cats. Restlessness and increased activity occur in previously quiet cats.[84,85]

Hyperthyroidism also occurs in association with bilateral multinodular ("adenomatous") hyperplasia in cats. These are multiple areas of hyperplasia of thyroid follicular cells that only slightly enlarge the affected lobe(s). In contrast to adenomas, the areas of nodular hyperplasia are not encapsulated and the adjacent thyroid parenchyma is not compressed. Hyperplastic nodules are composed of irregularly shaped, colloid-filled follicles lined

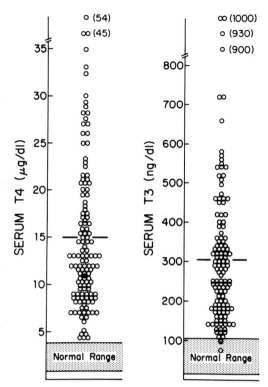

Fig. 3-23. Serum thyroid hormone levels in cats with hyperthyroidism. There is a marked elevation of serum thyroxine (mean: 15 μg/dl) and triiodothyronine (mean: 300 μg/dl) in cats with hyperthyroidism. (Courtesy of Dr. M. E. Peterson.[83])

by cuboidal follicular cells. The multiple foci of follicular cell hyperplasia may coalesce to form macroscopically observable thyroid adenomas.

Thyroid tumors in the dog only occasionally secrete sufficient thyroid hormone to overload the highly efficient excretory pathways for thyroid hormones in order to produce clinical signs of hyperthyroidism. It is surprising that hyperthyroidism occurs even with functional tumors since experimental induction of hyperthyroidism in the dog requires daily administration of about 25 times the normal replacement dose of thyroid hormone.[86] Dogs have an efficient enterohepatic excretory mechanism for thyroid hormones that is difficult to overload either from endogenous production by a tumor or exogenous administration of hormone. The clinical signs of

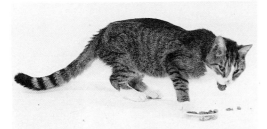

Fig. 3-24. Hyperthyroidism caused by a functional tumor derived from thyroid follicular cells that secreted thyroid hormones at an uncontrolled rate resulting in markedly elevated blood levels of T_4 and T_3. The cat had lost considerable body weight in spite of an increased appetite owing to the gluconeogenic effects of the long-standing elevation of thyroid hormones.

hyperthyroidism in dogs with functional thyroid tumors include weight loss, polyphagia, weakness and fatigue, intolerance to heat, and nervousness.[91]

Hyperplasia of Thyroid Follicular Cells ("Goiter")

Non-neoplastic and non-inflammatory enlargement of the thyroid develops in all domestic mammals, birds, and submammalian vertebrates. Certain forms of thyroid hyperplasia, especially nodular, may be difficult to differentiate from benign tumors (adenomas). The major pathogenic mechanisms responsible for the development of thyroid hyperplasia include iodine deficient diets, goitrogenic compounds that interfere with thyroxinogenesis, dietary iodide-excess, and genetic enzyme defects in the biosynthesis of thyroid hormones (Fig. 3-25). All of these seemingly divergent factors result in inadequate thyroxine/triiodothyronine synthesis and decreased blood levels of thyroid hormones. This is detected by the hypothalamus

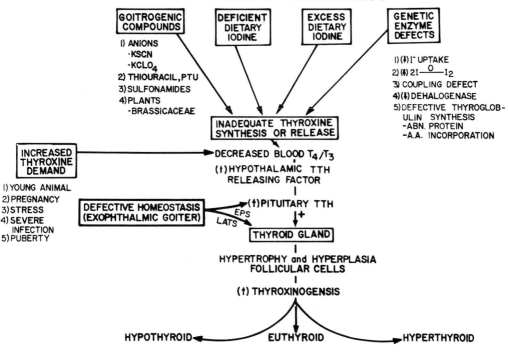

Fig. 3-25. Mechanisms of goitrogenesis. Multiple pathogenic factors (goitrogenic compounds, deficient and excess dietary iodine intake and genetic enzyme defects) result in inadequate thyroxine/triiodothyronine synthesis and leads to long-term stimulation of thyroid follicular cells by an increased secretion of pituitary thyrotrophin (TTH or TSH). LATS = Long Acting Thyroid Substance, an autoantibody that uses the TSH receptor to stimulate the synthetic and secretory activity of follicular cells. EPS = Exophthalmos Producing Substance; forward protrusion of the eyeball is part of this form of goiter in human patients.

and pituitary to increase the secretion of TSH, which results in hypertrophy and hyperplasia of follicular cells in the thyroid gland.

DIFFUSE HYPERPLASTIC GOITER. Iodine deficiency in the diet that resulted in diffuse thyroid hyperplasia was common in many goitrogenic areas throughout the world before the widespread addition of iodized salt to animal diets. Although iodine-deficient goiter still occurs worldwide in domestic animals, the outbreaks are sporadic and fewer animals are affected. Marginal iodine-deficient diets containing certain goitrogenic compounds may result in severe thyroid hyperplasia and clinical evidence of goiter. These substances include thiouracil, sulfonamides, anions of the Hofmeister series, and a number of plants from the family *Brassicacceae*. Young animals born to females on iodine-deficient diets are more likely to develop severe thyroid hyperplasia and have clinical signs of hypothyroidism. Both lateral lobes of the thyroid are uniformly enlarged in young animals with diffuse hyperplastic goiter. The enlargements may be extensive and result in palpable swelling in the cranial cervical area (Fig. 3-26). The affected lobes are firm and dark red because an extensive interfollicular capillary network develops under the influence of long-term TSH stimulation. The thyroid enlargements are the result of intense hyperplasia of follicular cells lining thyroid follicles with the formation of papillary projections into the lumens of follicles (Fig. 3-27). Endocytosis of colloid often proceeds at a rate greater than synthesis resulting in progressive depletion of colloid and partial collapse of follicles.

Iodine deficiency may be conditioned by other antithyroid compounds present in animal feeds and be responsible, in particular situations, for a high incidence of goiter. Prolonged low-level exposure to thiocyanates, which are produced by ruminal degradation of cyanogenic glucosides from plants such as white clover (*Trifolium*), couch grass, and linseed meal, and by degradation of glucosinolates of the Brassica crops, is associated with hyperplastic goiter in ruminants. Goitrin (5-vinyloxazolidine-2-thione) derived from the

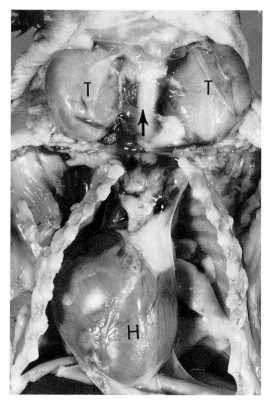

Fig. 3-26. Diffuse hyperplastic goiter in a pup resulting in prominent symmetrical enlargements of both thyroid (T) lobes. The hyperplastic thyroids were freely movable from the trachea (arrow) in the cervical region. H = heart.

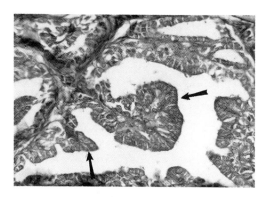

Fig. 3-27. Diffuse hyperplastic goiter illustrating papillary projections (arrows) into follicular lumens and partial collapse of follicles due to increased endocytosis of colloid in a pup.

glucosinolates of *Brassica* spp. inhibits organification of iodine (i.e., binding of I_2 to tyrosine residues in thyroglobulin molecule). *Leucaerna leucocephala* and other legumes of the genus are native or cultivated in many subtropical areas and contain the toxic amino acid mimosine.

Goiter in adult animals usually is of little clinical significance, and except for occasional local pressure influences, the general health of the animal is not impaired. It is of significance as a disease of the newborn, although the previous drastic losses in endemic areas are now controlled by the prophylactic use of iodized salt. Congenital hypothyroidism in domestic animals is associated with iodine-deficient hyperplastic goiter, even though the dam shows no evidence of thyroid dysfunction. Gestation is significantly prolonged, the larger goiters may cause dystocia (difficult birth), and there is a tendency to retain the fetal placenta. Affected foals are extremely weak and die within a few days after birth. The thyroids may be only moderately enlarged. Some calves with goiter are born partially or completely hairless. These calves either are born dead or die soon after birth. Newborn goitrous pigs, goats, and lambs frequently have myxedema and hair loss. The mortality rate is high, with the majority born dead or dying within a few hours of birth. Enlarged thyroid glands are readily palpable or visible in kids and lambs, but are not apparent in piglets because of the combination of short neck and myxedema. Asphyxiation may result also from pressure by the enlarged thyroid gland. Young goitrous animals that are treated and survive usually do not show permanent harmful effects.

COLLOID GOITER. Colloid goiter represents the involutionary phase of diffuse hyperplastic goiter in young adult and adult animals. The markedly hyperplastic follicular cells continue to produce colloid but endocytosis of colloid is decreased due to diminished pituitary TSH levels in response to the return of blood thyroxine and triiodothyronine back to the normal range. Both thyroid lobes are diffusely enlarged but are more translucent and lighter in color than with hyperplastic goiter.

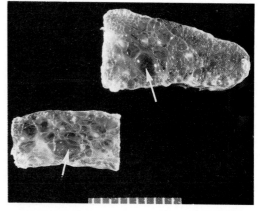

Fig. 3-28. Colloid goiter with macroscopically visible follicles filled with colloid (arrows). The scale represents 1 cm.

The differences in macroscopic appearances are the result of less vascularity in colloid goiter and development of macrofollicles distended with colloid (Fig. 3-28).

Colloid goiter may develop either after sufficient amounts of iodide have been added to the diet or after the requirements for thyroxine have diminished in an older animal. Blood thyroid hormone levels return to the normal range and the secretion of TSH by the pituitary gland is correspondingly decreased. Follicles are progressively distended (Figs. 3-28 and 3-29) with densely eosinophilic colloid due to diminished TSH-induced endocytosis. The follicular cells lining the macrofollicles are flattened and atrophic. The interface between the colloid and luminal surface of follicular cells is smooth and lacks the characteristic endocytotic vacuoles of actively secreting follicular cells (Fig. 3-30). Some involuted follicles in colloid goiter have remnants of the papillary projections of follicular cells extending into their lumen (Fig. 3-29).

The changes in diffuse hyperplastic and colloid goiters are consistent throughout the diffusely enlarged thyroid lobes. The follicles are irregular in size and shape in hyperplastic goiter because of varying amounts of lightly eosinophilic and vacuolated colloid in the lumen. Some follicles are collapsed due to lack of colloid (Fig. 3-27). The lining epithelial

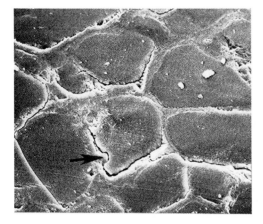

Fig. 3-29. Scanning electron micrograph of enlarged thyroid with colloid goiter illustrating large involuted follicles distended with colloid and remnants of papillary projections of hyperplastic follicular cells (arrow).

cells are columnar with a deeply eosinophilic cytoplasm and small hyperchromatic nuclei that often are situated in the basilar part of the cell. The follicles are lined by single or multiple layers of hyperplastic follicular cells that in some follicles may form papillary projections into the lumen (Fig. 3-29). Similar proliferative changes are present in ectopic thyroid parenchyma in the neck and mediastinum.

IODIDE-EXCESS GOITER. Although seemingly paradoxical, an excess of iodide in the diet also can result in thyroid hyperplasia in animals and man. Foals of mares fed dry seaweed containing excessive iodide may develop thyroid hyperplasia and clinically evident goiter.[5] The thyroid glands of the young are exposed to higher blood iodide levels than in the dam because of concentration of iodide, first by the placenta and then by the mammary gland. High blood iodide interferes with one or more steps of thyroxinogenesis, leading to lowered blood thyroid hormone levels, and a compensatory increase in pituitary TSH secretion. Excess iodine appears primarily to block the release of T_3 and T_4 from the follicle by interfering with proteolysis of colloid by lysosomes, but also interferes with the peroxidation of $2I$ to I_2, and disrupts the conversion of monoiodothyronine to diiodothyronine.

MULTIFOCAL ("NODULAR") HYPERPLASIA ("GOITER"). Nodular hyperplasia in thyroid

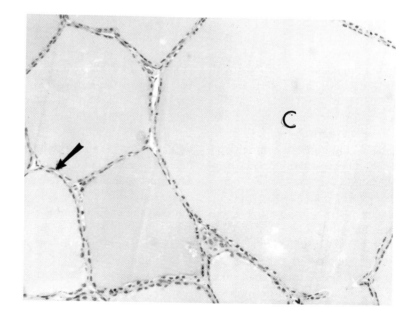

Fig. 3-30. Colloid goiter illustrating large distended thyroid follicles lined by flattened atrophic follicular cells (arrow). Distention of follicles with colloid (C) occurs due to diminished TSH-mediated endocytosis in a hyperplastic thyroid gland following return of blood T_4 and T_3 levels back into the normal range.

glands of old horses, cats, and dogs appears as multiple white to tan nodules of varying size (Fig. 3-31). The affected lobes are moderately enlarged and irregular in contour. Multinodular nodular goiter in most animals (except cats) is endocrinologically inactive and encountered as an incidental lesion at necropsy. However, there is evidence that functional thyroid adenomas in old cats with hyperthyroidism often develop in a gland with multinodular hyperplasia and that cerain cats with thyroid hormone excess only have multinodular hyperplasia in their thyroids. In contrast to thyroid adenomas, the areas of nodular hyperplasia are *not* encapsulated and result in minimal compression of adjacent parenchyma. Nodular goiter consists of multiple foci of hyperplastic follicular cells that are sharply demarcated but not encapsulated from the adjacent thyroid parenchyma. Some hyperplastic cells form small follicles with little or no colloid. Other nodules are formed by larger irregularly shaped follicles lined by one or more layers of columnar cells that form papillary projections into the lumen. Some of the follicles are involuted and filled with densely eosinophilic colloid. These changes appear to be the result of alternating periods of hyperplasia and colloid involution in the thyroid glands of old animals. The areas of nodular hyperplasia may be microscopic or grossly visible causing modest enlargement of the thyroid (Fig. 3-31). As a general rule, hyperplastic nodules are multiple, poorly or not at all encapsulated, variable in their histologic structure, and do not cause significant compression of adjacent thyroid parenchyma. Adenomas on the other hand tend to be solitary, well encapsulated, fairly uniform in histologic structure, and cause compression of the surrounding parenchyma owing to progressive expansive growth. Endocrinologically active thyroid adenomas result in colloid involution of follicles in the rim of surrounding thyroid due to inhibition of TSH secretion.

CONGENITAL DYSHORMONOGENETIC GOITER. An inability to synthesize and secrete adequate amounts of thyroid hormones beginning before or at birth has been documented in

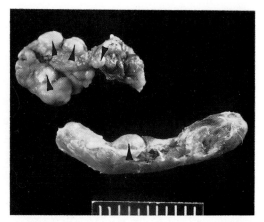

Fig. 3-31. Multinodular follicular cell hyperplasia (arrowheads) in both thyroid lobes from a cat with hyperthyroidism.

several animal species and in human infants.[28,32] The more prevalent forms of inherited goiter in man include defects in the iodination of tyrosines, deiodination of iodotyrosines, synthesis and proteolysis of thyroglobulin, coupling of iodotyrosines to form iodothyronines, and in iodide transport.

Congenital dyshormonogenetic goiter is inherited by an autosomal recessive gene in sheep (Corriedale, Dorset Horn, Merino, and Romney breeds),[88] Afrikander cattle,[81] and Saanen dwarf goats.[92] The subnormal growth rate, absence of normal wool development or a rough sparse hair coat, myxedematous swellings of the subcutis, weakness, and sluggish behavior suggest that the affected young are clinically hypothyroid. Most lambs with congenital goiter either die shortly after birth or are highly sensitive to the effects of adverse environmental conditions.

Thyroid glands are symmetrically enlarged at birth due to an intense diffuse hyperplasia of follicular cells.[18] Thyroid follicles are lined by tall columnar cells but follicles often have collapsed because of lack of colloid resulting from the marked endocytotic activity. The tall columnar follicular cells lining thyroid follicles have extensively dilated profiles of rough endoplasmic reticulum and large mitochondria, but there are relatively few dense granules associated with the Golgi apparatus and

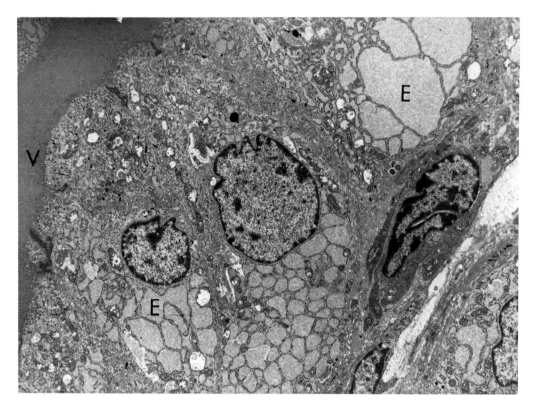

Fig. 3-32. Dyshormonogenetic goiter in a lamb illustrating hypertrophied thyroid follicular cells. Profiles of rough endoplasmic reticulum (E) are dilated by finely granular material and long microvilli (V) extend into the colloid. Few thyroglobulin-containing apical vesicles are present in the luminal aspect of the cell.

few thyroglobulin-containing apical vesicles near the luminal plasma membrane (Fig. 3-32). Numerous long microvilli extend into the follicular lumen.

Although thyroidal uptake and turnover of ^{131}I are greatly increased compared with erythroid controls, circulating thyroxine and triiodothyronine levels are consistently low. The lack of a defect in the iodide transport mechanism, organification or dehalogenation, plus an absence of normal 19S thyroglobulin in goitrous thyroids and only minute amounts of thyroglobulin-related antigens (0.01% of normal), suggest an impairment in thyroglobulin biosynthesis in animals with congenital goiter. A closely related or similar defect appears operational in the examples of congenital goiter in sheep, cattle, and goats.

The protein-bound iodine levels in animals with inherited congenital goiter are markedly elevated. This appears to be the result of iodination of albumin and other plasma proteins by the thyroid gland under long-term TSH stimulation, since hormonal iodide levels are significantly lower than in controls. The hypothyroid goats with congenital goiter can be returned to a state of euthyroidism by the addition of iodide (1.0 mg/day) to the diet. Although the goats remain unable to synthesize thyroglobulin, supplementation with additional iodide results in sufficient formation of triiodothyronine and thyroxine in the abnormal iodoproteins to make the animals euthyroid.

The presence of messenger RNA (mRNA) coding for thyroglobulin has been investigated to further elucidate the molecular basis for the impairment of thyroid hormone biosynthesis in congenital goiter.[113] Although thyroglobulin-mRNA sequences are present in the goitrous tissue, their concentration is markedly reduced (1/10 to 1/40 that of normal thyroid) and the intracellular distribution is abnormal (nuclear: 42% of normal, cytoplasmic: 7%, membrane fraction: 1 to 2%) (Table 3-1). The lack of thyroglobulin in these examples of congenital goiter in animals appears to be due to a defect in thyroglobulin-mRNA leading to aberrant processing of primary transcripts and/or transport of the thyroglobulin mRNA from the nucleus to the endoplasmic reticulum.

THYROID FUNCTION TESTS

Thyroid function tests frequently are needed in the diagnosis of thyroid diseases in animals. In hypothyroidism there is reduced metabolic activity and the most direct indicator of this change is the measurement of basal oxygen consumption. However, valid and satisfactorily reproducible measurements of oxygen consumption can only be made under carefully controlled laboratory conditions. Long and painstaking training of the animal is required to achieve the relaxation of mental and physical activity that is necessary for basal measurements. While the measurement of oxygen consumption is useful in experimental studies, it can not be employed successfully as a diagnostic procedure in clinical veterinary medicine.[19]

Cholesterol

Serum cholesterol concentration is an indirect and variable index of the peripheral action of thyroid hormone. For example, two-thirds of pet dogs with spontaneous hypothyroidism have fasting serum cholesterol concentration elevated above 300 mg/100 ml. However, hypercholesterolemia is probably as dependent upon the composition of the dog's diet as upon the severity and duration of hypothyroidism. Cholesterol values tend to be higher in the general pet dog population that is fed table scraps or home diets than in normal dogs maintained exclusively on commercially manufactured dry dog foods. Hypercholesterolemia also occurs in some dogs with cortisol-excess, a disease which must be considered in the differential diagnosis of hypothyroidism. The measurement of serum cholesterol is thus not a specific and dependable test of thyroid function, but fasting cholesterol values in excess of 600 mg/100 ml, which are often observed in hypothyroidism, infrequently occur in any other disease in the dog.[19]

Thyroidal Uptake of Radioiodine

The fraction of a tracer dose of radioiodine taken up by the thyroid primarily is dependent upon the functional integrity of the gland, the endogenous output of TSH, and the dietary intake of iodine. In dog breeds of European origin, peak uptake of radioiodine normally occurs between 48 and 96 hours after administration of the tracer, and radioiodine is released from the gland with a half-time of about 8 to 15 days. Peak uptake ranges from about 15% of the dose in dogs whose iodine

Table 3-1 *Subcellular distribution of thyroglobulin messenger RNA (mRNA) sequences in goats with congenital goiter and thyroglobulin deficiency as determined from hybridization between thyroglobulin complementary DNA and RNA.* *

	Distribution of Thyroglobulin mRNA Sequences (% of Recovered Sequences)		Concentration of Thyroglobulin mRNA Sequences in Goiter
	Normal Thyroid	Goiter	(% of Normal)
Nuclear RNA	5	35	42
Cytoplasmic RNA	25	38	7
Membrane-bound RNA	70	27	1–2

*From van Herle et al.[112]

intake is 500 μg per day to about 40% when iodine intake is 140 μg per day. Peak uptake occurs within 12 to 24 hours in the Basenji and the half-time of disappearance of radio-iodine from the gland is about 3 days. In addition, peak uptake in the Basenji is much lower (about one-half the value in European breeds) at the same level of iodine intake.[77]

The radioactivity in a duplicate dose of the tracer must be measured when thyroidal radioactivity is determined so that uptake may be expressed as a percentage of the administered dose. The duplicate dose ("or standard") must be placed in a phantom which provides both a radiation spectrum and a count rate per microcurie for the isotope of radioiodine similar to those that would occur in the thyroid of the dog in situ. Because the parotid salivary gland also clears iodide and is in close proximity to the thyroid, the uptake detector must be carefully positioned and appropriately collimated to exclude radioactivity from the parotid salivary gland, particularly if measurements are made within the first 48 hours. Under most circumstances, other extrathyroidal radioactivity in the neck does not contribute a significant error to the measurement.

In primary hypothyroidism, thyroidal uptake usually is less than 5% of the tracer dose, but uptake can also be depressed to this degree by dietary levels of iodine above 500 μg per day. If the iodine intake cannot be ascertained with reasonable certainty, it is advisable to utilize a low-iodine diet for 1 week prior to the measurement.[91] This can be accomplished by feeding fresh, cooked meat without salt or other additives or by the use of a canned, semisynthetic low-iodine diet.

Thyroidal uptake is elevated and the turnover of radioiodine from the gland is accelerated in iodine deficiency and in hyperthyroidism in dogs with functional thyroid tumors. When iodine intake is reduced to about 90 μg per day, peak uptake of 65 to 70% of the dose occurs within 24 hours; conversely, when iodine intake is lowered to 20 μg per day, peak uptake of 80 to 90% of the dose occurs within 4 to 12 hours after administration of the tracer.[11] The corresponding increase in the rate of disappearance of radioiodine from the gland is such that net thyroidal radioactivity may be well within the range for normal diets by 48 to 96 hours (Fig. 3-33). The increased uptake and turnover of radioiodine due to iodine deficiency can be distinguished from that of functional thyroid tumors by repetition of the tracer studies after a week or more following feeding a diet that provides a daily dose of iodine that is slightly in excess of the normal iodine requirement.

Protein-Bound Iodine

Because circulating thyroid hormone is almost exclusively bound to plasma proteins, protein-bound iodine (PBI) has been used as a measure of circulating thyroid hormone concentration in both man and animals. However, at the usual iodine intake level of about 500 μg per day in normal dogs, the concentration of nonhormonal iodine that is bound to plasma proteins is equal to or greater than the amount of hormonal iodine (in addition to the rela-

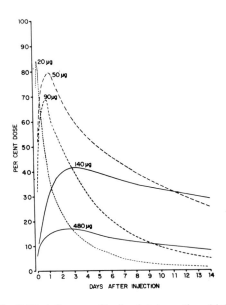

Fig. 3-33. Influence of iodine intake on thyroidal uptake and turnover of radioiodine. Each curve represents the averaged data for five adult beagles maintained at the designated level of iodine intake from 5 months (at 480 μg per day) to 1 year (at 20 μg per day). (Courtesy of Dr. Bruce Belshaw.[19])

tively large amount of free inorganic iodide in the plasma) (Fig. 3-7). The nonhormonal protein-bound iodine is not distinguished from hormonal iodine in the measurement of PBI, and its concentration is related not to thyroid function *per se* but to iodine intake. Thus, the measurement of PBI usually is unreliable in diagnosing hypothyroidism. However, Bullock[15] has shown that the PBI can be effectively employed as an index of the response to TSH stimulation. Twenty-four hours after a single intramuscular dose of 5 to 10 units of TSH, the average increase in PBI concentration is about 3 μg per 100 ml in normal dogs, compared with an average increase of only 0.4 μg per 100 ml in hypothyroid dogs. The normal values for protein-bound iodine for a variety of animal species and man are summarized in Table 3-2.

Thyroid Hormone by Radioimmunoassay

The most sensitive and accurate method for measurement of blood thyroxine (T_4) and triiodothyronine (T_3) levels is radioimmunoassay (RIA). The normal blood level of thy-

roxine in the dog ranges between 1.5 to 3.6 μg/dl (Fig. 3-34) (mean—2.48 μg/dl) and for triiodothyronine between 48 and 154 ng/dl (Fig. 3-35) (mean—95 ng/dl).[10] In dogs with hypothyroidism the thyroxine level usually is below 1.0 μg/dl (Fig. 3-36) and triiodothyronine is below 50 ng/dl (Fig. 3-37). When the levels are borderline, clearer separation of dogs with hypothyroidism from erythroid dogs can be made by injecting TSH. In the erythroid dog the thyroxine level will at least double 8 hours after IV or IM administration of TTH (Fig. 3-36). In dogs with primary hypothyroidism, the thyroxine and triiodothyronine levels do not change significantly after injection of TSH.[10] Plasma T_4 levels were no more than 0.2 μg/dl above control values at 8 hours post-TSH (Fig. 3-36) and plasma T_3 increased by no more than 10 ng/dl after TSH (Fig. 3-37).[4] The increase in serum T_3 after TSH was more variable in normal dogs than for T_4 but in dogs with primary hypothyroidism there was little (10 ng/dl or less) change in serum T_3 8 hours after TSH (Fig. 3-37).[10] Serum T_4 and T_3 values as determined by RIA in other animal species are summarized in Table 3-3.

Table 3-2 Normal Values for Protein-Bound Iodine (PBI) in Various Animals*

Species	PBI (μg %) ± Standard Error
Man	3.5–8.0 ± 0.4
Horse	3.6 ± 0.4
Monkey	6.6 ± 0.7
Rabbit	3.3 ± 0.5
Rabbit	2.16 ± 0.3
Rat	4.5 ± 0.4
Rat	3.50 ± 0.1
Guinea pig	2.5 ± 0.5
Hamster	3.5 ± 0.4
Opossum	0.4 ± 0.2
White Leghorn chicken	1.13 ± 0.1
Pekin duck	1.14 ± 0.1
Chicken	1.16 ± 0.3
Sheep	3.7 ± 0.3
Holstein cow	4.46 ± 0.3
Guernsey cow	3.91 ± 0.2
Calves, newborn	13.7 ± 5.0
Dogs	2.1 ± 0.5

*Adapted from Barker et al., Katsch and Windsor, Mellen and Hardy, and Zarrow et al.

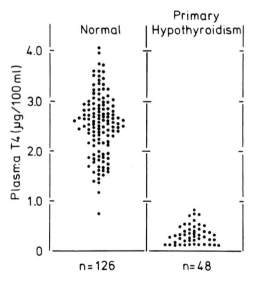

Fig. 3-34. Basal plasma thyroxine (T_4) values in 126 normal dogs and 48 dogs with primary hypothyroidism determined by radioimmunoassay. (From Belshaw and Rijnberk.[10])

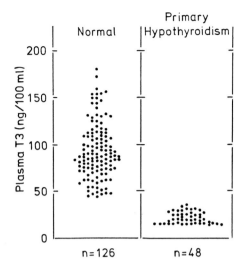

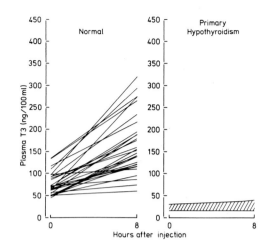

Fig. 3-35. Basal plasma triiodothyronine (T3) values in 126 normal dogs and 48 dogs with primary hypothyroidism determined by radioimmunoassay. (From Belshaw and Rijnberk.[10])

Fig. 3-37. Plasma triiodothyronine (T3) responses to TSH stimulation in 30 normal dogs and 28 dogs with primary hypothyroidism determined by radioimmunoassay. Only the highest and lowest response lines are shown for the hypothyroid dogs. (From Belshaw and Rijnberk.[10])

The peak increase in T_4 and T_3 are at 8 and 12 hours after TSH injection (1 unit/5 lb. body weight) and levels return to normal by 48 hours (Fig. 3-38).[39] Smaller doses (0.1 and 0.2 U) of TSH resulted in nonsignificant increases in serum T_4 but were able to increase serum T_3 to a similar degree as the larger dose (1.0 U) of TSH. It has been

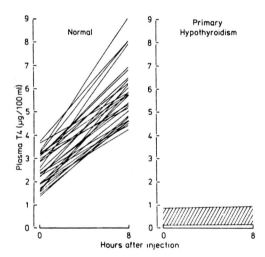

Fig. 3-36. Plasma thyroxine (T4) responses to TSH stimulation in 30 normal dogs and 28 dogs with primary hypothyroidism determined by radioimmunoassay. Only the highest and lowest response lines are shown for the hypothyroid dogs. (From Belshaw and Rijnberk.[10])

Table 3-3   Serum T4 and T3 Values by RIA

	T4 μg/dl	T3 ng/dl
Equine	1.63 ± 0.51 (0.95–2.38)	77.1 ± 45.75 (31–158)
Bovine	6.22 ± 2.03 (3.60–8.9)	92.50 ± 58.61 (41–170)
Caprine	3.45 ± 0.47 (3.0–4.23)	145.9 ± 29.32 (88–190)
Ovine	4.41 ± 1.13 (2.95–6.15)	99.6 ± 27.94 (63–150)
Porcine	3.32 ± 0.80 (1.70–4.68)	89.8 ± 36.17 (43–140)
Canine	1.51 ± 0.38 (0.70–2.18)	96.2 ± 21.39 (63–130)
Feline	2.02 ± 0.61 (1.18–2.95)	64.7 ± 20.62 (39–112)

From Reap, M., Cass, C., and Hightower, D.: Thyroxine and triiodo thyronine levels in ten species of animals. Southwestern Vet. *31*:31, 1978.
N = 10 in all species.

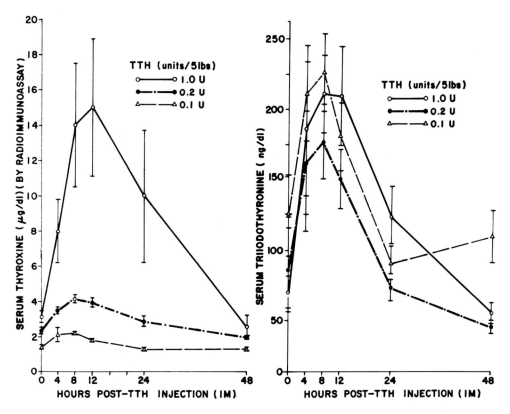

Fig. 3-38. Changes in serum thyroxine and triiodothyronine determined by radioimmunoassay following intramuscular injection of varying doses of thyrotrophic hormone (TSH) in normal dogs. The peak increase in circulating thyroid hormone levels occurs between 8 and 12 hours following TSH administration. (From Gosselin et al.[39])

reported that (3,5,3') triiodothyronine and reverse (3,3',5') triiodothyronine (rT$_3$) are secreted preferentially by the canine thyroid gland in response to thyrotrophin infusion, possibly due to local deiodination of thyroxine during secretion.[66]

Hyperthyroid cats usually have markedly elevated serum thyroxine and triiodothyronine levels.[83] Normal serum levels of T$_4$ in cats by radioimmunoassay are approximately 1.5 to 5.0 μg/dl and serum T$_3$ levels are 60 to 200 ng/dl. The serum T$_4$ levels in cats with hyperthyroidism range from 5.0 to over 50 μg/dl and serum T$_3$ levels range from 100 to 1,000 ng/dl (Fig. 3-23).

There are two additional considerations in the measurement of serum T$_4$ and T$_3$. First, there are significant diurnal oscillations in circulating thyroid hormone concentration in the dog, and for any of the above methods, the best separation between normal and hypothyroid dogs is obtained by measurements made at about noon, when hormone concentration in normal dogs usually is at its peak. The second consideration is that serum T$_4$ concentration declines in iodine deficiency in the dog, while serum T$_3$ remains within the normal range.

Thyroid Biopsy

The removal of the caudal one-fourth of either lobe of the thyroid for histologic examination is a simple surgical procedure without significant risk, even if the dog is hypothyroid. In most cases of primary hypothyroidism, there either is marked loss of thyroid follicles with replacement by adipose connective tissue (Fig. 3-39) or multifocal

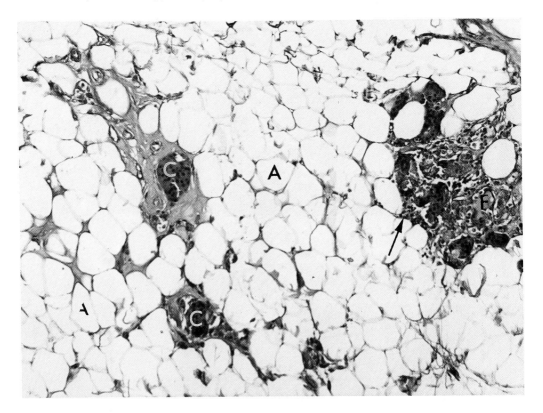

Fig. 3-39. Idiopathic atrophy ("follicular collapse") of the thyroid from a dog with hypothyroidism. There is extensive loss of follicular epithelium and replacement by adipose connective tissue (A). Only a few viable follicles (F) remain, together with small nests of C-cells (C).

lymphocytic thyroiditis which develops on an immunologic basis (Fig. 3-14). Histologic examination of a biopsy of the thyroid is a useful and reliable aid in the diagnosis of thyroid disease when either the results of serum assays for T_4 and T_3 are equivocal or a nodule is palpated in the thyroid area.

Since the scope of this book cannot include an exhaustive consideration of clinical problems in each of the animal species, the reader is referred to the following references for the details needed for clinical tests and interpretations.

Dogs:	Reid (1969); Hightower (1973); Bush (1969); Anderson (1971); Bullock (1970); Kallfelz (1969, 1973); Ekman (1972); Foreman (1970); Kyzar (1972); Scherzinger (1972); Terblanche (1970); Williams (1973).
Cattle:	Boitor (1970); Cowley (1971); Schneider (1973); Swanson (1973).
Horses:	Hightower (1971); Kallfelz (1970); Motley (1972).
Sheep:	Afiefy (1970); Herrington (1971); Draper (1969).
Swine:	Daburon (1970).
Cats:	Ling (1974).

REFERENCES

1. Afiefy, M. M., Zaki, K., Abul-Fadle, W., et al, (1970): Effects of season and sex on thyroid hormone level in the blood of Osimi sheep. Zentralb. Veterinaermed. [A] *17*:476.
2. Anderson. J. J. B., and Dorner, J. L. (1971): Total serum thyroxine in thyroidectomized Beagles, using ^{125}T-labeled thyroxine and comparison of T-3 and T-4 tests. J. Am. Vet. Med. Assoc. *159*:760.
3. Anderson, R. R. (1971): Secretion rates of thyroxine and triiodothyronine in dairy cattle. J. Dairy Sci. *54*:1195.
4. Auclair, R. F., Bonofiglio, R. A., and Rosenkrantz, H. (1970): Determination of serum thyroid hormone in laboratory animals. Am. J. Vet. Res. *31*: 1655.
5. Baker, H. J., and Lindsey, J. R. (1968): Equine

goiter due to excess dietary iodide. J. Am. Vet. Med. Assn. *153*:616.

6. Barker, S. B., Humphry, M. J., and Soley, M. H. (1951): The clinical determination of protein bound iodine, J. Clin. Invest. *30*:55.

7. Barlet, J. P. (1969): Variation of calcium and phosphate levels in the blood of the dairy cow at calving time: probable role of calcitonin in the etiology of the milk fever syndrome. Rech. Vet. *2*:93.

8. Bastenie, P. A., Ermans, A. M., Bonnyns, M., Neve, P., et al, (1975): Lymphocytic thyroiditis as an autoimmune disease. In Molecular Pathology, edited by R. A. Good. Springfield, Charles C Thomas.

9. Belshaw, B. E., and Becker, D. V. (1971): Necrosis of follicular cells and discharge of thyroidal iodine induced by administering iodide to iodine-deficient dogs. J. Clin. Endocrinol. Metab. *36*:466.

10. Belshaw, B. E., and Rijnberk, A. (1979): Radioimmunoassay of plasma T_4 and T_3 in the diagnosis of primary hypothyroidism in dogs. J.A.A.H.A. *15*:17.

11. Belshaw, B. E., Barandes, M., Becker, D. V., et al. (1974): A model of iodine kinetics in the dog. Endocrinology *95*:1078.

12. Belshaw, B. E., Cooper, T. B., and Becker, D. V. (1975): The iodine requirement and influence of iodine intake on iodine metabolism and thyroid function in the adult beagle. Endocrinology *96*: 1280.

13. Blaxter, K. L. (1946): Experiments with iodinated casein on farms in England and Wales. *36*:117.

14. Book, S. A. (1976): Influence of age on thyroidal ^{131}I uptake in Beagle pups. Lab. Anim. Sci. *26*:443.

15. Bullock, L. (1970): Protein bound iodine determination as a diagnostic aid for canine hypothyroidism. J. Am. Vet. Med. Assoc. *156*:892.

16. Bush, B. M. (1969): Thyroid disease in the dog, a review, J. Small Anim. Pract. *10*:95 and 185.

17. Bush, B. M. (1972). Thyroid function tests in a group of euthyroid dogs. Res. Vet. Sci. *13*:177.

18. Capen, C. C. (1980): Criteria for the development of animal models of diseases of the endocrine system. Am. J. Path. *101*:S141.

19. Capen, C. C., Belshaw, B. E., and Martin, S. L. (1975): Endocrine Diseases, In Textbook of Veterinary Internal Medicine–Diseases of the Dog and Cat, Section X, Chapter 50. Philadelphia, W. B. Saunders Co. 1351.

20. Caylor, H. D., Schlotthauer, C. F., and Pemberton, J. de J. (1927): Observations on the lymphatic connections of the thyroid gland. Anat. Rec. *36*:325.

21. Cheville, N. J. (1972): Ultrastructure of canine carotid body and aortic body tumors. Comparison with tissues of thyroid and parathyroid origin. Vet. Path. *9*:166.

22. Chopra, I. J., Solomon, D. H., and Chua Teco, G. N. (1973): Thyroxiine: Just a prohormone or a hormone too? J. Clin. Endocrinol. Metab. *36*:1050.

23. Clinton, L. T., Jr., and Adams, J. C. (1978): Radioimmunoassay of equine serum for thyroxine: reference values. Am. J. Vet. Res. *39*:1239.

24. Collins, W.T., Jr., and Capen, C.C. (1980): Ultrastructural and functional alterations in thyroid glands of rats produced by polychlorinated biphenyls compared with the effects of iodide excess and deficiency, and thyrotropin and thyroxine ad-

ministration. Virchows Arch [Cell Pathol] *33*: 213.

25. Crispin, S. M., and Barnett, K. C. (1978): Arcus lipoides corneae secondary to hypothyroidism in the Alsatian. J. Small Anim. Pract. *19*:127.

26. Curtis, R. J., and Abrams J. T. (1977): Circadian rhythms in the concentration of thyroid hormone in the plasma of normal calves. Br. Vet. J. *133*:134.

27. Davis, S. L., and Borger, M. L. (1973): Plasma levels of GH and TSH in rams. J. Anim. Sci. *36*:1204.

28. de Vijlder J. J. M., van Voorthuizen W. F., van Dijk, J. E., et al, (1978): Hereditary congenital goiter with thyroglobulin deficiency in a breed of goats. Endocrinology *102*:1214.

29. Ekholm, R., Engstrom, G., Ericson, L. E., et al. (1975): Exocytosis of protein into the thyroid follicle lumen. An early effect of TSH. Endocrinology *97*: 337.

30. Ekholm, R., and Wollman, S. H. (1975): Site of iodination in the rat thyroid gland deduced from electron microscopic autoradiographs. Endocrinology *97*:1432.

31. Ekman, L., Iwarsson, K., and Nyberg, J. A. (1972): Diagnosis of thyroid disorders in the dog. Kleintier-Praxis. *17*:70.

32. Falconer, I. R. (1966): Studies of the congenitally goitrous sheep: The iodinated compounds of serum and circulating thyroid-stimulating hormone. Biochem. J. *100*:190.

33. Foreman, R. E., Goodrich, R. M., and Bodcker, B. B. (1970): A monitor with a restraining unit for determining radio-iodine activity in canine thyroid glands. Am. J. Vet. Res. *31*:1303.

34. Godwin, M. C. (1936): The early development of the thyroid gland in the dog with special reference to the origin and position of accessory thyroid tissue within the thoracic cavity. Anat. Rec. *66*:233.

35. Gosselin, S., Capen, C. C., and Martin, S. L. (1977): Animal model of human disease: Lymphocytic thyroiditis in the dog. Am. J. Path. *90*:185.

36. Gosselin, S. J., Capen, C. C., and Martin, S. L. (1981): Histopathologic and ultrastructural evaluation of thyroid lesions associated with hypothyroidism in dogs. Vet. Path. *18*:299.

37. Gosselin, S. J., Capen, C. C., Krakowka, S., et al. (1981a): Lymphocytic thyroiditis in dogs: Induction with local graft-versus-host reaction. Am. J. Vet. Res. *42*:1856.

38. Gosselin, S. J., Capen, C. C., Martin, S. L., et al, (1981): Induced lymphocytic thyroiditis in dogs: Effect of intrathyroidal injection of thyroid autoantibodies. Am. J. Vet. Res. *42*:1565.

39. Gosselin, S. J., Martin, S. L., Capen, C. C., et al, (1980): Biochemical and immunological investigations of hypothyroidism in dogs. Canad. J. Comp. Med. *44*:158.

40. Griew, W. (1973): Histological changes in the thyroid glands of cattle and rabbits after feeding methylthiouracil. Berlin. Munch. Teriarytl. Wschr. *86*:50.

41. Guillemin, R. (1978): Peptides in the brain: The new endocrinology of the neuron. Science *202*:390.

42. Hammarström, S., Sterling, K., Milch, P. O., et al, (1977): Thyroid hormone action: The mitochondrial pathway. Science *197*:996.

43. Hatch, R. H., Kercher, C. J., and Roehrlasse, G. P. (1972): Response of hyperthyroid, euthyroid and

hypothyroid lambs to exogenous thyroxine. J. Anim. Sci. *34*:988.

44. Haensly, W. E., Jermier, J. A., and Getty, R. (1964): Age changes in the weight of the thyroid gland of the dog from birth to senescence. J. Gerontol. *19*:54.

45. Hernandez, M. V., Etta, K. M., Reineke, E. P., et al, (1972): Thyroid function in the prenatal and neonatal bovine. J. Anim. Sci. *34*:780.

46. Herrington, M. D., Elliott, R. C., and Brown, J. C. (1971): Diagnosis and treatment of thyroid dysfunction occurring in sheep fed on Cynodon plectostachyus. Rhodesian J. Agric. Res. *9*:87.

47. Hightower, D., Kyzar, J. R., Chester, D. K., et al, (1973): Replacement therapy for induced hypothyroidism in dogs. J. Am. Vet. Med. Assoc. *163*:979.

48. Hightower, D., Miller, L., and Kyzar, J. R. (1971): Comparison of serum and plasma thyroxine determinations in horses. J. Am. Vet. Med. Assoc. *159*:449.

49. Hoge, W. R., Lund, J. E., and Blakemore, J. C. (1974): Response to thyrotropin as a diagnostic aid for canine hypothyroidism. J. Am. Vet. Med. Assoc. *10*:167.

50. Holzworth, J., Theran, P., Carpenter, J. L., et al, (1980): Hyperthyroidism in the cat: Ten cases. J. Am. Vet. Med. Assoc. *176*:345.

51. Joyce, J. R., Thompson, R. B., Kyzar, J. R., et al. (1976): Thyroid carcinoma in a horse. J. Am. Vet. Med. Assoc. *168*:610.

52. Kallfelz, F. A. (1969): Determination of total serum thyroxine in the dog by competitive protein binding of labeled thyroxine. Am. J. Vet. Res. *30*:929.

53. Kallfelz, F. A. (1969): Comparison of the iodine-125 labelled triiodothyronine and iodine-125 labelled thyroxine tests in the diagnosis of thyroid gland function in the dog. J. Am. Vet. Med. Assoc. *154*:22.

54. Kallfelz, F. A. (1969): Determination of total serum thyroxine in the dog by competitive protein binding of labeled thyroxine. Am. J. Vet. Res. *30*:929.

55. Kallfelz, F. A. (1973): Observations on thyroid gland function in dogs: Response to thyrotropin and thyroidectomy and determination of thyroxine secretion rate. Am. J. Vet. Res. *34*:535.

56. Kallfelz, F. A., and Lowe, J. E. (1970): Some normal values of thyroid function in horses. J. Am. Vet. Med. Assoc. *156*:1888.

57. Kameda, Y. (1972): The accessory thyroid glands of the dog around the intrapericardial aorta. Arch. Histol. Jap. *34*:375.

58. Katovich, M., Evans, J. W., and Sanchez, O. (1974): Effects of season, pregnancy and lactation on thyroxine turnover in the mare. J. Anim. Sci. *38*:811.

59. Katsch, S., and Windsor, E. (1955): Unusual value for protein-bound iodine in the serum of the opossum. Science *121*:897.

60. Kelley, S. T., Oehme, F. W., and Brandt, G. W. (1974): Measurement of the thyroid gland function during the estrous cycle of nine mares. Am. J. Vet. Res. *35*:657.

61. Kelley, S. T., and Oehme, F. W. (1974): Circulating thyroid levels in dogs, horses, and cattle. V.M. /S.A.C. *69*:1531.

62. Kelley, S. T., Oehme, F. W., and Hoffman, S. B. (1974): Evaluation of selected commercial thyroid

function tests in dogs. Am. J. Vet. Res. *35*:733.

63. Kendall, E. C. (1915): Isolation in crystalline form a compound containing iodine which occurs in the thyroid; its chemical nature and physiological activity. Trans. Assoc. Am. Physicians *30*:402.

64. Kyzar, J. R., Chester, D. K., and Hightower, D. (1972): Comparison of T-3, T-4 tests and radioactive iodine uptake determinations in the dog V.M./ S.A.C. *67*:321.

65. Laurberg, D. (1976): T_4 and T_3 release from the perfused canine thyroid isolated in situ. Acta. Endocrinol. *83*:105.

66. Laurberg, P. (1978): Non-parallel variations in the preferential secretion of 3,5,3'-triiodothyronine (T_3) and 3,3',5'-triiodothyronine (rT_3) from dog thyroid. Endocrinology *102*:757.

67. Leav, I., Schiller, A. I., Rijnberk, A., et al, (1976): Adenomas and carcinomas of the canine and feline thyroid. Am. J. Path. *83*:61.

68. Ling, G. V., Lowenstine, L. J., and Kaneko, J. J. (1974): Serum thyroxine (T-4) and triiodothyronine (T-3) uptake values in normal adult cats. Am. J. Vet. Res. *35*:1247.

69. Lorenz, M. D., and Stiff, M. E. (1979): A comparison of serum thyroxine (T-4) content pre- and post-thyrotropin (TSH) stimulation in dogs.

70. Martin, S. L., and Capen, C. C. (1979): Hypothyroidism and the skin. In Symposium on Skin and Internal Diseases, Vol. 9, edited by G. H. Muller. Philadelphia, W. B. Saunders, Co. 29.

71. Mason, R., and Wilkinson, J. S. (1973): The thyroid gland—a review. Aust. Vet. J. *49*:44.

72. McCauley, E. H., Johnson, D. W., and Alhadji, I. (1972): Disease problems in cattle associated with rations containing high levels of iodide. Bovine Pract. *7*:22.

73. Mellen, W. S., and Hardy, L. B., Jr. (1957): Blood protein bound iodine in the fowl. Endocrinology *60*: 547.

74. Mizejewski, G. J., Baron, J., and Poissant, G. (1971): Immunologic investigations of naturally occurring canine thyroiditis. J. Immunol. *107*:1152.

75. Moore, L. A. (1958): Thyroprotein for dairy cattle. J. Dairy Sci. *41*:452.

76. Motley, J. S. (1972): Use of radioactive triiodothyronine in the study of thyroid function in normal horses. V.M./S.A.C. *67*:1225.

77. Nunez, E. A., Becker, D. V., Furth, E. D., et al. (1970): Breed differences and similarities in thyroid function in purebred dogs. Am. J. Physiol. *218*:1337.

78. Nunez, E. A., Belshaw, B. E., and Gershon, M. D. (1972): A fine structural study of the highly active thyroid follicular cell of the African Basenji dog. Am. J. Anat. *133*:463.

79. Oppenheimer, J. H. (1979): Thyroid hormone action at the cellular level. Science *203*:971.

80. Oppenheimer, J. H., Schwartz, H. L., Surks, M. I., et al. (1976): Nuclear receptors and the initiation of thyroid hormone action. Recent Prog Hormone Res *32*:529.

81. Pammenter, M., Albrecht, C., Liebenberg, W., et al. (1978): Afrikander cattle congenital goiter: Characteristics of its morphology and iodoprotein pattern. Endocrinology *102*:954.

82. Pelletier, G., Puviani, R., and Dussault, J. H. (1976):

Electron microscope immunohistochemical localization of thyroglobulin in the rat thyroid gland. Endocrinology *98*:1253.

83. Peterson, M. E. (1983): Diagnosis and treatment of feline hyperthyroidism. In Proc. 6th Kal Kan Symposium for Treatment of Small Animal Diseases, edited by E. van Marthens. Vet. Learning Systems, 63.

84. Peterson, M. E. (1984): Feline hyperthyroidism. Vet. Clin. N. A. (Sm. An. Pract.) *14*:809.

85. Peterson, M. E., Kintzer, P. P., Cavanagh, P. G., et al. (1983): Feline hyperthyroidism: Pretreatment clinical and laboratory evaluation of 131 cases. J. Am. Vet. Med. Assoc. *183*:103.

86. Piatnek, D. A., Olsen, R. E. (1961): Experimental hyperthyroidism in dogs and effect on salivariectomy. Am. J. Physiol. *201*:723.

87. Premachandra, B. N., and Lang, S. (1977): Circulating reverse triiodothyronine (rT$_3$) in the dog. Life Sci. *20*:1449.

88. Rac, R., Hill, G. N. Pain, R. W., et al. (1968): Congenital goitre in Merino sheep due to an inherited defect in the biosynthesis of thyroid hormone. Res. Vet. Sci. *9*:209.

89. Reap, M., Cass, C., and Hightower, D. (1978): Thyroxine and triiodothyronine levels in ten species of animals. Southwestern Vet. *31*:31.

90. Refetoff, S., Robin, N. I., and Fang, V. S. (1970): Parameters of thyroid function in serum of 16 selected vertebrate species: A study of PBI, serum T$_4$, free T$_4$, and the pattern of T$_4$ and T$_3$ binding to serum proteins. Endocrinology *86*:793.

91. Rijnberk, A. (1971): Iodine metabolism and thyroid disease in the dog. Thesis, University of Utrecht, Utrecht, The Netherlands.

92. Rijnberk, A., de Fijlder J. J. M., van Dijk, J. E., et al. (1977): Clinical aspects of iodine metabolism in goats with congenital goitre and hypothyroidism. Br. Vet. J. *133*:495.

93. Rodel, M. G. W. (1971): Neonatal goitre and skeletal deformities in autumn born lambs on star grass pasture. Rhodesia Agric. J. *68*:109.

94. Rogers, W. A., Donovan, E. F., and Kociba, G. J. (1975): Lipids and lipoproteins in normal dogs and in dogs with secondary hyperlipoproteinemia. J. Am. Vet Med. Assoc. *166*:1092.

95. Rojko, J. L., Hoover, E. A., and Martin, S. L. (1978): Histopathologic interpretation of cutaneous biopsies from dogs with various dermatologic disorders. Vet. Path. *15*:579.

96. Ryder, M. L. (1973): A note on the failure of thyroxine to restore wool growth to inactive follicles. Animal Prod. *16*:319.

97. Sage, J. M., Pond, W. G., Krook, L., O'Connor, J., et al. (1969): Bone metabolism in the thyroidectomized young pigs. Cornell Vet. *59*:547.

98. Scherzinger, E., Guzy, J. K., and Lorcher, K. (1972): Thyroid hormone concentration in the blood and thyroxine binding to serum proteins in various species. Zentralb. Veterinaermed. [A] *19*:585.

99. Schmidt, G. H., Warner, R. G., Tyrrell, H. F., et al. (1971): Effect of thyroprotein feeding on dairy cows. J. Dairy Sci. *54*:481.

100. Schneider, F., and Rosenmund, H. (1973): Determination of the thyroid function of cattle by the T-3 in-vitro test. Schweiz. Arch. Tierheilkd. *115*:135.

101. Seren, E., and Mora, A. (1973): Thyroid function in normal calves and in calves treated with methylthiouracil. Folia Vet. Lati. *3*:52.

102. Shively, J. N., Phemister, R. D., and Epling, G. P. (1969): Fine structure of thyroid epithelium of young dogs treated with thyrotropin hormone. Am. J. Vet. Res. *30*:229.

103. Siegel, E. T. (1977): Endocrine Diseases of the Dog. Philadelphia, Lea & Febiger.

104. Sihombing, D. T. H., Cromwell, G. L., and Hays, V. W. (1971): Effect of added thiocyanate and iodine to corn-soybean meal diets on performance and thyroid status of pigs. J. Anim. Sci. *33*:1154.

105. Spielman, A. A., Petersen, W. E., Fitch, J. B., et al. (1945): General appearance, growth and reproduction of thyroidectomized bovine. J. Dairy Sci. *28*:329.

106. Sterns, E. E. and Doris, P. (1968): Thyroid lymphography of the dog. Cancer *21*:468.

107. Stockard, C. R. (1941): The genetic and endocrine basis for differences in form and behavior. Philadelphia, Wistar Institute of Anatomy and Biology.

108. Sutherland, R. L., and Irvine, C. H. G. (1974): Effect of season and pregnancy on total plasma thyroxine concentrations in sheep. Am. J. Vet. Res. *35*:311.

109. Swanson, E. W., and Miller, J. K. (1973): Problems of estimating thyroxine secretion rates in cattle. J. Dairy Sci. *56*:92.

110. Swanson, E. W., and Miller, J. K. (1972): Restoration of normal lactation to hypothyroid cows. J. Dairy Sci. *56*:92.

111. Thake, D. C., Cheville, N. F., and Sharp, R. K. (1971): Ectopic thyroid adenomas at the base of the heart of the dog: Ultrastructural identification of dense tubular structures in endoplasmic reticulum. Vet. Path *8*:421.

112. van Herle A. J., Vassart, G., and Dunmont, J. E. (1979): Control of thyroglobulin synthesis and secretion. N. Engl. J. Med. *301*:239 and 307.

113. van Voorthuizen, W. F., Dinsort, C., Flavell R. A. et al. (1978): Abnormal cellular localization of thyroglobulin deficiency. Proc. Natl. Acad. Sci. (USA) *75*:74.

114. Vitover, J. (1976): Epithelial thyroid tumors in cows. Vet. Pathol. *13*:401.

115. Watson, J. W., and Sterns, E. E. (1969): Factors influencing distribution of ultrafluid lipiodol (U. F.L.) following intrathyroid injection. Cancer *23*:689.

116. Williams, W. B. (1973): Clinical symptoms of thyroid hormone deficiency in dogs. Gaceta Vet. *35* (271):17.

117. Zarrow, M. X., Yochim. J. M., and McCarthy, J. L. (1964): Experimental Endocrinology. New York, Academic Press, Inc.

The Calcium Regulating Hormones: Parathyroid Hormone, Calcitonin, and Cholecalciferol

CHARLES C. CAPEN

4

PARATHYROID glands are present in all air-breathing vertebrates. Phylogenetically, parathyroids first appear in amphibians coincidentally with the transition from an aquatic to a terrestrial life. It has been suggested that the appearance of parathyroid glands in tetrapods may have arisen from the need to protect against the development of hypocalcemia and the necessity to maintain skeletal integrity in terrestrial animals, which often are in a relatively low calcium-high phosphorus environment.[78,82]

The total concentration of calcium in the blood of mammals is approximately 10 mg/dl with some variation due to species, age, dietary intake of calcium, and analytical method used to quantitate blood levels. The total calcium in the blood is composed of protein-bound and diffusible fractions (Fig. 4-1). Diffusible calcium consists of calcium complexed to anions, such as phosphate and citrate, plus the biologically active free (ionic) calcium.[204]

Calcium ion plays a key role in many fundamental biologic processes, including muscle contraction, blood coagulation, enzyme activity, neural excitability, hormone release, and membrane permeability, in addition to being an essential structural component of the skeleton (Table 4-1). The precise control of calcium ion in extracellular fluids is vital, therefore, to the health of man and animals. To maintain a constant concentration of calcium, despite variations in intake and excretion, endocrine control mechanisms have evolved that primarily consist of the interactions of three major hormones.[198] Although the direct roles of parathyroid hormone

Table 4-1   Role of Calcium Ion in Extra-cellular Fluids

Neuronal excitability
Muscle contraction
Membrane structural integrity and permeability
Cell adhesion
Cell proliferation
Enzyme activity
Bone formation
Blood coagulation
Intercellular communication
Hormone release (stimulus-secretion coupling, e.g., insulin, epinephrine, TSH)

(PTH), calcitonin (CT), and vitamin D frequently are emphasized in the control of blood calcium, other hormones such as adrenal corticosteroids, estrogens, thyroxine, somatotropin, and glucagon may contribute to the maintenance of calcium homeostasis under certain conditions.[42,54]

PARATHYROID HORMONE

Macroscopic Anatomy of Parathyroid Glands

Parathyroid glands in most animal species consist of two pairs of glands situated in the

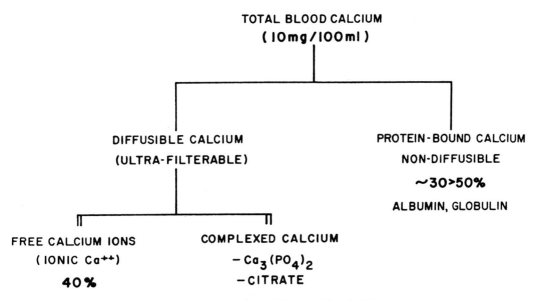

Fig. 4-1. Fractions of total blood calcium in blood.

MACROSCOPIC ANATOMY OF PARATHYROID GLANDS
IN DOMESTIC ANIMALS

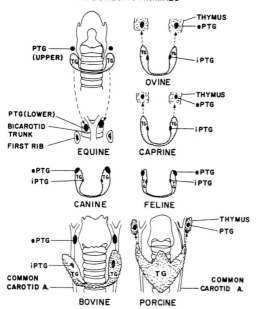

Fig. 4-2. Anatomic location of parathyroid glands in relation to the thyroids and related structures in several species of domestic animals. (Modified from Grau and Dellmann, 1958.)

anterior cervical region (Fig. 4-2). Embryologically parathyroids are of entodermal origin being derived from the III and IV pharyngeal pouches in close association with primordia of the thymus (Fig. 4-3). The entodermal bud that forms the thyroid gland arises on the midline at the level of the first pharyngeal pouch. This gives rise to the thyroglossal duct that migrates caudally. The proliferation of cell cords at the distal end of the thyroglossal duct forms the follicles of each thyroid lobe. The area at the base of the tongue marking the origin of the thyroid gland is referred to as the foramen cecum in postnatal life. Calcitonin-secreting C-cells of neural crest origin reach the postnatal thyroid gland by migrating into the ultimobranchial body. This last pharyngeal pouch moves caudally in mammals to fuse with the primordia of the thyroid gland and distributes C-cells into each thyroid lobe.

In the dog and cat both the external and internal parathyroids are close to the thyroid gland. The external parathyroid (III) in the dog is from 2 to 5 mm in length and is found

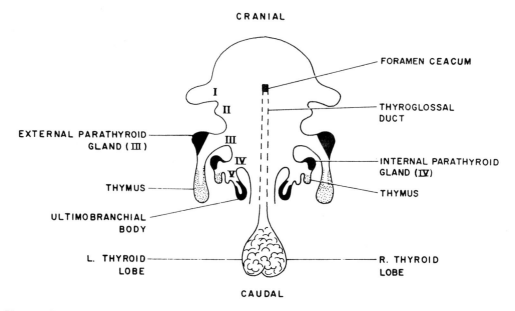

Fig. 4-3. Embryology of parathyroid glands and relationship to primordia for thyroid gland and ultimobranchial body.

in the loose connective tissue cranial and slightly lateral to the anterior pole of the thyroid. The internal parathyroid (IV) is smaller, flatter, and situated on the medial surface of the thyroid beneath the fibrous capsule. The blood supply of the two glands in the dog is separate, with the external parathyroid being supplied by a branch from the cranial thyroid artery and the internal parathyroid by minute ramifications of the arterial supply to the thyroid.[300]

In other species such as cattle and sheep the larger external parathyroid gland is located a considerable distance cranial to the thyroid in the loose connective tissue along the common carotid artery (Fig. 4-2). The smaller internal parathyroid is situated on the dorsal and medial surface of the thyroid gland. The larger lower parathyroid gland in horses is located a considerable distance from the thyroid in the caudal cervical region near the bifurcation of the bicarotid trunk at the level of the first rib (Fig. 4-2). Pigs have only a single pair of parathyroids found cranial to the thyroid, embedded either in thymus (young animals) or in adipose connective tissue (adult pigs). Rats also have a single pair of parathyroid glands that are located close to the thyroid.

Functional Cytology of Parathyroid Gland

Chief Cells

The parathyroid glands contain a single basic type of secretory cell concerned with the elaboration of one hormone.[55] The parathyroids of man and animals are composed of chief cells in different stages of secretory activity and in transition to oxyphil cells in certain species (Fig. 4-4).[40] Experimental and pathologic evidence has accumulated to suggest that certain fine structural characteristics of chief cells are associated with different stages of synthetic and secretory activity.[38,223,281]

Chief cells interpreted to be in an inactive (resting or involuted) stage of their secretory cycle predominate in the parathyroid glands of man and most animal species (Fig. 4-4). Inactive chief cells are cuboidal and have uncomplicated interdigitations between contiguous cells. The relatively electron-transparent cytoplasm contains poorly developed organelles and infrequent secretory granules. The cytoplasm has either numerous lipid bodies and lipofuscin droplets (e.g. bovine glands) or aggregations of glycogen granules (e.g. human and feline glands). The Golgi apparatus is small, composed of straight or curved stacks of agranular membranes, and associated with few prosecretory granules and vesicles in the process of formation. Individual profiles of granular endoplasmic reticulum, ribosomes, and small mitochondria are dispersed throughout the cytoplasm.

Chief cells in the active stage of the secretory cycle occur less frequently in the parathyroid glands of most species (Fig. 4-4). The cytoplasm of active chief cells has an increased electron-density due to the close proximity of organelles, secretion granules, overall density of the cytoplasmic matrix, and loss of glycogen particles and lipid bodies (Fig. 4-5).[278]

Oxyphil Cells and Transitional Forms

A second cell type in the parathyroid glands of certain animal species and human beings is the oxyphil cell (Fig. 4-6). Oxyphil cells are not present in the human fetal parathyroid gland and first appear in late childhood and increase in number with advancing age, often forming nodules in parathyroids of old individuals.[226] They are absent in parathyroids of the rat, chicken, and many species of lower animals.[78,84,110,158,228,271]

Oxyphil cells are observed either singly or in small groups interspersed between chief cells. They are larger than chief cells and their abundant cytoplasmic area is filled with numerous large, often bizarre-shaped, mitochondria (Fig. 4-6). Glycogen particles and free ribosomes are interspersed between the mitochondria. Granular endoplasmic reticulum, Golgi apparatuses, and secretory granules are poorly developed in oxyphil cells of

PARATHYROID GLAND CYTOLOGY

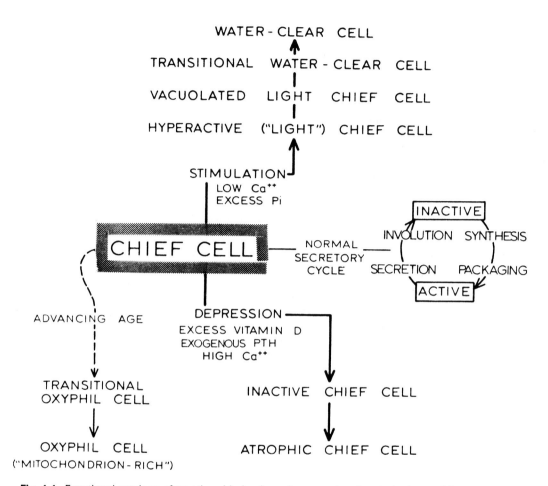

Fig. 4-4. Functional cytology of parathyroid glands under normal and pathologic conditions.

normal parathyroid glands,[38] suggesting that oxyphil cells do not have an active function in the biosynthesis of parathyroid hormone. Associated with the marked increase in mitochondria, oxyphil cells have been shown histochemically to have a higher oxidative and hydrolytic enzyme activity than chief cells.[15,132,322]

Cells are observed with cytoplasmic characteristics intermediate between those of chief and oxyphil cells. These transitional oxyphil cells have numerous mitochondria, but other organelles are present, including granular endoplasmic reticulum, Golgi apparatuses, and secretory granules. The significance of oxyphil cells in the pathophysiology of the parathyroid glands has not been elucidated completely. They are not altered in response to either short-term hypocalcemia or hypercalcemia in animals,[38] but both oxyphils and transitional forms may be increased in response to long-term stimulation of human parathyroid glands.[278] Occasional parathyroid adenomas composed predominately of oxyphil cells and transitional forms have been reported in man associated with excessive

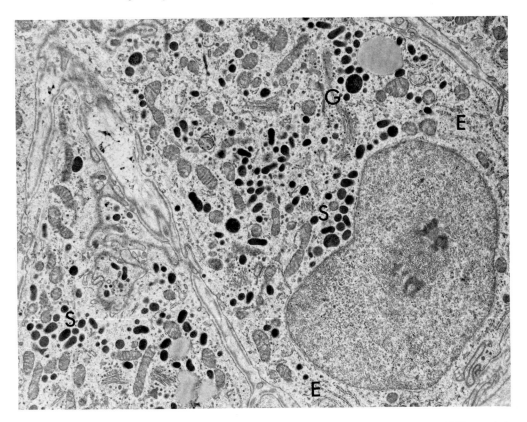

Fig. 4-5. Active chief cell from parathyroid gland of a cow. The cytoplasm contains many PTH-containing secretory granules (S) and well-developed organelles such as rough endoplasmic reticulum (E) and Golgi apparatus (G). 11,300 ×. (From Capen, 1971.)

parathyroid hormone secretion and a syndrome of primary hyperparathyroidism.[4,279] The transitional oxyphil cells comprising these neoplasms have many large mitochondria in their cytoplasm but a more extensive endoplasmic reticulum and well developed Golgi apparatus with more numerous secretory granules than oxyphil cells in normal parathyroid glands.[10] Therefore, oxyphil cells do not appear to be degenerate chief cells as previously thought but rather are derived from chief cells as the result of aging or some metabolic derangement (Fig. 4-4).

Chemistry of Parathyroid Hormone

A larger biosynthetic precursor of parathyroid hormone is first synthesized on ribosomes of the rough endoplasmic reticulum in chief cells.[9,71,75,76,103,126,166,188,250,296] Pre-

proparathyroid hormone (pre-proPTH) is the initial translation product synthesized on ribosomes.[73,171,272] It is composed of 115 amino acids and contains a hydrophobic signal or leader sequence of 25 amino acid residues that facilitate the penetration and subsequent vectorial discharge of the nascent peptide into the cisternal space of the rough endoplasmic reticulum (Fig. 4-7).[122,128] Preproparathyroid hormone is rapidly converted within 1 minute or less of its synthesis to proparathyroid hormone (ProPTH) by the proteolytic cleavage of the NH_2-terminal sequence of 25 amino acids (Fig. 4-7).[123,129]

The intermediate precursor, proPTH, is composed of 90 amino acids and moves within membranous channels of the endoplasmic reticulum to the Golgi apparatus (Fig. 4-7). Enzymes with trypsin-like and carboxypepti-

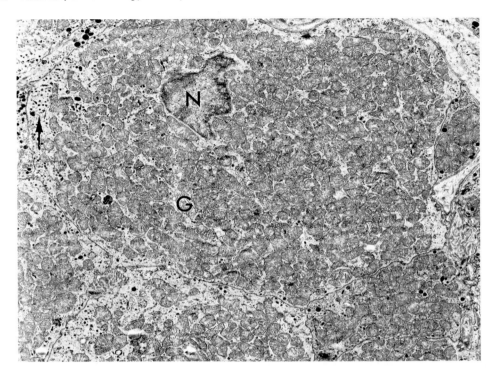

Fig. 4-6. Oxyphil cells in parathyroid of an adult cow. These metabolically altered parathyroid cells have a large cytoplasmic area packed with numerous mitochondria and a small irregular nucleus (N). The Golgi apparatus (G) is small and only a few small secretory granules (arrow) are present. 6,000 ×.

dase B-like activity within membranes of the Golgi apparatus cleave a hexapeptide from the NH_2-terminal (biologically active) end of the molecule forming active parathyroid hormone (PTH) (Fig. 4-8).[124,125,127,189] Active PTH is packaged into membrane-limited, macromolecular aggregates in the Golgi apparatus for subsequent storage in chief cells (Fig. 4-9). Under certain conditions of increased demand, PTH may be released directly from chief cells without being packaged into secretion granules (Fig. 4-8).

Biologically active parathyroid hormone secreted by chief cells is a straight chain polypeptide consisting of 84 amino acid residues with a molecular weight of approximately 9500.[33] The complete amino acid sequence has been reported for bovine and porcine PTH (Fig. 4-10). There are seven differences in amino acid residues between PTH molecules of the two species. Molecular fragments of PTH are formed in the peripheral circula-

tion and at the target cells of the hormone. The immunoheterogeneity created by the multiple circulating fragments of PTH caused significant problems in the development and application of highly specific radio-immunoassays to clinical diagnostic problems in human and animal patients.[8,116]

Biosynthesis of Parathyroid Hormone

In the early phases of secretory activity the endoplasmic reticulum of chief cells aggregates into large lamellar arrays and free ribosomes group into clusters.[281] It is presumably at this stage that a "batch" of pre-proparathyroid hormone is synthesized by the chief cells (Fig. 4-11). This is followed by a "packaging" phase in which the Golgi apparatus enlarges and often appears as multiple complexes in several parts of the chief cell associated with many prosecretory granules. As this occurs, the granular endoplasmic reticulum involutes

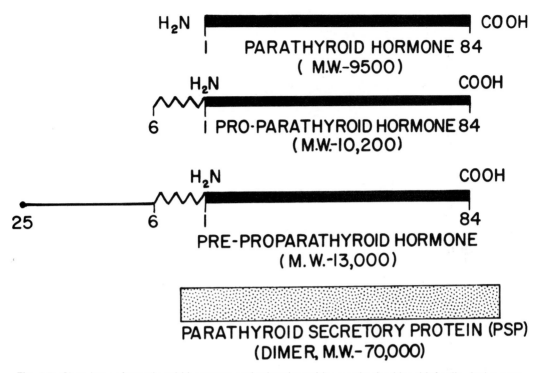

Fig. 4-7. Chemistry of parathyroid hormone and related peptides synthesized by chief cells. Active parathyroid hormone is first synthesized as part of larger biosynthetic precursor molecules. Pre-proparathyroid hormone (115 amino acids) is the initial translational product from ribosomes and is rapidly converted to proparathyroid hormone in the rough endoplasmic reticulum. Pro-parathyroid hormone (90 amino acids) is converted enzymatically to active parathyroid hormone (84 amino acids) in the Golgi apparatus as the hormone is packaged into secretory (storage) granules. Parathyroid secretory protein is a high molecular weight molecule synthesized by chief cells, incorporated into storage granules with active parathyroid hormone, and secreted in parallel with active hormone in response to changes in blood calcium. It probably functions as a binding protein during intracellular transport and secretion into the extracellular space.

and disperses. The secretory granules develop by sequential accumulation and condensation of finely granular material within cisternae of the Golgi apparatus. Prosecretory granules are concentrated in the vicinity of the Golgi apparatus and occasionally are observed in the process of becoming detached from the membranes of the Golgi complex.

It is at this stage in the Golgi apparatus that PTH (1-84 amino acid sequence) is cleaved enzymatically from proparathyroid hormone by an enzyme with trypsin- and carboxypeptidase B-like activity and packaged into mature secretory or storage granules.[8,75,103,124,189] As the Golgi apparatus subsequently involutes, acid phosphatase activity appears in membranes of portions of

the Golgi complex,[292] and acid phosphatase-positive lysosomal bodies are formed. During the involuting phase the packaged parathyroid hormone (1-84 amino acid sequence) moves from the Golgi region to the periphery of the cell where it is stored prior to secretion. The Golgi apparatus continues to involute, glycogen particles and lipid bodies accumulate in the cytoplasm, and the chief cell returns to the resting stage (Fig. 4-11). *In vitro* studies indicate that it is during the secreting and involuting phase that the ambient concentration of calcium exerts an effect on chief cells.[281] Low ambient calcium speeds up the rate of secretion and shortens the resting phase; conversely, high ambient calcium suppresses the rate of hormone secretion and

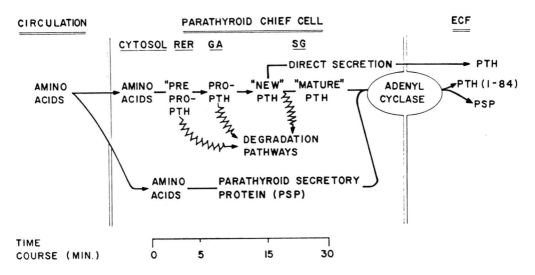

Fig. 4-8. Synthesis of parathyroid hormone (PTH) as part of larger biosynthetic precursors. Pre-preparathyroid hormone (pre-proPTH) is the initial translational product from ribosomes of the rough endoplasmic reticulum, which is rapidly converted to proparathyroid hormone (proPTH). ProPTH is converted enzymatically to biologically active ("New") PTH in the Golgi apparatus. A major portion of the biosynthetic precursors and active PTH is degraded and not secreted by chief cells. Parathyroid secretory protein (PSP) may function as a binding protein for PTH during intracellular storage in secretion granules and release into the extracellular space.

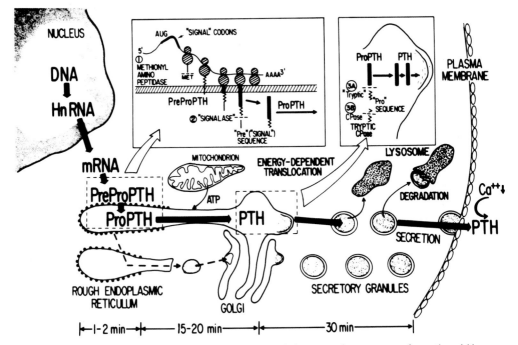

Fig. 4-9. Subcellular compartmentalization, transport, and cleavage of precursors of parathyroid hormone (PTH). Pre-proparathyroid hormone (pre-proPTH) is the initial translation product from ribosomes of the rough endoplasmic reticulum, which is rapidly converted to pro-parathyroid hormone (proPTH). The hydrophobic sequence on the amino-terminal end of the pre-proPTH facilitates penetration of the leading portion of the nascent peptide into the lumen of the endoplasmic reticulum. ProPTH is transported to the Golgi apparatus where it is converted enzymatically by a carboxypeptidase (CPase) to biologically active PTH. A major portion of the biosynthetic precursors and active PTH is degraded by lysosomal enzymes and is not secreted by chief cells under normal conditions. Parathyroid secretory protein (PSP) may function as a binding protein for PTH during intracellular storage in secretion granules and be released with PTH into the extracellular space. (From Habener and Potts, 1978.)

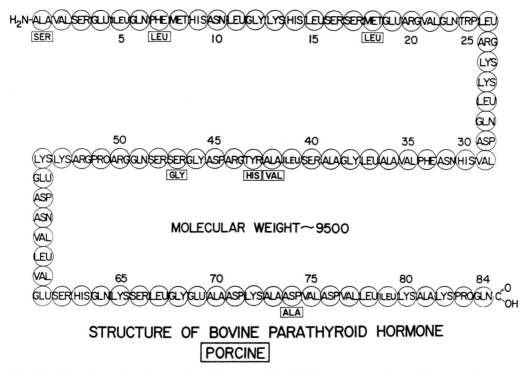

STRUCTURE OF BOVINE PARATHYROID HORMONE

Fig. 4-10. Chemistry of bovine parathyroid hormone. The 7 differences in amino acid sequence between bovine and porcine PTH are indicated by the squares beneath the 1 to 84 PTH molecule. (From Brewer et al., 1974.)

lengthens the resting phase of the secretory cycle.

Studies designed to elucidate the time-course of the parathyroid secretory cycle demonstrated by electron microscopic radio-autography that as early as 2 minutes after intravenous injection of ^{3}H-tyrosine in rats the label mainly was located over the rough endoplasmic reticulum.[225] By 5 to 10 minutes much of the label was present in the Golgi apparatus, after 20 to 30 minutes the label had migrated into secretory granules, and by 45 to 60 minutes the label content of the cells had decreased, suggesting release of synthesized material from chief cells. The rapid uptake and release of ^{3}H-tyrosine are consistent with the hypothesis that the turnover of parathyroid hormone is rapid (plasma half-life of 18 to 22 minutes) and that chief cells store relatively small amounts of preformed hormone but are capable of responding to fluctuations in blood calcium by rapidly altering the rates of synthesis and secretion.[13,295]

Storage of Parathyroid Hormone

Secretory ("storage") granules have been demonstrated at the level of ultrastructure within chief cells of the parathyroid glands in man and all animal species examined (Fig. 4-12).[2,55,278] The paucity of secretory granules in certain species (e.g. rat) has led some investigators to erroneously suggest that chief cells do not have a mechanism for the storage of preformed hormone.[251] Morphologically similar secretory granules isolated from other endocrine organs which produce polypeptide hormones (e.g. adenohypophysis, alpha and beta cells of pancreatic islets, parafollicular cells of thyroid) have been shown to contain hormonal activity.[19,85,150,156] Immunofluorescent studies using an antibody to parathyroid hormone demonstrated that fluorescein-labeled antibody was localized to the cytoplasm of chief cells in cattle, rats, and man.[133] Oxyphil cells which ultrastructurally appear to be nonsecretory did not have specific fluorescence.

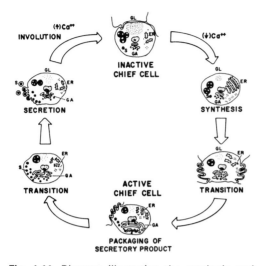

Fig. 4-11. Diagram illustrating the synthetic and secretory phases of the secretory cycle in parathyroid chief cells. In response to a reduction in ambient calcium concentration chief cells are stimulated to enter the active phase and synthesize a batch of pro-PTH on the rough endoplasmic reticulum. The pro-PTH is transported to the Golgi apparatus where it is packaged into secretory granules for storage and converted to PTH (1 to 84 amino acid sequence). Secretory granules are discharged from chief cells by exocytosis into perivascular spaces where the granules rapidly break up and PTH molecules enter the circulation. (Modified from Roth and Capen, 1974.)

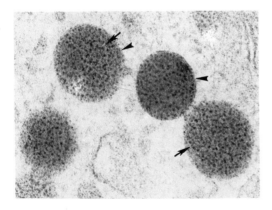

Fig. 4-12. Secretory granules within a chief cell composed of numerous small dense particles (arrows) and surrounded by a closely applied limiting membrane (arrow heads). These granules are believed to contain PTH (1 to 84 amino acid sequence) and probably parathyroid secretory protein. 82,500 ×.

L'Heureux and Melius initially demonstrated that parathyroid hormone activity resides within the particulate fraction of homogenized parathyroid glands in cattle.[182] MacGregor et al. reported that over 90% of parathyroid hormone (analyzed by bioassay, immunoassay, and chemical isolation) was in the particulate fraction of bovine parathyroids.[188] On electron microscopic examination those fractions containing the bulk of the parathyroid hormone contained numerous membrane-bound, electron-dense bodies that appeared to be identical to the secretory granules in intact chief cells.[75] Extraction of parathyroid homogenates with sodium deoxycholate (0.26%) and removal of proparathyroid hormone, but not PTH, left the mature membrane-bound secretory granules intact. It was also demonstrated that proparathyroid hormone represents only about 3% of the total hormonal content of the parathyroid gland, suggesting that the prohormone is rapidly converted to PTH before storage in secretion granules. Proparathyroid hormone appears to be associated with a second membrane-bound subcellular compartment, presumably the cisternal spaces of the endoplasmic reticulum, Golgi vesicles, or prosecretory granules.

Roth et al. localized PTH within chief cells of bovine parathyroids to the small membrane-limited secretory granules by immunocytochemical techniques using rabbit antiserum and peroxidase-labeled goat antirabbit globulin.[282] The rabbit antiserum used in these studies recognized multiple antigenic determinants of bovine PTH, including the biologically active N-terminal of the molecule. Reaction product was not deposited over the larger acid phosphatase-positive lysosomal bodies in chief cells.

In addition to parathyroid hormone (1 to 84 amino acid sequence), secretory granules in chief cells (Fig. 4-12) also contain a parathyroid secretory protein (PSP). Kemper et al. reported that bovine parathyroids incubated *in vitro* secrete a protein that is distinct from both proparathyroid hormone and PTH.[167] It is a large protein (two or more subunits of molecular weight 70,000) and comprises about 50% of the total protein secreted by the parathyroid. PSP appears to accompany PTH within the intracellular transport pathway through cytoplasmic organelles and is associated predominately with the particulate fractions of chief cells.[129] Secretion of PSP is stimulated or inhibited in parallel with that of PTH by varying the concentration of calcium in the incubation medium. The coordinated secretion of PSP and PTH in response to changes in ambient calcium suggests both molecules are present in the membrane-limited secretion granules in chief cells. Although the exact function of PSP is uncertain, it appears to be a "binding protein" for parathyroid hormone and to be analogous in function to the neurophysins secreted with oxytocin and vasopressin by the neurohypophyseal system.[99] The amino acid sequence of PSP is similar to chromagranin A present in catecholamine-containing secretory granules of the adrenal medulla.[73,77]

The secretory granules in chief cells usually are small, ranging from 100 to 300 mμ in their greatest diameter, and are composed of fine, dense particles (Fig. 4-12). They are electron-dense, surrounded by a delicate, closely applied limiting membrane, and are round to oval. Secretion granules are consistently smaller and more regular in shape than the acid phosphatase-positive lysosomal bodies (450 to 800 mμ) and lipofuscin granules present in chief cells.[292] The number of granules within chief cells varies considerably between species, with bovine parathyroids having consistently more secretory granules than man and other animals.[50] Chief cells in closely related species may vary considerably in the number of storage granules in their cytoplasm; for example, granules are infrequent in rats,[280] but are numerous in mouse parathyroids.[131,224]

Chief cells appear to have fewer storage granules than many other endocrine cells concerned with polypeptide hormone biosynthesis, e.g. adenohypophysis,[18] and calcitonin-secreting C- (parafollicular) cells of the thyroid (Fig. 4-13).[57,58] Correspondingly, the gland content of parathyroid hormone has

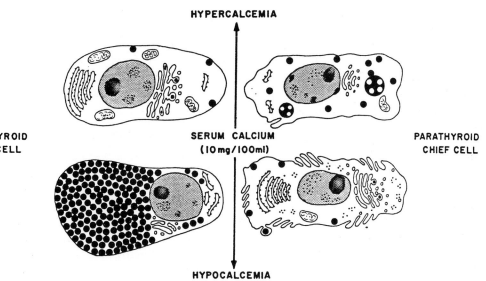

Fig. 4-13. Response of thyroid C-cells and parathyroid chief cells to hypercalcemia and hypocalcemia. C-cells accumulate secretory granules in response to hypocalcemia whereas chief cells are nearly degranulated but have an increased development of synthetic and secretory organelles. In response to hypercalcemia C-cells are degranulated and chief cells are predominantly in the inactive stage of the secretory cycle.

been reported to be low (0.004% of wet weight of bovine parathyroids).[12]

Secretion of Parathyroid Hormone

The secretory granules migrate peripherally in chief cells, and their limiting membrane fuses with the plasma membrane of the cell. An internal cytoskeleton composed of microtubules and contractile filaments has been reported to be important in the control of peripheral movement of secretory granules and liberation of secretory products from other endocrine cells (e.g. beta cells of the pancreatic islets).[178] The presence of peripheral microfilaments in chief cells, as well as the attachment of granules to the plasma membrane by stalklike condensations of cytoplasmic material in some species, suggests that a similar secretory mechanism exists in parathyroid glands.[354] The administration of colchicine, an inhibitor of intracellular transport and release of secretory products in a number of endocrine organs, also blocks the secretion of PTH from chief cells in rats.[263] Secretory granules increased 2- to 3-fold in chief cells of colchicine-treated rats compared to controls and the serum calcium level was lowered significantly. The dramatic reduction of assembled microtubules in the cytoplasm of chief cells after the administration of colchicine was interpreted to be responsible for the reduction in PTH secretion and accumulation of secretory granules. Stimulation of parathyroid glands by phosphate-induced hypocalcemia resulted in an increase of assembled microtubules, and few secretory granules accumulated in the cytoplasm. These findings suggest that microtubules also play an important role in the peripheral migration of secretory granules and secretion of PTH by chief cells as has been reported in other polypeptide hormone-secreting cells.

Secretory granules appear to be extruded from chief cells by exocytosis into perivascular spaces.[38,100,101] By scanning electron microscopy, numerous small spherules of similar size have been observed protruding from secretory surfaces of chief cells into perivascular spaces (Fig. 4-14).[38] Thiele and

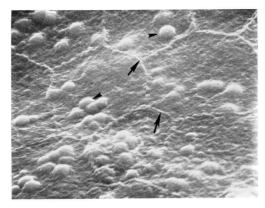

Fig. 4-14. Scanning electron micrograph of secretory surface of active chief cells in parathyroid gland illustrating secretory granules (arrow heads) budding into perivascular space. Chief cells are polyhedral and distinct cell boundaries can be visualized (arrows). 3,000 ×.

Wermbter utilized freeze-fracture techniques to demonstrate secretory granules being discharged from chief cells by exocytosis in the human parathyroid gland.[320] Secretion granules surrounded by their limiting membrane infrequently have been observed free in the narrow perivascular spaces of the parathyroids.[4,100] In the avian parathyroid a hiatus occasionally was observed at the site of fusion between the limiting membrane of the secretion granule and the plasma membrane of the chief cell.[354] A similar process, termed *emiocytosis*, for the liberation of insulin from secretion granules has been demonstrated in pancreatic beta cells.[178]

Control of Parathyroid Hormone Secretion

Secretory cells in the parathyroid gland store small amounts of preformed hormone but are capable of responding to minor fluctuations in calcium concentration rapidly by altering the rate of hormonal secretion,[252] and more slowly by altering the rate of hormonal synthesis.[280] In contrast to most endocrine organs that are under complex controls involving both long and short feedback loops, the parathyroids have a unique feedback control by the concentration of calcium (and to a lesser extent magnesium) ion in serum.[294,315]

If the blood calcium is elevated by the intravenous infusion of calcium, there is a rapid and pronounced reduction in circulating levels of immunoreactive parathyroid hormone (iPTH) (Fig. 4-15). Conversely, if the blood calcium is lowered by EDTA (ethylenediaminetetraacetic acid), there is a brisk and substantial increase in iPTH levels (Fig. 4-15).[237] The concentration of blood phosphorus has no direct regulatory influence on the synthesis and secretion of PTH; however, certain disease conditions with hyperphosphatemia in both animals and man are associated clinically with hyperparathyroidism. An elevated blood phosphorus level may lead indirectly to parathyroid stimulation by virtue of its ability to lower blood calcium.[174] If the blood phosphorus is elevated significantly by an infusion of phosphate and calcium administered simultaneously in amounts to prevent the accompanying reduction of blood calcium, plasma iPTH levels remain within the normal range (Fig. 4-15).

Magnesium ion has an effect on parathyroid secretory rate similar to that of calcium, but its effect is not equipotent to that of calcium.[196,199,211] The more potent effects of calcium ion in the control of PTH secretion, together with its preponderance over magnesium in the extracellular fluid, suggest a secondary role for magnesium in parathyroid control. However, the ultrastructural morphometric studies of Altenähr and Leonhardt suggested a quantitatively equal inhibition of parathyroid secretory activity by calcium and magnesium.[3]

Calcium ion not only controls the rate of biosynthesis and secretion of parathyroid hor-

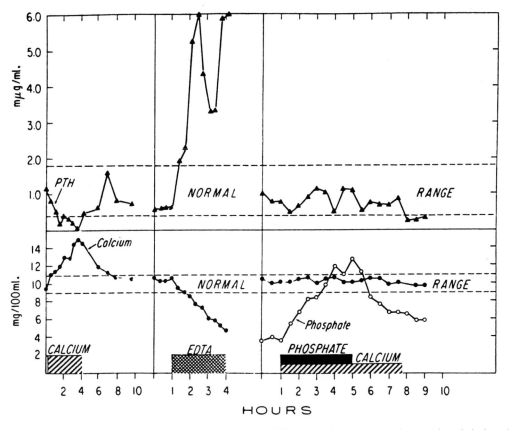

Fig. 4-15. Changes of plasma immunoreactive parathyroid hormone in response to hypercalcemia induced by calcium infusion, hypocalcemia produced by EDTA infusion, and hyperphosphatemia with normocalcemia in a cow. (From Aurbach and Potts, 1964.)

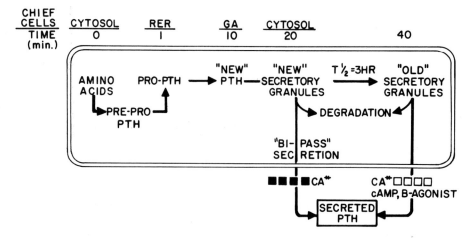

Fig. 4-16. Bypass secretion of parathyroid hormone in response to increased demand signaled by decreased blood calcium ion concentration. Recently synthesized and processed active PTH (1–84) may be released directly and not enter the storage pool of mature ("old") secretory granules in the cytoplasm of chief cells. PTH from the storage pool can be mobilized by cyclic adenosine monophosphate (cAMP) and beta (B)-agonists (such as epinephrine, norepinephrine, and isoproterenol) as well as by lowered blood calcium ion, whereas secretion from the pool of recently synthesized PTH can be stimulated only by a decreased calcium ion concentration. RER, rough endoplasmic reticulum; GA, Golgi apparatus. (Redrawn from Cohn and MacGregor, 1981.)

mone, but also other metabolic and intracellular degradative processes within chief cells (Fig. 4-16).[71] An increase of calcium ions in extracellular fluids rapidly inhibits the uptake of amino acids by chief cells, synthesis of proparathyroid hormone and conversion to PTH, and secretion of stored PTH.[75] The shifting of the percentage of flow of proparathyroid from the degradative pathways to the secretory route represents a key adaptive response of the parathyroid gland to a low calcium diet. Parathyroids from rats fed a low calcium (0.02%) diet convert approximately 40% of proparathyroid hormone to PTH compared to a 20% conversion in rats fed a control diet (Fig. 4-17).[72] During periods of long-term calcium restriction the enhanced synthesis and secretion of PTH would be accomplished by an increased capacity of the entire pathway in individual hypertrophied chief cells and through hyperplasia of active chief cells (Fig. 4-17).[75] Degradation of "mature PTH" by lysosomal enzymes occurs only after prolonged exposure of chief cells to a high calcium environment.

Recently synthesized and processed active PTH may be released directly in response to increased demand and bypass the chief cell's storage pool of mature secretory granules in the cytoplasm. Bypass secretion of calcium can be stimulated only by a low circulating concentration of calcium ion and not by other secretagogues for PTH (Fig. 4-16). Degrada-

ADAPTIVE RESPONSE OF PARATHYROID GLAND TO AMBIENT CALCIUM CONCENTRATION

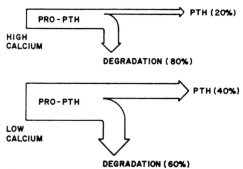

Fig. 4-17. Adaptive responses of parathyroid gland to low or high dietary calcium intake initially by increasing the efficiency of conversion of proPTH to PTH and secretion of PTH from chief cells. Hyperplasia of chief cells in response to long-term low calcium increases the overall capacity of the parathyroid to synthesize proPTH.

tion of "mature PTH" by lysosomal enzymes occurs after prolonged exposure of chief cells to a high-calcium environment.

Biologic Effects of Parathyroid Hormone

Parathyroid hormone is the principal hormone involved in the minute-to-minute fine regulation of blood calcium in mammals. It exerts its biologic actions by directly influencing the function of target cells primarily in bone and kidney, and indirectly in the intestine to maintain plasma calcium at a level sufficient to ensure the optimal functioning of a wide variety of body cells (Fig. 4-18).

In general the most important biologic effects of PTH are to (1) elevate the blood calcium concentration, (2) decrease the blood phosphorus concentration, (3) increase the urinary excretion of phosphorus by decreased tubular reabsorption, (4) increase tubular reabsorption of calcium, resulting in diminished calcium loss into the urine, (5) increase the rate of skeletal remodeling and the net rate of bone resorption, (6) increase osteolysis and the numbers of osteoclasts on bone surfaces, (7) increase the urinary excretion of hydroxyproline, (8) activate adenyl cyclase in target cells, and (9) accelerate the formation of the principal active vitamin D metabolite (1,25-dihydroxycholecalciferol) by the kidney through a tropic effect on the 1 α-hydroxylase in mitochondria of renal epithelial cells, in the proximal convoluted tubules.[259]

The action of PTH on bone is to mobilize calcium from skeletal reserves into extracellular fluids.[255,348] The administration of PTH causes an initial decline followed by a sustained increase in circulating levels of calcium. This transitory decrease in blood calcium is considered to be the result of a sequestration of calcium-phosphate in bone and soft tissues.[245] The subsequent increase in blood calcium results from an interaction of parathyroid hormone with osteoblasts and osteoclasts in bone.[144,145]

The response of bone to parathyroid hor-

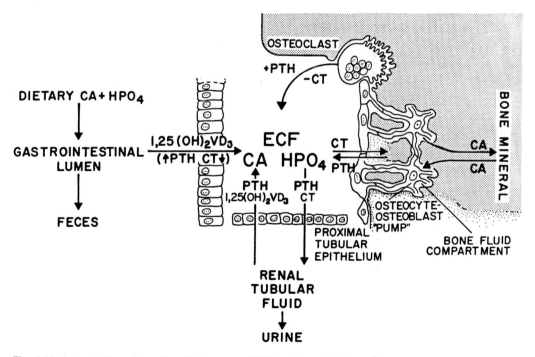

Fig. 4-18. Interrelation of parathyroid hormone (PTH), calcitonin (CT), and 1,25-dihydroxycholecalciferol (1,25-(OH)$_2$VD$_3$) in the hormonal regulation of calcium and phosphorus in extracellular fluids.

mone is biphasic. The immediate effects are the result of increasing the activity of existing osteocytes and osteoclasts present in bone. This rapid effect of parathyroid hormone depends upon the continuous presence of hormone and results in an increased flow of calcium from deep in bone to bone surfaces through the coordinated action of osteocytes and endosteal lining cells (inactive osteoblasts). This osteocyte-osteoblast "pump" is concerned with movement of calcium from the bone fluid to the extracellular fluid compartment (Fig. 4-19) in order to make fine adjustments in the blood calcium concentration under physiologic conditions (Parfitt, 1977).

The later effects of parathyroid hormone on bone are of a greater magnitude of response and not dependent upon the continuous presence of hormone. Osteoclasts appear to be primarily responsible for the long-term action of PTH on increasing bone resorption and overall bone remodeling.[63,64,67]

This is interesting in light of recent findings which have failed to demonstrate receptors for PTH on osteoclasts but receptors were present on osteoblasts.[249,293A] These cells normally are flat and cover bone surfaces. The initial binding of PTH to osteo-

blasts lining bone surfaces appears to cause the cells to contract thereby exposing the underlying mineral to osteoclasts.[270] If the increase in PTH is sustained, the size of the active osteoclast pool in bone is increased by activation of osteoprogenitor cells in the endosteal bone cell envelope.[260] The plasma membrane of osteoclasts in intimate contact with the resorbing bone surface is modified to form a series of membranous projections referred to as the brush "ruffled" border (Fig. 4-20). This area of active bone resorption is isolated from the extracellular fluids by adjacent transitional ("sealing") zones, thereby localizing the lysosomal enzymes and acidic environment to the immediate area undergoing dissolution. The mineral and organic components (e.g. hydroxyproline) released from bone are phagocytized by osteoclasts and transported across the cell in transport vesicles to be released into the extracellular fluid compartment (Fig. 4-20).

PTH-induced changes in osteoblasts appear rapidly as 1 hour after PTH administration to thyroparathyroidectomized (TXPTX) rat cells become more irregular. Compared with polyhedral lining cells in controls, PTH-stimulated osteoblasts are elongated due to extension of cytoplasmic processes along the orientation of the underlying collagen bundles. The cell bodies round up and there is some overlapping of cells. The intercellular spaces between osteoblasts are increased and blebs appear on the plasma membrane on the free surface. The change in shape of osteoblasts associated with PTH may be related to calcium entry into the cell and alteration in microtubule and microfilament function. PTH appears to inhibit microfilament function and the change in shape is blocked by drugs which prevent assembly of microtubules (Miller et al., 1976). Thus, PTH induced changes require a balance between microfilament and microtubular function. Increase in the calcium/phosphate ratio in the mitochondria of bone lining cells is associated with an increase in mitochondrial granules 5 minutes after injection of PTH into young rats (Norimatsu et al., 1982). In addition to alter-

OSTEOCYTE-OSTEOBLAST PUMP

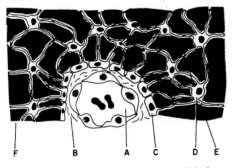

Fig. 4-19. Osteocyte-osteoblast "pump" is formed by the fusion of processes of endosteal lining (C) cells (inactive osteoblasts) and osteocytes (D) embedded in cortical bone (F). This functional cellular syncytium provides a mechanism for transcellular transport of calcium from the bone-fluid compartment around osteocytes (E) to the extracellular fluid compartment (B) and capillaries (A).

OSTEOCLASTIC OSTEOLYSIS

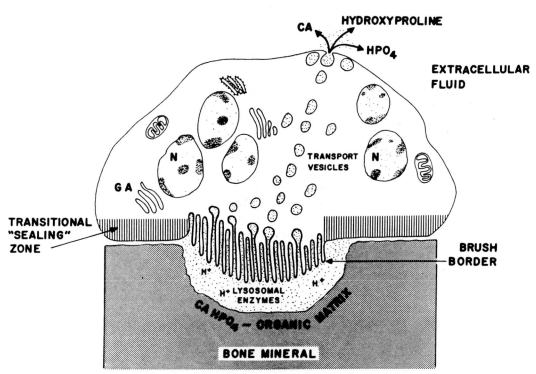

Fig. 4-20. Osteoclastic osteolysis on a bone surface with release of calcium, phosphorus, and hydroxyproline (from organic matrix of bone) into extracellular fluids. The brush border is a specialized area of the plasma membrane of osteoclasts that is in intimate contact with the underlying bone mineral. Adjacent transitional zones isolate the area undergoing active resorption and provide a mechanism for the concentration of lysosomal enzymes and acidic environment required for the dissolution of bone mineral.

ations in microfilaments, microtubules and mitochondrial granules, PTH is able to increase endocytosis in lining cells. The increased mitochondrial granules and endocytic activity of bone lining cells in response to PTH may be exaggerated morphologic reflections of the role these cells play in calcium homeostasis between bone and extracellular fluid.

The change in shape of osteoblasts in response to PTH also may be critical to mediation of osteoclastic bone resorption stimulated by the hormone. Since there is general agreement that osteoblasts but not osteoclasts have receptors for PTH,[270] PTH-induced osteoclasis may be mediated by changes in shape of osteoblasts. The alteration of osteoblast shape would expose matrix to wandering osteoclasts. Bone resorption products, parti-

cularly osteocalcin, can attract osteoclast precursors and enhance the resorption process. Alternatively, osteoblasts directly may elaborate chemical mediators to stimulate osteoclasts.

A long-term increase in PTH secretion also may result in the formation of greater numbers of osteoblasts and an increase in bone formation and resorption. However, since resorption by osteoclasts usually is greater than bone formation by osteoblasts, there is a net negative skeletal balance. Osteoblasts in TXPTX rats given exogenous PTH were active and had a prominent rough endoplasmic reticulum and Golgi apparatus and large mitochondria. The plasma membranes of osteoblasts were extensively convoluted and associated with numerous initial loci of mineralization.[341] The addition of

PTH to bone cultures *in vitro* has been shown to inhibit collagen synthesis and diminish the uptake of proline and glycine by osteoblasts and to reduce incorporation into organic matrix.[111,243]

The major effect of PTH under physiologic conditions is exerted on bone cells on endosteal surfaces and in the haversian cell envelope.[260] In disease states of hyperparathyroidism, the activation of osteoprogenitor cells occurs in the periosteal bone cell envelope as well, leading to the formation of active bone metabolic units on the periosteal surface. This process results in the characteristic subperiosteal areas of bone resorption seen radiographically in both primary and secondary hyperparathyroidism (Fig. 4-21).

Parathyroid hormone has a rapid (within 5 to 10 minutes) and direct effect on renal tubular function leading to decreased reabsorption of phosphate and phosphaturia. The site of action of PTH on blocking tubular reabsorption of phosphate has been localized by micropuncture methods to the proximal tubule of the nephron (Fig. 4-22). In addition, PTH leads to an increased urinary excretion of potassium, bicarbonate, sodium, cyclic adenosine monophosphate, and amino acids.

Although the effect of PTH on the tubular reabsorption of phosphorus has been considered to be of major importance, evidence has accumulated suggesting that the ability of PTH to enhance the renal reabsorption of calcium is of considerable importance in the maintenance of calcium homeostasis. This effect of PTH upon tubular reabsorption of calcium appears to be due to a direct action on the distal convoluted tubule.[308] The urinary excretion of magnesium, ammonia, and

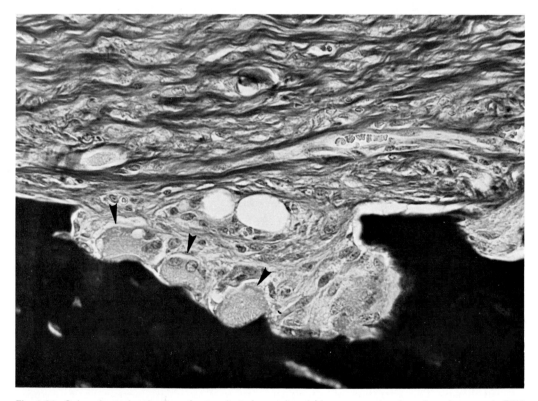

Fig. 4-21. Subperiosteal activation of osteoclasts (arrow heads) in response to a long-term increase in PTH secretion in an animal with hyperparathyroidism. The increased bone resorption may disrupt tendinous insertions of muscles elevating the periosteum and result in bone pain.

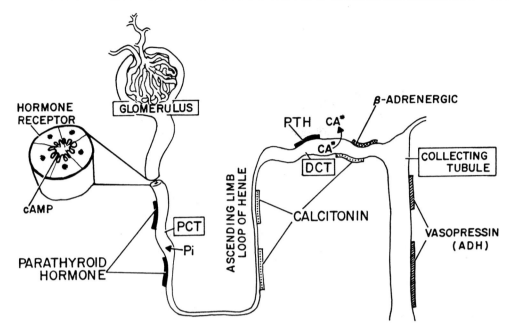

Fig. 4-22. Distribution of target cells for parathyroid hormone and calcitonin in the nephron. The parathyroid hormone-mediated diminished tubular reabsorption of phosphorus occurs in the proximal convoluted tubules (PCT), whereas the increased calcium reabsorption results in cells located in the distal convoluted tubules (DCT). Cells with receptors for calcitonin that are situated in the ascending limb of the loop of Henle and distal convoluted tubule (DCT) also diminish tubular reabsorption of phosphorus and cause phosphaturia.

titratable acidity also are decreased by PTH. The other important effect of PTH on the kidney is in the regulation of the conversion of 25-hydroxycholecalciferol to 1,25-dihydroxycholecalciferol and other metabolites of vitamin D. The role of PTH as a tropic hormone in the metabolic activation of cholecalciferol will be discussed further in the section of this chapter on vitamin D.

Parathyroid hormone has been shown to promote the absorption of calcium from the gastrointestinal tract in animals under a variety of experimental conditions.[227] This effect is not as rapid as the action on the kidney and is not observed in vitamin D-deficient animals. It is uncertain whether this increased intestinal calcium transport is a direct effect of PTH on absorptive cells or more likely an indirect effect of PTH by its action of stimulating the renal synthesis of the biologically active metabolite of vitamin D.

Parathyroid hormone is secreted continuously from chief cells under normal condi-

tions. In the liver and possibly elsewhere, PTH (straight chain 1 to 84 amino acid sequence) is cleaved into a smaller (approximately one third of the molecule) amino terminal (biologically active portion) and a larger (approximately two thirds of the molecule) carboxy terminal (biologically inactive portion) fragments.[152] The kidney is a major organ for the degradation of PTH (Fig. 4-23). Biologically active PTH from peritubular capillaries is degraded by specific proteases on the surface of renal tubular cells. In addition, both biologically active (NH_2-1-34) and inactive (34—84 COOH) fragments are degraded intracellularly by lysosomal enzymes within renal tubular cells (Fig. 4-23).

Mechanism of Action of Parathyroid Hormone

The calcium-mobilizing and phosphaturic activities of parathyroid hormone are mediated through the intracellular accumulation

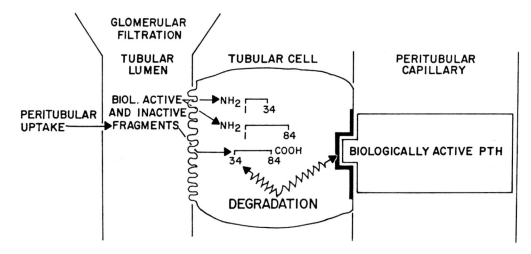

Fig. 4-23. Metabolic degradation of parathyroid hormone by the kidney. Biologically active parathyroid hormone (PTH) is degraded by specific proteases on the surface of renal tubular epithelial cells. Biologically active (NH_2-1–34) and inactive (34–84 COOH) fragments may be degraded intracellularly by lysosomal enzymes within renal tubular cells.

of 3′,5′-adenosine monophosphate (cAMP) in target cells (Fig. 4-24).[257,259] Binding of PTH to specific isoreceptors on target cells results in the activation of adenylate cyclase in the plasma membrane. The adenylate cyclase stimulates the conversion of ATP to cAMP in target cells. The accumulation of cyclic 3′,5′ AMP in target cells functions as an intracellular mediator or second messenger of parathyroid hormone action to increase permeability for calcium ion (Fig. 4-25). The resultant increase in cytosol calcium content in combination with the cAMP accumulation initiates the synthesis and release of lysosomal enzymes, and triggers other biochemical reactions in bone resorbing cells that result

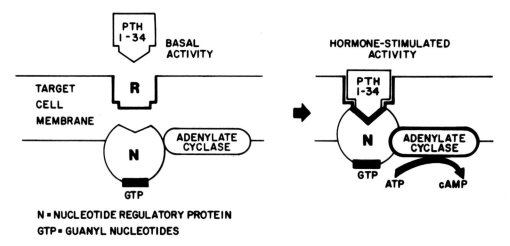

Fig. 4-24. Mechanism of parathyroid hormone action. The biologically active end of the hormone (PTH 1–34) binds to specific receptors (R) on the surface of target cells. The receptor-hormone complex is coupled to the catalytic subunit of adenylate cyclase in the cell membrane by a nucleotide regulatory (N-) protein. This results in the intracellular accumulation of cyclic adenosine monophosphate (cAMP), which serves as the "second messenger" for polypeptide hormones such as PTH in target cells and results in expression of the biologic response of the hormone.

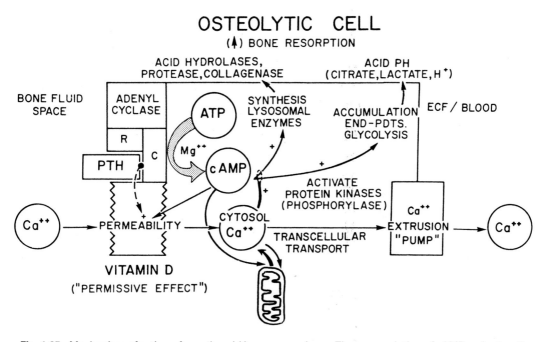

Fig. 4-25. Mechanism of action of parathyroid hormone on bone. The accumulation of cAMP and cytosolic calcium under the influence of PTH appears to trigger the physiologic reactions within osteolytic cells that results in bone resorption. The local release of lysosomal enzymes and end products of glycolysis creates an environment that favors the dissolution of bone.

eventually in breakdown of both the inorganic and organic phases of bone.[258]

In addition, parathyroid hormone contributes to the regulation of the rate of formation of 1,25-dihydroxycholecalciferol, the principal metabolically active form of vitamin D_3, by mitochondria in renal tubular epithelial cells.[89] The active metabolites of vitamin D make bone cells more sensitive to the direct effects of PTH ("permissive effect") and greatly enhance the gastrointestinal absorption of calcium, thereby amplifying the effect of PTH upon plasma calcium concentration.[260]

Certain similarities exist in the homeostatic control of the blood calcium and glucose concentration in extracellular fluids (Fig. 4-26). A common feature of both homeostatic mechanisms is the duality of control. The first level is of limited magnitude but capable of rapid response and sensitive to small changes in control signal concentration. Stimulation of the osteocyte-osteoblast pump and the renal conservation of calcium function in this

capacity as an immediate reservoir to maintain the levels of blood calcium within narrow limits. Glycogenolysis serves as a similar mechanism for maintaining the blood glucose concentration. The second level of control has a greater potential magnitude but responds more slowly and is less sensitive to slight changes in control signal concentration. Osteoclastic osteolysis and increased absorption of calcium in the intestine serve a similar function as gluconeogenesis in maintaining a sustained supply of calcium or glucose for the extracellular fluids.[260]

CALCITONIN

Calcitonin (thyrocalcitonin, CT) is a more recently discovered hormone than PTH.[83] Phylogenetically, the early appearance of calcitonin in primitive elasmobranch fish precedes the first appearance of PTH in amphibians. Copp et al.,[83] in experiments designed to test the McLean-Urist hypothesis of negative feedback control of blood calcium by parathyroid hormone, perfused the parathy-

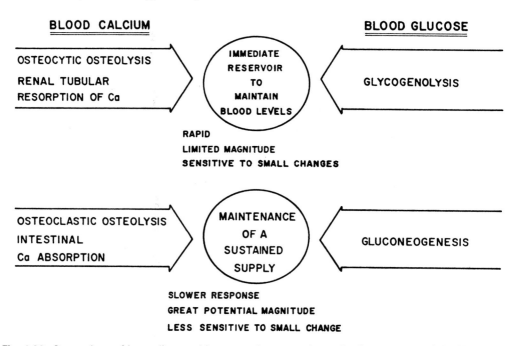

Fig. 4-26. Comparison of immediate and long-term homeostatic mechanisms to control the blood concentration of calcium and glucose.

roid-thyroid complex of dogs with alternating intervals of blood with a low (−CA) and high (+CA) calcium concentration and measured the effects on calcium levels in peripheral blood (Fig. 4-27). Two findings from these experiments were difficult to explain by the existing concept of a single hormone controlling the concentration of blood calcium. First, the fall in systemic calcium following perfusion of the thyroid-parathyroid complex was more rapid and of greater magnitude than expected from only an inhibition of PTH secretion. Second, thyroparathyroidectomy following the last low calcium perfusion resulted in a continued progressive rise in blood calcium rather than the expected fall after removal of the source of PTH. These and subsequent experiments led to development of the hypothesis of a second calcium-regulating hormone secreted by the parathyroid-thyroid complex in response to hypercalcemia which lowered plasma calcium.

Conflicting views on the origin of calcitonin were resolved by definitive studies in the goat whose parathyroid glands, unlike

those of the dog, can be perfused with blood having a high or low calcium content independent of the thyroid glands. Hypercalcemic perfusion of the external parathyroid gland alone failed to induce a fall in systemic plasma calcium. However, when the thyroid was included in the perfusion area, a striking hypocalcemia could be elicited (Fig. 4-28). The presence of a calcium-lowering hormone within the mammalian thyroid gland was further confirmed by the demonstration that a thyroid extract would produce a similar fall in plasma calcium (Fig. 4-28). It is now well established that calcitonin is of thyroid rather than parathyroid origin in mammals and that calcitonin and thyrocalcitonin are one and the same hormone.

C (Parafollicular)-Cells in Thyroid or Ultimobranchial Glands

Calcitonin has been shown to be secreted by a second endocrine cell population in the mammalian thyroid gland. C-cells are distinct from follicular cells in the thyroid that secrete thyroxine and triiodothyronine.[162]

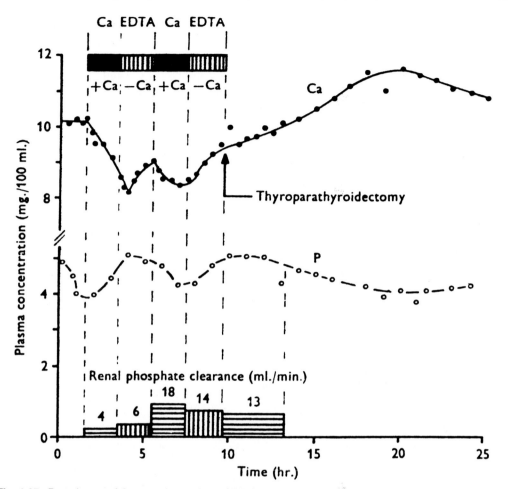

Fig. 4-27. Experiment of Copp and associates (1962) that led to the discovery of calcitonin. Perfusion of the thyroid-parathyroid complex in dogs with high calcium concentration in blood resulted in a more rapid and greater decline in peripheral calcium concentration than was expected only by the inhibition of PTH secretion. Thyroidectomy following the last low calcium infusion resulted in a progressive hypercalcemia rather than the expected decline in blood calcium following removal of the source of PTH.

They are situated either within the follicular wall immediately beneath the basement membrane or between follicular cells (Fig. 4-29) and as small groups of cells between thyroid follicles. C-cells do not border the follicular colloid directly and their secretory polarity is oriented toward the interfollicular capillaries (Fig. 4-29). The distinctive feature of C-cells is the presence of numerous small membrane-limited secretory granules in the cytoplasm. Immunocytochemical techniques have localized the calcitonin activity of C-cells to these secretory granules.[87]

Calcitonin-secreting C-cells have been shown to be derived embryologically from cells of the neural crest. Primordial cells from the neural crest migrate ventrally and become incorporated within the last (ultimobranchial) pharyngeal pouch. They move caudally with the ultimobranchial body to the point of fusion with the midline primordia that gives rise to the thyroid gland (Fig. 4-30). The ultimobranchial body fuses with and is incorporated into the thyroid near the hilus in mammals, and C-cells subsequently are distributed throughout the gland. Although C-cells are present throughout the thyroid gland in postnatal life of man and

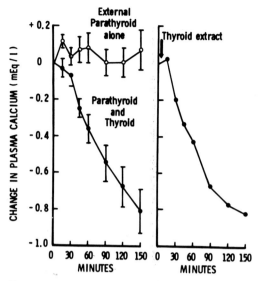

Fig. 4-28. Demonstration of thyroid rather than parathyroid origin of calcitonin in mammals. Hypercalcemic perfusion of the external parathyroid gland alone in the goat had no effect on systemic plasma calcium; however, when the thyroid gland was included in the area perfused there was a striking fall in plasma calcium. Administration of a thyroid extract produced a similar hypocalcemic response. (From Foster et al., 1972.)

most other mammals, they often remain more numerous near the hilus and point of fusion with the ultimobranchial body. In submammalian species C-cells and calcitonin activity remain segregated in the ultimobranchial gland which is anatomically distinct from both the thyroid and the parathyroid glands (Fig. 4-31). In the avian ultimobranchial gland a network of stellate cells with long cytoplasmic processes supports the C-cells.[355]

Chemistry of Calcitonin

Calcitonin is a polypeptide hormone composed of 32 amino acid residues arranged in a straight chain with a 1-7 disulfide linkage.[82] It is a smaller molecule than parathyroid hormone (84 amino acids) and is synthesized as part of a larger biosynthetic precursor molecule.[347] Pre-procalcitonin is the initial translational product formed in the rough endoplasmic reticulum (Fig. 4-32). It is transported to the Golgi apparatus where it is converted to calcitonin prior to packaging in membrane-limited secretory granules. De-

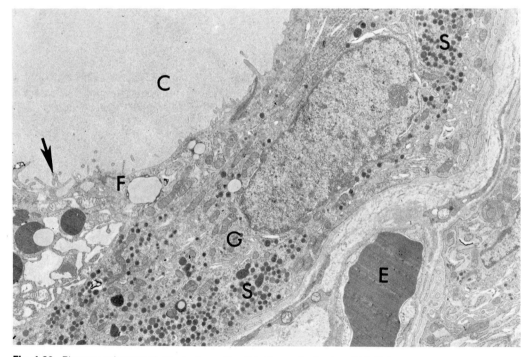

Fig. 4-29. Electron micrograph illustrating a C-cell in the wall of a thyroid follicle wedged between several follicular cells (F). The cytoplasm of C-cells has many calcitonin-containing secretion granules (S) and a prominent Golgi apparatus (G). Follicular cells (F) line the follicle and extend microvilli (arrow) into the colloid (C). The secretory polarity of C-cells is directed toward interfollicular capillaries (E) rather than toward the follicle lumen as with follicular cells. 7,700 ×.

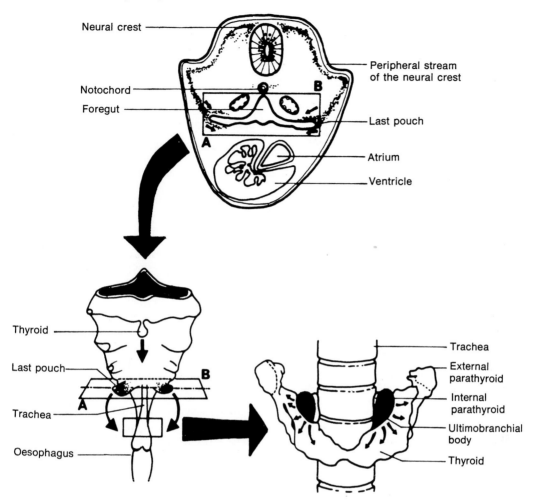

Fig. 4-30. Schematic representation of neural crest origin of calcitonin-secreting C-cells. Primordial cells arising from neural crest migrate ventrally during embryonic life to become incorporated in the last (ultimobranchial) pharyngeal pouch. The ultimobranchial body fuses with primordia of the thyroid and distributes C-cells throughout the mammalian thyroid gland. (From Foster et al., 1972.)

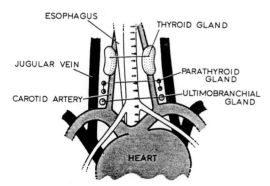

Fig. 4-31. Calcitonin-secreting C-cells in submammalian vertebrates remain in an anatomically distinct endocrine organ. The ultimobranchial gland in chickens is situated caudal to the 2 pairs of parathyroids and thyroid gland along the carotid artery.

pending upon the need for calcitonin, a proportion of the precursors and active hormone undergo degradation prior to release from C-cells. Under certain pathologic conditions (e.g. neoplasia) these neural crest-derived C-cells may secrete other humoral factors including serotonin, bradykinin, ACTH, prostaglandins, amongst others (Fig. 4-32).

The calcitonin gene is expressed differently in thyroid (C-cells) and neural tissues.[159,301] In thyroid C-cells the mRNA encodes primarily for pre-procalcitonin (molecular weight: 17,400 daltons), whereas in neural tissues there is alternative RNA processing and encoding for pre-procalcitonin gene-

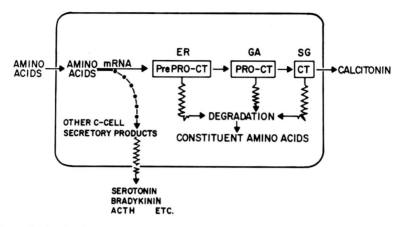

Fig. 4-32. Biosynthesis of calcitonin in thyroid C-cells. Preprocalcitonin (Pre PRO-CT) and pro-calcitonin (PRO-CT) are biosynthetic precursors that undergo post-translational processing to form biologically active calcitonin (CT). Some of the precursor molecules and calcitonin may undergo enzymatic degradation prior to secretion from C-cells. Neuroendocrine cells, as thyroid C-cells, may secrete other products (e.g. serotonin, bradykinin, ACTA) under certain disease conditions.

related peptide (CGRP) (15,900 daltons). CGRP is a neuropeptide composed of 37 amino acids and is concerned with nociception, ingestive behavior, and modulation of the nervous and endocrine systems.

The complete amino acid sequence of porcine, bovine, ovine, and salmon calcitonin, other animal species and human calcitonin has been determined. Synthetic human calcitonin has been prepared and shown to be bio-

logically active. The structure of calcitonin differs considerably between species. The calcitonin molecules of 5 selected species share only 9 of the 32 amino acid residues (Fig. 4-33). However, the amino terminal of the calcitonin molecule is similar in all species. It consists of a seven-membered ring enclosed by an intrachain disulfide bridge. The complete sequence of 32 amino acids and the disulfide bond are essential for full biologic

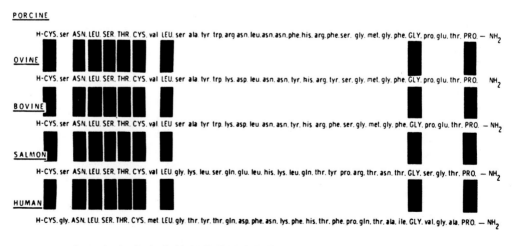

Fig. 4-33. Amino acid sequence of the calcitonin molecule from 5 species. The 9 residues in the chain of 32 amino acids shared by the calcitonin molecule in all 5 species are indicated by the vertical bars. (From Foster et al., 1972.)

activity. It is surprising that salmon calcitonin is more potent in lowering blood calcium on a weight basis than any of the other calcitonins when administered to mammals, including man. The reason for the greater biologic potency of salmon calcitonin in mammals is uncertain but probably is related to an increased resistance to metabolic degradation or a greater affinity for receptor sites in bone and other target tissues.[130]

Regulation of Calcitonin Secretion

The concentration of calcium ion in plasma and extracellular fluids is the principal physiologic stimulus for the secretion of calcitonin by C-cells.[82] Calcitonin is secreted continuously under conditions of normocalcemia, but the rate of secretion of calcitonin increases greatly in response to an elevation in blood calcium. Magnesium ion has a similar effect on calcitonin secretion as calcium, but these effects are observed only under experimental conditions with nonphysiologic levels of magnesium.

C-cells under normal conditions store substantial amounts of calcitonin in their cytoplasm in the form of membrane-limited secretory granules (Fig. 4-29). In response to hypercalcemia, stored hormone from C-cells is discharged rapidly into interfollicular capillaries (Fig. 4-13).[58] If the hypercalcemic stimulus is sustained, this is followed by an increased development of cytoplasmic organelles concerned with the synthesis and secretion of calcitonin (Fig. 4-13). The endoplasmic reticulum with attached ribosomes is hypertrophied and the Golgi apparatus is enlarged and associated with prosecretory granules in the process of formation. Hyperplasia of C-cells occurs in response to long-term hypercalcemia.[58,79] When the blood calcium is lowered, the stimulus for calcitonin secretion is diminished and numerous secretory granules accumulate in the cytoplasm of C-cells (Fig. 4-13). The storage of large amounts of preformed hormone in C-cells and rapid release in response to moderate elevations in blood calcium probably are a reflection of the physiologic role of calcitonin as an emergency hormone to protect against the development of hypercalcemia.

Calcitonin secretion is increased in response to a high calcium meal often before a significant rise in plasma calcium can be detected. The cause of this increase in calcitonin secretion is either a small undetectable rise in plasma ionized calcium or a direct stimulation of certain gastrointestinal hormones by the oral calcium load which in turn act as secretagogues for calcitonin release from the thyroid gland.[80] Gastrin, pancreozymin, and glucagon all have been demonstrated to stimulate calcitonin release under experimental conditions in animals.[59,104] These findings suggest that gastrointestinal hormones may be important in triggering the early release of calcitonin to prevent the development of hypercalcemia following the ingestion of a high calcium meal. (Fig. 4-34).[121]

Biologic Effects of Calcitonin

The administration of calcitonin or stimulation of endogenous secretion results in the development of varying degrees of hypocal-

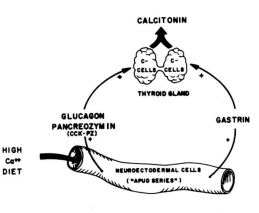

Fig. 4-34. Gastrointestinal hormone-thyroid C-cell axis provides a mechanism for rapid release of calcitonin from the thyroid in response to a high calcium diet before a significant elevation in blood calcium.

cemia and hypophosphatemia. These effects of calcitonin on plasma calcium and phosphorus are most evident in young animals or older animals with increased rates of skeletal turnover. Calcitonin exerts its function by interacting with target cells, primarily in bone and kidney, and to a lesser extent in the intestine. The action of PTH and CT is antagonistic on bone resorption (Fig. 4-18) but synergistic on decreasing the renal tubular reabsorption of phosphorus (Fig. 4-22). The hypocalcemic effects of calcitonin are primarily the result of decreased entry of calcium from the skeleton into plasma due to a temporary inhibition of PTH-stimulated bone resorption.[1,107] The hypophosphatemia develops from a direct action of calcitonin on increasing the rate of movement of phosphate out of plasma into soft tissue and bone,[311] as well as from the inhibition of bone resorption. The action of CT is not dependent on vitamin D, since it acts both in vitamin D-deficient animals and after the administration of large doses of vitamin D.

The action of calcitonin on inhibiting bone resorption stimulated by PTH and other factors is from blockage of osteoclastic osteolysis (Fig. 4-18). Osteoclasts have receptors for calcitonin, and specific structural alterations are produced in osteoclasts by calcitonin.[65,66] Osteoclasts withdraw from resorptive surfaces and the brush border and transitional zone become atrophic.[164,297,339] In addition, the rate of activation of osteoprogenitor cells to preosteoclasts and osteoclasts decreases, resulting in decreased osteoclast numbers. Although CT can block bone resorption completely, the inhibition is a transitory effect. The continuous administration of CT in vivo and in vitro in the presence of PTH leads to an "escape phenomenon" whereby the effects of PTH on increasing bone resorption become manifest in the presence of CT.[107]

The effects of calcitonin on bone formation are less dramatic. Initially there appears to be an increase in the rate of bone formation, but the long-term administration of calcitonin appears to lead to a reduction in both bone resorption and formation. Calcitonin-secreting C-cell neoplasms in both bulls and human beings are associated with a low rate of skeletal turnover and densely mineralized bone.[25,260] Unfortunately, calcitonin has not proven to be an effective therapeutic agent to induce a long-term increase in bone formation in human patients with post-menopausal osteoporosis.

Calcitonin and PTH both decrease renal tubular reabsorption of phosphate to cause phosphaturia; however, the adenylate cyclase-linked receptors for calcitonin are found in the ascending limb of Henle and the distal convoluted tubule (Fig. 4-22). In addition, calcitonin results in diuresis of sodium, chloride, and calcium.[259] The physiologic significance of calcitonin on renal electrolyte excretion in mammals is uncertain and this function as a regulator of ionic balance may be more important in primitive vertebrates such as fish. Likewise, the physiologic importance of calcitonin on gastrointestinal absorption of calcium is equivocal. Olson et al. reported that low doses of calcitonin markedly inhibit calcium absorption in isolated, vascularly perfused preparations of small intestine.[238] Parathyroid hormone was shown to stimulate calcium absorption in this system under similar conditions.

Physiologic Significance of Calcitonin

Calcitonin and parathyroid hormone acting in concert provide a dual negative feedback control mechanism to maintain the concentration of calcium in extracellular fluids within narrow limits. Present evidence suggests that parathyroid hormone is the major factor concerned with the minute-to-minute regulation of blood calcium under normal conditions. This probably is related to the fact that protection against the development of hypocalcemia by PTH in most higher mammals living in a relatively low calcium-high phosphorus environment is a life-sustaining function.

Calcitonin appears to function more as an emergency hormone to (1) prevent the development of "physiologic" hypercalcemia during the rapid postprandial absorption of calcium and (2) protect against excessive loss of calcium and phosphorus from the maternal skeleton during pregnancy. For example, thyroidectomized cows without a source of calcitonin develop a significant hypercalcemia following a high calcium meal (40 g/day) compared to intact control cows fed a similar diet (Fig. 4-35).[17]

In hibernating vertebrates the alternating secretion of CT and PTH permits the cyclic withdrawal of calcium from the skeleton to maintain plasma calcium homeostasis during hibernation and bone structure after arousal.[236] The effects of calcitonin on renal electrolyte excretion may be of physiologic importance in the regulation of osmotic balance in certain lower vertebrates residing in a high ionic environment.

CHOLECALCIFEROL (VITAMIN D)

The third major hormone involved in the regulation of calcium metabolism and skeletal remodeling is cholecalciferol (vitamin D_3) or irradiated ergosterol (vitamin D_2). Al-

though these compounds have been considered to be vitamins for a long time, they can equally be considered hormones (Table 4-2).[105,169,231] Cholecalciferol is ingested in small amounts in the diet and can be synthesized in the epidermis from precursor molecules (e.g. 7-dehydrocholesterol) through a previtamin D_3 intermediate form (Fig. 4-36). This reaction is catalyzed by ultraviolet irradiation (wavelength 290 to 320 mμ) from the sun. A high-affinity vitamin D-binding protein transports cholecalciferol from its site of synthesis in the skin by the blood to the liver.[148,149]

In response to prolonged exposure to sunlight, previtamin D_3 is converted to lumisterol and tachysterol (Fig. 4-37). Because the DBP has no affinity for lumisterol and minimal affinity for tachysterol, the translocation of these photoisomers into the circulation is negligible and they are sloughed off with the natural turnover of the skin (Holick, 1981).

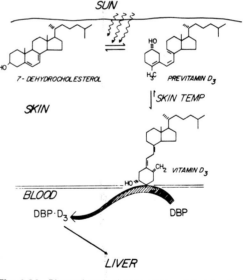

Fig. 4-36. Photochemical conversion of 7-dehydrocholesterol to previtamin D_3 in the epidermis following exposure to ultraviolet radiation from sunlight. Previtamin D_3 subsequently undergoes thermal conversion to vitamin D_3 (cholecalciferol), which enters dermal capillaries and binds to a specific vitamin D_3-binding protein (DBP). Protein-bound vitamin D_3 is transported to the liver for the initial step of metabolic activation. (From Holick, 1981.)

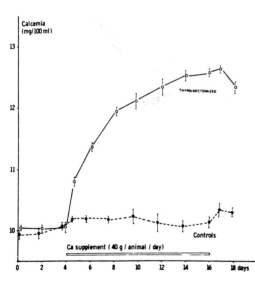

Fig. 4-35. Hypercalcemic response to an oral calcium load in thyroidectomized cows without an endogenous source of calcitonin compared to that of control cows with intact thyroid glands. (From Barlet, 1972.)

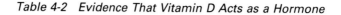

Table 4-2   Evidence That Vitamin D Acts as a Hormone

1. Chemical structure resembling that of steroid hormones
2. Very small quantities (ng) of active form required for full biologic activity
3. Synthesized by one organ (skin) from precursor molecules (provitamins) by photoactivation, lesser amounts from dietary sources
4. Transported by blood in bound form to target cells primarily in intestine and bone
5. Enhances rate of existing reactions in target cells to elicit a physiologic response
6. Mechanism of action:
    —similar to steroid hormones, enters cell and binds to cytosol receptor
    —hormone-receptor complex transported to nucleus
    —binds to specific nuclear receptors
    —facilitates transcription of mRNA from DNA
    —increases protein synthesis in target cells (e.g. CaBP)
7. Toxic in excessive amounts

Metabolic Activation of Vitamin D

Vitamin D must be metabolically activated before it can produce its known physiologic functions in target cells.[88,91,170] Vitamin D_3 from dietary sources is absorbed by facilitated diffusion and bound to an alpha-2 globulin in the blood for transport. Cholecalciferol from endogeneous sources is synthesized in the skin from 7-dehydrocholesterol by a photochemi-

cal reaction in the presence of ultraviolet irradiation (Fig. 4-38).[148] It is also bound to an alpha-2 globulin in the blood and transported to the liver.

The first step in the metabolic activation of vitamin D is the conversion of cholecalciferol to 25-hydroxycholecalciferol (25-OH-CC) in the liver.[136] The enzyme responsible for controlling this reaction is a hepatic microsomal

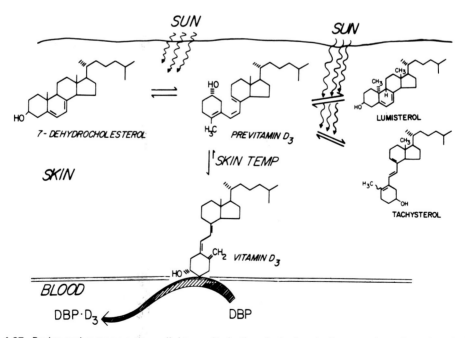

Fig. 4-37. Prolonged exposure to sunlight results in the photochemical conversion of previtamin D_3 to lumisterol and tachysterol. These photoisomers remain primarily in the epidermis and are lost with the natural turnover of the skin since the vitamin D_3-binding protein has a low affinity for these isomers. (From Holick, 1981.)

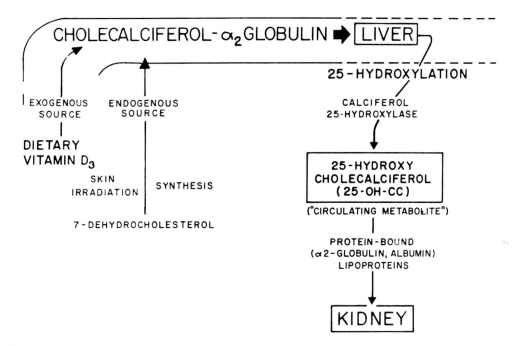

Fig. 4-38. Metabolism of vitamin D. The initial step of metabolic activation of vitamin D_3 from endogenous and dietary sources is in the liver to form 25-hydroxycholecalciferol.

enzyme referred to as calciferol-25-hydroxylase associated with the endoplasmic reticulum.[21] Although 25-OH-CC may exert biologic effects when substantial amounts are present, it primarily serves as a precursor for the formation of more active vitamin D metabolites. Considerably larger amounts of protein-bound 25-OH-CC circulate than with the more hydroxylated active metabolites of vitamin D, such as 1,25-dihydroxycholecalciferol, which are present in extremely low levels in the blood. The high circulating levels of 25-OH-CC serve as a reservoir of precursor vitamin D for the synthesis of the active form of vitamin D by the kidney.

This first metabolite of cholecalciferol (25-OH-CC) is transported to the kidney and undergoes further transformation to a more polar and active metabolite (Fig. 4-39).[135] The principal active metabolite of 25-OH-CC formed in the kidney is 1,25-dihydroxycholecalciferol (1,25-DiOH-CC), but additional metabolites are formed such as 24,25-DiOH-CC and others (Fig. 4-39).[32,89,92,233,235] The rate of formation of 1,25-DiOH-CC is cat-

alyzed by 25-hydroxycholecalciferol-1α-hydroxylase in mitochondria of renal epithelial cells in the proximal convoluted tubules.[36,209] It has been shown that the 1α-hydroxylase enzyme system is a mixed function steroid hydroxylase similar to those in the adrenal cortex, contains cytochrome P-450, and requires molecular oxygen. 1,25-dihydroxycholecalciferol exerts strong product feedback inhibition on the 1α-hydroxylase in the kidney.[120] The conversion of 25-OH-CC to 1,25-DiOH-CC is the rate-limiting step in vitamin D metabolism and is the primary reason for the delay between administration of vitamin D and expression of its biologic effects.[93,233]

The control of this final step in the metabolic activation of vitamin D is complex and appears to be regulated by the plasma calcium concentration and its influence on the rates of secretion of PTH and possibly CT (Fig. 4-37).[106,113,262] The two other major hormones controlling calcium metabolism appear to have opposite effects on this 1α-hydroxylase and formation of 1,25-DiOH-CC. Parathyroid hormone and conditions

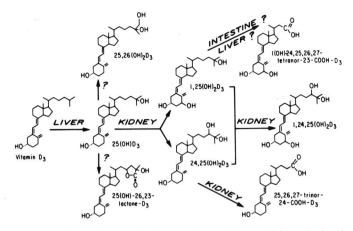

Fig. 4-39. Two-step metabolic activation of cholecalciferol (vitamin D_3) beginning in the liver to form 25-hydroxycholecalciferol. This first metabolite is subsequently released from the liver and transported in a protein-bound form to the kidney, where it is converted to 1,25-dihydroxycholecalciferol (its principal biologically active metabolite) and several other metabolites. (From Norman, 1979.)

that stimulate PTH secretion increase the conversion of 25-OH-CC to 1,25-DiOH-CC, whereas calcitonin under certain conditions inhibits the conversion. A low concentration of phosphorus in the blood increases the formation of 1,25-DiOH-CC, whereas a high phosphorus concentration suppresses the activity of the 1α-hydroxylase (Fig. 4-40). Minute-to-minute changes in 1α-hydroxylase activity may result from changes in the ionic environment of renal mitochondria caused by the accumulation or release of calcium and inorganic phosphate.

The rates of synthesis of 24,25-DiOH-CC and 1,25-DiOH-CC appear to be reciprocally related and controlled by similar factors.[89,314] When 1,25-DiOH-CC synthesis increases, the formation of 24,25-DiOH-CC declines and vice versa (Fig. 4-40). For example, feeding a high calcium diet decreases the formation of 1,25-DiOH-CC and 25-OH-CC is diverted to form primarily 24,25-DiOH-CC, a metabolite that is much less active in stimulating intestinal calcium transport. 24,25-DiOH-CC may play a role in bone formation,[241] egg hatchability, and with 1,25-DiOH-CC exert negative feedback control on the parathyroid gland (Fig. 4-48).[141]

Other hormones under certain conditions may increase the activity of renal 1α-hydroxy-

lase and the formation of 1,25-DiOH-CC. Prolactin, estradiol, placental lactogen, and possibly STH enhance 1α-hydroxylase activity.[190] Increased secretion of these hormones, either alone or in combination, appears to be important in the efficient adaptation to the major calcium demands during life. The physiologic adjustments in calcium homeostasis imposed by pregnancy, lactation, and growth are mediated primarily by an increased intestinal absorption of calcium stimulated by 1,25-DiOH-CC.

1,25-DiOH-CC is the major biologically active metabolite of cholecalciferol that interacts with target cells in the intestine and bone under physiologic conditions to enhance the rates of existing reactions and increase calcium mobilization (Fig. 4-39).[92] Its onset of action is more rapid and the degree of potency is much greater than with either cholecalciferol or 25-OH-CC. A similar two-step process of metabolic activation also occurs with irradiation ergosterol (vitamin D_2).

A disease of cattle known as Enteque seco in the Argentine and Espichamento in Brazil is characterized by widespread mineralization of the cardiovascular system, lung, kidney, and other soft tissues.[62,94] A similar disease affects cattle and horses in many other countries worldwide, including the United States. Af-

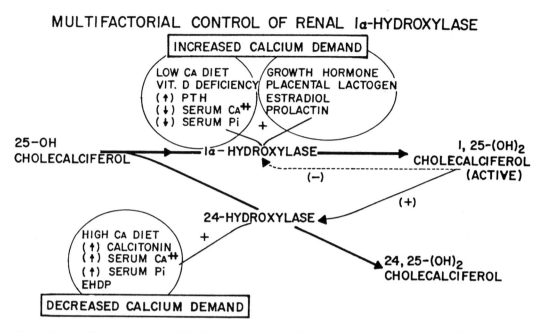

MULTIFACTORIAL CONTROL OF RENAL Iα-HYDROXYLASE

Fig. 4-40. Multifactorial control of the final step of metabolic activation of vitamin D in the kidney. Several conditions associated with increased calcium demand result in a stimulation of 1,25-(OH)₂ cholecalciferol production from 25-OH cholecalciferol by increasing the activity of 1 α-hydroxylase in mitochondria of renal tubular epithelial cells. Under conditions of decreased calcium demand the production of 1,25-(OH)₂ is diminished, but 24,25-(OH)₂ cholecalciferol (an inactive metabolite in calcium mobilization) is formed by activation of a 24-hydroxylase.

fected cattle develop a chronic debilitating disease characterized by weight loss, painful gait, kyphosis, polyuria, and dyspnea. The lesions of soft tissue mineralization are remarkably similar to those produced experimentally with large doses of vitamin D.[49,134,186] Studies have shown that ingestion of small amounts of dried leaves from an indigenous plant (*Solanum malacoxylon*) greatly increased the rate of intestinal calcium and phosphorus absorption to produce hypercalcemia and hyperphosphatemia (Fig. 4-41),[286] osteosclerosis,[60] parathyroid atrophy, and hyperplasia of thyroid C-cells.[61] Extracts of the leaves of *Solanum malacoxylon* contain an extremely potent, water-soluble, active principle which stimulates the intestinal calcium transport system.[329] The active principle has been shown to be 1,25-DiOH-CC conjugated to a glycoside. *Cestrum diurnum* ("day-blooming jessamine") also contains substantial amounts of 1,25-DiOH-CC and has caused a similar debilitating disease in cattle and horses in the southeastern part of the United States.[330–332]

Chemistry of Vitamin D and Metabolites

The chemical structure of cholecalciferol (vitamin D₃) resembles that of other steroid hormones. It is a seco-steroid in which the B ring of the basic steroid nucleus has been opened by cleavage of the 9 carbon-10 carbon bond.[234] Photoactivation by ultraviolet irradiation (290 to 320 mμ) of 7-dehydrocholesterol in the epidermis of the skin results in a cleavage between the 9 and 10 carbons and unfolding of the B ring of the basic steroid nucleus (Fig. 4-42).[138] During metabolic activation of cholecalciferol (or irradiation ergosterol), hydroxyl groups are successively attached at positions 1 and 25 of the steroid nucleus by specific hydroxylases in the liver and kidney to form the hormonal or biologically active form of vitamin D (Fig. 4-42). In

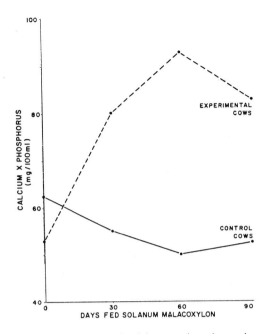

Fig. 4-41. Elevation of calcium × phosphorus ion product following ingestion of *Solanum malacoxylon.* The leaves of this calcinogenic plant contain large quantities of the principal active metabolite (1,25 dihydroxycholecalciferol) of vitamin D. The chronic debililating disease associated with ingestion of calcinogenic plants results in a major economic loss in cattle in several regions of the world.

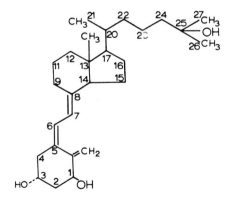

1, 25 - DIHYDROXYCHOLECALCIFEROL

Fig. 4-42. Chemistry of the "hormonal" form of vitamin D. The chemical structure of 1,25-dihydroxycholecalciferol resembles that of steroid hormones. Molecular weight of the principal active metabolite of vitamin D is 416.

other natural metabolites of cholecalciferol, the two hydroxyl groups are attached at either 25 and 25 or 25 and 26 positions.

There are a number of other sterols closely related to cholecalciferol. Vitamin D_2 is formed by the irradiation of the plant sterol referred to as ergosterol. When irradiated ergosterol is ingested and absorbed from the intestine, it undergoes a series of similar steps of metabolic activation as those described for cholecalciferol (vitamin D_3). However, the more active metabolites of ergosterol are 25-hydroxyergosterol and 1,25-dihydroxyergosterol synthesized by the liver and kidney, respectively. Another related sterol of considerable therapeutic interest is dihydrotachysterol. The A ring of the steroid nucleus in this compound is rotated so that the hydroxyl in position 3 occupies a position sterically equivalent to the hydroxyl position 1 of 1,25-dihydroxycholecalciferol. Dihydroxytachysterol undergoes metabolic transformation to 25-dihydrotachysterol, but subsequent hydroxylation of position 1 does not occur. Therefore, the major biologically active metabolite of dihydrotachysterol is 25-dihydrotachysterol and not a dihydroxylated metabolite as with cholecalciferol and ergosterol.

Biologic Effects and Mechanism of Action of Active Vitamin D Metabolites

Vitamin D and its active metabolites function to increase the absorption of calcium and phosphorus from the intestine, thereby maintaining adequate levels of these electrolytes in the extracellular fluids in order to permit the appropriate mineralization of bone matrix (Fig. 4-18).[239] From a functional point of view vitamin D can be thought to act in such a way as to cause the retention of sufficient mineral ions to ensure mineralization of bone matrix, whereas PTH maintains the proper ratio of calcium to phosphate in extracellular fluids. In addition, a small amount of active vitamin D is needed to permit PTH to exert its action on bone ("permissive effect") (Fig. 4-25).

The major target tissue for 1,25-dihydroxycholecalciferol is the mucosa of the small intestine. In the proximal part it increases the active transcellular transport of calcium and in the distal part the transport of phosphorus. Following synthesis in the kidney 1,25-DiOH-CC is transported in a protein-bound form to specific target cells in the intestine and bone (Fig. 4-39). Circulating levels of this hormonal form of cholecalciferol are extremely low. Free 1,25-DiOH-CC penetrates the plasma membrane of target cells and initially binds to a cytoplasmic receptor in cells of the intestine (Fig. 4-43).[35] Subsequently, the hormone-receptor complex is transferred to the nucleus and 1,25-DiOH-CC binds to specific receptors in the nuclear chromatin where it stimulates gene expression leading to increased synthesis of vitamin D-dependent proteins such as calcium-binding protein (CaBP) by intestinal cells.[136,137,170,336]

Intestinal absorptive cells are responsive to 1,25-DiOH-CC and are concerned with the transport of calcium from the lumen to the blood stream. The projection of villi from the floor into the lumen of the intestine greatly increases the effective surface area for absorption of nutrients (Fig. 4-44). The luminal surface (brush border) of intestinal absorptive cells is highly specialized and has numerous microvilli which further increase the intestinal surface area (Figs. 4-45 and 4-46).[137]

In response to 1,25-dihydroxycholecalciferol intestinal absorptive cells synthesize and secrete a specific calcium-binding protein (CaBP).[318,334] Calcium-binding protein has been isolated from several tissues (e.g. small intestine, kidney, parathyroid gland, bone, mammary gland, and the shell gland of laying hens) across which significant amounts of calcium are transported. A vitamin D-dependent calcium-binding protein also has been demonstrated in bone, particularly in the spongiosa and cartilagenous growth plate.[70]

The absorptive capacity of the intestine for calcium is a direct function of the amount of CaBP present.[157,335,336] The administration of vitamin D or feeding low calcium and low phosphorus diets has been shown to stimulate the synthesis of CaBP, which contributes to the increased intestinal absorption of calcium. The physiologic functions of CaBP appear to be related to the transcellular transport of calcium from the luminal to basilar border of intestinal absorptive cells and the regulation intracellular calcium concentration (Thorens et al., 1982). At the basilar aspect of intestinal absorptive cells, calcium is exchanged for sodium and enters the extracellular fluids. Vitamin D may also exert an effect on mitochondrial membranes and increase the accumulation of calcium granules within mitochondria of intestinal cells.[285] At the basilar aspect of absorptive cells calcium is exchanged for sodium and enters the extracellular fluids.

The active metabolites of cholecalciferol also act on bone.[89,145] In young animals vita-

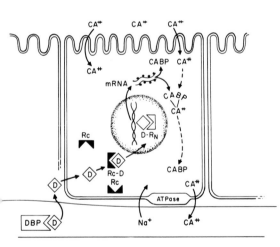

Fig. 4-43. Molecular mechanism of action of 1,25-dihydroxycholecalciferol in the intestine. The active metabolite of vitamin D is transported to the intestine by a vitamin D-binding protein (DBP). The hydrophilic steroid penetrates the plasma membrane, binds to a cytoplasmic receptor, and is transported to the nucleus where it interacts with the nuclear chromatin to increase the formation of mRNA. The mRNA becomes associated with ribosomes on the endoplasmic reticulum and directs the synthesis of new proteins such as calcium-binding protein (CABP). The CABP is involved in the transcellular transport of calcium to the basilar aspects of the intestinal absorptive cells where calcium is exchanged for sodium and enters the extracellular fluid compartment.

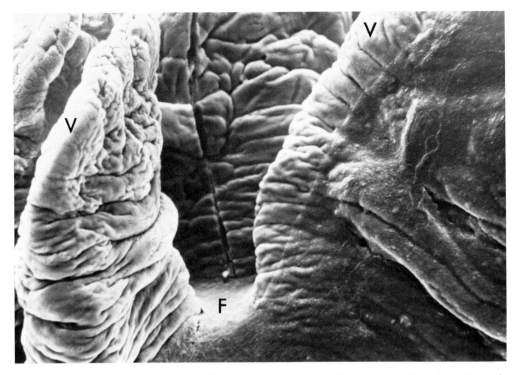

Fig. 4-44. Scanning electron micrograph illustrating the structure of the small intestine where absorption of calcium occurs from dietary sources. Villi (V) project from the floor (F) of the intestine into the lumen and greatly increase the surface area. The surface of the intestinal villi appears relatively smooth at low magnification. 300 ×.

min D is required for the orderly growth and mineralization of cartilage in the growth plate (Fig. 4-47). Young animals fed diets deficient in vitamin D and housed indoors without exposure to ultraviolet irradiation develop rickets. In the absence of vitamin D, mineral granules do not accumulate within mitochondria of hypertrophied chondrocytes in the growth plates of long bones. Mineralization of the cartilaginous matrix fails to occur and the formation of woven bone on spicules of cartilage and subsequent remodeling to lamellar bone are blocked in this disease. The epiphyseal plate is irregularly thickened as progressively more primordial cartilaginous matrix accumulates and fails to mineralize. The administration of either cholecalciferol, 25-OH-CC or 1,25-DiOH-CC leads to reestablishment of a normal calcification front in the osteoid on bone surfaces and at the growth plate, often before there is a change in the mineral ion product of extracellular fluids.

In addition to this effect on mineralization of bone matrix, vitamin D is necessary for osteoclastic resorption and calcium mobilization from bone. Small amounts of vitamin D or its active metabolite are necessary to permit osteolytic cells to respond to PTH ("permissive effect") under physiologic conditions (Fig. 4-25). Both 1,25-DiOH-CC, 25-OH-CC, and cholecalciferol in pharmacologic doses will stimulate osteoclastic proliferation and the resorption of bone *in vitro* and *in vivo*. 1,25-dihydroxycholecalciferol is about 100 times more potent on a weight basis in stimulating bone resorption *in vitro* as 25-OH-CC.[256,265] Pharmacologic amounts of vitamin D_3 in adult thyroparathyroidectomized (TXPTX) rats increase osteoclastic resorption and stimulate osteoblastic hyperplasia in the absence of PTH and CT.[340] 1,25-DiOH-CC induces hyperplasia of osteoblasts

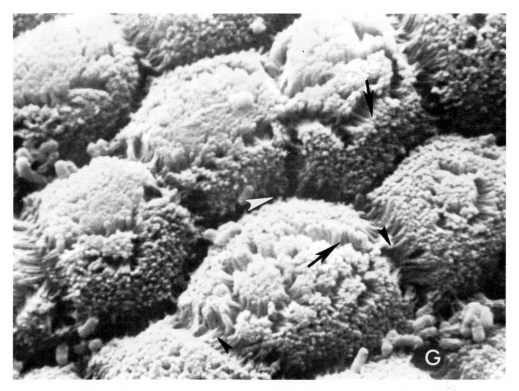

Fig. 4-45. Surface architecture of the intestinal villi illustrated in Figure 4-44 at high magnification. Junctions can be visualized between individual absorptive cells (arrow heads) and orifices of goblet cells (G). The luminal surface of absorptive cells in modified by the presence of numerous microvilli (arrows) which greatly increase the intestinal surface area. 3,000 ×.

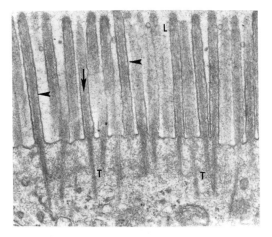

Fig. 4-46. Microvilli on absorptive cells extending into the intestinal lumen (L). The trilaminar membrane of microvilli (arrow heads) contains the vitamin D-dependent enzymes thought to be concerned with the translocation of calcium into absorptive cells. Fine filaments in the cores of microvilli extend into the terminal web (T) of absorptive cells. 21,750 ×.

in TXPTX rats fed either high or low calcium diets but increases osteoclast numbers only in rats with a low dietary calcium intake.[342,343] These results suggest that exogenous 1,25-DiOH-CC with appropriate dietary calcium supplementation may selectively stimulate osteoblastic activity without increasing bone destruction and may be useful in treating certain osteopenic diseases.

Deficiency of vitamin D results not only from simple dietary lack or inadequate exposure to sunlight, but also from a deficiency of the 1α-hydroxylase enzyme essential for metabolic activation of precursor molecules. Vitamin D-dependent rickets in both pigs and human beings is a familiar disease inherited by an autosomal recessive gene. Newborn pigs appear healthy and have normal blood calcium and phosphorus concentrations. At 4 to 6 weeks of age blood

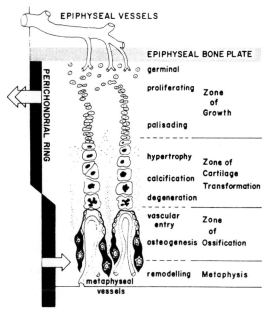

Fig. 4-47. Metaphyseal growth plate from a long bone. Vitamin D provides an adequate concentration of calcium and phosphorus in extracellular fluids to permit the mineralization of cartilagenous matrix that results in an orderly degeneration of chondrocytes and eventual ingrowth of osteoblasts into the scaffold provided by the degenerating cartilage cells with formation of osteoid.

calcium and phosphorus decrease, alkaline phosphatase activity increases (Fig. 4-48), and clinically detectable rickets develops during the following 3 to 4 weeks. The pigs develop deformities of bone in the axial and abaxial skeleton, severe pain, and classical lesions of rickets.

In response to the hypocalcemia, plasma immunoreactive parathyroid hormone levels (ng/ml) in pigs with vitamin D-dependent rickets are elevated (mean 1.94) compared with control pigs (mean 0.51, range 0.27 to 0.75 ng/ml) (Fig. 4-49). Serum 25-hydroxy-cholecalciferol (25-OH-D3) levels are strikingly elevated in pigs with clinical rickets (75 ng/ml) compared with control pigs (8 ng/ml), whereas serum 1,25-DiOH-CC is markedly depressed in rachitic pigs (17 pg/ml) compared with normal pigs (47 pg/ml). Repeated administration of either 5 or 10 μg 25-OH-D$_3$/day to pigs with vitamin D-dependent rickets for 2 to 3 weeks will not significantly change the plasma concentrations of calcium, phosphorus, and immunoreactive parathyroid hormone; however, small (1 to 4 μg) doses of 1,25-DiOH-CC daily for 3 to 4 weeks

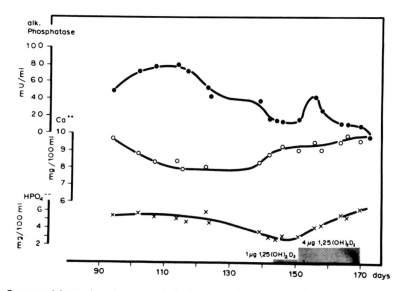

Fig. 4-48. Serum calcium, phosphorus, and alkaline phosphatase levels in pigs with vitamin D-dependent rickets before and following administration of 1 and 4 μg 1,25-dihydroxycholecalciferol. (Courtesy of Dr. R. Wilke, 1979.)

results in increased plasma calcium, decreased phosphorus, and a return of immunoreactive parathyroid hormone and alkaline phosphatase levels to near the normal range (Fig. 4-49).

Less is known regarding the action of cholecalciferol and its active metabolites on the kidney. Present evidence suggests that active metabolites of vitamin D stimulate the retention of calcium and phosphorus by increasing proximal tubular reabsorption (Fig. 4-18).

Recent evidence suggests that the active metabolites of vitamin D also have a direct effect on the parathyroid gland, in addition to their well-characterized action on intestine and bone. The parathyroids selectively localize 1,25-DiOH-CC and contain specific cytoplasmic and nuclear receptors for the active metabolite of vitamin D.[153,337] Under experimental conditions, the administration of either 1,25-DiOH-CC or cholecalciferol decreases parathyroid weight and the DNA content of stimulated glands. Lower doses of 1,25-DiOH-CC require 24,25-DiOH-CC to significantly lower parathyroid weight in vitamin D-deficient chicks (Fig. 4-50). Therefore, a negative feedback loop exists whereby vitamin D metabolites (either alone or in combination) directly interact with parathyroid cells to diminish the secretion of PTH, which in turn diminishes the formation of 1,25-DiOH-CC (Fig. 4-50).

DISORDERS OF PARATHYROID FUNCTION

Hyperparathyroidism

Hyperparathyroidism is a metabolic disorder in which excessive amounts of PTH secreted by pathologic parathyroid glands cause disturbances of mineral and/or skeletal homeostasis. The predominant clinical features are the result of disturbances of serum calcium and bone metabolism due to prolonged hypersecretion of PTH.[44,45] The skeletal lesion of generalized fibrous osteodystrophy (osteitis fibrosa) is characterized by increased bone resorption, decreased radiographic density, and incomplete fractures.[52]

Primary Hyperparathyroidism

Parathyroid hormone is produced in excess of normal in primary hyperparathyroidism by a functional lesion in the parathyroid gland for no useful purpose. This disease is encountered less frequently in older dogs

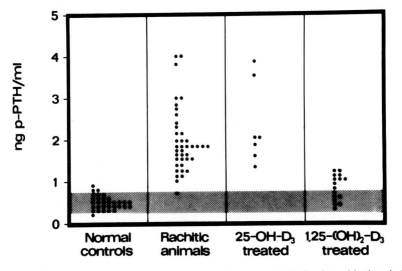

Fig. 4-49. Elevated plasma immunoreactive parathyroid hormone levels in pigs with vitamin D-dependent rickets compared with control pigs. Parathyroid hormone levels returned to the normal range following administration of 1,25-dihydroxycholecalciferol (25-OH-D₃). (Courtesy of Dr. R. Wilke, 1979.)

PARATHYROID-VITAMIN D INTERACTIONS

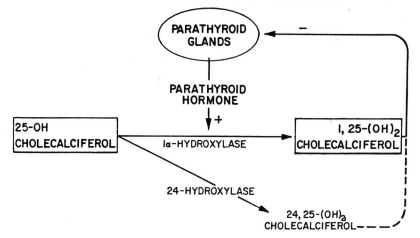

Fig. 4-50. Negative feedback exerted by vitamin D metabolites on parathyroid chief cells to decrease the rate of parathyroid hormone secretion, which in turn diminishes the rate of formation of additional 1,25-dihydroxycholecalciferol.

than is the relatively common secondary hyperparathyroidism.

The normal control mechanisms for PTH secretion by the concentration of blood calcium ion are lost in primary hyperparathyroidism. Hormone secretion is autonomous and the parathyroid gland produces excessive amounts of hormone in spite of a sustained increase of blood calcium. Cells of the renal tubules are particularly sensitive to alterations in the amount of circulating PTH. The hormone acts on these cells initially to promote the excretion of phosphorus and the retention of calcium (Fig. 4-51). A prolonged increased secretion of PTH results in accelerated osteocytic and osteoclastic bone resorption. Mineral is removed from the skeleton and replaced by immature fibrous connective tissue. The bone lesion of fibrous osteodystrophy is generalized throughout the skeleton but is accentuated in local areas.

The lesion responsible for the excessive secretion of PTH in dogs usually is an adenoma composed of active chief cells with interspersed oxyphil and water-clear cells.[53,172,179,345] Chief cell adenomas usually are single and result in considerable enlargement of the parathyroid gland (Fig. 4-52). They can be located either in the cervical region near the thyroid or infrequently within the thoracic cavity near the base of the heart.[68] Other lesions occasionally associated with primary hyperparathyroidism are chief cell hyperplasia, and chief cell carcinoma.[55,246] C-cells in the thyroid gland are usually hyperplastic (Fig. 4-52) but are unable to return the blood calcium to normal.

The functional disturbances observed clinically are the result of weakening of bones by excessive resorption. Lameness due to fractures of long bones may occur after relatively minor physical trauma. Compression fractures of vertebral bodies can exert pressure on the spinal cord and nerves resulting in motor and/or sensory dysfunction. Excessive resorption of cancellous bone of the skull resulting in a loosening or loss of teeth from alveolar sockets and hyperostosis of the mandible and maxilla due to proliferation of woven bone have been observed in dogs with primary hyperparathyroidism. Radiographic evaluation reveals areas of subperiosteal cortical resorption, loss of lamina dura around the teeth (Fig. 4-53), soft tissue mineralization, bone cysts (Fig. 4-54), and a generalized decrease in bone density with multiple fractures. Mineralization of renal tubules (Fig. 4-55) and formation of multiple calculi[168] (Fig. 4-56)

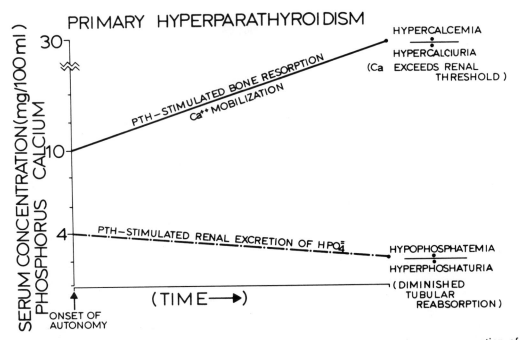

Fig. 4-51. Alterations in serum calcium and phosphorus in response to an autonomous secretion of parathyroid hormone in primary hyperparathyroidism.

may occur in advanced cases of primary hyperparathyroidism in the dog with substantial elevations of blood calcium. Hypercalcemia results in anorexia, vomiting, constipation, depression, and generalized muscular weakness due to decreased neuromuscular excitability.[242]

The most important and practical laboratory test to aid in establishing the diagnosis of primary hyperparathyroidism is quantitation of total blood calcium. Although other laboratory findings may be variable, hypercalcemia is a consistent finding and results from accelerated release of calcium from bone (Fig. 4-51). The blood calcium of normal animals is near 10 mg/dl with some variation, de-

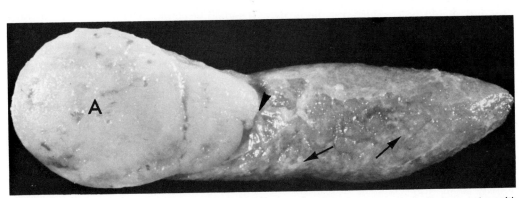

Fig. 4-52. Parathyroid adenoma (A) in the external parathyroid gland removed surgically from a dog with primary hyperparathyroidism. The neoplasm is sharply demarcated (arrow head) from the adjacent thyroid parenchyma. The focal light areas in the thyroid represent areas of C-cell hyperplasia (arrows) stimulated by the long-term hypercalcemia.

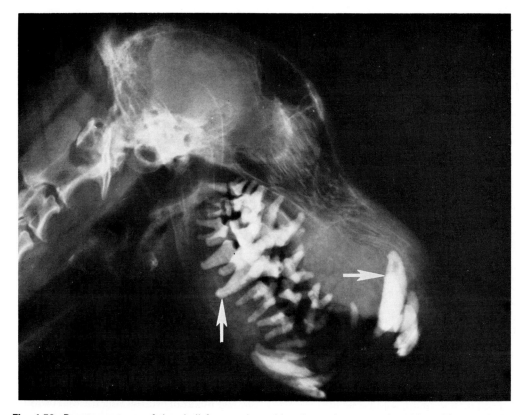

Fig. 4-53. Roentgenogram of the skull from a dog with primary hyperparathyroidism (Fig. 4-52). As a result of the chronic hypersecretion of PTH the cancellous bone of the maxilla, mandible, and skull is nearly resorbed completely and replaced by an extensive proliferation of fibrous connective tissue, unmineralized osteoid, and neocapillaries. Lamina dura dentes and alveolar socket bone are extensively resorbed and the teeth are loosely embedded in connective tissue (arrows).

pending upon the analytical method employed as well as the age and diet of the animal. Calcium values consistently above 12 mg/dl should be considered to be in the hypercalcemic range. The blood phosphorus is low (4 mg/dl or less) or in the low-normal range due to inhibition of renal tubular reabsorption of phosphorus by the excess PTH. Alkaline phosphatase activity (an enzyme involved in both apposition and resorption of bone) may be elevated in the serum of animals with overt bone disease. The increased activity of this enzyme is thought to result from a compensatory increase in osteoblastic activity along trabeculae as a response to mechanical stress in bones weakened by excessive resorption.

Successful removal of the functional para-thyroid lesion results in a rapid decrease in circulating PTH levels because the half-life of PTH in plasma is approximately 20 minutes. It should be emphasized that plasma calcium levels in patients with overt bone disease may decrease rapidly and be subnormal within 12 to 24 hours after operation, resulting in severe hypocalcemic tetany. Serum calcium levels should be monitored frequently following surgical removal of a parathyroid neoplasm. Postoperative hypocalcemia (5 mg/dl and lower) can be the result of (1) depressed secretory activity of chief cells due to long-term suppression by the chronic hypercalcemia or injury to the remaining parathyroid tissue during surgery, (2) abruptly decreased bone resorption due to lowered PTH levels, and (3) accelerated mineralization of osteoid matrix

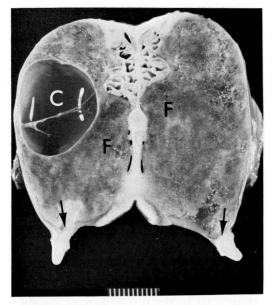

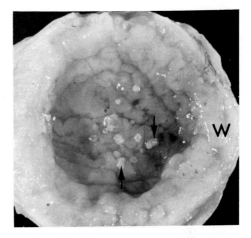

Fig. 4-56. Multiple small calculi (arrows) in lumen of the urinary bladder from a dog with primary hyperparathyroidism. The wall of the urinary bladder (W) is thickened in response to the chronic irritation of the cystic calculi.

Fig. 4-54. Cross section of maxilla of a dog with primary hyperparathyroidism illustrating severe hyperostotic fibrous osteodystrophy. Extensive proliferation of woven bone consisting of fibroblasts and osteoblasts with deposition of unmineralized osteoid (F) partially occlude the nasal cavity. A cystic area (C) with extensive bone resorption is present in one side of the maxilla that contains blood and fibrin strands. The teeth are embedded in connective tissue and are freely movable in the sockets (arrows). The scale represents 1 cm.

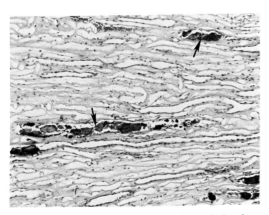

Fig. 4-55. Mineralization of collecting tubules (arrows) in the kidney of a dog with long-term hypercalcemia caused by primary hyperparathyroidism. 62 ×.

formed by the hyperplastic osteoblasts but previously prevented from undergoing mineralization by the elevated PTH levels. Infusions of calcium gluconate to maintain the serum calcium between 7.5 and 9.0 mg/dl, feeding high calcium diets, and supplemental vitamin D therapy will correct this serious postoperative complication.

Primary hyperparathyroidism also has been described in young German shepherds associated with autonomous chief cell parathyroid hyperplasia. The pups develop hypercalcemia, hypophosphatemia, increased immunoreactive parathyroid hormone, and increased fractional clearance of inorganic phosphate in the urine.[321] Clinical signs include stunted growth, muscular weakness, polyuria, polydipsia, and a diffuse reduction in bone density. Intravenous infusion of calcium failed to suppress the autonomous secretion of parathyroid hormone by the diffuse hyperplasia of chief cells in all parathyroids. Other lesions include nodular hyperplasia of thyroid C-cells and widespread mineralization of lungs, kidney, and gastric mucosa. The disease appears to be inherited as an autosomal recessive trait in dogs.

Renal Secondary Hyperparathyroidism

Secondary hyperparathyroidism as a complication of chronic renal failure is a metabolic disease characterized by an excessive, but not autonomous, rate of PTH secretion. This disorder is encountered most frequently in dogs but also occurs in cats and other animal species. The secretion of hormone by the hyperplastic parathyroid glands in this disorder usually remains responsive to fluctuations in blood calcium.

The primary etiologic mechanism in renal hyperparathyroidism is a long-standing, progressive renal disease resulting in severely impaired function. Chronic renal insufficiency in older dogs results from interstitial nephritis, glomerulonephritis, nephrosclerosis, or amyloidosis. Several congenital anomalies such as cortical hypoplasia,[165] polycystic kidneys, and bilateral hydronephrosis may result in renal insufficiency in younger dogs. When the renal disease progresses to the point where there is significant reduction in glomerular filtration rate, phosphorus is retained and progressive hyperphosphatemia develops (Fig. 4-57). Although the concentration of blood phosphorus has no direct regulatory influence on the synthesis and secretion of PTH, it may, when elevated, contribute to parathyroid stimulation by virtue of its ability to lower blood calcium.

Parathyroid stimulation in patients with chronic renal disease can be attributed directly to the hypocalcemia that develops during the pathogenesis of the disease. As the phosphorus concentration increases, blood calcium decreases reciprocally.[172,174] Impaired intestinal absorption of calcium due to an acquired defect in vitamin D metabolism also plays a significant role in the development of hypocalcemia in chronic renal insufficiency and uremia.[14,34] Chronic renal disease impairs the production of 1,25-dihydroxycholecalciferol (biologically active metabolite of vitamin D) by the kidney thereby diminishing intestinal calcium transport and leading to the development of hypocalcemia.[194,232] Initially, the elevated blood phosphorus depresses the activity of the 1α-hydroxylase in the kidney. In the later stage of chronic renal disease there are decreased numbers of tubular epithelial cells with 1α-hydroxylase activity to form the active metabolite of vitamin D.

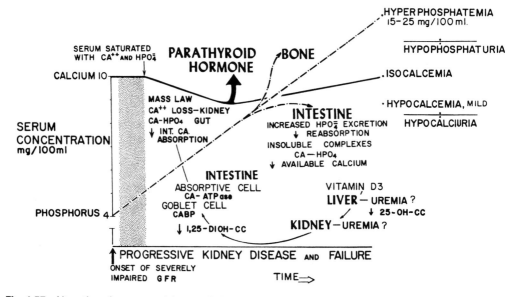

Fig. 4-57. Alterations in serum calcium and phosphorus during the pathogenesis of secondary hyperparathyroidism associated with progressive renal failure.

All four parathyroid glands are enlarged due to organellar hypertrophy initially and cellular hyperplasia later as compensatory mechanisms to increase hormonal synthesis and secretion in response to the hypocalcemic stimulus (Fig. 4-58). Since the parathyroid gland stores comparatively little preformed hormone, the rate of peptide synthesis appears to be rate-limiting for hormonal secretion. Although the parathyroids are not autonomous, the concentration of PTH in the peripheral blood in patients with chronic renal failure may exceed that of primary hyperparathyroidism. A greatly increased number and size of chief cells are required, therefore, to sustain the vastly increased rates of hormonal secretion in patients with long-standing renal disease.

Parathyroid hormone accelerates osteocytic and osteoclastic resorption, results in release of stored calcium from bone, and returns the blood calcium toward normal (Fig. 4-57). The long-lasting increase in bone resorption eventually results in the metabolic bone disease associated with chronic renal insufficiency. Progressive glomerular and tubular dysfunction with loss of target cells interferes with expression of the phosphaturic response by the increased circulating PTH in renal disease. Phosphorus is retained and the blood concentration continues to rise in spite

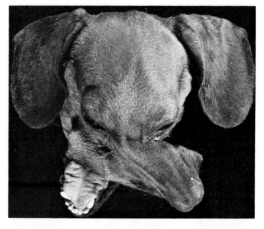

Fig. 4-59. Renal secondary hyperparathyroidism in a 5-year-old Dachshund illustrating extensive resorption of cancellous bone. The maxilla and mandible were both extremely pliable and could be displaced considerably with minimal pressure.

of the secondary hyperparathyroidism (Fig. 4-57).

Although skeletal involvement is generalized with hyperparathyroidism, it does not affect all parts uniformly. Bone lesions become apparent earlier and reach a more advanced degree in certain areas. Resorption of alveolar socket bone and loss of lamina dura dentes occur early in the course of the disease. This results in loose teeth which may be dislodged easily and interfere with mastication. Cancellous bones of the maxilla and mandible also are sites of predilection in hyperparathyroidism. Due to the accelerated resorption the bones become softened and, readily pliable (i.e. "rubber-jaw disease"), and the jaws fail to close properly (Figs. 4-59 and 4-60). Long bones of the abaxial skeleton are less dramatically affected. Lameness, stiff gait, and fractures after relatively minor trauma may result from the increased bone resorption. Areas of subperiosteal resorption by numerous osteoclasts may disrupt the osseous attachment of tendons, leading to elevation and stretching of the periosteum, bone pain, and an inability to support the body's weight.

A small percentage of dogs with chronic kidney disease will have moderate hypercalcemia.[102] Although the exact mechanism for

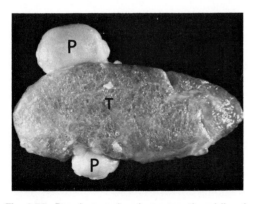

Fig. 4-58. Renal secondary hyperparathyroidism in a dog illustrating enlargement of external and internal parathyroids (P) due to hypertrophy and hyperplasia of active chief cells. The adjacent thyroid gland (T) appears normal.

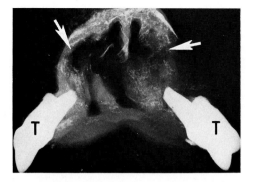

Fig. 4-60. Roentgenogram of cross section of maxilla from the dog with renal secondary hyperparathyroidism illustrated in Fig. 4-59. Under the influence of a long-term excess of PTH the cancellous bone of the maxilla is nearly completely resorbed and partially replaced by immature fibrous connective tissue, neocapillaries, and spicules of poorly mineralized osteoid (arrows). Alveolar socket bone has been resorbed and the teeth (T) are loose.

the development of hypercalcemia with renal disease is uncertain, it may be the result of diminished PTH degradation by the damaged kidney,[108,151] decreased urinary calcium excretion, or hypercitricemia with the increased formation of calcium-citrate complexes.

Nutritional Secondary Hyperparathyroidism

The increased secretion of parathyroid hormone with this metabolic disorder is a compensatory mechanism directed against a disturbance in mineral homeostasis induced by nutritional imbalances. The disease occurs commonly in cats,[283,290] dogs, certain non-human primates,[155] and laboratory animals, as well as in many farm animal species.[41,114,174,202]

Dietary mineral imbalances of etiologic importance in the pathogenesis of nutritional secondary hyperparathyroidism are (1) a low content of calcium, (2) excessive phosphorus with normal or low calcium, and (3) inadequate amounts of vitamin D_3. The significant end result is hypocalcemia which results in parathyroid stimulation. A diet low in calcium fails to supply the daily requirement even though a greater proportion of ingested

calcium is absorbed and hypocalcemia develops (Fig. 4-61). Ingestion of excessive phosphorus results in increased intestinal absorption and elevation of blood phosphorus. Hyperphosphatemia does not stimulate the parathyroid gland directly but does so indirectly by virute of its ability to lower blood calcium when the serum becomes saturated with respect to these two ions. Diets containing inadequate amounts of vitamin D_3 (even with normal levels of vitamin D_2) cause diminished intestinal calcium absorption and hypocalcemia in certain New World monkeys.

In response to the nutritionally induced hypocalcemia all parathyroid glands undergo cellular hypertrophy and hyperplasia.[50] Active chief cells stimulated by diet-induced hypocalcemia become larger and more tightly arranged together (Fig. 4-62) compared to those in parathyroids of normal animals (Fig. 4-63). Since kidney function is normal, the increased levels of PTH result in diminished renal tubular reabsorption of phosphorus, increased reabsorption of calcium, and blood levels return toward normal (Fig. 4-61). In addition, bone resorption is accelerated and release of calcium elevates blood calcium levels to the low-normal range. Continued ingestion of the imbalanced diet sustains the state of compensatory hyperparathyroidism, which leads to progressive development of the metabolic bone disease.

Nutritional secondary hyperparathyroidism develops in young cats fed a predominantly meat diet.[247] For example, beef heart or liver contains minimal amounts of calcium (7 to 9 mg/100 g) and has a markedly imbalanced calcium to phosphorus (Ca : P) ratio (1 : 20 to 1 : 50). An adequate diet for kittens up to 6 months of age should supply 200 to 400 mg calcium and approximately 200 μg iodine daily, and from 10,000 to 15,000 IU of vitamin A weekly.[290]

Kittens fed beef heart or liver develop functional disturbances within approximately 4 weeks. Clinical signs are dominated by disturbances in locomotion manifested by a reluctance to move, posterior lameness, and an incoordinated gait (Fig. 4-64).[283] The cor-

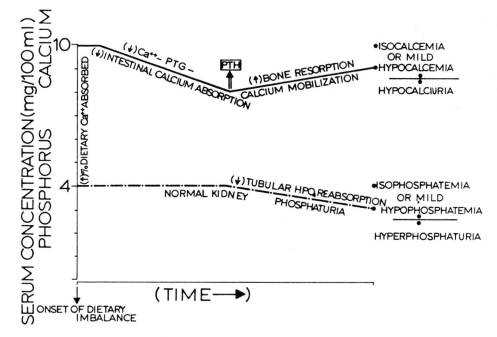

Fig. 4-61. Alterations in serum calcium and phosphorus in the pathogenesis of nutritional secondary hyperparathyroidism caused by feeding a diet low in calcium or deficient in cholecalciferol but with normal amount of phosphorus.

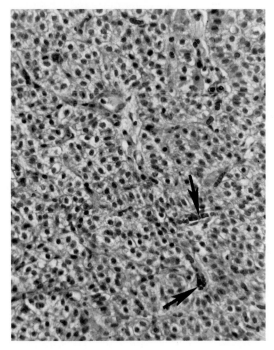

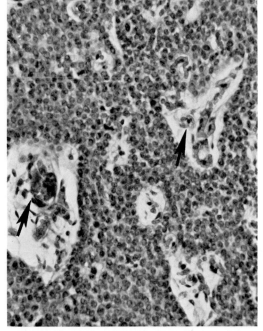

Fig. 4-62. Chief cell hyperplasia in the parathyroid of a cat with nutritional hyperparathyroidism. The hyperactive chief cells are enlarged, lightly eosinophilic, closely packed together with narrow perivascular spaces. 315 ×.

Fig. 4-63. Chief cells in parathyroid of a cat fed a balanced control diet at same magnification as Fig. 4-62. Chief cells are smaller (especially in the cytoplasmic area), more loosely arranged, and perivascular spaces are more prominent. 315 ×.

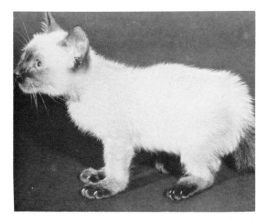

Fig. 4-64. Kitten with secondary hyperparathyroidism of nutritional origin. The kitten was reluctant to move, owing to bone pain, and there was lateral deviation of the paws.

tex of long bones is progressively thinned due to increased reabsorption, and the medullary cavity is widened. Affected kittens become quiet, are reluctant to play, and assume a sitting position or are in sternal recumbency. Normal activities may result in sudden onset of severe lameness due to incomplete or folding fractures of one or more bones. The high content of digestible protein (over 50% on a wet basis) and fat promotes rapid growth in kittens fed beef heart. They appear well-nourished and their hair coat maintains a good luster.

Synonyms used to describe this metabolic disorder in cats have included osteogenesis imperfecta, juvenile osteoporosis, and paperbone or Siamese cat disease. In general, kittens are more susceptible and develop more severe skeletal lesions than adult cats fed a similar diet. The disease develops rapidly because the dietary imbalance is wide and the skeletal metabolic rate of kittens is high. Vertebral fractures with compression of spinal cord and paralysis are common complications in kittens but are infrequent in adult cats (Fig. 4-65).

The feeding of a monotonous meat diet to dogs of any age results in secondary hyperparathyroidism with the development of skeletal disease of varying severity by similar

mechanisms as described previously.[175,289] The low calcium content and unfavorable Ca : P of nonsupplemented all-meat diets are unable to fulfill the daily requirements either for growing pups (240 mg calcium and 200 mg phosphorus/lb body weight/day) or adult dogs (120 mg calcium and 100 mg phosphorus/lb body weight/day).

Lameness is the initial functional disturbance in growing dogs and may vary from a slight limp to complete inability to walk. The bones are painful on palpation and folding fractures of long bones and vertebrae are not uncommon.[115,210] Clinical signs often are related to resorption of jaw bones in adult dogs. Parathyroid hormone-stimulated resorption of alveolar socket bone results in loss of lamina dura dentes, loosening and subsequent loss of teeth from their sockets, and recession of gingiva with partial root exposure in advanced cases.[117,175,254,288,323]

Secondary hyperparathyroidism of nutritional origin also occurs in collections of aviculturists (domestic and captive birds),[11,186,326] zoological parks (caged lions and tigers, green iguanas, crocodiles, etc.),[5,6,269,325,327,359] and laboratory animals used for research (ground squirrels, nonhuman primates, etc.).[155,173,181,269]

In horses the most frequent nutritional imbalance involves the ingestion of excessive phosphorus. This results in an increased intestinal absorption of phosphorus and elevation of the blood phosphorus concentration. Hyperphosphatemia does not stimulate the parathyroid gland directly but does so indirectly by virtue of its ability to lower blood

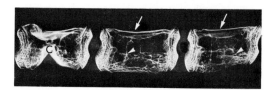

Fig. 4-65. Roentgenogram of lumbar vertebrae from a kitten with nutritional hyperparathyroidism. Note the loss of trabecular bone (arrow heads), thinning of the cortex (arrows), and cavitation (C) of the body of the vertebrae.

calcium. Horses that develop the disease usually have been fed high-grain diets with below-average quality roughage. Evidence of high phosphorus intake may be difficult to establish inasmuch as the excess phosphorus may be fed by the owner in the form of a bran supplement added to a grain diet in order to improve the health of the horse. The diet usually is palatable and nutritious except for the unbalanced phosphorus (excessive amounts) and calcium (marginal or deficient) content. A diet deficient in calcium fails to supply the daily requirement even though a greater proportion of ingested calcium is absorbed and hypocalcemia develops. Occasionally, horses may develop nutritional hyperparathyroidism after pasturing on grasses with a high oxalate content. This results in intestinal malabsorption of calcium.[328] The oxalates appear to form insoluble complexes with calcium in the intestine resulting in an elevated fecal calcium: phosphorus ratio (2.35 : 1) compared with horses on a similar calcium and phosphorus intake but without the oxalate-rich plants (fecal calcium: phosphorus ratio 1.2 : 1). The interference in intestinal calcium absorption results in the development of progressive hypocalcemia that leads to parathyroid stimulation and development of the metabolic bone disease.

Initial clinical signs in horses with nutritional secondary hyperparathyroidism usually include a transitory shifting lameness in one or more limbs, generalized tenderness of joints, and a stilted gait.[174] The lameness develops as a result of increased osteoclastic resorption of outer circumferential lamellae with disruption of tendinous insertions and bone trabeculae supporting the articular cartilage resulting in disruption of joint cartilage on weight-bearing. Resorption of alveolar socket bone and loss of lamina dura dentes occur early and may result in loose teeth. Later in the course of the disease, severe lesions develop in bones of the skull, especially the maxilla and mandible, resulting in bilateral firm enlargements of the facial bones immediately above and anterior to the facial crests. The horizontal rami of the mandibles

are irregularly thickened by a progressive hyperostotic fibrous osteodystrophy ("big head") that develops in horses with nutritional secondary hyperparathyroidism. The hyperostosis of skull bones results from osteoid and fibrous connective tissue deposition in excess of the volume of bone resorbed. The chronic excess intake of phosphorus and increased secretion of PTH result in stimulation of osteoblasts to form osteoid in excess of the amount of bone resorbed by osteoclasts and progressive enlargement of skeletal bones. The hyperostotic fibrous osteodystrophy may impinge upon the nasal cavity, resulting in dyspnea, especially after exertion.

Changes in urine calcium and phosphorus are more consistent and useful in the clinical diagnosis of nutritional secondary hyperparathyroidism in horses. The increased secretion of PTH acts on the normal kidneys to markedly increase urinary phosphorus excretion but decrease calcium loss in the urine compared to normal horses.[161] Blood urea nitrogen, serum creatinine, and other parameters used to assess renal function are within normal limits in horses with nutritional hyperparathyroidism. Serum alkaline phosphatase levels often are in the high normal range or are elevated in horses with overt bone disease, reflecting the increased osteoblastic and osteoclastic activity in hyperparathyroidism. Under experimental conditions, horses fed a high phosphorus diet (phosphorus, 1.4%; calcium 0.7%) are able to more rapidly normalize their blood calcium following an ethylene-diaminetetra-acetic acid (EDTA)-induced hypocalcemia than controls fed a balanced diet (phosphorus, 0.6%; calcium 0.7%) owing to the increased parathyroid activity.[7]

This metabolic disorder has been recognized in primates for many years and has received numerous appellations, including cage paralysis, simian bone disease, and osteomalacia. Hypocalcemia resulting from either inadequate dietary vitamin D_3 intake in New World laboratory primates housed indoors or excessive phosphorus in the diet of pet monkeys leads to long-term stimulation of the

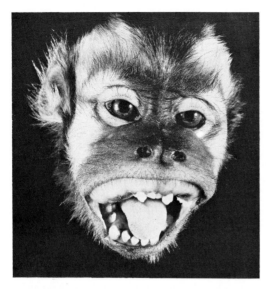

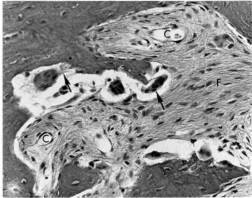

Fig. 4-67. Osteoclastic resorption (arrows) of trabecular bone in the rib of a New World primate with nutritional hyperparathyroidism. The long-term excess of PTH stimulates the activation of increased numbers of osteoclasts that break down bone which is subsequently replaced by a proliferation of immature fibrous connective tissue (F) and neocapillaries (C). 62 ×.

Fig. 4-66. Nutritional secondary hyperparathyroidism in a pet monkey with severe maxillary hyperostosis causing distortion of the face, partial displacement of the teeth, and difficulty in mastication of food. The mouth could not be closed completely because of the proliferation of fibrous tissue and deposition of poorly mineralized osteoid (i.e. woven bone).

parathyroid glands. The monkeys become inactive, offer less resistance to handling, and have difficulty masticating their food. In the more advanced stages there is maxillary hyperostosis due to osteoid deposition and proliferation of fibrous connective tissue (Fig. 4-66), joint pain, and distortion of limbs by palpable fractures without mineralized calluses. There is radiographic evidence of generalized skeletal demineralization, loss of lamina dura dentes, subperiosteal cortical bone resorption, bowing deformities, and multiple folding fractures of long bones. Cortical bone is thinned due to the activity of increased numbers of osteoclasts (Fig. 4-67). The resorbed bone is partially replaced by the proliferation of immature fibroblasts and neocapillaries.

Hypercalcemia of Malignancy (Pseudohyperparathyroidism)

Pseudohyperparathyroidism is a metabolic disorder in which PTH-like proteins or other bone-resorbing substances are secreted in excessive amounts by malignant tumors of nonparathyroid origin. Tumor cells in human beings and animals have been shown to produce several humoral substances that induce calcium mobilization from bone, including PTH-like protein(s),[37,213,230,253,298] prostaglandins (PG E2),[112,291,316,324] osteoclast-activating factor, colony-stimulating activity, and transforming growth factor.[220,221]

There are three different pathogenic mechanisms of cancer-associated hypercalcemia: (1) humoral hypercalcemia of malignancy (HHM), (2) hypercalcemia induced by metastases of solid tumors to bone, and (3) hematologic malignancies.[217] Humoral hypercalcemia of malignancy is a syndrome associated with diverse animal and human malignant neoplasms.[216] Characteristic clinical findings in patients with HHM include hypercalcemia, hypophosphatemia, hypercalciuria (often with decreased fractional calcium excretion), increased fractional excretion of phosphorus, increased nephrogenous cAMP, and increased osteoclastic bone resorption.[216,302] The clinical disturbances of HHM are due to the release of humoral factors from the neoplasms which have effects distant to the site of the tumor, viz., bone, kidney, and intestine.[218]

Malignancies that are associated with HHM and have been well studied include the adenocarcinoma derived from apocrine glands of the anal sac of the dog,[208,273] the Rice-500 Leydig cell tumor[266] and Walker carcinosarcoma of the rat,[219] and squamous cell carcinoma and renal cell carcinoma of human beings.[306] However, there exist multiple other neoplasms that induce HHM in animals and humans. Current evidence suggests that the humoral factors associated with HHM are parathyroid hormone-like peptides and/or transforming growth factors.[218] Parathyroid hormone (PTH)-like factors bind to the PTH receptor of bone and kidney, but do not cross-react immunologically with native PTH. Recently, PTH-related proteins have been purified from three human tumors associated with HHM.[37,213,230] The PTH-related proteins have identical N-terminal sequences and share sequence homology to native PTH at the amino-terminal end of the molecule.

Hypercalcemia Associated with Apocrine Adenocarcinoma

Rijnberk and co-workers[267,268] described a syndrome of pseudohyperparathyroidism in elderly female dogs associated with perirectal adenocarcinomas. The dogs had persistent hypercalcemia and hypophosphatemia that returned to normal following surgical excision of the neoplasm in the perirectal area. The hypercalcemia persisted following removal of the parathyroid gland. Immunoreactive PTH levels were within the normal range for the dog but were inappropriately high for the degree of hypercalcemia.

Meuten et al.[205] reported detailed clinical, macroscopic, and histopathologic features of adenocarcinomas arising from the apocrine gland of the anal sac in dogs. This unique clinical syndrome occurred in aged (mean 10 years), predominantly female (92%) dogs, and was characterized by persistent hypercalcemia and hypophosphatemia (Table 4-3). Serum calcium values ranged from 11.4 to 24.0 mg/dl. Tumor ablation resulted in a prompt return to normocalcemia, but the hypercalcemia recurred with tumor regrowth, suggesting the neoplastic cells were producing a humoral substance that increased calcium mobilization. All tumors had histopathologic features of malignancy and 96% had metastasized to iliac and sublumbar lymph nodes.

Functional disturbances in dogs with pseudohyperparathyroidism include generalized muscular weakness, anorexia, vomiting,

Table 4-3 Serum and Urine Data From Dogs with Apocrine Gland Adenocarcinoma and Control Dogs.*

	Control Dogs (n = 15)	Normocalcemic Tumor-Control Dogs (n = 6)	Apocrine Ca Hypercalcemia (n = 10)
Serum calcium (mg/dl)	9.7 ± 0.13	9.4 ± 0.14	15.7 ± 0.56[†]
Serum phosphorus (mg/dl)	4.1 ± 0.13	4.2 ± 0.31	3.0 ± 0.42
Serum albumin (g/dl)	3.1 ± 0.12	2.8 ± 0.08	3.1 ± 0.13
Serum creatinine (mg/dl)	0.9 ± 0.05	1.0 ± 0.07	1.6 ± 0.25
Serum ALP (IU/liter)	40 ± 4	54 ± 9	116 ± 34
Urine phosphorus (mg/dl GF)	0.76 ± 0.07	0.54 ± 0.12	2.00 ± 0.72
Serum 1,25-DiOH-CC (pg/ml)	26 ± 5	16 ± 4	23 ± 5
Plasma PGE$_2$M	19.0 ± 4.2	22.2 ± 9.9	21.0 ± 4.8

* Values are expressed as mean ± standard error.
[†] Significant difference (P < 0.05) compared with control dogs and normocalcemic control dogs.
++ Different number of dogs.

n, number; *apocrine CA*, apocrine gland adenocarcinoma and hypercalcemia; *ALP*, alkaline phosphatase; *GF*, glomerular filtrate; *1,25-DiOH-CC*, 1,25-dihydroxyvitamin D; PGE$_2$M; 13,14-dihydro-15-retro-prostaglandin E2.

From Meuten, D. G., Segre, G.V., Capen, C. C. et al. (1983)

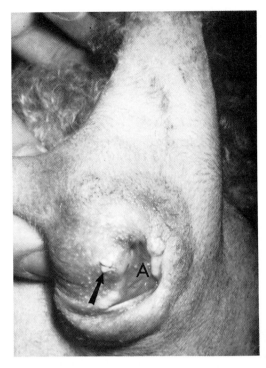

Fig. 4-68. Cancer-associated hypercalcemia. Perirectal region of a dog with hypercalcemia and a small adenocarcinoma (arrow) derived from apocrine glands of the anal sac. (A, anus; T, tail).

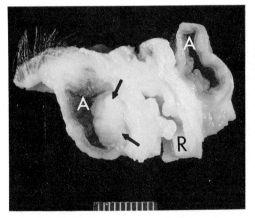

Fig. 4-69. Transverse section of perineum from a female dog with hypercalcemia and an adenocarcinoma derived from apocrine glands of the anal sac. Anal sacs (A) are present on both sides of the rectum (R). A tumor nodule (arrows) 1 cm in diameter arising in the wall of the left anal sac protrudes into its lumen. The scale represents 1 cm. (From Meuten DJ, Cooper BJ, Capen CC et al., 1983.)

bradycardia, depression, polyuria, and polydipsia. These clinical signs are the result primarily of severe hypercalcemia and complicate the problems associated with the malignant neoplasm.

Apocrine adenocarcinomas develop as a firm mass in the perirectal area, ventral-lateral to the anus, in close association with the anal sac, but are not attached to the overlying skin (Figs. 4-68 and 4-69). This unique neoplasm develops from apocrine glands of the anal sac (Fig. 4-70) and forms distinctive glandular acini with projections of apical cytoplasm extending into a lumen (Fig. 4-71). It is histologically distinct from the more common perianal (circumanal) gland tumor that develops primarily in male dogs. The major-

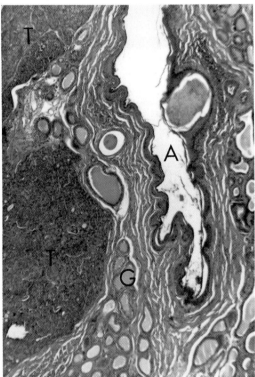

Fig. 4-70. A close anatomical relationship exists between the apocrine adenocarcinoma (T) and normal apocrine glands (G) in the wall of the anal sac. The anal sac (A) is lined by stratified squamous epithelium (H&E, × 125) (From Meuten DJ, Cooper BJ, Capen CC et al., 1981.)

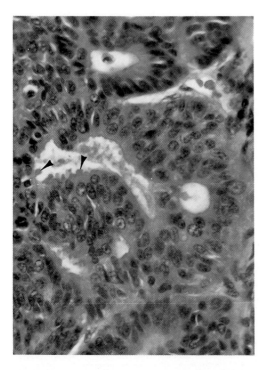

Fig. 4-71. Biopsy of an adenocarcinoma arising from apocrine glands in the wall of the anal sac from a dog with persistent hypercalcemia. The glandular acini are lined by single or multiple layers of columnar neoplastic cells with characteristic apical projection of cytoplasm into the lumen (arrowheads). The acini contain varying amounts of colloid-like material and occasional inflammatory cells (H&E, × 315) (From Meuten DJ, Cooper BJ, Capen CC et al., 1981.)

PTH-containing storage granules in chief cells of normal parathyroid glands; however, additional studies are required to determine if they contain hormonal activity.

The parathyroid glands are small and difficult to locate or not visible macroscopically in dogs with cancer-associated hypercalcemia.[205] Atrophic parathyroid glands in dogs with apocrine adenocarcinomas were characterized by narrow cords of inactive chief cells with an abundant fibrous connective tissue stroma and widened perivascular spaces (Fig. 4-75). The inactive chief cells have a markedly reduced cytoplasmic area, prominent hyperchromatic nuclei, and are closely packed together. These findings are interpreted to suggest that the apocrine adenocarcinomas do not produce a susbstance that stimulates PTH secretion but rather the parathyroid glands are responding to the persistent hyper-

ity of neoplasms are histologically bimorphic with glandular and solid areas (Fig. 4-72). The solid pattern of arrangement of neoplastic cells is characterized by sheets, microlobules, and packets separated by a thin fibrovascular stroma. Pseudorosettes are common in solid areas adjacent to small blood vessels.

The tumor cells in adenocarcinomas derived from apocrine glands of the anal sac ultrastructurally contain a well-developed rough endoplasmic reticulum, clusters of free ribosomes, large mitochondria, and prominent Golgi apparatuses (Fig. 4-73). Small membrane-limited secretory granules are present occasionally in the apical cytoplasm of neoplastic cells (Fig. 4-74). These granules are of similar size and electron density as

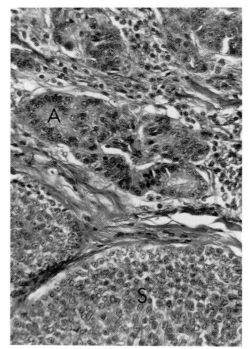

Fig. 4-72. Characteristic bimorphic growth pattern in adenocarcinoma derived from apocrine glands of the anal sac with adjacent solid areas (S) and acini (A) formed by neoplastic cells. (H&E, × 125) (From Meuten DJ, Cooper BJ, Capen CC et al., 1981.)

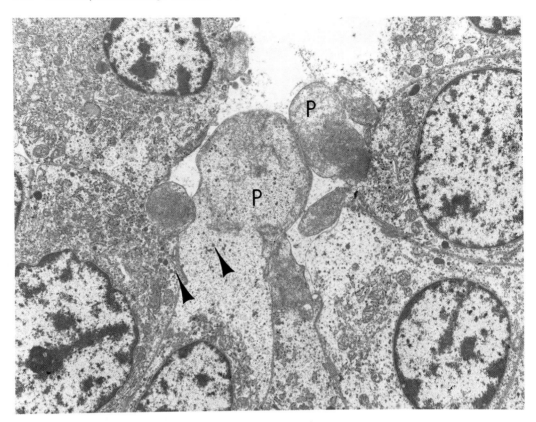

Fig. 4-73. Apical projections (P) of cytoplasm into glandular acini in a dog with persistent hypercalcemia associated with an adenocarcinoma arising from apocrine glands of the anal sac. Small, electron-dense granules (arrowheads) are present in the cytoplasm of neoplastic cells. These granules are similar morphologically to parathyroid hormone-containing secretory granules in chief cells of the parathyroid gland. 4,000 ×.

calcemia by undergoing trophic atrophy. Thyroid parafollicular (C) cells often respond to the persistent elevation in blood calcium levels by undergoing diffuse or nodular hyperplasia.[205]

Skeletal demineralization in dogs with pseudohyperparathyroidism is mild in comparison with some other causes of hypercalcemia (e.g. primary hyperparathyroidism) and usually undetectable by conventional roentgenographic methods. Neoplastic cells from the perirectal adenocarcinomas rarely metastasize to bone and caused osteolysis.[205] Variable numbers of osteoclasts have been detected on bone surfaces in dogs with marked hypercalcemia, possibly reflecting different states in the course of the disease

and phases of bone remodeling activity (Fig. 4-76).

Histomorphometric analysis indicates that dogs with apocrine adenocarcinomas and hypercalcemia have significantly decreased trabecular bone volume as compared with age-matched control dogs. Total resorptive surface (Howship's lacunae with and without osteoclasts) is increased significantly, as are the number of osteoclasts per millimeter of trabecular bone. By comparison, dogs with primary hyperparathyroidism also have significantly increased total resorptive surface and numbers of osteoclasts.[207]

The mean concentration of immunoreactive parathyroid hormone (iPTH) in the plasma of dogs with hypercalcemia and apo-

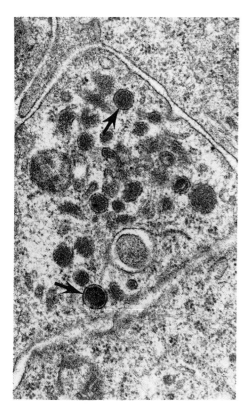

Fig. 4-74. Cancer-associated hypercalcemia. Small (200 to 400 nm in diameter) electron-dense secretory granules (arrows) in neoplastic cells with an electron-dense core, closely applied limiting membrane, and narrow submembranous space in a dog with hypercalcemia associated with an adenocarcinoma derived from apocrine glands of the anal sac (original magnification × 34,300). (From Meuten DJ, Capen CC, Kociba GJ et al., 1983.)

crine adenocarcinomas was 168 ± 40 pg/ml with a range of undetectable to 266 pg/ml (Fig. 4-77).[207,208] The concentration of iPTH in dogs with apocrine adenocarcinomas is not significantly different from the concentration in control dogs (322 ± 33 pg/ml) or normocalcemic tumor controls (264 ± 33 pg/ml) or normocalcemic tumor controls (264 ± 46 pg/ml) but is decreased significantly compared with that of dogs with primary hyperparathyroidism. The concentration of iPTH in dogs with renal failure is markedly increased compared with that of control dogs (Fig. 4-77). Plasma iPTH levels are undetectable in dogs with primary hypoparathyroidism but in-

creased in dogs with primary hyperparathyroidism (mean: 1540 pg/ml) (Fig. 4-78).[208]

Urea-hydrochloric acid extracts from apocrine adenocarcinoma, tumors from normocalcemic control dogs, and lymph nodes from control dogs without tumors have been assayed for iPTH before and after precipitation with trichloroacetic acid. Immunoreactive PTH was not detected in tissue extracts from any tumor or lymph node. The iPTH concentrations in extracts of parathyroid glands from adult dogs were greater than 200 μg/g.[208]

The mean serum concentration of 1,25-dihydroxyvitamin D(1,25-DiOH-CC) in dogs with apocrine adenocarcinomas and hypercalcemia was 23 pg/ml with a range of 7 to

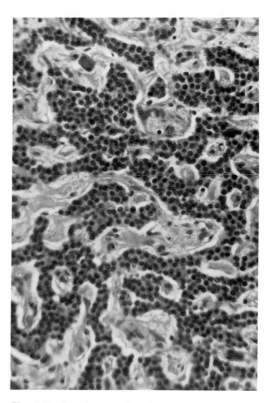

Fig. 4-75. Inactive parathyroid gland of a dog with hypercalcemia (15.8 mg/dl) and adenocarcinoma derived from apocrine glands of the anal sac. Inactive chief cells have a reduced cytoplasmic area and clumped nuclear chromatin. Narrow cords of chief cells are separated by wide bands of collagen and prominent perivascular spaces. (H&E, × 315) (From Meuten DJ, Segre GV, Capen CC et al., 1983.)

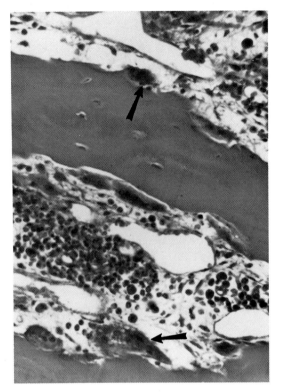

Fig. 4-76. Biopsy of iliac crest of a dog with cancer-associated hypercalcemia. The bone surfaces have numerous closely associated osteoclasts (arrowheads). (H&E, × 315) (From Meuten DJ, Segre GV, Capen CC et al., 1981.)

58 pg/ml (Table 4-3).[208] Although these dogs had hypercalcemia and normophosphatemia, the mean serum 1,25-DiOH-CC concentration is not significantly different from either group of normocalcemic control dogs. The concentration of 1,25-DiOH-CC decreased 2-fold to 8-fold following excision of the apocrine adenocarcinomas (Fig. 4-78). The mean preoperative serum calcium level was 16.5 mg/dl, and the mean preoperative serum 1,25-DiOH-CC concentration was 32 pg/ml, whereas postoperative values were 10 mg/dl and 6 pg/ml, respectively.

Dogs with carcinomas derived from apocrine glands of the anal sac have a significantly greater urine calcium excretion than either control dogs or normocalcemic tumor-control dogs and have higher urine calcium levels than dogs with primary hyperparathyroidism (Fig.

4-79).[208] In addition, the results for fractional excretion of calcium indicate that the urinary excretion of calcium in dogs with apocrine carcinomas is significantly greater than that of clinically normal dogs.

Urinary cyclic adenosine monophosphate (cAMP) per deciliter glomerular filtrate (GF) is increased significantly in dogs with carcinomas derived from apocrine glands of the anal sac compared with that of clinically normal dogs but not compared with that of tumor-control dogs (Fig. 4-79).[208] Urinary excretion of phosphorus and hydroxyproline has been reported to be higher in dogs with apocrine carcinomas than in control dogs, but the differences were not significant (Fig. 4-79).[208] Significant differences have not been demonstrated in the concentrations of serum albumin, urea nitrogen, alkaline phosphatase, or phosphorus in dogs with apocrine adenocarcinomas.

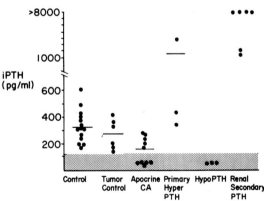

Fig. 4-77. Plasma iPTH concentrations in dogs with hypercalcemia associated with adenocarcinomas derived from apocrine glands of the anal sac compared to other parathyroid diseases. Plasma iPTH levels were decreased in dogs with apocrine carcinomas compared with control dogs. Dogs with hypoparathyroidism (hypo-PTH) had undetectable concentrations of iPTH, whereas dogs with primary (hyperPTH) and secondary (renal hyperPTH) hyperparathyroidism had increased concentrations of iPTH compared with control dogs. Four of five dogs with chronic renal disease had iPTH values greater than 8,300 pg/ml. The limit of detectability for the iPTH assay (112 pg/ml) is indicated by the shaded area. Horizontal lines indicate the mean for the respective groups. (From Meuten DJ, Segre GV, Capen CC et al., 1983.)

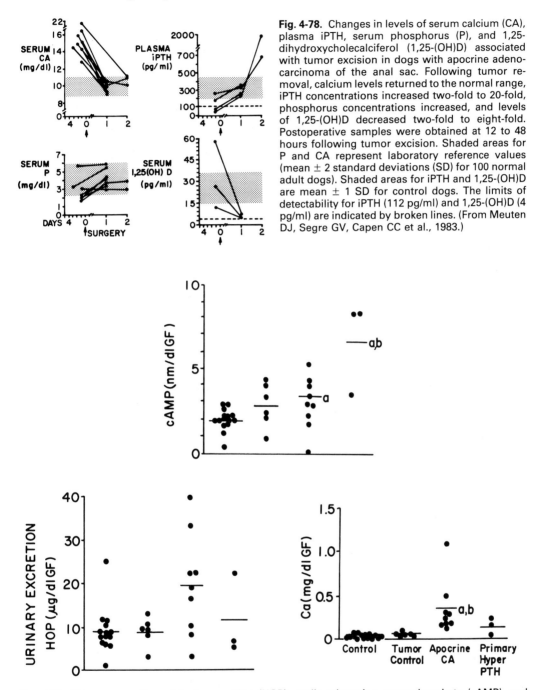

Fig. 4-78. Changes in levels of serum calcium (CA), plasma iPTH, serum phosphorus (P), and 1,25-dihydroxycholecalciferol (1,25-(OH)D) associated with tumor excision in dogs with apocrine adenocarcinoma of the anal sac. Following tumor removal, calcium levels returned to the normal range, iPTH concentrations increased two-fold to 20-fold, phosphorus concentrations increased, and levels of 1,25-(OH)D decreased two-fold to eight-fold. Postoperative samples were obtained at 12 to 48 hours following tumor excision. Shaded areas for P and CA represent laboratory reference values (mean ± 2 standard deviations (SD) for 100 normal adult dogs). Shaded areas for iPTH and 1,25-(OH)D are mean ± 1 SD for control dogs. The limits of detectability for iPTH (112 pg/ml) and 1,25-(OH)D (4 pg/ml) are indicated by the broken lines. (From Meuten DJ, Segre GV, Capen CC et al., 1983.)

Fig. 4-79. Urinary excretion of hydroxyproline (HOP), cyclic adenosine monophosphate (cAMP), and calcium (Ca) in dogs with apocrine adenocarcinoma of the anal sac compared with that in normocalcemic controls with and without tumors and in dogs with primary hyperparathyroidism. Levels of calcium and cAMP excretion were significantly increased in dogs with apocrine carcinomas compared with those in control dogs without tumors but not compared with those of control dogs with tumors. cAMP excretion was significantly greater in hyperparathyroid dogs than in any other group. Hydroxyproline excretion in dogs with apocrine carcinomas was greater than in controls but this difference was not significant. Horizontal lines indicate mean for the group. Significant differences (P < 0.05) from control dogs are indicated by a and from tumor-controls by b. (From Meuten DJ, Segre GV, Capen CC et al., 1983.)

Biopsy specimens from apocrine adenocarcinomas usually have histologic evidence of malignancy, and 96% metastasize to iliac or lumbar lymph nodes.[205] Invasion of tumor cells usually is present into adjacent tissues and endothelial-lined vessels forming emboli. Tumor cell emboli appear to be more common in lymphatic vessels than in blood vessels (Fig. 4-80).

Renal mineralization has been detected histologically in 90% of dogs with pseudohyperparathyroidism associated with apocrine adenocarcinomas particularly when the ion product for calcium and phosphorus was 50 or greater.[205] Tubular mineralization is most pronounced near the corticomedullary junction (Fig. 4-81) but also is present in cortical and deep medullary tubules, Bowman's cap-

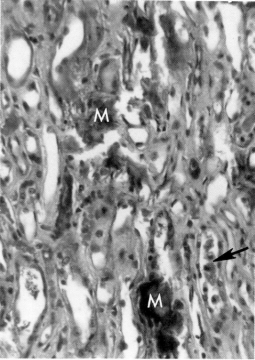

Fig. 4-81. Renal tubular mineralization (M) in a dog with cancer-associated hypercalcemia. Desquamated epithelial cells (arrow) are present in the lumen of some tubules. (H&E, × 315) (From Meuten DJ, Cooper BJ, Capen CC et al., 1981.)

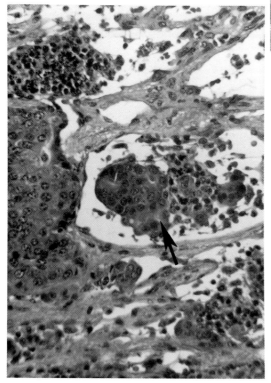

Fig. 4-80. Biopsy of adenocarcinoma arising from apocrine glands of anal sac illustrating tumor cell emboli (arrow) in lymphatic. Dogs with this tumor often have metastases in sublumbar lymph nodes. (H&E, × 315) (From Meuten DJ, Cooper BJ, Capen CC et al., 1981.)

sule, and glomerular tuft. Mineralization is present less frequently in the fundic mucosa of the stomach and endocardium.[205]

Dogs with adenocarcinomas derived from apocrine glands of the anal sac develop hypercalcemia secondary to the production of humoral factor that appears to be distinct from iPTH or prostaglandin E2.[208] This factor(s) increases bone resorption and the urinary excretion of calcium and phosphorus. The inappropriate serum concentration of 1,25-dihydroxycholecalciferol for the degree of hypercalcemia in tumor-bearing dogs and the rapid decrease following excision of the tumor suggests that the tumor may secrete a substance or substances that alter(s) the activity of the 1α-hydroxylase in the kidney. The persistent hypercalcemia causes secretory inactivity of the parathyroid glands and decreased production of iPTH. Surgical removal of the tumor usually is followed by an increased secretion of iPTH that prevents the development of postoperative hypocalcemia. The humoral factor(s) secreted by this unique adenocarcinoma in dogs are different from PTH in that they are not recognized by an immunoassay that detects canine iPTH; but similar in that they both induce osteoclastic osteolysis, hyperphosphaturia, and maintain normal serum 1,25-DiOH-CC levels in spite of the persistent hypercalcemia.

Nude Mouse Model of Canine Apocrine Adenocarcinoma

An animal model of humoral hypercalcemia of malignancy in nude mice has been developed utilizing a serially transplantable apocrine adenocarcinoma (CAC-8) derived from a hypercalcemic dog.[273] The hypercalcemic tumor line (CAC-8) is presently in passage 14, has a latent period of 2 to 4 weeks before onset of tumor growth, and has a tumor

doubling rate of approximately 10 days. The tumor initially grows in an exponential manner and then continues slow volume expansion to a total of 4 to 10 cm³. Mortality due to large tumor size or hypercalcemia is not a common occurrence due to the transplanted carcinomas. Most nude mice with transplanted CAC-8 survive for greater than 200 days. Histologic evaluation of CAC-8 in nude mice revealed a consistent pattern of a carcinoma with the formation of glandular acini containing eosinophilic secretory product and interspersed solid areas. This pattern closely resembles the primary tumor from the hypercalcemic dog.

Nude mice with transplanted CAC-8 develop severe hypercalcemia (mean of 16.3 ± 0.6 mg/dl; controls 8.6 ± 0.2 mg/dl) and hypophosphatemia (mean of 4.4 ± 0.4 mg/dl; controls 6.7 ± 0.6 mg/dl) when tumor volume is greater than 1 cm³ (Fig. 4-82).[268] The serum calcium concentration returned to the normal

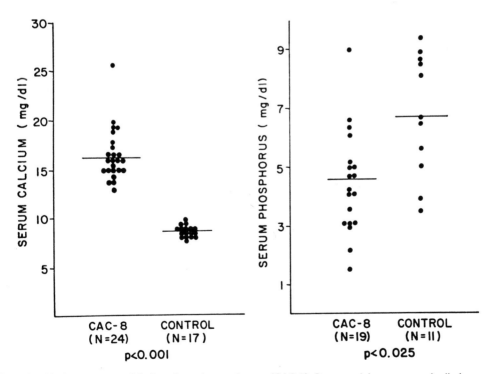

Fig. 4-82. Nude mouse model of canine adnocarcinoma (CAC-8). Serum calcium was markedly increased and serum phosphorus was decreased in tumor-bearing (CAC-8) nude mice compared to controls. (From Rosol TJ et al., 1986.)

range 2 days after surgical removal of the tumors (Fig. 4-83). Serum 1,25-dihydroxycholecalciferol (1,25-DiOH-CC) levels are significantly increased to 82 ± 8.8 pg/ml in nude mice with marked hypercalcemia (mean: 15.7 mg/dl) compared to 64 ± 15.3 pg/ml in nude mice with mild hypercalcemia (mean 11.3 mg/dl) and to 43 ± 1.8 pg/ml in control nude mice (mean serum calcium: 8.6 mg/dl) (Fig. 4-84). Serum 1,25-DiOH-CC levels were significantly correlated to serum calcium levels with a correlation coefficient of 0.55.[273]

Urinary excretion of calcium is significantly increased in tumor-bearing nude mice with a range of 0.25 to 2.75 mg calcium (Ca)/mg creatinine (Cr) and a mean of 0.89 ± 0.27 mg Ca/mg Cr compared to a mean of 0.09 ± 0.02 mg Ca/mg Cr in controls. Urinary phosphorus excretion is not significantly altered in tumor-bearing nude mice.[273] Maintenance

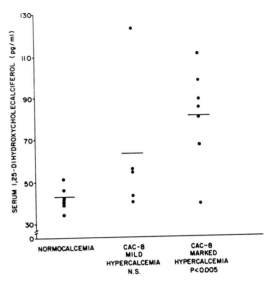

Fig. 4-84. Serum 1,25-dihydroxycholecalciferol (1,25(OH)2D) levels in nude mice with marked hypercalcemia (mean: 15.7 mg/dl), mild hypercalcemia (mean: 11.3 mg/dl), and normocalcemic non-tumor-bearing control nude mice (mean: 8.65 mg/dl). Serum 1,25(OH)2D levels were increased significantly in CAC-8-bearing nude mice with marked hypercalcemia; N.S. not significant. (From Rosol TJ, et al., 1986.)

of a phosphorus excretion rate similar to control nude mice suggests a relative phosphaturia which may be due to a PTH-like effect from the transplanted adenocarcinoma. The degree of phosphaturia also may have been reduced by inhibition of renal adenylate cyclase by the hypercalcemia. Urinary cAMP and hydroxyproline excretion are increased 1.4-fold and 2.3-fold, respectively, in tumor-bearing nude mice compared to control nude mice.[273] The nude mice are exposed to CAC-8 tumor-related effects for greater than 15 weeks and may have a blunted rise in urinary cAMP due both to desensitization of surface receptors and hypercalcemia-associated inhibition of renal adenylate cyclase.[20,312]

Histomorphometric analysis of bone revealed decreased total and cortical bone area in tumor-bearing nude mice with no significant difference in total vertebral or percent (%) trabecular areas.[273] Trabecular surfaces in CAC-8-bearing nude mice have numerous osteoclasts in lacunae and prominent osteoid

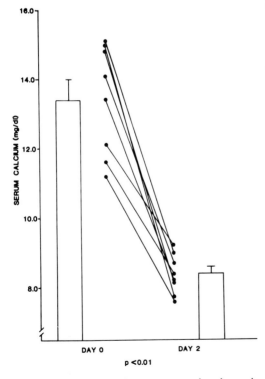

Fig. 4-83. Serum calcium concentration in nude mice bearing transplanted canine adenocarcinoma (CAC-8) before and 2 days after removal of subcutaneously transplanted CAC-8 tumors.

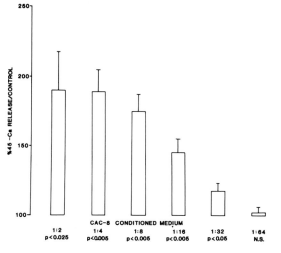

Fig. 4-85. In vitro bone resorption induced by conditioned cell culture medium from hypercalcemic canine adenocarcinoma (CAC-8). The data is expressed as % 45 Ca released from treatment calvaria as a percentage of controls (± SEM). (From Rosol TJ, et al., 1986.)

seams covered with hypertrophied osteoblasts compared to controls. Dynamic histomorphometric studies using lumbar vertebrae from nude mice indicate that double-labeled surface area and mineralization rate are increased which resulted in a 2.5-fold increase in bone formation rate at the tissue level.[273] Tissue level parameters evaluate the basic multicellular units (BMU) of bone remodeling which have quantum properties, whereas cellular level parameters evaluate the rates of function of individual cells (i.e., osteoblasts or osteoclasts).[109] Bone resorption rate is increased 3.3-fold at the tissue level and is not significantly increased at the cellular level. Bone formation has been reported to be reduced in most human patients with HHM[304] and in rats with the Leydig cell tumor;[312] however, osteoblastic surface and mineral apposition rate were increased in hypercalcemic nude mice bearing a human renal carcinoma.[307] The increase in bone formation at the tissue level in nude mice with CAC-8 may represent a tumor-related stimulation (PTH-like effect), an endogenous coupling of bone formation which was unable to completely compensate for the enhanced bone

resorption, or a 1,25-DiOH-CC-mediated effect.

Tumor extracts and conditioned culture medium from primary tumor explants stimulate ^{45}calcium (Ca) release from neonatal mouse calvaria in a dose-dependent manner[275] (Fig. 4-85). Fractionation of CAC-8 extract using gel filtration chromatography revealed peak bone resorbing activity at an approximate molecular mass of 28,000. A PTH receptor antagonist (^{8,18}norleucine, ^{34}tyrosine) bovine PTH (3-34) amide (bPTH [3-34] amide) antagonized in vitro bone resorption in mouse calvaria induced by bPTH (1-34) at a molar ratio of 1:10,000 (native PTH:antagonist).[276] Bovine PTH (3-34) amide also significantly reduces bone resorption induced by CAC-8 tumor extract up to 70% (Fig. 4-86). These data indicated that bone resorption stimulated in vitro by the CAC-8 model of HHM is due, at least partially, to binding of humoral factors to the PTH receptor. The PTH receptor antagonist, bPTH (3-34) amide, has been reported not to inhibit in vitro bone resorption induced by the rat

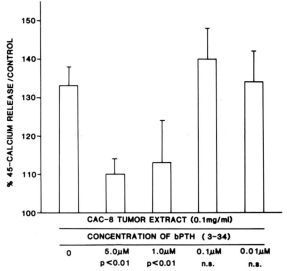

Fig. 4-86. Parathyroid hormone receptor antagonist [8,18 Nle, 34Tyr] bPTH (3-34) amide partially blocks in vitro bone resorption stimulated by an extract (0.10 mg/ml) from the hypercalcemic canine adenocarcinoma (CAC-8). (From Rosol TJ and Capen CC, 1988.)

Leydig cell or Walker tumor models of HHM.[96] Treatment with indomethacin, heating at 56°C for 30 minutes or 100°C for 3 minutes, did not significantly inhibit [45]Ca release from CAC-8 extract or CM-treated calvaria. However, indomethacin completely inhibited bone resorption induced by epidermal growth factor.

Parathyroid hormone stimulates adenylate cyclase and cyclic adenosine monophosphate (cAMP) production in both kidney and bone cells by binding to specific cell membrane receptors.[96] Tumor extracts from the canine adenocarcinoma (CAC-8) grown in nude mice derived from a hypercalcemic dog significantly stimulate adenylate cyclase (AC) of ROS 17 /2.8 cells (an osteoblast-like cloned cell line derived from a rat osteosarcoma).[191,277] The PTH receptor antagonist, bPTH (3-34) amide, significantly reduced AC stimulation by bPTH and CAC-8 extract in ROS, UMR and opossum kidney (OK) cell lines that have PTH receptors. This indicates that CAC-8 extract may stimulate AC of the cell lines by binding to the PTH receptor. However, CAC-8 extract appears to bind to the PTH receptors of the ROS, UMR, and OK cells with different affinities or activate the receptors with different magnitudes since tumor extract did not stimulate AC of the cell lines to equal levels.[277]

The AC-stimulating activity of CAC-8 is stable to treatment by heat (60°C for 1 hour and 100°C for 3 minutes), sensitive to enzymatic digestion by trypsin, inactivated by chemical reduction with dithiothreitol, and has a relative molecular weight of 34,000 by gel exclusion chromatography.[277] The results of these studies suggest that the hypercalcemic tumor line (CAC-8) contains a protein factor which stimulates adenylate cyclase of bone and kidney cells in a similar manner to PTH (1-34).

Transforming growth factors (TGF) are a family of proteins present in neoplastic and normal tissues.[118] There are two classes of TGF: (1) TGF-α, which is present predominantly in neoplastic tissues and binds to the receptor for epidermal growth factor (EGF), and (2) TGF-β, which is present in many normal and neoplastic tissues and binds to a separate receptor distinct from the EGF and TGF-α receptor. Transforming growth factor activity is defined as the ability to stimulate the growth of specific indicator cell lines as colonies in soft agar. In addition, both TGF-α and TGF-β have been shown to stimulate in vitro bone resorption.[317] Therefore, it has been hypothesized that TGF may be one of the factors involved in the pathogenesis of hypercalcemia in human and animal models of HHM.[218]

Tumor extract from the hypercalcemic adenocarcinoma (CAC-8) stimulates the formation of colonies in soft agar of NRK (clone 49F) cells (a continuous cell line derived from normal rat kidney fibroblasts).[274] NRK cells form large colonies in the presence of EGF and serum. It has been demonstrated that NRK cells require both TGF-α and TGF-β for stimulation of colony growth. The neonatal calf serum used in the assay is likely the source of TGF-β necessary to form colonies in the presence of EGF. Tumor (CAC-8) extract induces colony formation in soft agar which is not dependent on the addition of EGF, suggesting the presence of TGF-α activity. The addition of EGF with tumor extract increased the size and number of colonies formed by NRK cells (Fig. 4-87). These characteristics are similar to other TGF previously described.[118] The relationship of the TGF activity in CAC-8 extract to the in vitro bone resorption activity or AC-stimulating activity is not known at present.

Humoral hypercalcemia of malignancy in human patients is associated with multiple tumor types, i.e. squamous cell carcinoma (most commonly from the head and neck or lung), renal cell carcinoma, pheochromocytoma, breast carcinoma, ovarian carcinoma, and other less common tumors.[217,306] Stewart et al.[303] have demonstrated that the different tumor types associated with HHM in humans contain AC-stimulating activity. There are two well characterized cell lines derived from human tumors: (1) renal carcinoma cell line 786-0, and (2) squamous cell carcinoma.[229,309]

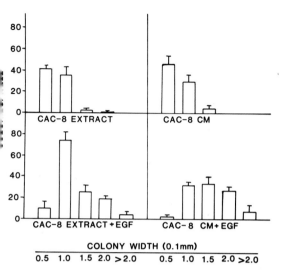

Fig. 4-87. Transforming growth factor activity demonstrated in extracts of hypercalcemic canine adenocarcinoma (CAC-8). Number and size of NRK colonies induced in soft agar by CAC-8 tumor extract (0.5 mg/ml) or CAC-8 conditioned medium (CM) with or without epidermal growth factor (EGF) (10 ng/ml).

A parathyroid hormone-related protein (PTH-rP) has been purified from the conditioned medium of a human lung carcinoma cell line (BEN).[213] The protein has a molecular weight of 18,000 and 8 of the first 16 amino acid residues share sequence homology with hPTH. This protein also was purified on the basis of its ability to stimulate adenylate cyclase (AC) of bone cell lines. The gene encoding PTH-rP has been cloned and encodes a prepro-peptide of 36 amino acids and a mature protein of 141 amino acids.[309] A similar protein (17,000 daltons) with an identical N-terminal amino acid sequence has been isolated from a human breast carcinoma.[37] The three PTH-related proteins appear to be similar or identical proteins isolated on the basis of their ability to stimulate adenylate cyclase. The protein isolated from the renal cell carcinoma is smaller than the other two proteins but may be only a small part of the larger molecule. Antisera produced to the N-terminal region of PTH-rP demonstrated little cross-reactivity to native PTH; however, PTH-rP appears to stimulate PTH-depen-

dent adenylate cyclase since PTH receptor antagonists will block AC stimulation.[213] PTH-rP may bind to the PTH receptor in bone and kidney to increase bone resorption and renal tubular reabsorption of calcium (Fig. 4-88).

It is not known if HHM is the result of a single humoral factor or multiple factors. The PTH-rP may require the presence of another factor to induce hypercalcemia in vitro such as a transforming growth factor or interleukin-1β.[216,287] It is hypothesized that the hypercalcemic adenocarcinoma in dogs also contains a PTH-rP since the AC-stimulating and in vitro bone resorbing activity present are in a similar molecular weight range and can be inhibited by PTH receptor antagonists.[275-277]

Hypercalcemia Associated with Lymphosarcoma

Lymphosarcoma is the most common neoplasm associated with hypercalcemia in dogs and cats.[242,338] Estimates of the prevalence of hypercalcemia in dogs with lymphoma vary from 10 to 40%. Peripheral lymph node enlargement may or may not be detected, but there usually is evidence of anterior mediastinal or visceral involvement. It is not completely resolved whether the hypercalcemia develops from the production of humoral substances by neoplastic cells (e.g. PTH-related

MECHANISM OF ACTION OF PTH-RELATED PEPTIDE

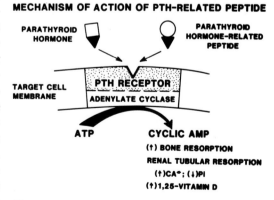

Fig. 4-88. Parathyroid hormone-related protein produced by tumor cells appears to result in hypercalcemia by binding to PTH receptors in bone and kidney. The stimulation of increased bone resorption and renal tubular reabsorption of calcium results in the persistent elevation of blood calcium.

protein, prostaglandins, osteoclast-activating factor) or from physical disruption of trabecular bone due to frequent marrow involvement, or both.

Heath and co-workers[140] reported that serum iPTH levels were subnormal in hypercalcemic dogs with lymphosarcoma and that plasma immunoreactive PG E2 levels did not differ from those of controls. Culture media from normal lymphoid tissue and control media had no effect on release of ^{45}Ca from prelabeled fetal mouse forelimb bones; however, media from tumor tissue increased ^{45}Ca release. These findings suggest that the local production of bone-resorbing factors (e.g. osteoclast-activating factor) is important in stimulating calcium from bone in certain dogs with lymphosarcoma and hypercalcemia.

Dogs with lymphosarcoma and hypercalcemia have decreased trabecular bone volume

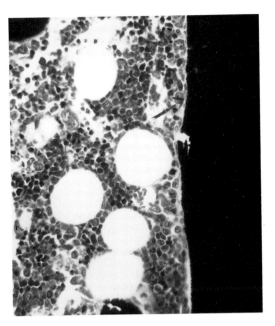

Fig. 4-90. Lumbar vertebra of a control dog with a bone trabeculum that has smooth surfaces, no osteoclasts, and flattened osteoblasts (arrow). (von Kossa-tetrachrome, × 700). (From Meuten DJ, Kociba GJ, Capen CC et al., 1983.)

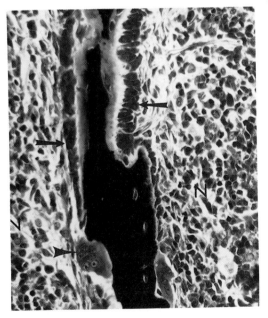

Fig. 4-89. Lumbar vertebra of a dog with hypercalcemia and lymphosarcoma. Several large osteoclasts (arrowheads) are present in lacunae along a thin bone trabecula. Hyperplastic osteoblasts (arrows) and prominent osteoid seams are present adjacent to the resorptive surfaces. The marrow contains neoplastic lymphoid cells (N). (von Kossa-tetrachrome, × 700). (From Meuten DJ, Kociba GJ, Capen CC et al., 1983.)

and increased osteoclastic osteolysis compared with control dogs and dogs with normocalcemia and lymphosarcoma.[206] Dogs with neoplastic cells in bone marrow consistently have increased osteoclastic bone resorption. Dogs with hypercalcemic lymphosarcoma often have osteoclasts on trabecular bone surfaces opposite a surface lined by osteoid and large columnar osteoblasts (Fig. 4-89). Bone surfaces in normocalcemic control dogs are smooth and lined by flattened osteoblasts but only rarely by osteoclasts (Fig.4-90). Dogs with lymphosarcoma that are normocalcemic did not have increased bone resorption.[206] Hypercalcemic dogs with lymphosarcoma have decreased concentrations of plasma iPTH and serum 1,25-DiOH-CC compared with normocalcemic dogs with lymphosarcoma and control dogs (Fig. 4-91) The plasma concentration of 13, 14-dihydro-15-keto-prostaglandin E_2 (PG E2M) is elevated (approximately 2-fold) significantly in hypercalcemic dogs with lymphosarcoma compared to con-

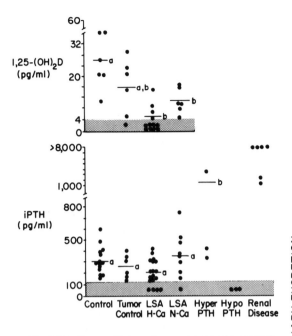

Fig. 4-91. Dogs with lymphosarcoma and hypercalcemia (LSA H-Ca) have lower concentrations of plasma iPTH and serum 1,25-(OH)$_2$D than normocalcemic lymphosarcoma dogs (LSA N-Ca). Dogs with hypoparathyroidism (HypoPTH) had undetectable concentrations of iPTH, while dogs with primary (hyperPTH) and secondary renal hyperparathyroidism (renal disease) had increased concentrations of iPTH compared with control dogs. Four of six dogs with chronic renal disease had plasma iPTH concentrations greater than 8,300 pg/ml. The limits of detectability for the iPTH assay (112 pg/ml) and the 1,25-(OH)$_2$D assay (4 pg/ml) are indicated by the shaded areas. Horizontal lines indicate the mean for the respective groups. Different letters indicate significantly different means (P < 0.05). (From Meuten DJ, Kociba GJ, Capen CC et al., 1983.)

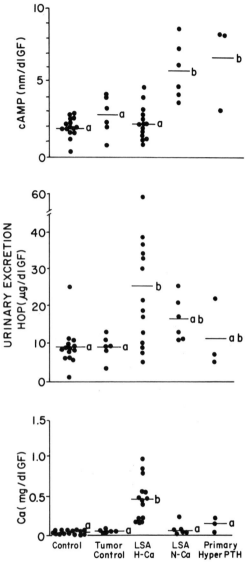

Fig. 4-92. Urinary excretion of calcium, cAMP, and hydroxyproline in five groups of dogs. Urine calcium levels were significantly greater in hypercalcemic dogs with lymphosarcoma (LSA H-Ca) than in normocalcemic dogs with lymphosarcoma (LSA N-Ca). Hydroxyproline excretion was significantly increased in dogs with lymphosarcoma and hypercalcemia compared with control dogs and was greater in hypercalcemic dogs with lymphosarcoma than in normocalcemic dogs with lymphosarcoma. Urine cAMP was significantly greater in primary hyperparathyroid dogs than in control dogs and in dogs with lymphosarcoma and hypercalcemia. Horizontal lines indicate mean values. Different letters indicate significant differences (P < 0.05). (From Meuten DJ, Kociba GJ, Capen CC et al., 1983.)

trols. Immunoreactive PTH is not detected in lymphosarcoma tissue.[206]

Urinary excretion of calcium, phosphorus, and hydroxyproline is increased in hypercalcemic dogs with lymphosarcoma (Fig. 4-92).[206] Light and electron microscopic examination of parathyroid glands revealed inactive or atrophic chief cells and evidence of secretory inactivity in dogs with lymphosarcoma and hypercalcemia. Ultrastructurally, lymphosarcomas are composed of tumor cells with large nuclei and a paucity of cytoplasmic organelles. Lymphosarcoma in dogs with hypercalcemia appears to produce a bone-resorbing substance that is immunologically distinct from iPTH and 1,25-DiOH-CC.

Weir et al.[338] recently reported that hypercalcemic dogs with lymphosarcoma had increased urinary calcium (fractional and 24-hour) and phosphorus (fractional) excretion. Acid-urea extracts of tumor tissue from hypercalcemic dogs contained adenylate cyclase-stimulating activity in vitro, whereas extracts from normocalcemic lymphosarcomas did not. Further purification of tumor extract yielded an adenylate cyclase-stimulating protein which appeared to interact specifically with the PTH receptor. These findings suggest that hypercalcemia in some dogs with lymphosarcoma may be mediated by a tumor-derived circulating bone-resorbing factor which is distinct from PTH.

Other causes of hypercalcemia that must be differentiated from pseudohyperparathyroidism and primary hyperparathyroidism are vitamin D intoxication and malignant neoplasms with osseous metastases. The hypercalcemia of hypervitaminosis D may be of similar magnitude as in primary hyperparathyroidism but usually is accompanied by hyperphosphatemia and normal serum alkaline phosphatase activity. Skeletal disease is not a consistent feature, since the increased concentrations of blood calcium and phosphorus are derived principally from augmented intestinal absorption rather than from bone resorption. Malignant neoplasms with osseous metastases may cause moderate to severe hypercalcemia and hypercalciuria, but the alkaline phosphatase activity and serum phosphorus are usually normal or moderately elevated. These changes are believed to be due to release of calcium and phosphorus into the blood from areas of bone destruction at rates greater than can be cleared by the kidney and intestine. Bone involvement can be multifocal but usually is sharply demarcated and localized to the area of metastasis. Osteolysis associated with tumor metastases has been shown to be the result of a physical disruption not only of bone by neoplastic cells but also to the local production of humoral substances that stimulate bone resorption, such as prostaglandins and osteoclast-activating factor.

Hypercalcemia may be detected occasionally in dehydrated animals. The magnitude of elevation in blood usually is mild and is attributed to fluid volume contraction that results in hyperproteinemia and an increased relative concentration of ionized and nonionized calcium. The hypercalcemia rapidly resolves following fluid therapy. The majority of dehydrated animals do not develop hypercalcemia. Prolonged immobilization can lead to hypercalcemia as a consequence of continued bone resorption associated with diminished bone accretion. Hypercalcemia of this type occurs infrequently in animals that cannot move around freely because of extensive musculoskeletal or neurologic injury.

Hypercalcemia has been reported in experimentally adrenalectomized dogs and in some cases of naturally occurring Addison's-like disease in dogs (Musselman, 1975; Walser et al., 1963). The magnitude of elevation in serum calcium values may exceed 26 mg/dl under experimental conditions, whereas dogs with Addison's-like disease evaluated in our hospital have had blood calcium values up to 15 mg/dl. Experimental evidence suggests that the type of hypercalcemia associated with hypoadrenocorticism is unusual in that the ionized calcium fraction remains normal while the nonionized calcium fraction increases. If the ionized calcium does indeed remain normal, it follows that this type of hypercalcemia should not be deleterious to the animal. The elevated calcium value rapidly returns to normal following treatment for hypoadrenocorticism.

Many clinical signs of hypercalcemia are similar regardless of underlying cause. Hypercalcemia affects primarily the urinary, gastrointestinal, and nervous systems although other systems also may be affected.

Anorexia, vomiting, and constipation result from the decreased excitability of gastrointestinal smooth muscle caused by hypercalcemia. Generalized weakness of skeletal muscle develops as a result of decreased neuromuscular excitability. Decreased neuromuscular excitability also causes depression of lower motor neuron reflexes (e.g. hyporeflexia of patellar, gastrocnemius, and triceps reflexes). Behavioral changes, depression, stupor, coma, seizures, and muscle twitching have been observed in dogs with hypercalcemia. Lameness and bone pain from demineralization of bone or pathologic fractures can be major signs. Cardiac arrhythmia, shortening of the Q-T interval, and prolongation of the P-R interval (first-degree heart block) may be detected by electrocardiographic evaluation. Ventricular fibrillation develops in extreme hypercalcemia.[69]

Polyuria and polydipsia are encountered early in the course of most diseases characterized by hypercalcemia and often are major reasons causing client concern. Initially, the polyuria and polydipsia are independent of uremic signs from primary renal failure; however, the syndrome of uremia may develop as a result of the toxic effects of persistent hypercalcemia on the kidney. Severe dehydration often occurs from the combined effects of polyuria, emesis, and lack of oral water intake.

The severity of clinical signs often is related to the magnitude of the hypercalcemia and the rapidity of elevation in blood calcium. Animals with serum calcium values in excess of 16.0 mg/dl generally have the most severe clinical signs. Exceptions to this rule occur and occasionally animals with severe hypercalcemia have mild clinical signs. Concomitant electrolyte and acid-base imbalances may modulate the severity of clinical signs. Most notably, metabolic acidosis will increase the ionized fraction of serum calcium and magnify the severity of clinical signs. The magnitude of simultaneous phosphorus retention appears to influence the degree of soft-tissue mineralization in the kidney and elsewhere.

Other clinical signs not directly attributable to hypercalcemia may be associated with the underlying cause of the elevation in blood calcium concentration. Since neoplasms of several types are commonly associated with hypercalcemia, tumor growth in lymph nodes and various organs may be detected as enlargement or dysfunction of the particular organ involved.

Hypoparathyroidism

In hypoparathyroidism either subnormal amounts of parathyroid hormone are secreted by pathologic parathyroid glands or the hormone secreted is unable to interact normally with target cells. Hypoparathyroidism has been recognized occasionally in dogs, particularly in the smaller breeds such as schnauzers and terriers.[97,154,160,248,293] However, the incidence of occurrence is much less than hyperparathyroidism in both dogs and cats.

Several pathogenic mechanisms can result in an inadequate secretion of parathyroid hormone (Table 4-4). The parathyroid glands may be damaged or inadvertently removed during the course of operation on the thyroid gland. If the glands or their vascular supply have only been damaged but not removed, functional parenchyma often regenerates and clinical manifestations subsequently disappear.

Agenesis of both pairs of parathyroids is a rare cause of congenital hypoparathyroidism in pups. Idiopathic hypoparathyroidism in adult dogs usually is associated with diffuse lymphocytic parathyroiditis resulting in extensive degeneration of chief cells with partial replacement by fibrous connective tissue. In the early stages of lymphocytic parathyroiditis, there is extensive infiltration of the gland with lymphocytes and plasma cells, and nodular regenerative hyperplasia of the remaining chief cells. Later, the parathyroid gland is completely replaced by lymphocytes,

Table 4-4 Pathogenic Mechanisms of Hypoparathyroidism

Congenital (agenesis, hypoplasia)
Idiopathic (degeneration)
Immune-mediated parathyroiditis
Iatrogenic (neck surgery, irradiation)
Metastatic neoplasms
Trophic atrophy from hypercalcemia
Inability of target cells to respond
    lack of adenyl cyclase in bone and/or kidney
    ("pseudohypoparathyroidism")

fibroblasts, and neocapillaries with only an occasional viable chief cell (Fig. 4-93). The lymphocytic parathyroiditis may develop by means of an immune-mediated mechanism, since a similar destruction of secretory paren- chyma and lymphocytic infiltration has been produced experimentally in dogs by repeated injections of parathyroid tissue emulsions.[187] Other possible causes of hypoparathyroidism include invasion and destruction of para- thyroids by primary (thyroid, salivary, etc.) or metastatic neoplasms in the anterior cerv- ical area. Trophic atrophy of parathyroids occurs associated with severe hypercalcemia resulting from vitamin D intoxication, ectopic production of parathyroid hormone- related protein by nonendocrine neoplasms, and multifocal osteolytic lesions with release of calcium associated with tumor metastases.

In human beings a variant of the syndrome of hypoparathyroidism has been reported in which target cells in kidney and bone are un- able to respond to the secretion of normal amounts of parathyroid hormone.[22,95] This is due to a lack of the nucleotide regulatory (N-) protein that couples the hormone-receptor complex to the catalytic subunit of adenylate cyclase in the plasma membrane, resulting in an inability to form cAMP in target cells (Fig. 4-25) (Farfel et al., 1980). Severe hypo- calcemia develops in patients with pseudo- hypoparathyroidism even though para- thyroid glands are hyperplastic,[278] and immunoreactive parathyroid hormone levels are elevated.[22]

The functional disturbances and clinical manifestations of hypoparathyroidism pri- marily are the result of increased neuromus-

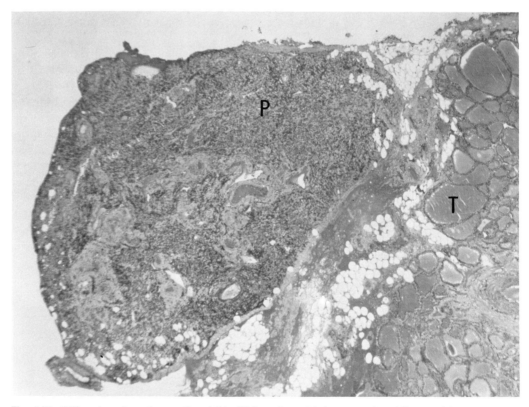

Fig. 4-93. Diffuse lymphocytic parathyroiditis (P) in a dog with hypoparathyroidism and hypocalcemia. The external parathyroid gland has been completely replaced by lymphocytes, plasma cells, fibroblasts, and neocapillaries. T = thyroid gland × 32.

cular excitability and tetany. Bone resorption is decreased and blood calcium levels diminish progressively (4 to 6 mg/dl) due to the lack of parathyroid hormone (Fig. 4-94). Affected dogs are restless, nervous, and ataxic with intermittent tremors of individual muscle groups that progress to generalized tetany and convulsive seizures. Concurrently, blood phosphorus levels are substantially elevated due to increased renal tubular reabsorption.

DISORDERS OF C-CELL FUNCTION

Clinical syndromes associated with abnormalities in secretion of calcitonin are recognized much less frequently than disorders of parathyroid hormone secretion in both animals and man.[358] The syndromes identified so far have been the result of excess secretion of calcitonin rather than a lack of secretion.

Hypercalcitoninism

A hypersecretion of calcitonin has been reported in human beings[139,299] and bulls[25,46] with thyroid C-cell neoplasms (medullary or ultimobranchial). In human patients the syndrome often is familial and affects many individuals in a kindred.

Calcitonin-secreting C-cell neoplasms occur frequently in populations of adult to aged bulls (Fig. 4-95). The chronic stimulation of ultimobranchial derivatives in the thyroid by the high calcium diets fed to bulls may be related to the pathogenesis of the neoplasm.[176,177] Cows do not develop proliferative C-cell lesions under similar dietary conditions, probably because of the high physiologic requirements for calcium imposed by pregnancy and lactation. The higher plasma immunoreactive calcitonin levels in bulls than in cows may be related to their greater intake of dietary calcium relative to physiologic requirements (Fig. 4-96).

C-cell (medullary) thyroid carcinomas also occur in dogs and horses sporadically as a firm mass in the anterior cervical region.[179] Calcitonin activity can be localized to the cyto-

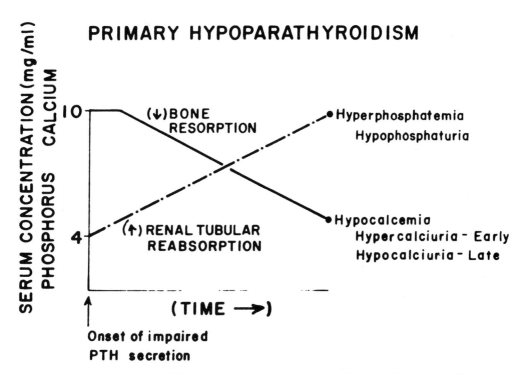

PRIMARY HYPOPARATHYROIDISM

(↓)BONE RESORPTION

●Hyperphosphatemia
Hypophosphaturia

(↑) RENAL TUBULAR REABSORPTION

●Hypocalcemia
Hypercalciuria - Early
Hypocalciuria - Late

SERUM CONCENTRATION (mg/ml) PHOSPHORUS   CALCIUM

10

4

(TIME →)

↑
Onset of impaired
PTH secretion

Fig. 4-94. Alterations in serum calcium and phosphorus in response to an inadequate secretion of parathyroid hormone. There are a progressive increase in serum phosphorus levels and a marked decline in serum calcium levels that result in neuromuscular tetany.

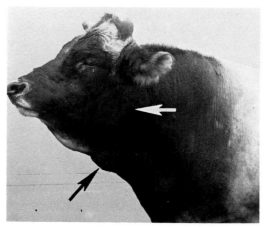

Fig. 4-95. Calcitonin-secreting C-cell (ultimobranchial) neoplasm in thyroid gland of an adult bull. The tumor has resulted in a prominent enlargement in the anterior cervical region (arrows) and has metastasized to several anterior cervical lymph nodes.

plasm of tumor cells by immunoenzymatic techniques. In addition to calcitonin, medullary (C-cell) carcinomas in man may secrete other humoral substances, such as prostaglandins, serotonin, and bradykinin, that result in a wide spectrum of clinical manifestations.[203] The incidence of occurrence of C-cell tumors in dogs is uncertain, but Zarrin reported that 7 of 200 thyroid tumors in dogs were derived from C-cells.[356] They often are firm on palpation due to the presence of large amounts of amyloid in the stroma (Fig. 4-97). Thyroid neoplasms of C-cell origin can be readily differentiated ultrastructurally by the presence of numerous membrane-limited secretory granules in the cytoplasm. Small granules of this type are not present in thyroid tumors derived from follicular cells.

C-cell tumors in both human beings and bulls frequently are associated with the simultaneous occurrence of pheochromocytomas in the adrenal medulla and neoplasms in other endocrine organs of neural crest origin.[46,299] Serum calcium and phosphorus levels in adults with a chronic excessive secretion of calcitonin usually remain in the low normal range due to the relatively slow turnover rate of bone. Osteosclerotic changes have been reported in

bulls with this syndrome of long-term and excessive calcitonin secretion (Fig. 4-98).

Hypocalcitoninism

Specific disease syndromes resulting from a lack of calcitonin secretion have not been recognized in either man or animals. However, experimentally thyroidectomized animals are less able than normal to handle a calcium load and may develop hypercalcemia (Fig. 4-35).[81,310]

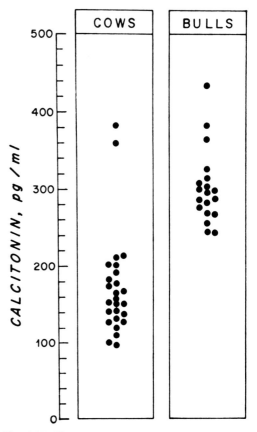

Fig. 4-96. The higher plasma immunoreactive calcitonin levels in bulls (303 ± 13 pg/ml) than in cows (165 ± 12 pg/ml) may be related to the high dietary intake of calcium relative to physiologic requirements. This prolonged stimulation of calcitonin-secreting C-cells by the high calcium intake in the diet has been suggested to be important in the pathogenesis of the high incidence of C-cell (ultimobranchial) neoplasms in older bulls. (From Deftos et al., 1972.)

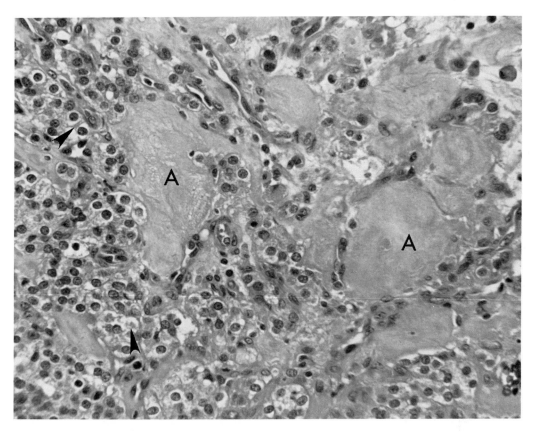

Fig. 4-97. Calcitonin-secreting C-cell neoplasm in the thyroid gland of a dog. The cytoplasmic area of C-cells stains lightly eosinophilic. The large accumulations of amyloid (A) in the interstitium gives this type of thyroid tumor a characteristically firm consistency on palpation. H & E; × 315.

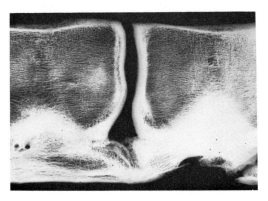

Fig. 4-98. Radiograph of lumbar vertebrae illustrating osteosclerosis in a bull with a calcitonin-secreting thyroid C-cell neoplasm. Trabeculae are radiodense and have minimal evidence of osteoclastic resorption.

HYPOCALCEMIC SYNDROMES IN ANIMALS

A number of metabolic disorders characterized primarily by the development of hypocalcemia and associated manifestations occur in several different animal species (Table 4-5). Many of these hypocalcemic syndromes develop near the time of the increased calcium demand associated with parturition and probably are a reflection of a temporary failure of calcium homeostatic mechanisms. A comparable hypocalcemic syndrome associated with parturition does not occur in human beings. The eclampsia that develops in women is related to a toxemia of pregnancy with degenerative changes in the liver, kidney, and placenta rather than disturbances in mineral homeo-

Table 4-5 Hypocalcemic Syndromes in Animals

Species	Disease
Cow	Parturient hypocalcemia ("milk fever")
Bitch	Puerperal tetany, eclampsia
Queen	Puerperal tetany, eclampsia
Ewe	Pre- and postparturient paresis ("moss ill or staggers"; "lambing sickness")
Nanny goat	Hypocalcemia
Mare	Parturient eclampsia, postpartum tetany
Sow	Eclampsia
Chinchilla	Hypocalcemia

stasis. Parturient hypocalcemia in dairy cows and puerperal tetany of bitches are examples of hypocalcemic syndromes of major economic significance and will be discussed in greater detail.

Parturient Hypocalcemia in Dairy Cows

Parturient hypocalcemia is a metabolic disease of high-producing dairy cows characterized by the development of severe hypocalcemia, hypophosphatemia, and paresis near the time of parturition. The pathogenic mechanisms responsible for the rapid and precipitous decrease in calcium and phosphorus levels in the blood are complex and involve several interrelated factors.[39] Total and ionized calcium levels decrease progressively beginning several days before parturition (Fig. 4-99). Serum magnesium may increase reciprocally as calcium declines. The blood glucose concentration often is increased in response to hypocalcemia due to an interference with the secretion of insulin from beta cells. An adequate amount of calcium ion in extracellular fluids is required for insulin secretion in response to glucose and other secretagogues for insulin.[346] The uptake of calcium by beta cells appears to stimulate the contraction of microfilaments which triggers the peripheral migration of storage granules and release of insulin. Infusion of glucose in a cow with severe hypocalcemia fails to increase blood levels of insulin; however, if calcium is administered before the injection of glucose, there is a rapid and substantial increase in insulin secretion (Fig. 4-100).

The development of parturient hypocalcemia in dairy cows for a number of years was considered to be the result of an inadequate response of the parathyroid glands to the substantial demands for calcium imposed by the mineralization of fetal bones and the initiation of lactation. Ultrastructural studies indicated that parathyroid chief cells in cows with parturient hypocalcemia were capable of re-

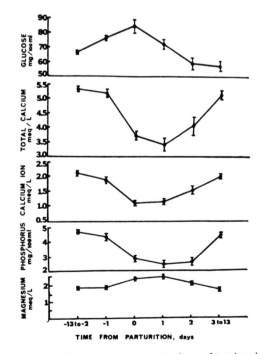

Fig. 4-99. Mean plasma concentrations of total and ionized calcium and inorganic phosphorus decrease rapidly near parturition whereas magnesium and glucose levels increase with the development of hypocalcemia in cows. (From Blum et al., 1972.)

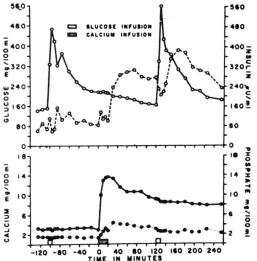

Fig. 4-100. Failure of insulin release in response to glucose infusion in cows with severe hypocalcemia. The ability to release insulin can be restored if calcium is injected to elevate blood calcium levels 2 hours before the second glucose infusion. (From Littledike et al., 1969.)

sponding to the increased demands for calcium by the secretion of stored hormone and hypertrophy of secretory organelles concerned with the synthesis of new hormone.[57] Chief cells were primarily in the active stage of their secretory cycle and were depleted of storage granules or the secretory granules had migrated peripherally and were fused with the plasma membrane (Fig. 4-101). These structural findings suggested an active secretory response by parathyroid glands in cows with parturient hypocalcemia and were in agreement with the biochemical studies of Mayer et al.[200,201] They used a sensitive immunoassay to measure plasma levels of parathyroid hormone and detected equal or greater levels of hormone in cows with parturient hypocalcemia than in normal parturient cows (Fig. 4-102). The immunoreactivity in the plasma of hypocalcemic cows is composed partially of biologically active intact parathyroid hormone in addition to hormone fragments which do not possess biologic activity.[198] The ability of parathyroid glands to respond to the challenge for extra calcium mobilization with increased

hormonal synthesis and secretion does not appear to be defective in cows that develop parturient hypocalcemia.

Target cells in bone and skeletal calcium reserves of cows with parturient hypocalcemia appear to be temporarily refractive to the action of the elevated levels of parathyroid hormone. Investigations have shown that the elevation of serum calcium in response to exogenous parathyroid extract is less when administered prepartum than postpartum.[192] Bone turnover, particularly resorption, is low in cows with parturient hypocalcemia and only a few osteoclasts are present on smooth inactive trabecular bone surfaces (Fig. 4-103).[284] The urinary excretion of hydroxyproline, derived from the breakdown of bone matrix, does not increase significantly during late gestation in cows that develop the disease, as occurs in cows that maintain their serum calcium near normal through parturition and early lactation.[23] A secretion of calcitonin prepartum in certain cows, especially those fed high calcium diets, may be one factor that contributes to the inability of increased parathyroid hormone levels to mobilize calcium rapidly from skeletal reserves and maintain blood levels during the critical period near parturition. The thyroid content of calcitonin is reduced (14% of control cows) and many C- (parafollicular) cells are degranulated.[353] Elevated plasma levels of calcitonin have been reported in cows prior to the development of profound hypocalcemia by some investigators,[25,183] but not by others.[196] Barlet has been able to induce a syndrome of hypocalcemia analogous to parturient paresis by the long-term intravenous infusion of calcitonin in lactating cows.[17]

The decline in blood calcium may be rapid in certain high-producing dairy cows near parturition and the initiation of lactation. Since bone resorption during the prepartal period often is relatively low due to a substantial intake of dietary calcium, there is a relatively small pool of active bone-resorbing cells capable of responding to PTH. Therefore, when PTH secretion increases because of the rapidly developing hypocalcemia, the

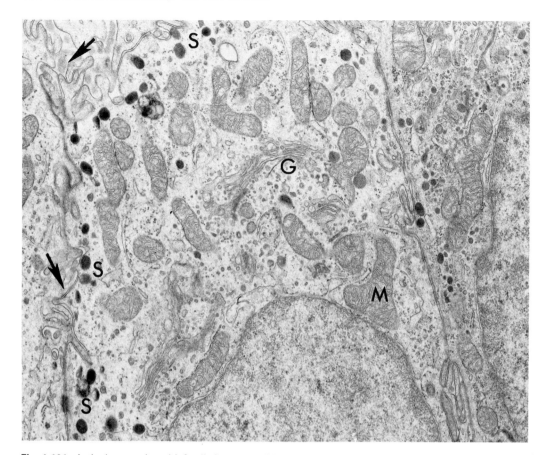

Fig. 4-101. Actively secreting chief cells in a cow with parturient hypocalcemia. PTH-containing secretory granules (S) have moved to the periphery of the cell and are aligned along the plasma membrane in response to the hypocalcemic stimulus. Secretory organelles such as mitochondria (M) and the Golgi apparatus (G) are hypertrophied and plasma membranes of adjacent active chief cells are interdigitated (arrows). The ability of parathyroid glands to respond to the challenge for calcium mobilization by increased PTH synthesis and secretion does not appear to be defective in cows that develop parturient hypocalcemia. 20,000 ×. (From Capen and Young, 1967.)

increase in activity of the few active osteoclasts present is insufficient to restore the plasma calcium concentration to normal. The activation of osteoprogenitor cells and the subsequent conversion of preosteoclasts to osteoclasts under the influence of increased PTH with expansion of the pool of active bone-resorbing cells require time (as long as 48 to 72 hours in an adult cow) and an adequate concentration of calcium in extracellular fluids.[259] If the extracellular fluid calcium falls below a critical level, the increased circulating concentration of PTH may be ineffective in causing an elevation of cytosol calcium in target cells to activate new bone-resorbing cells. Neither an increased endogenous secretion of PTH nor the exogenous administration of parathyroid extract to cows will restore homeostasis once the hypocalcemia is profound. Only the administration of calcium and elevation of calcium in extracellular fluids will restore the responsiveness to PTH, trigger bone resorption, and correct the hypocalcemia.

The composition of the prepartal diet fed to dairy cows is known to be a significant factor in the pathogenesis of parturient hypocalcemia. High calcium diets have been

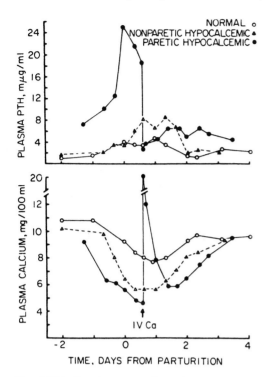

Fig. 4-102. Development of varying degrees of hypocalcemia in cows near parturition with corresponding increase in plasma PTH levels. The cow developing severe hypocalcemia (below 5 mg/100 ml) had a considerably greater increase in plasma PTH than the moderate rise detected in nonparetic, hypocalcemic, and normal cows. Note that PTH levels decline rapidly following treatment of the paretic cow with intravenous calcium. (From Mayer, 1970.)

ing chief cells are most numerous in parathyroids of cows fed balanced prepartal diets.[47,48] In response to the elevated blood calcium in cows fed high calcium prepartal diets, thyroid stores of calcitonin are diminished and C-cells are partially degranulated and appear to be actively synthesizing more hormone.[27] This stimulation of C-cells is accompanied by a decrease in bone turnover near parturition. Trabecular bone surfaces are inactive and few osteoclasts are resorbing bone.

A test of the immediately available calcium reserves by ethylenediaminetetraacetic acid (EDTA)-induced hypocalcemia compares the long-term effects of high calcium and balanced prepartal diets on the function of parathyroid glands and bone. Cows fed balanced diets respond to the experimental hypocalcemic challenge with a more rapid and greater increase in plasma PTH levels (Fig. 4-104) and the return of blood calcium to preinfusion levels was faster than in cows fed a high calcium diet. This was accompanied by a marked increase in urinary hydroxyproline excretion, suggesting increased bone matrix catabolism in response to the PTH secretion.[23,25] These findings suggest that the long-term feeding of a high calcium diet prepartum will partially suppress chief cells in the parathyroid glands, so that they are less able to respond rapidly by increased PTH synthesis and secretion to a hypocalcemic challenge either induced by EDTA infusion or associated with parturition and the initiation of lactation (Fig. 4-105).

Calcium homeostasis in pregnant cows fed a high calcium diet appears to be maintained principally by intestinal calcium absorption (Fig. 4-106). This greater reliance on intestinal absorption rather than on PTH-stimulated bone resorption probably is a significant factor in the more frequent development of profound hypocalcemia near parturition in cows fed high calcium prepartal diets. These cows would be more susceptible to the decreased calcium available for absorption as a result of the anorexia often associated with the high blood estrogen levels at parturition.[215]

Calcium homeostasis in cows fed balanced or relatively low calcium diets prepartum ap-

incriminated in significantly increasing the incidence of the disease.[98,305] Conversely, low calcium diets or prepartal diets supplemented with pharmacologic doses of vitamin D have been reported to reduce the incidence of the disease.[30,142,143,214]

Although cows fed a high calcium diet (CA 150 g:P 25 g/day) have higher blood calcium levels prepartum, they are less able to maintain serum calcium near the critical time of parturition. Plasma immunoreactive parathyroid hormone levels are lower prepartum than in cows fed a balanced diet (CA 25 g: P 25 g/day) and decline further at 48 hours postpartum.[27] Chief cells in the inactive stage of the secretory cycle predominate in cows fed high calcium diets, whereas actively synthesiz-

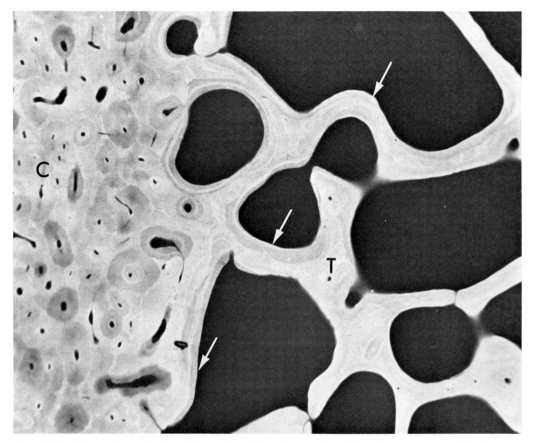

Fig. 4-103. Microradiograph of inactive cortical (C) and trabecular (T) bone from a cow with parturient hypocalcemia. The majority of trabecular bone surfaces are smooth, radiodense, and have few resorption cavities where osteoclasts are breaking down bone in order to mobilize calcium from skeletal reserves. (From Rowland, et al., 1972.)

pears to be more under the fine control of PTH secretion with the approach of parturition.[350] The higher levels of PTH secreted during the prepartal period by an expanded population of actively synthesizing chief cells results in a larger pool of active bone-resorbing cells to fulfill the increased needs for calcium mobilization at the critical time near parturition and the initiation of lactation. These cows would be less susceptible to the influence of decreased calcium absorption and flow into the extracellular calcium pool resulting from the anorexia and intestinal stasis associated with parturition (Fig. 4-107).

A syndrome biochemically and clinically resembling naturally occurring parturient paresis has been produced experimentally in

cows by the prepartal administration of diphosphonates.[352] These compounds are synthetic analogues of pyrophosphate and are proven inhibitors of bone resorption. When cows with no known history of parturient paresis were fed a low calcium diet and administered dichloromethane diphosphonate (CL_2MDP) postpartum, they consistently developed hypocalcemia and hypophosphatemia with muscular weakness, incoordination, and eventually sternal or lateral recumbency.[351] These studies suggest an important role for the skeleton in the maintenance of calcium homeostasis at parturition in dairy cows.[349] Following an intravenous EDTA infusion given 10 days prepartum, CL_2MDP-treated cows developed a severe

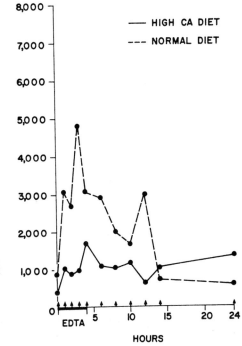

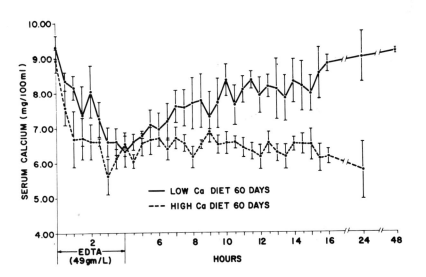

Fig. 4-104. Test of parathyroid gland response to experimental hypocalcemia induced by EDTA in pregnant cows fed high calcium and normal balanced diets. Cows fed the normal prepartal diet responded to the hypocalcemia with a more rapid and greater increase in immunoreactive PTH than cows fed a high calcium diet. (From Black, Capen, and Arnaud, 1973.)

Fig. 4-105. Immediately available calcium reserves in pregnant cows fed a low calcium compared to a high calcium diet prior to parturition. In response to a hypocalcemic challenge provided by a EDTA infusion, cows fed the low calcium diet are able to mobilize calcium from skeletal reserves and return the blood calcium level to the normal range more rapidly than cows fed a high calcium diet thereby preventing the development of hypocalcemia. In cows fed the high calcium diet chief cells in the parathyroid gland are inactive and there are few osteoclasts on bone surfaces. Cows fed the low calcium diet have predominately actively secreting chief cells in the parathyroids and frequent osteoclasts on bone surfaces.

HIGH CALCIUM PREPARTAL DIET

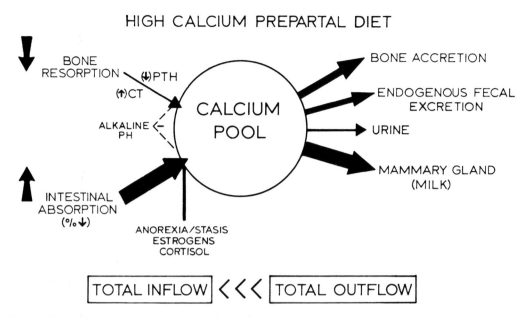

Fig. 4-106. Calcium homeostasis in cows fed a high calcium prepartal diet is primarily dependent upon intestinal calcium absorption. The rate of bone resorption is low and parathyroid glands are inactive. Anorexia and gastrointestinal stasis that often occur near parturition interrupt the major inflow into the extracellular fluid calcium pool. Outflow of calcium with the onset of lactation exceeds the rate of inflow into the calcium pool and the cows develop a progressive hypocalcemia and paresis. (Modified from Mayer, 1971.)

LOW CALCIUM PREPARTAL DIET

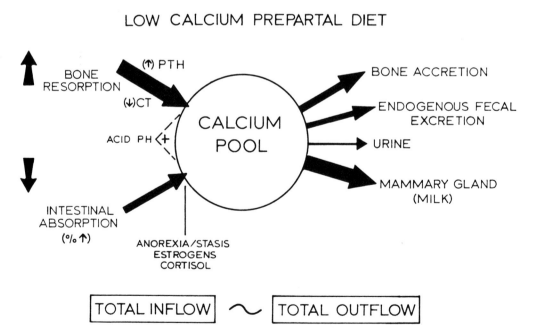

Fig. 4-107. Calcium homeostasis in cows fed a low calcium prepartal diet. Bone resorption and intestinal absorption both contribute substantially to the inflow of calcium to the pool in extracellular fluids. The anorexia and gastrointestinal stasis that often occur near parturition may temporarily interrupt one inflow pathway. However, there is more likely to be an adequate pool of active bone resorbing cells capable of responding to the increased PTH secretion under these dietary conditions to maintain an approximate balance between calcium inflow and outflow, thereby preventing the development of progressive hypocalcemia. (Modified from Mayer, 1971.)

and prolonged hypocalcemia despite elevated levels of parathyroid hormone. Urinary excretion of hydroxyproline was low and remained relatively unchanged during the 24 hours of the EDTA study. The rapid mobilization of calcium reserves in cows administered CL_2MDP prepartum was impaired because of diminished resorption of bone even though secretion of parathyroid hormone increased in response to severe hypocalcemia induced by parturition or EDTA. These results suggest that the CL_2MDP-treated cows that developed parturient hypocalcemia were similar to cows fed a high calcium diet in that they were more dependent upon calcium absorption from the gastrointestinal tract than upon skeletal calcium mobilization for the maintenance of calcium homeostasis.

Pharmacologic doses of vitamin D_2 have been administered to dairy cows prepartum to develop an effective method for the prevention of parturient hypocalcemia and paresis. High levels of the parent vitamin D compound are known to increase the rate and quantity of calcium and phosphorus absorbed from the intestinal tract in cattle, to progressively elevate the blood calcium and phosphorus levels after 3 to 5 days, and to increase the net calcium deposition and retention in areas of new bone growth. The calcium mobilization rate and the immediately available calcium reserve increase in cattle after vitamin D injection. Hibbs and Pounden reported that 20 to 30 million IU of vitamin D_2 fed daily for at least 3 but not more than 7 days before parturition prevented approximately 80% of the cases of parturient hypocalcemia.[143] Due to the inherent difficulty in accurately predicting the date of parturition, however, clinical and pathological evidences of toxicity have been observed in cattle given vitamin D in large doses for an extended period.[49] These included gastrointestinal stasis, diuresis and anorexia, abnormal cardiac function, reduced rumination, weight loss, and extensive mineralization of the cardiovascular system. Cardiovascular mineralization was not present after 7 days of administration of the parent vitamin D compound but was observed after 10 days and

became extensive and widespread after 21 days. The 3- to 5-day delay preceding a significant elevation in blood calcium and phosphorus and the cardiovascular toxicity following administration for extended periods have limited the usefulness of the parent vitamin D compound in preventing the development of hypocalcemia in susceptible cows.

Active vitamin D metabolites appear to be promising in the prevention of parturient hypocalcemia and paresis.[54] The more rapid onset of action (6 to 8 hours), greater potency (up to several hundredfold), and ability to regulate more precisely the magnitude of elevation in blood calcium, thereby minimizing potential toxic effects, are distinct advantages of the principal active metabolite of vitamin D_3 (1,25-dihydroxcholecalciferol) over the parent vitamin D compound in the development of an effective prophylactic regimen for parturient paresis-susceptible dairy cows. The administration of 1,25-dihydroxyvitamin D by the intramuscular route results in a dose-related increase in serum calcium (Fig. 4-108). The earliest significant increase occurred at 18 hours in cows receiving 600 and 270 μg of steroid, and blood levels remained elevated during the 5-day experimental period.[147] A peak increase of 4.2 mg. in calcium up to 12.1 mg/dl occurred in cows administered 600 μg at 48 hours (Fig. 4-108). Serum phosphorus was increased significantly by 12 hours following injection of 600 μg of 1,25-dihydroxyvitamin D and remained elevated during the experimental period. A peak increase of 3.1 mg in phosphorus up to 8.8 mg/dl occurred in cows receiving 600 μg of steroid at 66 hours. Urinary hydroxyproline was significantly elevated by 12 hours following injection of 60 μg of 1,25-dihydroxyvitamin D and remained elevated for 48 hours. The principal active metabolite of vitamin D appeared to increase bone resorption in adult cows, in addition to its well-known effect on stimulating intestinal calcium transport.

Studies in parturient paresis-susceptible pregnant cows indicate that the intramuscular administration of 600 μg of 1,25-dihydroxyvitamin D between 24 and 48 hours prepar-

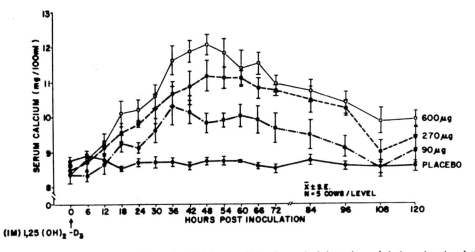

Fig. 4-108. Changes in serum calcium for 120 hours following administration of 4 dose levels of the principal active metabolite of vitamin D_3 (1,25-dihydroxycholecalciferol). Serum calcium was significantly elevated by 18 hours following intramuscular injection of 270 and 600 μg of 1,25-$(OH)_2D_3$ and remained elevated above placebo-injected control cows during the 5 day experimental period. (From Hoffsis, G. F., et al.: The use of 1,25-dihydroxycholecalciferol in the prevention of parturient hypocalcemia in dairy cows. Bovine Pract., 13 : 88, 1978.)

tum, before a decline in serum calcium and phosphorus had occurred, was effective in maintaining blood levels near the time of parturition. Blood calcium and phosphorus were stable or increasing at parturition and during initiation of lactation.[43] If the actual time of parturition was not predicted, the initial 600-μg dose of 1,25-dihydroxyvitamin D was administered from 3.5 to 11 days before parturition. Blood calcium and phosphorus were stabilized by the injection of a smaller (270 μg) dose of steroid at 48- to 96-hour intervals until the actual time of parturition. Figure 4-109 illustrates the effects in a Jersey

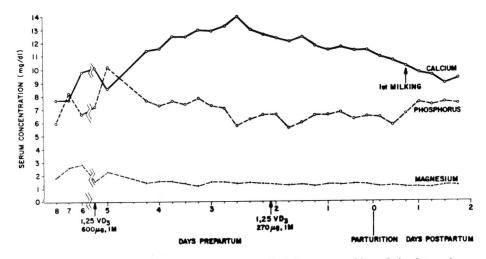

Fig. 4-109. Effect of two doses (600 μg, 270 μg) of 1,25-$(OH)_2D_3$ separated by a 3-day interval on serum calcium, phosphorus, and magnesium in a parturient paresis-susceptible Jersey cow. (From Capen, C. C., et al.: 1,25-Dihydroxycholecalciferol and the prevention of parturient hypocalcemia and paresis ("milk fever") in pregnant dairy cows. *In* Proceedings of 4th Workshop on Vitamin D, edited by A. W. Norman, et al. Berlin/New York, Walter de Gruyter., Inc., 1979.)

cow in which the 600-μg dose was administered at 5.5 days prepartum followed after 72 hours by 270 μg of 1,25-$(OH)_2D_3$. The serum calcium increased progressively for 60 hours following the 600-μg injection, was 10.9 mg/dl at parturition, and remained at 9.3 mg/dl 42 hours postpartum. The serum phosphorus was 6.2 mg/dl at parturition and had increased to 7.2 mg/dl at 42 hours postpartum.

Puerperal Tetany in the Bitch

Less is known about the development of hypocalcemic syndromes in other animal species than in the cow. Puerperal tetany is most frequently encountered in the small, hyperexcitable breeds of dogs. The clinical course is rapid and the bitch may proceed from premonitory signs of restlessness, panting, and nervousness to ataxia, trembling, muscular tetany, and convulsive seizures in 8 to 12 hours.[163,264]

Functional disturbances associated with hypocalcemia in the bitch are primarily the result of neuromuscular tetany (Fig. 4-110), whereas in cows the clinical signs are related to paresis (Fig. 4-111). The occurrence of either tetany or paresis in response to hypo-calcemia appears to be the result of basic physiologic differences in the function of the neuromuscular junction of the cow and the bitch.[31] The release of acetylcholine and transmission of nerve impulses across neuromuscular junctions are blocked by hypocalcemia in cows (but not in bitches) leading to muscle paresis (Fig. 4-111). The dog appears to have a higher margin of safety in neuromuscular transmission in that the degree the endplate potential exceeds the firing threshold is greater in the dog than in the cow. Excitation-secretion coupling is maintained at the neuromuscular junction in the bitch with hypocalcemia. Tetany occurs in the bitch as a result of spontaneous repetitive firing of motor nerve fibers (Fig. 4-110). Due to the loss of stabilizing membrane-bound calcium, nerve membranes become more permeable to ions and require a stimulus of lesser magnitude to depolarize.

There is no evidence to suggest that puerperal tetany (eclampsia) in heavily lactating bitches is the result of an interference in parathyroid hormone secretion. Severe hypocalcemia and often hypophosphatemia develop near the time of peak lactation (approximately 1 to 3 weeks postpartum), probably the result

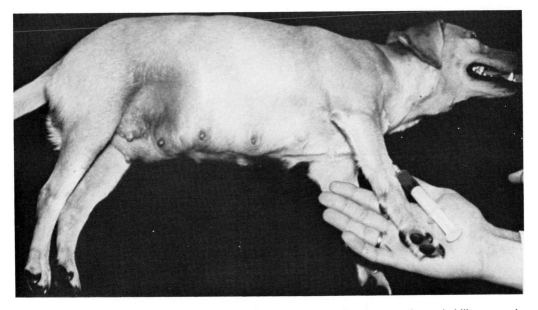

Fig. 4-110. Puerperal tetany in a bitch with hypocalcemia. Increased neuromuscular excitability occurs in the bitch with hypocalcemia, since excitation-secretion coupling is maintained at the motor endplate.

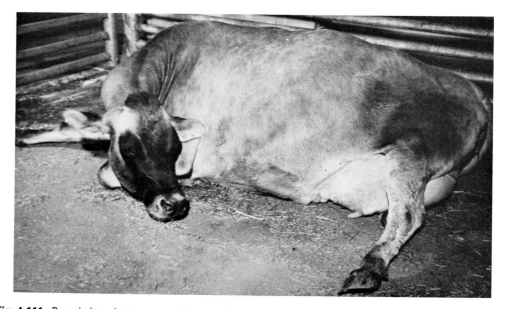

Fig. 4-111. Paresis in a Jersey cow with parturient hypocalcemia owing to a blockage in neuromuscular transmission.

of temporary failure in homeostasis resulting in an imbalance between the rates of inflow to and outflow from the extracellular fluid calcium pool. The administration of intravenous calcium to stop the tetany combined with temporarily decreasing the lactational drain of calcium by removing the pups usually corrects the disruption of calcium homeostasis in the majority of bitches. Supplemental dietary calcium and vitamin D have proven useful in preventing relapses in certain bitches with puerperal tetany.[193]

REFERENCES

1. Aliapoulios, M. A., Goldhaber, P., and Munson, P. L. (1966): Thyrocalcitonin inhibition of bone resorption induced by parathyroid hormone in tissue culture. Science *151:*330.
2. Altenähr, E. (1972): Ultrastructural pathology of parathyroid glands. Curr. Top. Pathol. *56:*1.
3. Altenähr, E., and Leonhardt, F. (1972): Suppression of parathyroid gland activity by magnesium. Morphometric ultrastructural investigation. Virchows Arch. [Pathol. Anat.] *335:*297.
4. Altenähr, E., and Seifert, G. (1971): Ultrastruktureller Vergleich menschlicher Epithelkörperchen ber sekundärem Hyperparathyreodismus und primärem Adenom. Virchows Arch. [Pathol. Anat.] *353:*60.
5. Anderson, M. P., and Capen, C. C. (1976): Nutritional osteodystrophy in captive green iguanas (*Iguana iguana*). Virchows Arch. [Cell Pathol.] *21:*229.
6. Anderson, M. P., and Capen, C. C. (1976): Ultrastructural evaluation of parathyroid and ultimobronchial glands in iguanas with experimental nutritional osteodystrophy. Gen. Comp. Endocrinol. *30:*209.
7. Argenzio, R. A., Lowe, J. E., Hintz, H. F., et al. (1974): Calcium and phosphorus homeostasis in horses. J. Nutr. *104:*18.
8. Arnaud, C. D. (1973): Parathyroid hormone: Coming of age in clinical medicine. Am. J. Med. *55:*577.
9. Arnaud, C. D., Sizemore, G. W., Oldham, S. B., et al. (1971): Human parathyroid hormone: Glandular and secreted molecular species. Am. J. Med. *50:*630.
10. Arnold, B. M., Kovacs, K., Horvath, E., et al. (1974): Functioning oxyphil cell adenoma of the parathyroid gland: Evidence for parathyroid secretory activity of oxyphil cells. J. Clin. Endocrinol. Metab. *38:*458.
11. Arnold, S. A., Kram, M. A., Hintz, H. F., et al. (1974): Nutritional secondary hyperparathyroidism in the parakeet. Cornell Vet. *64:*37.
12. Aurbach, G. D., and Potts, J. T., Jr. (1964): The Parathyroids. *In* Advances in Metabolic Diseases, Vol. 1, edited by R. Levine and R. Luft. New York, Academic Press, pp. 45–93.
13. Aurbach, G. D., Potts, J. T., Jr., Chase, L. R., et al. (1969): Polypeptide hormone and calcium metabolism. Ann. Int. Med. *70:*1243.
14. Avioli, L. V., and Haddad, J. G. (1973): Vitamin D: Current concepts. Metabolism *22:*507.
15. Balogh, K., and Cohen, R. B. (1961): Oxidative enzymes in the epithelial cells of normal and patho-

logical human parathyroid glands. Lab. Invest. *10:* 354.

16. Barlet, J. P. (1968): Induction expérimentale d'un syndrome analogue á la fiévre vitulaire par administration de thyrocalcitonine á des vaches en cours de lactation. C. R. Acad. Sci. (Paris) *267:*2010.

17. Barlet, J. P. (1972): Calcium homeostasis in the normal and thyroidectomized bovine. Horm. Metab. Res. *4:*300.

18. Barnes, B. G. (1963): The fine structure of the mouse adenohypophysis in various physiologic states. *In* Cytologic de L'Adenohypophyse, edited by J. Benoit and C. da Lage. Paris, Centre National de la Récherche Scientifique, pp. 91–109.

19. Bauer, W. C., and Teitelbaum, S. L. (1966): Thyrocalcitonin activity of particulate fractions of the thyroid gland. Lab. Invest. *15:*323.

20. Beck N., Singh H., Harbans S., et al. (1974): Direct inhibitory effects of hypercalcemia on renal actions of parathyroid hormone. J. Clin. Invest. *53:*717.

21. Bhattacharyya, M. H., and DeLuca, H. F. (1974): Subcellular location of rat liver calciferol-25-hydroxylase. Arch. Biochem. Biophys. *160:*58.

22. Birkenhäger, J. C., Seldenrath, H. J., Hackeng, W. H. L., et al. (1973): Calcium and phosphorus metabolism, parathyroid hormone, calcitonin and bone histology in pseudohypoparathyroidism. Eur. J. Clin. Invest. *3:*27.

23. Black, H. E., and Capen, C. C. (1971): Urinary and plasma hydroxyproline during pregnancy, parturition and lactation in cows with parturient hypocalcemia. Metabolism *20:*337.

24. Black, H. E., and Capen, C. C. (1973): Plasma calcitonin-like activity and urinary cyclic adenosine monophosphate during pregnancy, parturition, and lactation in cows with parturient hypocalcemia. Horm. Metab. Res. *5:*297.

25. Black, H. E., Capen, C. C., and Arnaud, C. D. (1973): Ultrastructure of parathyroid glands and plasma immunoreactive parathyroid hormone in pregnant cows fed normal and high calcium diets. Lab. Invest. *29:*173.

26. Black, H. E., Capen, C. C., and Young, D. M. (1973): Ultimobranchial thyroid neoplasms in bulls. A syndrome resembling medullary thyroid carcinoma in man. Cancer *32:*865.

27. Black, H. E., Capen, C. C., Yarrington, J. T., et al. (1973): Effect of a high calcium prepartal diet on calcium homeostatic mechanisms in thyroid glands, bone, and intestine of cows. Lab. Invest. *29:*437.

28. Blum, J. W., Mayer, G. P., and Potts, J. T., Jr. (1974): Parathyroid hormone responses during spontaneous hypocalcemia and induced hypercalcemia in cows. Endocrinology *95:*84.

29. Blum, J. W., Ramberg, C. F., Jr., Johnson, K. G., et al. (1972): Calcium (ionized and total), magnesium, phosphorus, and glucose in plasma from parturient cows. Am. J. Vet. Res. *33:*51.

30. Boda, J. M., and Cole, H. H. (1956): Studies on parturient paresis in dairy cattle. Ann. N.Y. Acad. Sci. *64:*370.

31. Bowen, J. M., Blackmon, D. M., and Heavner, J. E. (1970): Neuromuscular transmission and hypocalcemic paresis in the cow. Am. J. Vet. Res. *31:*831.

32. Boyle, I. T., Omdahl, J. L., Gray, R. W., et al.

(1973): The biological activity and metabolism of 24,25-dihydroxyvitamin D_3. J. Biol. Chem. *248:* 4174.

33. Brewer, H. B., Fairwell, T., Rittel, W., et al. (1974): Recent studies on the chemistry of human, bovine and porcine parathyroid hormone. Am. J. Med. *56:* 759.

34. Brickman. A. S., Coburn, J. W., Massry, S. G., et al. (1974): 1,25 dihydroxy-vitamin D_3 in normal man and patients with renal failure. Ann. Intern. Med. *80:*161.

35. Brumbaugh, P. F., and Haussler, M. R. (1973): Nuclear and cytoplasmic receptors for 1,25-dihydroxycholecalciferol in intestinal mucosa. Biochem. Biophys. Res. Commun. *51:*74.

36. Brunette, M. G., Chan, M., Ferriere, C., et al. (1978): Site of 1,25 $(OH)_2$ vitamin D_3 synthesis in the kidney. Nature *276:*287.

37. Burtis, W. J., Wu, T., Bunch, C., et al. (1987): Identification of a novel 17,000-dalton parathyroid hormone-like adenylate cyclase-stimulating protein from a tumor associated with humoral hypercalcemia of malignancy. J. Biol. Chem. *262:*7151.

38. Capen, C. C. (1971): Fine structural changes of parathyroid glands in response to experimental and spontaneous alterations of extracellular fluid calcium. Am. J. Med. *50:*598.

39. Capen, C. C. (1972): Endocrine control of calcium metabolism and parturient hypocalcemia in dairy cattle. *In* Proc. 4th Ann. Conv. Am. Assoc. Bovine Pract., edited by E. I. Williams, Stillwater, Heritage Press, pp. 189–198.

40. Capen, C. C. (1975): Functional and fine structural relationships of parathyroid glands. *In* Advances in Veterinary Sciences and Comparative Medicine. New York, Academic Press, pp. 249–286.

41. Capen, C. C. (1982): Nutritional secondary hyperparathyroidism in horses. *In*: Current Therapy in Equine Medicine. (N. E. Robinson, Editor) Philadelphia, W. B. Saunders Co., pp. 160–163.

42. Capen, C. C. (1983): Structural and biochemical aspects of parathyroid gland function in animals. *In*: Monograph on Pathology of Laboratory Animals: Volume 1, Endocrine System. (T. C. Jones, U. Mohr, and R. D. Hunt, Editors). International Life Sciences Institute Series. New York, Springer-Verlag, Inc., pp. 217–247.

43. Capen, C. C. (1985): The Endocrine Glands. Chapter 3. *In*: Pathology of Domestic Animals. Third Edition, Volume III. (K. V. F. Jubb, P. C. Kennedy and N. Palmer, Editors). New York, Academic Press Inc, pp. 237–303.

44. Capen, C. C. (1985): Calcium-regulating hormones and metabolic bone disease. *In*: Textbook of Small Animal Orthopaedics. Chapter 59, Philadelphia, J. B. Lippincott Co. (C. D. Newton and D. M. Nunamaker, Editors). pp. 673–722.

45. Capen, C. C. (1988): The Endocrine System. *In*: Textbook of Special Veterinary Pathology. Chapter 9, (R. G. Thomson, Editor), Philadelphia, B. C. Decker Publisher.

46. Capen, C. C., and Black, H. E. (1974): Calcitonin-secreting ultimobranchial neoplasms of the thyroid gland in bulls: An animal model for medullary thyroid carcinoma in man (Sipple's syndrome). Am. J.

Pathol. *74:*377.

47. Capen, C. C., and Black, H. E. (1975): Fine-structural evaluation of parathyroid glands of cows fed high, normal, and low-calcium diets. *In* Electron Microscopic Concepts of Secretion: Ultrastructure of Endocrinal and Reproductive Organs, edited by M. Hess, New York, pp. 379–398.

48. Capen, C. C., Black, H. E., and Arnaud, C. D. (1973): Fine structural evaluation of parathyroid glands from cows fed low and high calcium diets. *In* 31st Ann. Proc. Electron Microscopy Soc. Amer., edited by C. J. Arceneaux. Baton Rouge, Claitor's Publishing, pp. 678–679.

49. Capen, C. C., Cole, C. R., and Hibbs, J. W. (1966): The pathology of hypervitaminosis D in cattle. Pathol. Vet *3:*350.

50. Capen, C. C., Cole, C. R., and Hibbs, J. W. (1968): The influence of vitamin D on calcium metabolism and the parathyroid glands of cattle. Fed. Proc. *27:* 142.

51. Capen, C. C., Hoffsis, G. F., and Norman, A. W. (1979): 1,25-dihydroxycholecalciferol and the prevention of parturient hypocalcemia and paresis ("milk fever") in pregnant diary cows. *In* Proceedings of 4th Workshop on Vitamin D, edited by A. W. Norman, et al. Berlin/New York, Walter de Gruyter.

52. Capen, C. C., and Martin, S. L. (1974): Hyperparathyroidism in animals. *In* Current Veterinary Therapy, V, edited by R. W. Kirk. Philadelphia, W. B. Saunders Co., pp. 797–805.

53. Capen, C. C., and Martin, S. L. (1977): Calcium metabolism and disorders of parathyroid glands. Vet. Clin. North Am. *7:*513.

54. Capen, C. C., and Martin, S. L. (1982): Calcium regulating hormones and diseases of the parathyroid glands, Chapter 66. *In*: Textbook of Veterinary Internal Medicine. Second Edition. (S. J. Ettinger, Editor) Philadelphia, W. B. Saunders Co., pp. 1550–1592.

55. Capen, C. C., and Roth, S. I. (1973): Ultrastructural and functional relationships of normal and pathologic parathyroid cells. *In* Pathobiology Annual, edited by H. L. Ioachim. New York, Appleton-Century-Crofts, pp. 129–175.

56. Capen, C. C., and Rowland, G. N. (1968): Ultrastructural evaluation of the parathyroid glands of young cats with experimental hyperparathyroidism. Z. Zellforsch. Mikrosk. Anat. *90:*495.

57. Capen, C. C., and Young, D. M. (1967): The ultrastructure of the parathyroid glands and thyroid parafollicular cells of cows with parturient paresis and hypocalcemia. Lab. Invest. *17:*717.

58. Capen, C. C., and Young, D. M. (1969): Fine structural alterations in thyroid parafollicular cells of cows in response to experimental hypercalcemia induced by vitamin D. Am. J. Pathol. *57:*365.

59. Care, A. D., Bates, R. F. L., Phillippo. M., et al. (1970): Stimulation of calcitonin release from bovine thyroid by calcium and glucagon. J. Endocrinol. *48:*667.

60. Carrillo, B. J. (1973): Efecto de la intoxicación de *Solanum malacoxylon* en el sistema óseo. Rev. Invest. Agropecuarias, INTA, Serie 4. *10:*65.

61. Carrillo, B. J. (1973): Efecto de la intoxicación de *Solanum malacoxylon* en la morfologia de las células parafoliculares de la tiroides. Rev. Invest. Agropecuarias, INTA, Serie 4. *10:*41.

62. Carrillo, B. J., and Worker, N. A. (1967): Enteque seco: arteriosclerosis y calcificación metastásica de origen tóxico en anímales a pastoreo. Rev. Invest. Agropecuarias, INTA, Serie 4, *4:*9.

63. Chambers, T. J. (1980): The cellular basis of bone resorption. Clin. Orthop. Rel. Res. *151:*283.

64. Chambers, T. J., and Fuller, K. (1985): Bone cells predispose bone surfaces to resorption by exposure of mineral to osteoclastic contact. J. Cell Sci. *76:*155.

65. Chambers, T. J., and Mangus, C. J. (1982): Calcitonin alters behavior of isolated osteoclasts. J. Pathol. *136:*27.

66. Chambers, T. J., and Moore, A. (1983): The sensitivity of isolated osteoclasts to morphological transformation by calcitonin. J. Clin. Endocrinol. Metab. *57:*819.

67. Chambers, T. J., Revell, P. A., Fuller, K., et al. (1984): Resorption of bone by isolated rabbit osteoclasts. J. Cell. Sci. *66:*383.

68. Cheville, N. F. (1972): Ultrastructure of canine carotid body and aortic body tumors. Comparison with tissues of thyroid and parathyroid origin. Vet. Pathol. *9:*166.

69. Chew, D. J., and Capen, C. C. (1980): Hypercalcemic nephropathy and associated disorders. *In*: Current Veterinary Therapy VII. (R. W. Kirk, Editor), Philadelphia, W. B. Saunders Co., pp. 1067–1072.

70. Christakos, S., and Norman, A. W. (1978): Vitamin D_3-induced calcium binding protein in bone tissue. Science *202:*70.

71. Chu, L. L. H., MacGregor, R. R., Anast, C. S., et al. (1973): Studies on the biosynthesis of rat parathyroid hormone and proparathyroid hormone: Adaptation of the parathyroid gland to dietary restriction of calcium. Endocrinology *93:*915.

72. Chu, L. L. H., MacGregor, R. R., Liu, P. I., et al. (1973): Biosynthesis of proparathyroid hormone and parathyroid hormone by human parathyroid glands. J. Clin. Invest. *52:*3089.

73. Cohn, D. V., and Elting, J. (1983): Biosynthesis, processing, and secretion of parathormone and secretory protein-I. Recent Progress Hormone Res. *39:*181.

74. Cohn, D. V., and MacGregor, R. R. (1981): The biosynthesis, intracellular processing, and secretion of parathormone. Endocrine Rev. *2:*1.

75. Cohn, D. V., MacGregor, R. R., Chu, L. L. H., et al. (1974): Biosynthesis of proparathyroid hormone and parathyroid hormone. Chemistry, physiology and role of calcium in regulation. Am. J. Med. *56:* 767.

76. Cohn, D. V., MacGregor, R. R., Chu, L. L., et al. (1972): Calcemic fraction-A: Biosynthetic peptide precursor of parathyroid hormone. Proc. Natl. Acad. Sci. USA *69:*1521.

77. Cohn, D. V., Zangerle, R., Fischer-Colbrie, R., et al. (1982): Similarity of secretory protein I from parathyroid gland to chromogranin A from adrenal medulla. Proc. Natl. Acad. Sci. (USA) *79:*6056.

78. Coleman, R. (1969): Ultrastructural observations on the parathyroid glands of *Xenopus laevis* Daudin.

Z. Zellforsch. *100:*201.

79. Collins, W. T. Jr., Capen, C. C., Dobereiner, J., et al. (1977): Ultrastructural evaluation of parathyroid glands and thyroid C cells of cattle fed *Solanum malacoxylon.* Am. J. Pathol. *87:*603.

80. Cooper, C. W., Schwesinger, W. H., Ontjes, D. A., et al. (1972): Stimulation of secretion of pig thyrocalcitonin by gastrin and related hormonal peptides. Endocrinology *91:*1079.

81. Copp, D. H. (1969): Endocrine control of calcium homeostasis. J. Endocrinol. *43:*137.

82. Copp, D. H. (1970): Endocrine regulation of calcium metabolism. Ann. Rev. Physiol. *32:*61.

83. Copp, D. H., Cameron, E. C., Cheney, B. A., et al. (1962): Evidence for calcitonin—a new hormone from the parathyroid that lowers blood calcium. Endocrinology *70:*638.

84. Cortelyou, J. R., and McWhinnie, D. J. (1967): Parathyroid glands of amphibians. I. Parathyroid structure and function in the amphibians, with emphasis on regulation of mineral ions in body fluids. Am. Zoologist *7:*843.

85. Costoff, A., and McShan, W. H. (1969): Isolation and biological properties of secretory granules from rat anterior pituitary granules. J. Cell Biol. *43:*564.

86. Deftos, L. J., Murray, T. M., Powell, D. et al. (1972): Radioimmunoassays for parathyroid hormones and calcitonins. *In* Calcium, Parathyroid Hormone and the Calcitonins, edited by R. V. Talmage and P. L. Munson. Amsterdam, Excerpta Medica pp. 140–151.

87. DeGrandi, P. B., Kraehenbuhl, J. P., and Campiche, M. A. (1971): Ultrastructural localization of calcitonin in the parafollicular cells of the pig thyroid gland with cytochrome c-labeled antibody fragments. J. Cell Biol. *50:*446.

88. DeLuca, H. F. (1973): The kidney as an endocrine organ for the production of 1,25-dihydroxyvitamin D_3, a calcium-mobilizing hormone. N. Engl. J. Med. *289:*359.

89. DeLuca, H. F. (1974): Vitamin D—1973. Am. J. Med. *56:*871.

90. DeLuca, H. F. (1976): Recent advances in our understanding of the vitamin D endocrine system. J. Lab. Clin. Med. *87:*7.

91. DeLuca, H. F. (1977): Vitamin D as a prohormone. Biochem. Pharmacol. *26:*563.

92. DeLuca, H. F. (1978): Vitamin D and calcium transport. Ann. N.Y. Acad. Sci. *307:*356.

93. DeLuca, H. F., and Schnoes, H. K. (1983): Vitamin D: Recent advances. Ann. Rev. Biochem. *52:* 411.

94. Döbereiner, J., Tokarnia, C. H., DaCosta, J. B. D., et al. (1971): "Espichamento", intoxicacão de bovinos por *Solanum malacoxylon*, no pantanal de mato grosso. Pesq. Agropec. Bras., Sér. Vet. 91.

95. Drezner, M., Neelon, F. A., and Lebovitz, H. E. (1973): Pseudohypoparathyroidism type II. A possible defect in the reception of the cyclic AMP signal. N. Engl. J. Med. *289:*1056.

96. D'Souza, S. M., Ibbotson, K. J., and Mundy, G. R. (1984): Failure of parathyroid hormone antagonists to inhibit *in vitro* bone resorbing activity produced by two animal models of the humoral hypercalcemia of malignancy. J. Clin. Invest. *74:*1104.

97. Elissalde, G. S., Wooldridge, J. B., Steel, E. G., et al. (1980): Treatment of a seizuring hypoparathyroid dog. Canine Pract. *7:*14.

98. Ender, F., Dishington, I. W., and Helgebostad, A. (1962): Parturient paresis and related forms of hypocalcemic disorders induced experimentally in dairy cows. Acta Vet. Scand. *3*(Suppl. 1):1.

99. Fawcett, C. P., Powell, A. E., and Sachs, H. (1968): Biosynthesis and release of neurophysin. *83:*1299.

100. Fetter, A. W., and Capen, C. C. (1968): Ultrastructural evaluation of the parathyroid glands of pigs with naturally occurring atrophic rhinitis. Pathol. Vet. *5:*481.

101. Fetter, A. W., and Capen, C. C. (1970): The ultrastructure of the parathyroid glands of young pigs. Acta Anat. *75:*359.

102. Finco, D. R., and Rowland, G. N. (1978): Hypercalcemia secondary to chronic renal failure in the dog: A report of four cases. J. Am. Vet. Med. Assoc. *173:*990.

103. Fischer, J. A., Oldham, S. B., Sizemore, G. W., et al. (1972): Calcium-regulated parathyroid hormone peptidase. Proc. Natl. Acad. Sci. USA *69:*2341.

104. Foster, G. V., Byfield, P. G. H., and Gudmundsson, T.V. (1972): Calcitonin. *In* Clinics in Endocrinology and Metabolism, *Vol. I,* edited by I. MacIntyre. Philadelphia, W. B. Saunders Co., pp. 93–124.

105. Fraser, D. R. (1983): The physiological economy of vitamin D. Lancet *833:*969.

106. Fraser, D. R., and Kodicek, E. (1973): Regulation of 25-hydroxycholecalciferol-1-hydroxylase activity in kidney by parathyroid hormone. Nature (London) *241:*163.

107. Freitag, J., Martin, K. J., Hruska, D. A., et al. (1978): Impaired parathyroid hormone metabolism in patients with chronic renal failure. N. Engl. J. Med. *298:*29.

108. Friedman, J., Au, W. Y. W., and Raisz, L. G. (1968): Responses of fetal rat bone to thyrocalcitonin in tissue culture. Endocrinology. *82:*149.

109. Frost, H. M. (1983): The skeletal intermediary organization. Metab. Bone Dis. & Rel. Res. *4:*281.

110. Fujii, H., and Isono, H. (1972): Ultrastructural observations on the parathyroid glands of the hen (*Gallus domesticus*). Arch. Histol. Jpn. *34:*155.

111. Gaillard, P. J. (1965): Observations on the effect of parathyroid products on explanted mouse limbbone rudiments. *In* The Parathyroid Glands. Ultrastructure, Secretion, and Function, edited by P. J. Gaillard, R. V. Talmage and A. M. Budy. Chicago, University of Chicago Press, pp. 145–169.

112. Galasko, C. S. B., Bennett, A. (1976): Relationship of bone destruction in skeletal metastases to osteoclast activation and prostaglandins. Nature *263:*508.

113. Garabedian, M., Holick, M. F., DeLuca, H. F., et al. (1972): Control of 25-hydroxycholecalciferol metabolism by parathyroid glands. Proc. Natl. Acad. Sci. USA *69:*1673.

114. Gilka, F., and Sugden, E. A. (1984): Ectopic mineralization and nutritional hyperparathyroidism in boars. Canad. J. Comp. Med. *48:*102.

115. Goddard, K. M., Williams, G. D., Newberne, P. M., et al. (1970): A comparison of all-meat, semimoist, and dry-type dog foods as diets for growing beagles. J. Am. Vet. Med. Assoc. *157:*1233.

116. Goltzman, D., Bennett, H. P. J., Koutsilieris, M., et al. (1986): Studies of the multiple molecular forms of bioactive parathyroid hormone and parathyroid hormone-like substances. Recent Prog. Hormone Res. *42:*665.

117. Gorham, J. R., Peckham, J. C., and Alexander, J. (1970): Rickets and osteodystrophia fibrosa in foxes fed a high horsemeat ration. J. Am. Vet. Med. Assoc. *156:*1331.

118. Goustin, A. S., Leof, E. B., Shipley, G. D., et al. (1986): Growth factors and cancer. Cancer Res. *46:* 1015.

119. Grau, H., and Dellmann, H. D. (1958): Über tierartliche Unterschiede der Epithelkörperchen unserer Haussäugetiere. Z. Mikros-Anat. Forsch. *64:* 192.

120. Gray, R. W., Omdahl, J. L., Ghazarian, J. G., et al. (1972): 25-hydroxycholecalciferol-1-hydroxylase: Subcellular location and properties. J. Biol. Chem. *247:*7528.

121. Gray, T. K. and Ontjes, D. A., (1975): Clinical aspects of thyrocalcitonin. Clin. Orthop. *111:*238.

122. Habener, J. F. (1976): New concepts in the formation, regulation of release, and metabolism of parathyroid hormone. *In* Polypeptide Hormones: Molecular and Cellular Aspects, Ciba Fnd. Symp. 41. Amsterdam, Elsevier/Excerpta Medica, pp. 197–224.

123. Habener, J. F. (1981): Recent advances in parathyroid hormone research. Clin. Biochem. *14:*223.

124. Habener, J. F., Chang, H. T., and Potts, J. T., Jr. (1977): Enzymatic processing of proparathyroid hormone by cell-free extracts of parathyroid glands. Biochemistry *16:*3910.

125. Habener, J. F., and Kronenberg, H. M. (1978): Parathyroid hormone biosynthesis: structure and function of biosynthetic precursors. Fed. Proc. *37:* 2561.

126. Habener, J. F., Powell, D., Murray, T. M., et al. (1971): Parathyroid hormone: Secretion and metabolism *in vitro*. Proc. Natl. Acad. Sci. USA *68:*2986.

127. Habener, J. F., and Potts, J. T., Jr. (1976): Chemistry, biosynthesis, secretion and metabolism of parathyroid hormone. *In* Handbook of Physiology, Endocrinology VII—Parathyroid Gland. Washington, D. C., American Physiology Society, Chapter 13, pp. 313–342.

128. Habener, J. F., and Potts, J. T., Jr. (1978): Biosynthesis of parathyroid hormone. N. Engl. J. Med. *299:*580, 635.

129. Habener, J. F., and Potts, J. T., Jr. (1979): Subcellular distribution of parathyroid hormone, hormonal precursors, and parathyroid secretory protein. Endocrinology *104:*265.

130. Habener, J. F., Singer, F. R., Neer, R. M., et al. (1972): Metabolism of salmon and porcine calcitonin: An explanation for the increased potency of salmon calcitonin. *In* Calcium, Parathyroid Hormone and the Calcitonins, edited by R. V. Talmage and P. L. Munson. Amsterdam, Exerpta Medica, pp. 152–156.

131. Hara, J., and Nagatsu-Ishibashi, I. (1964): Electron microscopic study of the parathyroid gland of the mouse. Nagoya J. Med. Sci. *26:*119.

132. Harcourt-Webster, J. N., and Truman, R. F. (1969): Histochemical study of oxidative and hydrolytic enzymes in the abnormal human parathyroid. J. Pathol. *97:*687.

133. Hargis, G. K., Yakulis, V. J., Williams, G. A., et al. (1964): Cytological detection of parathyroid hormone by immunofluorescence. Proc. Soc. Exp. Biol. Med. *117:*836.

134. Harrington, D. D. (1982): Acute vitamin D_2 (ergocalciferol) toxicosis in horses: Case report and experimental studies. J. Am. Vet. Med. Assoc. *180:* 867.

135. Haussler, M. R., Boyce, D. W., Littledike, E. T., et al. (1971): A rapidly acting metabolite of vitamin D_3. Proc. Natl. Acad. Sci. USA *68:*177.

136. Haussler, M. R., and McCain, T. A. (1977): Basic and clinical concepts related to vitamin D metabolism and action. N. Engl. J. Med. *297:*974, 1041.

137. Haussler, M. R., Nagode, L. N., and Rasmussen, H. (1970): Induction of intestinal brush border alkaline phosphatase by vitamin D and identity with CA-ATPase. Nature (London) *228:*1199.

138. Havinga, E. (1973): Vitamin D, example and challenge. Experientia *29:*1181.

139. Hazard, J. B. (1977): The C cells (parafollicular cells) of the thyroid gland and medullary thyroid carcinoma. Am. J. Pathol. *88:*214.

140. Heath, H., Weller, R. E., and Mundy, G. R. (1980): Canine lymphosarcoma: A model for study of the hypercalcemia of cancer. Calcif. Tissue Int. *30:*127.

141. Henry, H. L., and Norman, A. W. (1978): Vitamin D: two dihydroxylated metabolites are required for normal chicken egg hatchability. Science *201:*835.

142. Hibbs, J. W., and Conrad, H. R. (1960): Studies of milk fever in dairy cows. VI Effect of three prepartal dosage levels of vitamin D on milk fever incidence. J. Dairy Sci. *43:*1124.

143. Hibbs, J. W., and Pounden, W. D. (1956): Effect of parturient paresis and the oral administration of large prepartal doses of vitamin D on blood calcium and phosphorus in dairy cattle. Ann. N.Y. Acad. Sci. *64:*375.

144. High, W. B., Black, H. E., and Capen, C. C. (1981A): Histomorphometric evaluation of the effects of low dose parathyroid hormone administration on cortical bone remodeling in adult dogs. Lab. Invest. *44:*449.

145. High, W. B., Capen, C. C., and Black, H. E. (1981B): Histomorphometric evaluation of the effects of intermittent 1,25-dihydroxycholecalciferol administration on cortical bone remodeling in adult dogs. Am. J. Pathol. *104:*41.

146. High, W. B., Capen, C. C., and Black, H. E. (1981C): Effects of 1,25-dihydroxycholecalciferol, parathyroid hormone and thyroxine on trabecular bone remodeling in adult dogs: A histomorphometric study. Am. J. Pathol. *105:*1856.

147. Hoffsis, G. F., Capen, C. C., and Norman, A. W. (1978): The use of 1,25-dihydroxycholecalciferol in the prevention of parturient hypocalcemia in dairy cows. Bovine Pract. *13:*88.

148. Holick, M. F., and Clark, M. B. (1978): The photobiogenesis and metabolism of vitamin D. Fed. Proc. *37:*2567.

149. Holick, M. F., Frommer, J. E., McNeill, S. C., et al. (1977): Photometabolism of 7-dehydrocholesterol to

previtamin D₃ in skin. Bioch. Biophys. Res. Commun. *76:*107.

150. Howell, S. L., Fink, C. J., and Lacy, P. E. (1969): Isolation and properties of secretory granules from rat islets of Langerhans, I. Isolation of a secretory granule fraction. J. Cell Biol. *41:*154.

151. Hruska, K. A., Kopelman, R., Rutherford, W. E., et al. (1975): Metabolism of immunoreactive parathyroid hormone in the dog. The role of the kidney and the effects of chronic renal disease. J. Clin. Invest. *56:*39.

152. Hruska, K. A., Martin, K., Mennes, P., et al. (1977): Degradation of parathyroid hormone and fragment production by the isolated perfused dog kidney. The effect of glomerular filtration rate and perfusate Ca⁺⁺ concentrations. J. Clin. Invest. *60:* 501.

153. Hughes, M. R., and Haussler, M. R. (1978): 1,25-dihydroxyvitamin D₃ receptors in parathyroid glands. J. Biol. Chem. *253:*1065.

154. Hulter, H. N., Toto, R. D., Bonner, E. L., Jr., et al. (1981): Renal and systemic acid-base effects of chronic hypoparathyroidism in dogs. Am. J. Physiol. *241:*495.

155. Hunt, R. D., Garcia, F. G., and Hegsted, D. M. (1967): A comparison of vitamin D₂ and D₃ in new world primates. I. Production and regression of osteodystrophia fibrosa. Lab. Anim. Care *17:*222.

156. Hymer, W. C., and MeShan, W. H. (1963): Isolation of rat pituitary granules and the study of their biochemical properties and hormonal activities. J. Cell Biol. *17:*67.

157. Ingersoll, R. J., and Wasserman, R. H. (1971): Vitamin D₃-induced calcium-binding protein. J. Biol. Chem. *246:*2808.

158. Isono, H., Sakurai, S., Fujii, H., et al. (1971): Ultrastructural change in the parathyroid gland of the phosphate treated newt. *Triturus pyrrhogaster* (Boié). Arch. Histol. Jpn. *33:*357.

159. Jacobs, J. W. (1985): Calcitonin gene expression. Bone Mineral Res. *3:*151.

160. Jones, B. R. and Alley, M. R. (1985): Primary idiopathic hypoparathyroidism in St. Bernard dogs. New Zealand Vet. J. *33:*94.

161. Joyce, J. R., Pierce, K. R., Romane, W. M., et al.: (1971): Clinical study of nutritional secondary hyperparathyroidism in horses. J. Am. Vet. Med. Assoc. *158:*2033.

162. Kalina, M., and Pearse, A. G. E. (1971): Ultrastructural localization of calcitonin in C-cells of dog thyroid: an immunocytochemical study. Histochemie *26:*1.

163. Kallfelz, F. A. (1968): Puerperal tetany. In Current Veterinary Therapy III, edited by R. W. Kirk. Philadelphia, W. B. Saunders Co., pp. 64–65.

164. Kallio, D. M., Garant, P. R., and Minkin, C. (1972): Ultrastructural effects of calcitonin on osteoclasts in tissue culture. J. Ultrastruct. Res. *39:*205.

165. Kaufman, C. F., Soirez, R. F., and Tasker, J. P. (1969): Renal cortical hypoplasia with secondary hyperparathyroidism in the dog. J. Am. Vet. Med. Assoc. *155:*1679.

166. Kemper, B., Habener, J. F., Potts, J. T., Jr., et al. (1972): Parathyroid hormone: Identification of a biosynthetic precursor to parathyroid hormone.

Proc. Natl. Acad. Sci. USA *69:*643.

167. Kemper, B., Habener, J. F., Rich, A., and Potts, J. T., Jr. (1974): Parathyroid secretion: Discovery of a major calcium-dependent protein. Science *184:*167.

168. Klausner, J. S., Fernandez, F. R., O'Leary, T. P., et al.: (1986): Canine primary hyperparathyroidism and its association with urolithiasis. Vet. Clin. N. Am. *16:*227.

169. Kodicek, E. (1974): The story of vitamin D from vitamin to hormone. Lancet. *2:*325.

170. Kodicek, E., Lawson, D. E. M., and Wilson, P. W. (1970): Biological activity of a polar metabolite of vitamin D₃. Nature (London) *228:*763.

171. Kronenberg, H. M., Igarashi, T., Freeman, M. W., et al.: (1986): Structure and expression of the human parathyroid hormone gene. Recent Prog. Hormone Res. *42:*641.

172. Krook, L. (1957): Spontaneous hyperparathyroidism in the dog. Acta Pathol. Microbiol. Scand. *41* (Suppl. 122):1.

173. Krook, L., and Barrett, R. B. (1962): Simian bone disease—a secondary hyperparathyroidism. Cornell Vet. *52:*459.

174. Krook, L., and Lowe, J. E. (1964): Nutritional secondary hyperparathyroidism in the horse. Pathol. Vet. *1*(Suppl. 1):1.

175. Krook, L., Lutwak, L., Henrickson, P. A., et al.: (1971): Reversibility of nutritional osteoporosis: Physicochemical data on bones from an experimental study in dogs. J. Nutr. *101:*233.

176. Krook, L., Lutwak, L., and McEntee, K. (1969): Dietary calcium, ultimobranchial tumors and osteopetrosis in the bull. A syndrome of calcitonin excess? Am. J. Clin. Nutr. *22:*115.

177. Krook, L., Lutwak, L., McEntee, K., et al.: (1971): Nutritional hypercalcitoninism in bulls. Cornell Vet. *61:*625.

178. Lacy, P. E., Howell, S. L., Young, D. A., et al.: (1968): New hypothesis of insulin secretion. Nature (London) *219:*1177.

179. Leav, I., Schiller, A. L., Rijnberk, A., et al.: (1976): Adenomas and carcinomas of the canine and feline thyroid. Am. J. Pathol. *83:*61.

180. Legendre, A. M., Merkley, D. F., Carrig, C. G., et al.: (1976): Primary hyperparathyroidism in a dog. J. Am. Vet. Med. Assoc. *168:*694.

181. Lehner, N. D. M., Bullock, B. C., Clarkson, T. B., et al.: (1976): Biological activities of vitamin D₂ and D₃ for growing squirrel monkeys. Lab. Anim. Care *17:*483.

182. L'Heureux, M. V., and Melius, P. (1956): Differential centrifugation of bovine parathyroid tissue. Biochem. Biophys. Acta *20:*447.

183. Littledike, E. T., Arnaud, C. D., Schroeder, L., et al.: (1971): Calcitonin, parathyroid hormone and parturient hypocalcemia of dairy cows. Abst. 53rd Meeting of the Endocrine Society, A67.

184. Littledike, E. T., Whipp, S. C., and Schroeder, L. (1969): Studies on parturient paresis. J. Am. Vet. Med. Assoc. *155:*1955.

185. Long, G. G. (1984): Acute toxicosis in swine associated with excessive dietary intake of vitamin D. J. Am. Vet. Med. Assoc. *184:*164.

186. Long, P., Choi, G., and Rehmel R. (1983): Oxyphil cells in a red-tailed hawk (*Buteo jamaicensis*) with

nutritional secondary hyperparathyroidism. Avian Dis. *27*:839.

187. Lupelescu, A., Potorac, E., Pop, A., et al.: (1968): Experimental investigation on immunology of the parathyroid gland. Immunology *14*:475.

188. MacGregor, R. R., Chu, L. L. H., Hamilton, J. W., et al. (1973): Studies on the subcellular localization of proparathyroid hormone and parathyroid hormone in the bovine parathyroid gland: Separation of newly synthesized from mature forms. Endocrinology *93*:1387.

189. MacGregor, R. R., Hamilton, J. W., and Cohn, D. V. (1978): The mode of conversion of proparathormone to parathormone by a particulate converting enzymic activity of the parathyroid gland. J. Biol. Chem. *253*:2012.

190. MacIntyre, I., Colston, K. W., Szelke, M., et al.: (1978): A survey of the hormonal factors that control calcium metabolism. Ann. N. Y. Acad. Sci. *307*: 345.

191. Majeska, R. J., Rodan, S. B., and Rodan, G. A. (1980): Parathyroid hormone-responsive clonal cell lines from rat osteosarcoma. Endocrinology 107: 1494.

192. Martig, J., and Mayer, G. P. (1973): Diminished hypercalcemic response to parathyroid extract in prepartum cows. J. Dairy Sci. *56*:1042.

193. Martin, S. L., and Capen, C. C. (1980): Puerperal tetany. *In*: Current Veterinary Therapy VII, (R. W. Kirk, Editor). Philadelphia, W. B. Saunders Co., pp. 1027–1029.

194. Mawer, E., B., Backhouse, J., Taylor, C. M., et al.: (1973): Failure of formation of 1,25-dihydroxycholecalciferol in chronic renal insufficiency. Lancet *2*: 626.

195. Mayer, G. P. (1970): The roles of parathyroid hormone and thyrocalcitonin in parturient paresis. *In* Parturient Hypocalcemia, edited by J. J. B. Anderson. New York, Academic Press, pp. 177–193.

196. Mayer, G. P. (1971): A rational basis for the prevention of parturient paresis. Bovine Pract. *6*:2.

197. Mayer, G. P. (1974): Relative importance of calcium and magnesium in the control of parathyroid secretion. Abst. 56th Annual Meeting of The Endocrine Society, pp. A-181.

198. Mayer, G. P., Habener, J. F., and Potts, J. T., Jr. (1973): Significance of plasma immunoreactive parathyroid hormone in hypocalcemic cows. *In* Production Diseases in Farm Animals, edited by J. M. Payne, K. G. Hibbitt, and B. F. Sansom. London, Baillaire Tindall, pp. 217–220.

199. Mayer, G. P., and Hurst, J. G. (1978): Comparison of the effects of calcium and magnesium on parathyroid hormone secretion rate in calves. Endocrinology *102*:1803.

200. Mayer, G. P., Ramberg, C. F., Jr., and Kronfeld, D. S. (1969): Calcium homeostasis in the cow. Clin. Orthop. *62*:79.

201. Mayer, G. P., Ramberg, C. F., Jr., Kronfeld, D. S., et al. (1969): Plasma parathyroid hormone concentration in hypocalcemic parturient cows. Am. J. Vet. Res. *30*:1587.

202. McKenzie, R. A., Gartner, R. J. W., Blaney, B. J. et al. (1981): Control of nutritional secondary hyperparathyroidism in grazing horses with calcium plus phosphorus supplementation. Aust. Vet. J. *57:* 554.

203. Melvin, K. E. W., Tashjian, A. H., Jr., et al. (1972): Studies in familial (medullary) thyroid carcinoma. Recent Prog. Hormone Res. *28*:399.

204. Meuten, D. J., Chew, D. J., Capen, C. C., et al. (1982): Relationship of serum total calcium to albumin and total protein in dogs. J. Am. Vet. Med. Assoc. *180*:63.

205. Meuten, D. J., Cooper, B. J., Capen, C. C., et al. (1981): Hypercalcemia associated with an adenocarcinoma derived from the apocrine glands of the anal sac. Vet. Pathol. *18*:454.

206. Meuten, D. J., Kociba, G. J., Capen, C. C. et al. (1983): Hypercalcemia in dogs with lymphosarcoma: Biochemical, ultrastructural and histomorphometric investigation. Lab. Invest. *49*:553.

207. Meuten, D. J., Segre, G. V., Capen, C. C. et al. (1983): Hypercalcemia in dogs with adenocarcinoma derived from apocrine glands of the anal sac. Biochemical and histomorphometric investigations. Lab. Invest. *48*:428.

208. Meuten, D. J., Capen, C. C., Kociba, G. J., et al. (1983): Hypercalcemia associated with malignancy. In Proceedings of VI Kal-Kan Symposium – Clinical Endocrinology. Edited by C. C. Capen and S. L. Martin. Princeton Junction, NJ. Veterinary Learning Systems, Inc. pp, 95–100.

209. Midgett, R. J., Spielvogel, A. M., Coburn, J. W., et al. (1973): Studies on calciferol metabolism. VI. The renal production of the biologically active form of vitamin D, 1,25-dihydroxycholecalciferol; species, tissue and subcellular distribution. J. Clin. Endocrinol. Metab. *36*:1153.

210. Morris, M. L., Teeter, S. M., and Collins, D. R., (1971): The effects of the exclusive feeding of an all-meat dog food. J. Am. Vet. Med. Assoc. *158*:477.

211. Morrissey, J. J., and Cohn, D. V. (1978): The effects of calcium and magnesium on the secretion of parathormone and parathyroid secretory protein by isolated porcine parathyroid cells. Endocrinology *103*:2081.

212. Morrissey, R. L., Zolock, D. T., Bucci, T. J., et al. (1978): Immunoperoxidase localization of vitamin D-dependent calcium binding protein. J. Histochem. Cytochem. *26*:628.

213. Moseley, J. M., Kubota, M., Diefenbach-Jagger, H., et al. (1987): Parathyroid hormone-related protein purified from a human lung cancer cell line. Proc. Natl. Acad. Sci. (U. S. A.) *84*:5048.

214. Muir, L. A., Hibbs, J. W., and Conrad, H. R. (1968): Effect of vitamin D on the ability of cows to mobilize blood calcium. J. Dairy Sci. *51*:1046.

215. Muir, L. A., Hibbs, J. W., and Conrad, H. R., et al. (1972): Effect of estrogen and progesterone on feed intake and hydroxyproline excretion following induced hypocalcemia in dairy cows. J. Dairy Sci. *55*:1613.

216. Mundy, G. R. (1987): The hypercalcemia of malignancy. Kidney International *31*:142.

217. Mundy, G. R., Ibbotson, K. J., D'Souza, S. M., et al. (1984): The hypercalcemia of cancer. Clinical implications and pathogenic mechanisms. N. Engl. J. Med. *310*:1718.

218. Mundy, G. R., Ibbotson, K. J., and D'Souza, S. M. (1985): Tumor products and the hypercalcemia of malignancy. J. Clin. Invest. *76*:391.

219. Mundy, G. R., Jacobs, J. W., Ibbotson, K. J., et al. (1984): Hypercalcemia of malignancy. In Endocrine Control of Bone and Calcium Metabolism., edited by D. V. Cohn, T. Fujita, J. T. Potts, Jr., et al.: Amsterdam, Elsevier Science Publications. pp. 278–283.

220. Mundy, G. R., Laben, R. A., Raisz, L. G., et al. (1974): Bone-resorbing activity in supernatants from lymphoid cell lines. N. Engl. J. Med. *290*:867.

221. Mundy, G. R., Luben, R. A., Raisz, L. G., et al. (1974): Bone-resorbing activity in supernatants from lymphoid cell lines. N. Engl. J. Med. *290*:867.

222. Mundy, G. R., Raisz, L. G., Cooper, R. A., et al. (1974): Evidence for the secretion of an osteoclast stimulating factor in myeloma. N. Engl. J. Med. *291*:1041.

223. Munger, B. L., and Roth, S. I. (1963): The cytology of the normal parathyroid glands of man and Virginia deer. J. Cell Biol. *16*:379.

224. Nakagami, K. (1967): Comparative electron microscopic studies of the parathyroid glands. II. Fine structure of the parathyroid gland of the normal and the calcium chloride treated mouse. Arch. Histol. Jpn. *28*:185.

225. Nakagami, K., Warshawsky, H., and LeBlond, C. P. (1971): The elaboration of protein and carbohydrate by rat parathyroid cells as revealed by electron microscope radioautography. J. Cell Biol. *51*:596.

226. Nakagami, K., Yamazaki, Y., and Tsunoda, Y. (1968): An electron microscopic study of the human fetal parathyroid gland. Z. Zellforsch. Mikrosk. Anat. *85*:89.

227. Nemere, I., and Norman, A. W. (1986): Parathyroid hormone stimulates calcium transport in perfused duodena from normal chicks: Comparison with the rapid (transcaltachic) effect of 1,25-dihydroxyvitamin D₃. Endocrinology *119*:1406.

228. Nevalainen, T. (1969): Fine structure of the parathyroid gland of the laying hen. Gen. Comp. Endocrinol. *12*:561.

229. Nissenson, R. A., Strewler, G. J., Williams, R. D., et al. (1985): Activation of the parathyroid hormone receptor-adenylate cyclase system in osteosarcoma cells by a human renal carcinoma factor. Cancer Res. *45*:5358.

230. Nissenson, R. A., Leung, S., Diep, D., et al. (1987): Purification of a low molecular weight form of the tumor-derived parathyroid hormone-like protein. J. Bone Min. Res. *2*:Suppl. 1:388A.

231. Norman, A. W. (1980): 1,25-(OH)₂-D₃ as a steroid hormone. *In*: Vitamin D: Molecular Biology and Clinical Nutrition (A. W. Norman, Editor). New York, Marcel Dekker, Inc., pp. 197–250.

232. Norman, A. W., and Henry, H. (1974): The role of the kidney and vitamin D metabolism in health and disease. Clin. Orthop. *98*:258.

233. Norman, A. W., and Henry, H. (1974): 1,25-Dihydroxycholecalciferol—a hormonally active form of vitamin D₃. Recent Prog. Horm. Res. *30*:43.

234. Norman, A. W., and Henry, H. L. (1979): Vitamin D to 1,25-dihydroxycholecalciferol: evolution of a steroid hormone. Trends Biochem. Sci. January: 14.

235. Norman, A. W., Johnson, R. L., Osborn, T. W., et al. (1976): The chemistry, conformational and biological analysis of vitamin D₃, its metabolites and analogues. Clin. Endocrinol. *5*(Suppl):121.

236. Nunez, E. A., Whalen, J. P., and Krook, L. (1972): An ultrastructural study of the natural secretory cycle of the parathyroid gland of the bat. Am. J. Anat. *134*:459.

237. Oldham, S. B., Fischer, J. A., Capen, C. C., et al. (1971): Dynamics of parathyroid hormone secretion *in vitro*. Am. J. Med. *51*:650.

238. Olson, E. B., Jr., DeLuca, H. F., and Potts, J. T., Jr. (1972): The effect of calcitonin and parathyroid hormone on calcium transport of isolated intestine. In Calcium, Parathyroid Hormone and the Calcitonins, edited by R. V. Talmage and P. L. Munson. Amsterdam, Excerpta Medica, pp. 240–246.

239. Omdall, J. L., and DeLuca, H. F. (1973): Regulation of vitamin D metabolism and function. Physiol. Rev. *53*:327.

240. Omen, G. S. (1973): Pathobiology of ectopic hormone production by neoplasms in man. In Pathobiology Annual, Vol. 3, edited by H. L. Ioachim. New York, Appleton-Century-Crofts, pp. 177–216.

241. Ornoy, A., Goodwin, D., Noff, D., et al. (1978): 24,25-Dihydroxyvitamin D is a metabolite of vitamin D essential for bone formation. Nature *276*:517.

242. Osborne, C. A., and Stevens, J. B. (1973): Pseudohyperparathyroidism in the dog. J. A. V. M. A. *162*:125.

243. Owen, M., and Bingham, P. J. (1968): The effect of parathyroid extract on RNA synthesis in osteogenic cells *in vivo*. *In* Parathyroid Hormone and Thyrocalcitonin (Calcitonin), edited by R. V. Talmage and L. F. Bélanger. Amsterdam, Excerpta Medica, pp. 216–225.

244. Parfitt, A. M. (1977): The cellular basis of bone turnover and bone loss. Clin. Orthop. *127*:236.

245. Parsons, J. A., and Robinson, C. J. (1971): Calcium shift into bone causing transient hypocalcemia after injection of parathyroid hormone. Nature (London) *230*:581.

246. Pearson, P. T., Dellman, H. D., Berrier, H. H., et al. (1965): Primary hyperparathyroidism in a beagle. J. Am. Vet. Med. Assoc. *147*:1201.

247. Pedersen, N. C. (1983): Nutritional secondary hyperparathyroidism in a cattery associated with the feeding of a fad diet containing horsemeat. Feline Pract. *13*:19.

248. Peterson, M. E. (1982): Treatment of canine and feline hypoparathyroidism. J. Am. Vet. Med. Assoc. *181*:1424.

249. Pliam, N. B., Nyiredy, K. O., and Arnaud, C. D. (1982): Parathyroid hormone receptors in avian bone cells. Proc. Natl. Acad. Sci. (USA) *79*:2061.

250. Potts, J. T., Jr. (1976): Chemistry and physiology of parathyroid hormone. Clin. Endocrinol. *5*(Suppl): 307.

251. Potts, J. T., Jr., and Deftos, L. J. (1969): Parathyroid hormone, thyrocalcitonin, vitamin D and bone mineral metabolism. *In* Duncan's Diseases of Metabolism, Endocrinology and Nutrition, 6th edition, Vol. 2, edited by P. K. Bondy. Philadelphia, W. B.

Saunders Co., pp. 904–1082.

252. Potts, J. T., Jr., Murray, T. M., Peacock, M., et al. (1971): Parathyroid hormone: Sequence synthesis, immunoassay studies. Am. J. Med. *50*:639.

253. Powell, D., Singer, F. R., Murray, T. M., Minkin, C., and Potts, J. T., Jr. (1973): Nonparathyroid humoral hypercalcemia in patients with neoplastic diseases. N. Engl. J. Med. *289*:176.

254. Price, D. A. (1970): Dogs need more than meat. J. Am. Vet. Med. Assoc. *156*:681.

255. Raisz, L. G., and Kream, B. E. (1983): Regulation of bone formation. N. Engl. J. Med. *309*:29.

256. Raisz, L. G., Trummel, C. L., Holick, M. F., et al. (1972): 1,25-dihydroxycholecalciferol: A potent stimulator of bone resorption in tissue culture. Science *175*:768.

257. Rasmussen, H. (1971): Ionic and hormonal control of calcium homeostasis. Am. J. Med. *50*:567.

258. Rasmussen, H. (1972): The cellular basis of mammalian calcium homeostasis, *In* Clinics in Endocrinology and Metabolism, edited by I. MacIntyre. Philadelphia, W. B. Saunders Co., pp. 3–20.

259. Rasmussen, H. (1974): Parathyroid hormone, calcitonin, and the calciferols. *In* Textbook of Endocrinology, edited by R. H. Williams. Philadelplia, W. B. Saunders Co., pp. 660–773.

260. Rasmussen, H., and Bordier, P. (1974): The Physiological and Cellular Basis of Metabolic Bone Disease. Baltimore, Williams & Wilkins Co.

261. Rasmussen, H., and Gustin, M. C. (1978): Some aspects of the hormonal control of cellular calcium metabolism. Ann. N. Y. Acad. Sci. *307*:391.

262. Rasmussen, H., Wong, M., Bikle, D., et al. (1972): Hormonal control of the renal conversion of 25-hydroxycholecalciferol to 1,25-dihydroxycholecalciferol. J. Clin. Invest. *51*:2502.

263. Reaven, E. P., and Reaven, G. M. (1974): A quantitative ultrastructural study of microtubule assembly and granule accumulation in parathyroid glands of control, phosphate, and colchicine treated rats. *In* Abst. (No. 252) 56th Annual Meeting of The Endocrine Society, pp. A–182.

264. Resnick, S. (1972): Hypocalcemia and tetany in the dog. Vet. Med. Small Anim. Clin. *67*:637.

265. Reynolds, J. J., Holick, M. F., and DeLuca, H. F. (1973): The role of vitamin D metabolites in bone resorption. Calcif. Tissue Res. *12*:295.

266. Rice, B. F., Roth, L. M., Cole, F. E. et al. (1975): Hypercalcemia and neoplasia. Biologic, biochemical and ultrastructural studies of a hypercalcemia-producing Leydig cell tumor of the rat. Lab. Invest. *33*:426.

267. Rijnberk, A. (1970): Pseudohyperparathyroidism in the dog. T. Diergenessk. *95*:515.

268. Rijnberk, A., Elsinhorst, Th. A. M., Kolman, J. P., et al. (1978): Pseudohyperparathyroidism associated with perirectal adenocarcinomas in elderly female dogs. T. Diergeneesk. *103*:1069.

269. Rings, R. W., Doyle, R. E., Hooper, B. E., et al. (1969): Osteomalacia in the golden-mantled ground squirrel (*Citellus lateralis*). J. Am. Vet. Med. Assoc. *155*:1224.

270. Rodan, G. A., and Martin, T. J. (1981): The role of osteoblasts in hormonal control of bone resorption – A hypothesis. Calcif. Tis. Int. *33*:349.

271. Rogers, D. C. (1965): An electron microscope study of the parathyroid gland of the frog (*Rana clamitans*). J. Ultrastruct. Res. *13*:478.

272. Rosenblatt, M. (1982): Pre-preparathyroid hormone, proparathyroid hormone, and parathyroid hormone. Clin. Orthopaed. Rel. Res. *170*:260.

273. Rosol, T. J., Capen, C. C., Weisbrode, S. E., et al. (1986): Humoral hypercalcemia of malignancy: Nude mouse model of a canine adenocarcinoma derived from apocrine glands of the anal sac. Biochemical, histomorphometric and ultrastructural studies. Lab. Invest. *54*:679.

274. Rosol, T. J., and Capen, C. C. (1986): In vitro bone resorption and transforming growth factor (TGF) activities in hypercalcemic canine adenocarcinoma tumor-line (CAC-8) in nude mice. J. Bone Min. Res. 1 (suppl.1): 180.

275. Rosol, T. J., Capen, C. C., and Minkin, C. (1986): In vitro bone resorption activity produced by a hypercalcemic adenocarcinoma tumor line (CAC-8) in nude mice. Calcif. Tissue Int. *39*:334.

276. Rosol, T. J., and Capen, C. C. (1988): Inhibition of *in vitro* bone resorption by a parathyroid hormone receptor antagonist in the canine adenocarcinoma model of humoral hypercalcemia of malignancy. Endocrinology. *122*:2098.

277. Rosol, T. J., Capen, C. C. and Brooks, C. L. (1987): Bone and kidney adenylate cyclase-stimulating activity produced by a hypercalcemic canine adenocarcinoma line (CAC-8) maintained in nude mice. Cancer Res. *47*:690.

278. Roth, S. I., and Capen, C. C. (1974): Ultrastructural and functional correlations of the parathyroid glands. *In* International Review of Experimental Pathology, Vol. 13, edited by G. W. Richter and M. A. Epstein, New York, pp. 162–221.

279. Roth, S. I., and Munger, B. L. (1962): The cytology of the adenomatous, atrophic, and hyperplastic parathyroid glands of man. A light- and electron-microscopic study. Virchows Arch. [Path. Anat.] *335*:389.

280. Roth, S. I., and Raisz, L. G. (1964): Effect of calcium concentration on the ultrastructure of rat parathyroid in organ culture. Lab. Invest. *13*:331.

281. Roth, S. I., and Raisz, L. G. (1966): The course and reversibility of the calcium effect on the ultrastructure of the rat parathyroid gland in organ culture. Lab. Invest. *15*:1187.

282. Roth, S. I., Su, S. P., Segre, G. V., et al. (1974): The immunocytochemical localization of parathyroid hormone in the bovine. Fed. Proc. *33*:241.

283. Rowland, G. N., Capen, C. C., and Nagode, L. N. (1968): Experimental hyperparathyroidism in young cats. Pathol. Vet. *5*:504.

284. Rowland, G. N., Capen, C. C., Young, D. M., et al. (1972): Microradiographic evaluation of bone from cows with experimental hypervitaminosis D, diet-induced hypocalcemia, and naturally occurring parturient paresis. Calcif. Tissue Res. *9*:179.

285. Sampson, H. W., Matthews, J. L., Martin, J. H., et al. (1970): An electron microscopic localization of calcium in the small intestine. Calcif. Tissue Res. *5*:305.

286. Sansom, B. F., Vagg, M. J., and Döbereiner, J. (1971): The effects of *Solanum malacoxylon* on calcium metabolism in cattle. Res. Vet. Sci. *12*:604.

287. Sato, K., Fujii, Y., Kasono, K., et al. (1987): Interleukin-1 and PTH-like factor are responsible for humoral hypercalcemic associated with esophageal carcinoma cells (EC-G1). J. Bone Min. Res. 2:Suppl 1:387A.
288. Saville, P. D., and Krook, L. (1969): Gravimetric and isotopic studies in nutritional hyperparathyroidism in beagles. Clin. Orthop. 62:15.
289. Saville, P. D., Krook, L., Gustafsson, P., et al. (1969): Nutritional secondary hyperparathyroidism in a dog. Morphologic and radioisotope studies with treatment. Cornell Vet. 59:155.
290. Scott, P. P. (1968): The special features of nutrition of cats, with observations on wild felidae nutrition in the London zoo. Symp. Zool. Soc. London 21:21.
291. Seyberth, H. W., Segre, G. V., Morgan, J. L., et al. (1975): Prostaglandins as mediators of hypercalcemia associated with certain types of cancer. N. Engl. J. Med. 293:1278.
292. Shannon, W. A., and Roth, S. I. (1971): Acid phosphatase activity in mammalian parathyroid glands. In 29th Ann. Proc. Electron Microscopy Soc. Amer., edited by C. J. Arceneaux. Baton Rouge, Claitor's Publishing, pp. 516–517.
293. Sherding, R. G., Meuten, D. J., Chew, D. J., et al. (1980): Primary hypoparathyroidism in the dog. J. N. Am. Vet. Med. Assoc. 176:439.
293A. Silve, C. M., Hradek, G. T., Jones, A. L. et al. (1982): Parathyroid hormone receptor in intact embryonic chicken bone: Characterization and cellular localization. J. Cell Biol. 94:379.
294. Sherwood, L. M., Lundberg, W. B., Targovnik, et al. (1971): Synthesis and secretion of parathyroid hormone in vitro. Am. J. Med. 50:658.
295. Sherwood, L. M., Mayer, G. P., Ramberg, C. F., et al. (1968): Regulation of parathyroid hormone secretion: Proportional control by calcium, lack of effect of phosphate. Endocrinology 83:1043.
296. Sherwood, L. M., Rodman, J. S., and Lundberg, W. B. (1970): Evidence for a precursor to circulating parathyroid hormone. Proc. Natl. Acad. Sci. (USA) 67:1631.
297. Singer, F. R., Melvin, K. W., and Mills, B. G. (1976): Acute effects of calcitonin on osteoclasts in man. Clin. Endocrinol. 5(Suppl):333.
298. Singer, F. E., Powell, D., Minkin, C., Bethune, J. E., Brickman, A., and Coburn, J. W. (1973): Hypercalcemia in reticulum cell sarcoma without hyperparathyroidism or skeletal metastases. Ann. Intern. Med. 78:365.
299. Sipple, J. F. (1961): Association of pheochromocytoma with carcinoma of the thyroid gland. Am. J. Med 31:163.
300. Smithcors, J. F. (1964): The Endocrine System. In Anatomy of the Dog, edited by M. E. Miller, G. C. Christensen and H. E. Evans. Philadelphia, W. B. Saunders Co., pp. 822–826.
301. Steenbergh, P. H., Hoppener, J. W. M., Zandberg, J., et al. (1984): Calcitonin gene related peptide coding sequence is conserved in the human genome and is expressed in medullary thyroid carcinoma. J. Clin. Endocrinol. Metab. 59:358.
302. Stewart, A. F., Horst, R., Deftos, L. J., et al. (1980): Biochemical evaluation of patients with cancer-associated hypercalcemia. N. Engl. J. Med. 303:1377.
303. Stewart, A. F., Insogna, K. L., Burtis, W. J., et al. (1986): Frequency and partial characterization of adenylate cyclase-stimulating activity in tumors associated with humoral hypercalcemia of malignancy. J. Bone Min. Res. 1:267.
304. Stewart, A. F., Vignery, A., Silverglate, A., et al. (1982): Quantitative bone histomorphometry in humoral hypercalcemia of malignancy: Uncoupling of bone cell activity. J. Clin. Endocrinol. Metab. 55:219.
305. Stott, G. H. (1968): Dietary influence on the incidence of parturient paresis. Fed. Proc. 27:156.
306. Strewler, G. J., and Nissenson, R. A. (1987): Nonparathyroid hypercalcemia. Adv. Intern. Med. 32: 235.
307. Strewler, G. J., Wronski, T. J., Halloran, B. P., et al. (1986): Pathogenesis of hypercalcemia in nude mice bearing a human renal carcinoma. Endocrinology 119:303.
308. Sutton, R. A. L., and Dirks, J. H. (1978): Renal handling of calcium. Fed. Proc. 37:2112.
309. Suva, L. J., Winslow, G. A., Wettenhall, R. E. H., et al. (1987): A parathyroid hormone-related protein implicated in malignant hypercalcemia: Cloning and expression. Science 237:893.
310. Swaminathan, R., Bates, R. F. L., and Care, A.D. (1972): Fresh evidence for a physiological role of calcitonin in calcium homeostasis. J. Endocrinol. 54:525.
311. Talmage, R. V., Anderson, J. J. B., and Cooper, C. W. (1972): The influence of calcitonins on the disappearance of radiocalcium and radiophosphorus from plasma. Endocrinology 90:1185.
312. Tam, C. S., Heersche, J. N. M., Santora, A., et al. (1984): Skeletal response in rats following the implantation of hypercalcemia-producing Leydig cell tumors. Metabolism 33:50.
313. Tamayo, J., Bellorin-Fort, E., and Martin, K. J. (1983): Effects of dietary-induced hyperparathyroidism on the parathyroid hormone-receptor-adenylate cyclase system of canine kidney. Evidence for postreceptor mechanism of desensitization. J. Clin. Invest. 72:422.
314. Tanaka, T., and DeLuca, H. F. (1974): Stimulation of 24,25-dihydroxyvitamin D_3 production by 1,25-dihydroxyvitamin D_3. Science 183:1198.
315. Targovnik, J. H., Rodman, J. S., and Sherwood, L. M. (1976): Regulation of parathyroid hormone secretion in vitro: Quantitative aspects of calcium and magnesium ion control. Endocrinology 88:1477.
316. Tashjian, A. H., Jr. (1978): Role of prostaglandins in the production of hypercalcemia by tumors. Cancer Res. 38:4138.
317. Tashjian, A. H., Jr., Voelkel, E. F., Lazzaro, M., et al. (1985): Alpha and beta human transforming growth factors stimulate prostaglandin production and bone resorption in cultured mouse calvaria. Proc. Natl. Acad. Sci. (USA) 82:4535.
318. Taylor, A. N., and Wasserman, R. H. (1970): Immunofluorescent localization of vitamin D-dependent calcium-binding protein. J. Histochem. Cytochem. 18:107.
319. Teitelbaum, A. P., and Strewler, G. J. (1984): Parathyroid hormone receptors coupled to cyclic adenosine monophosphate formation in an established

renal cell line. Endocrinology *114*:980.

320. Thiele, J., and Wermbter, G. (1974): Die Feinstruktur der akivierten Hauptzelle der menschlichen Parathyroidea. Eine Darstellung mit Hilfe de Gefrierätztechnik. Virchows Arch. [Cell. Pathol.] 15: 251.

321. Thompson, K. G., Jones, L. P., Smylie, W. A., et al. (1984). Primary hyperparathyroidism in German shepherd dogs: A disorder of probable genetic origin. Vet. Pathol. *21*:370.

322. Trembly, G., and Pearse, A. G. E. (1959): A cytochemical study of oxidative enzymes in the parathyroid oxyphil cell and their functional significance. Br. J. Exp. Pathol. *40*:66.

323. Van Pelt, R. W., and Caley, M. T. (1974): Nutritional secondary hyperparathyroidism in Alaskan red fox kits. J. Wildlife Dis. *10*:47.

324. Voelkel, E. F., Tashjian, A. H., Jr., Franklin, R., et al. (1985): Hypercalcemia and tumor-prostaglandins: The VX2 carcinoma model in the rabbit. Metabolism *24*:973.

325. Wallach, J. D. (1971): Environmental and nutritional diseases of captive reptiles. J. Am. Vet. Med. Assoc. *159*:1632.

326. Wallach, J. D., and Flieg, G. M. (1969): Nutritional secondary hyperparathyroidism in captive birds. J. Am. Vet. Med. Assoc. *155*:1046.

327. Wallach, J. D., and Hoessle, C. (1968): Fibrous osteodystrophy in green iguanas. J. Am. Vet. Med. Assoc. *153*:863.

328. Walthall, J. C., and McKenzie, R. A. (1976): Osteodystrophia fibrosa in horses at pasture in Queensland: Field and laboratory observations. Aust. Vet. J. *52*:11.

329. Wasserman, R. H. (1974): Calcium absorption and calcium-binding protein synthesis: *Solanum malacoxylon* reverses strontium inhibition. Science *183*: 1092.

330. Wasserman, R. H. (1975): Metabolism, function and clinical aspects of vitamin D. Cornell Vet. *65*:3.

331. Wasserman, R. H. (1978): Physiological regulation of calcium metabolism: The consequences of excess intake of 1,25-dihydroxycholecalciferol from natural sources. Ann. N. Y. Acad. Sci. *307*:442.

332. Wasserman, R. H., Corradino, R. A., and Krook, L. (1975): *Cestrum diurnum*: a domestic plant with 1,25-Dihydroxycholecalciferol-like activity. Biochem. Biophys. Res. Commun. *62*:85.

333. Wasserman, R. H., Corradino, R. A., Krook, L., et al. (1976): Studies on the 1α,25-dihydroxycholecalciferol-like activity in a calcinogenic plant, *Cestrum diurnum*, in the chick, J. Nutr. *106*:457.

334. Wasserman, R. H., Corradino, R. A., and Taylor, A. N. (1968): Vitamin D-dependent calcium-binding protein. J. Biol. Chem. *243*:3978.

335. Wasserman, R. H. and Fullmer, C. S. (1983): Calcium transport proteins, calcium absorption, and vitamin D. Ann. Rev. Physiol. *45*:375.

336. Wasserman, R. H., and Taylor, A. N. (1972): Metabolic roles of fat-soluble vitamins D. E., and K. Ann. Rev. Biochem. *41*:179.

337. Wecksler, W. R., Henry, H. L., and Norman, A. W. (1977): Studies on the mode of action of calciferol: Subcellular localization of 1,25-dihydroxyvitamin D_3 in chicken parathyroid glands. Arch.

338. Weir, E. C., Norrdin, R. W., Matus, R. E., et al. (1988): Humoral hypercalcemia of malignancy in canine lymphosarcoma. Endocrinology *122*:602.

339. Weisbrode, S. E., and Capen, C. C. (1974): Ultrastructural evaluation of the effects of calcitonin on bone in thyroparathyroidectomized rats administered vitamin D. Am. J. Pathol. *77*:395.

340. Weisbrode, S. E., Capen, C. C., and Nagode, L. N. (1973): Fine structural and enzymatic evaluation of bone in thyroparathyroidectomized rats receiving various levels of vitamin D. Lab. Invest. *28*:29.

341. Weisbrode, S. E., Capen, C. C., and Nagode, L. N. (1974): Effects of parathyroid hormone on bone of thyroparathyroidectomized rats. Am. J. Pathol. *75*: 529.

342. Weisbrode, S. E., Capen, C. C., and Norman, A. W. (1978): Ultrastructural evaluation of the effects of 1,25-dihydroxyvitamin D_3 on bone of thyroparathyroidectomized rats fed a low-calcium diet. Am. J. Pathol. *92*:459.

343. Weisbrode, S. W., Capen, C. C., and Norman, A. W. (1979): Influence of diet in the response of bone cells to 1,25-dihydroxcholecalciferol in thyroparathyroidectomized rats. In Proc. 4th Workshop on Vitamin D, edited by A. W. Norman, et al. Berlin/New York, Walter de Gruyter.

344. Weymouth, R. J., and Seibel, H. R. (1969): An electron microscopic study of the parathyroid glands in man: Evidence of secretory material. Acta Endocrinol. *61*:334.

345. Wilson, J. W., Harris, S. G., Moore, W. D., et al. (1974): Primary hyperparathyroidism in a dog. J. Am. Vet. Med. Assoc. *164*:942.

346. Witzel, D. A., and Littledike, E. T. (1973): Suppression of insulin secretion during induced hypocalcemia. Endocrinology *93*:761.

347. Wolfe, H. J. (1982): Calcitonin: perspectives and current concepts. J. Endocrinol. Invest. *5*:423.

348. Wong, G. L. (1986): Skeletal effects of parathyroid hormone. Bone Mineral Res. *4*:103.

349. Yarrington, J. T., Capen, C.C., Black, H. E., (1977): Inhibition of bone resorption: An important mechanism in the pathogenesis of parturient hypocalcemia. Bovine Pract. *12*:30.

350. Yarrington, J. T., Capen, C. C., Black, H. E. et al. (1977): Effects of low calcium prepartal diet on calcium homeostatic mechanisms in the cow: Morphologic and biochemical studies. J. Nutr. *107*:2244.

351. Yarrington, J. T., Capen, C. C., Black, H. E., et al. (1977): Effect of dichloromethane diphosphonate on calcium homeostatic mechanisms in pregnant cows. Am. J. Pathol. *87*:165.

352. Yarrington, J. T., Capen, C. C., Black, H. E., et al. (1976): Experimental parturient hypocalcemia in cows following prepartal chemical inhibition of bone resorption. Am. J. Pathol. *83*:569.

353. Young, D. M., and Capen, C. C. (1970): Thyrocalcitonin content in the thyroid glands of cows with vitamin D-induced hypercalcemia. Endocrinology *86*:1463.

354. Youshak, M. S., and Capen, C. C. (1970): Fine structural alterations in parathyroid glands of chickens with osteopetrosis. Am. J. Pathol. *60*:257.

355. Youshak, M. S., and Capen, C. C. (1971): Ultra-

Biochem. Biophys. *183*:168.

structural evaluation of ultimobranchial glands from normal and osteopetrotic chickens. Gen. Comp. Endocrinol. *16*:430.

356. Zarrin, K. (1977): Naturally occurring parafollicular cell carcinoma of the thyroids in dogs. A histological and ultrastructural study. Vet. Pathol. *14*:556.

357. Zenoble, R. D., and Rowland, G. N. (1979): Hypercalcemia and proliferative, myelosclerotic bone reaction associated with feline leukovirus infection in a cat. J. Am. Vet. Med. Assoc. *175*:591.

358. Ziegler, R., Deutschle, U., and Raue, F. (1984): Calcitonin in human pathophysiology. Hormone Res. *20*:65.

359. Zwart, P., and van de Watering, C. C., (1969): Disturbance of bone formation in the common iguana, *Iguana iguana* I: Pathology and etiology. Acta Zool. Pathol. Antwerp. *48*:333.

The Endocrine Pancreas

W. H. Hsu and M. H. Crump

5

THE pancreas is a glandular organ which has exocrine and endocrine roles in the regulation of adequate nutrition of most cells of an animal during the pre- and postprandial states. As an exocrine gland, the pancreas secretes pancreatic juice which consists of digestive enzymes, electrolytes and water. The digestive enzymes of pancreatic juice are required for the digestion of complex substrates in food so they may be absorbed across the epithelial cells of the small intestine. These breakdown products then enter the systemic circulation. As an endocrine gland, the pancreas secretes peptide hormones, such as insulin, glucagon, somatostatin, and pancreatic polypeptide. Insulin and glucagon maintain fairly stable concentrations of glucose and other nutrients in the blood. Insulin, secreted by the B cells of the islets of Langerhans, facilitates the movement of glucose across cell membranes, thereby lowering the concentrations of blood glucose. Conversely, glucagon, secreted by the A cells of islets, raises the concentrations of glucose in the blood by increasing hepatic glycogenolysis and gluconeogenesis. The endocrine regulation of glucose metabolism is of utmost importance in mammalian homeostasis because every cell requires an adequate supply of energy for survival. Insulin and glucagon are key hormones for the regulation of glucose metabolism. Pancreatic somatostatin, a paracrine hormone, inhibits the release of insulin and glucagon. Paracrine refers to the diffusion of a hormone locally to adjacent cells where an effect takes place. The role of pancreatic polypeptide has not been clearly established, but it appears to participate in the regulation of food intake. Thus, pancreatic polypeptide may indirectly contribute to the control of levels of glucose in the blood. In addition to these pancreatic hormones, other endocrine secretions such as growth hormone, catecholamines, ACTH, and glucocorticoids play important roles in the regulation of glucose metabolism by increasing glycogenolysis and/or gluconeogenesis.

The concentration of blood glucose varies among the domestic animals (Table 5-1). Monogastric animals have concentrations of blood glucose which is in the range of 80 to 120 mg/dl, regardless of age. The concentration of glucose in the blood of ruminants varies with the age and development of their gastrointestinal tract. Adult ruminants have a well-developed multi-compartmental stomach, which acts as a fermentation vat. Most of the carbohydrate fraction of the diet is incom-

Table 5-1 Blood Glucose in the Normal, Depancreatized, and Diabetic Animals

Species	Normal Blood Glucose (mg/dl)	Treatment*	Post-treatment Blood Glucose (mg/dl)
Pigeon	160	A	300 (with ensuing death)
Duck	108 (97–133)	A	126, 123, 118
Mouse	94	A	111–371
Rat	90–160	A	396–933
Rat	105	P	185
Rabbit, fasting	60–120	A	476–581
		P	400–500
Sheep	30–50	A	140–200
Goat	35	P	75–165
Cat	108	P	592 (338–1050)
Dog fasting	100–110	P	475–510
		P + Insulin	100–150
Monkey	75–80	P	200–400

*A = alloxan diabetes; P = pancreatectomy.
From Zarrow et al.: 1964.

pletely oxidized to short-chain fatty acids. These fatty acids are absorbed passively from the gastrointestinal tract and converted into glucose and fats. Glucose in the feed never reaches the small intestine because microbes in the forestomach compartments of the ruminant stomach metabolize all available carbohydrates. Almost no glucose is absorbed in the small intestine. Thus, the adult ruminant is in a constant state of gluconeogenesis and has a blood glucose concentration of 40 to 60 mg/dl. Young ruminants, such as the bovine, have blood concentrations of glucose which resemble those in monogastric animals before their stomachs become fully functional. These blood levels decrease as the bovine gastrointestinal tract changes with age and adult levels are obtained by 6 months of age.

Diabetes mellitus, which is caused by a deficiency in insulin and results in hyperglycemia, is an important disease in veterinary medicine. Cells of diabetic animals do not receive adequate nutrition because insulin is not present to aid cellular uptake of glucose and amino acids. Hyperglycemia results in high levels of glucose in the glomerular filtrate which exceed the absorptive maximum of the kidney tubules. Excretion of glucose along with water and electrolytes in the urine results in an osmotic diuresis. The clinical sequelae include faulty glucose and fat metabolism,

water and electrolyte loss, and metabolic acidosis. These metabolic disturbances will eventually lead to death unless insulin is administered therapeutically.

The main purpose of this chapter is to describe the role of the endocrine pancreas in maintaining adequate cellular nutrition during fasting and feeding. The four peptide hormones of the pancreas, which are insulin, glucagon, somatostatin and pancreatic polypeptide, will be discussed.

ANATOMY

The pancreas is located in the upper right quadrant of the abdominal cavity in close association with the duodenum. The pancreas, which is composed primarily of parenchymal or functional tissue with very little stroma or connective tissue, is supplied with an extensive neural and vascular network. The endocrine cells of the pancreas constitute 2 to 3% of the total pancreatic mass and are located in clusters of cells, which are called islets of Langerhans. The cells of the pancreatic islets are innervated by sympathetic and parasympathetic fibers which influence hormone release.

Four functional cell types have been described in the islets (Fig. 5-1). These cells and the peptide hormones they synthesize and release are listed on page 188.

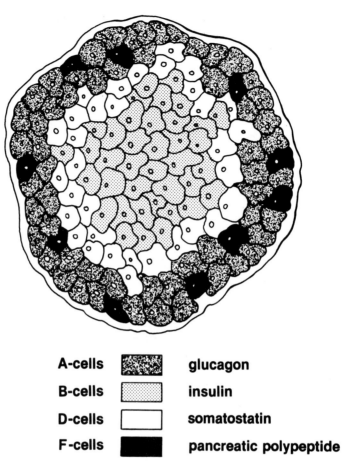

A-cells	glucagon
B-cells	insulin
D-cells	somatostatin
F-cells	pancreatic polypeptide

Fig. 5-1. The pancreatic islet.

These cell types are not randomly distributed within each islet. The B cells which are located in the center of each islet account for 60% of the total cell number. The A cells are located in the periphery or outer part of the islet and comprise 30% of the islet cells. The D cells are located between the A and B cells and account for approximately 10% of the islet cells. The F cells are few in number and are not always found in the islets. When found, they are located with the A cells. The islets do not have ducts so the hormones diffuse into capillaries and are carried to all parts of the body.

INSULIN

Insulin is synthesized and secreted by the B cells in the islets of Langerhans and con-

sists of two peptide chains, A and B, which are linked by two disulfide bridges. The amino acid sequence of insulin is shown in Figure 5-2 along with individual species differences. Canine and porcine insulin have the same structure. The major functions of insulin are to control the movement of glucose into cells and the intracellular metabolism of glucose.

Biosynthesis of Insulin

The synthesis of insulin in the B cells is stimulated by feeding and an increase in the plasma concentration of glucose reaching the islets. In addition to supplying glucose, feeding causes neural stimulation of the pancreas and the release of gastrointestinal hormones which in turn stimulate insulin release. The transcription of mRNA for the biosynthesis of

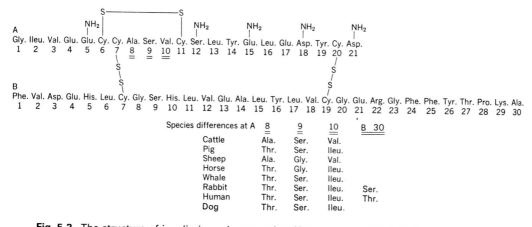

Fig. 5-2. The structure of insulin in various species. (Sanger, F.: Br. Med. Bull., *16*:183, 1960.)

insulin takes place in the nucleus. Translation begins in the rough endoplasmic reticulum with the formation of preproinsulin *de novo* on cytosolic polysomes. This molecule consists of an N-terminal prepeptide, the B-chain of insulin, a connecting peptide, and the A-chain of insulin. Proinsulin is formed when the 23 amino acids of the N-terminal prepeptide are cleaved in the rough endoplasmic reticulum and the disulfide bonds form between the two chains. After the proinsulin molecule is transferred from the rough endoplasmic reticulum to the Golgi apparatus, the connecting peptide is detached in the granules. Insulin is stored in the cytosol of the B cell in membrane-bound granules.

Human insulin has recently been synthesized by a genetically engineered *E. coli* bacterium. The A and B chains are produced separately and then combined to form the active molecule. This procedure will most likely be the future source of insulin (and other protein hormones) for therapeutic uses, since ten pounds of animal pancreas are required to provide every human diabetic with an annual supply of insulin. The purity of the synthetic hormone is preferred because antibodies may be produced by patients treated with heterologous insulin, due to structural variations of insulin in different species (Fig. 5-2).

Regulation of Insulin Release

Release takes place when the membrane-bound granules are displaced from the cytosol to the plasma membrane of the B cells. The membrane of the granule fuses with the plasma membrane of the B cell and the insulin contained in the granules is freed from the cell by exocytosis. The insulin molecules then diffuse into capillaries and enter the portal system.

The release of insulin from the B cells is regulated by a number of factors which include natural compounds such as glucose, amino acids, free fatty acids, gastrointestinal hormones, and glucagon, as well as the autonomic nervous system. Release is stimulated by parasympathetic stimulation while adrenergic stimulation normally inhibits release.

Glucose plays an important role in the control of insulin synthesis and release from the cell. The blood glucose level of normal animals varies little. When a large amount of glucose is given intravenously to these animals, there is a moderate and short-lived elevation of blood glucose. This is referred to as the glucose tolerance curve (Fig. 5-3). This curve is greatly extended in both amplitude and duration in diabetic animals. As the blood glucose level rises, the B cells release additional insulin which stimulates storage of glycogen by the liver and/or glucose utilization by the extrahepatic tissues.

The effects of glucose on insulin release are believed to be mediated via elevation of cytosolic Ca^{++}. Initially, the effects of glucose are due to the redistribution of cellular Ca^{++}, whereas the sustained effects are due to an increased Ca^{++} influx attributed to activation

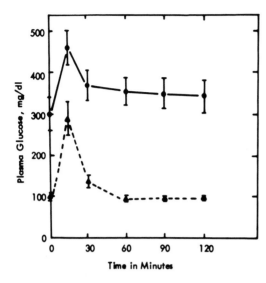

Fig. 5-3. Intravenous glucose tolerance test in normal (broken line) and in diabetic (solid line) dogs. Diabetes mellitus was induced with streptozotocin (30 mg/kg) and alloxan (50 mg/kg). (From Martin, S. L., and Capen, C. C., *In* Canine Medicine, edited by E. J. Catcott, Courtesy American Veterinary Publications, Inc., 1979)

of the plasma membrane calcium channels. Calcium is an effective modulator of insulin release. Hypercalcemia or the administration of calcium ionophores promotes insulin release, while hypocalcemia or the administration of calcium channel blockers decreases insulin release.

Glucose causes an increase in cAMP levels in the B cells. Increased cellular cAMP promotes insulin release only when glucose is present. Therefore, cAMP may contribute to glucose-dependent insulin stimulation, but cAMP alone will not activate the secretory processes.

In the canine, the B cells release insulin when stimulated with long-chain fatty acids and butyrate. Ruminants obtain approximately 70% of their energy from short-chain fatty acids of microbial origin. Butyrate and to a lesser degree, propionate, are potent stimulators of insulin release in ruminants.

Dietary amino acids also promote insulin release by a direct action on the B cells and indirectly through the release of gastrointestinal hormones (discussed later). In humans, most of the essential amino acids stimulate insulin release while non-essential amino acids do not. Some amino acids (e.g., arginine and lysine) stimulate insulin release only in the presence of glucose, while others (e.g., leucine) do not require glucose for stimulation and can directly stimulate the release of insulin. The mechanisms by which these amino acids act directly on the B cells to promote insulin release are unknown.

Administration of oral glucose causes a greater insulin release than parenteral administration of glucose. Although it has been known for over 70 years that intravenous injection of large doses of glucose provokes glycosuria more effectively than oral glucose, it was only recently recognized that this difference was due to a greater capacity of oral glucose to evoke insulin release. This suggests that some sort of anticipatory signal or signals, termed incretin, from the gastrointestinal tract stimulate the pancreas to release insulin. Therefore, the gastrointestinal tract and the pancreas form an enteropancreatic axis not only for the digestion and absorption of nutrients but also by controlling the utilization of these substances within the body. Several gastrointestinal hormones, including secretin, cholecystokinin, gastrin, vasoactive intestinal polypeptide, enteroglucagon, and gastric inhibitory polypeptide, have been shown to directly stimulate B cells to release insulin. These hormones share some similarities in chemical structure. Gastric inhibitory polypeptide is thought to be the most important gastrointestinal hormone in the stimulation of insulin release. Both glucose and fat in the gut stimulate the release of gastric inhibitory polypeptide. Cholecystokinin may play a similar role as a protein- and amino acid-sensitive hormone.

Insulin, glucagon and somatostatin modulate the release of one another through a paracrine relationship (Fig. 5-4). Glucagon and related peptides stimulate insulin release, while the release of glucagon by A cells is inhibited when insulin is released from B cells in their vicinity. Isolated B cells are less responsive to glucose than when they are in

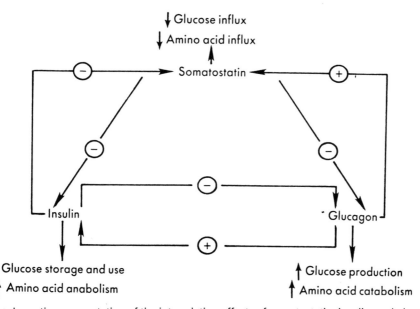

Fig. 5-4. A schematic representation of the interrelating effects of somatostatin, insulin, and glucagon on release and their effects on glucose and amino acid metabolism. (From Genuth, S. M., *In* Physiology, edited by R. M. Berne and M. N. Levy, 1983. Courtesy C. V. Mosby Co.)

contact with other islet cells. Somatostatin inhibits the release of both insulin and glucagon while glucagon stimulates somatostatin release. The effect of insulin on somatostatin release is unclear, but insulin probably is inhibitory in this respect.

Both the sympathetic and parasympathetic nervous systems richly innervate the islets and control the release of insulin. The predominant effect of catecholamines is to inhibit insulin release, a response mediated by α_2-adrenergic receptors. Exercise and other states of stress associated with activation of the sympathetic nervous system, including body burns, hypothermia, hypoxia, and surgery can lead to a suppression of insulin release via catecholamines acting on these α_2-adrenergic receptors. In the presence of drugs that block the α_2-adrenergic receptors, catecholamines activate β_2-adrenergic receptors to increase insulin release. This activation is mediated by the adenylate cyclase system to increase cAMP levels.

The parasympathetic nervous system also exerts a positive influence on insulin release. Stimulation of the vagus nerve increases insulin release by activating the cholinergic (muscarinic) receptors of B cells.

The hypothalamus regulates the autonomic input to the islets. Electrical stimulation of the ventrolateral hypothalamus leads to a rapid increase in insulin release, via a vagal pathway, while electrical stimulation of the ventromedial hypothalamus produces a decrease in insulin release mediated by the splanchnic (sympathetic) nerves. The hypothalamus also controls appetite and integrates feeding behavior and is, therefore, an important and indirect regulator of the B cell secretion.

Effects of Insulin

The major function of insulin is to facilitate the transport or flux of glucose across the plasma membrane of cells of most tissues. The exceptions are the red and white blood cells, as well as some of the neural, renal and intestinal tissues which do not require insulin for glucose transport (Fig. 5-5). Insulin stimulates the entry of amino acids into cells while glucose supplies energy for the synthesis of amino acids into protein. The metabolic ef-

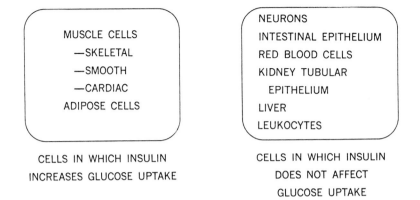

Fig. 5-5. The role of insulin.

fects of insulin are depicted in Figure 5-6. The transport of glucose and amino acids into the cells may occur immediately while other cellular changes are more subtle and occur over larger time frames (i.e., hours to days). These latter changes include transcriptional and translational changes of enzymes which regulate cellular metabolism.

Insulin reduces the plasma concentration of glucose and inhibits the release of glucose from the liver (Fig. 5-6). Glucose uptake by skeletal muscle and adipose tissue is enhanced by insulin. Insulin inhibits "hormone sensitive lipase" in adipocytes to prevent further fat degradation by increasing intracellular glucose. Levels of free fatty acids in the plasma decrease as lipolysis is decreased and fat synthesis is stimulated in the adipocytes.

Insulin hyperpolarizes cell membranes by facilitating influx of K^+. In clinical situations, insulin therapy may result in hypokalemia and hypolgycemia. Hypokalemia may result in cardiovascular disturbances due to the exogenously administered insulin. The exact mechanism of action on the membrane potential is not known but there is speculation that the Na^+/K^+-ATPase system is acted on directly by insulin.

Mechanism of Insulin Action

Insulin is an anabolic hormone which controls carbohydrates, fat, and protein metabolism (Fig. 5-6). The exact mechanisms by which insulin exerts this control remain to be determined. These effects are initiated when insulin binds to a receptor on the plasma membrane. The cellular events may be subdivided into those events which result from internalization of the insulin receptor complex. The interaction of insulin with the receptor in the plasma membrane of cells triggers an increase in glucose-transporting proteins in the plasma membrane. There is speculation that two subunits of the receptor protein, one acting as a protein kinase to phosphorylate another subunit, cause the number of glucose-transporting proteins to increase. The molecular events, which cause these protein carriers to increase, are being intensively investigated.

Insulin increases glycogen and fat synthesis (Fig. 5–7). Intracellular concentrations of cAMP are low when synthesis is taking place in cells exposed to insulin. This may be due to an inhibition of adenylate cyclase, which decreases the converison of ATP to cAMP. Insulin also increases phosphodiesterases which enhance the breakdown of cAMP. Conversely, catabolic hormones such as glucagon and catecholamines increase cAMP concentrations in cells (Fig. 5-7). So anabolic hormones decrease cAMP while catabolic hormones increase cAMP concentrations.

Cyclic AMP activates cAMP-dependent protein kinases in cells by binding to the regulatory unit of the kinases (Fig. 5-7). The catalytic unit of the protein kinase molecule is activated to phosphorylate the inactive de-

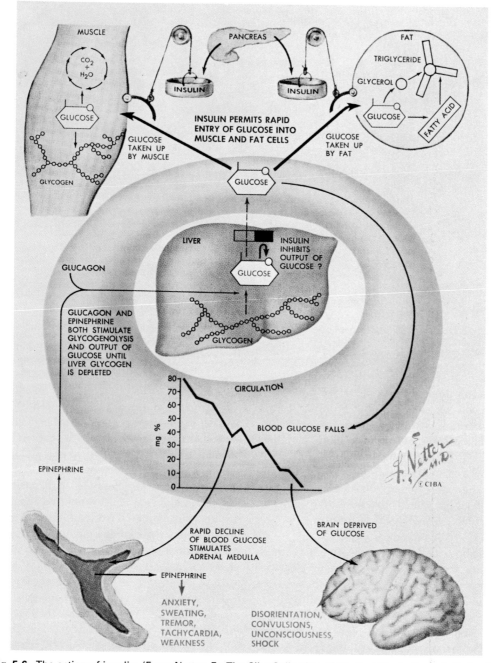

Fig. 5-6. The action of insulin. (From Netter, F.: The Ciba Collection of Medical Illustrations, 4, Endocrine System and Metabolic Diseases. 1963. Also Clinical Symposia, 1963. Ciba.)

phosphophosphorylase enzyme molecule to form phosphorylase, the active enzyme. The enzyme undergoes a conformational change with the addition of phosphate and glycogen breakdown procedes. Phosphatases dephosphorylate the active enzyme, phosphorylase, to form dephosphophosphorylase, the inactive molecule. Phosphatases are widespread in low

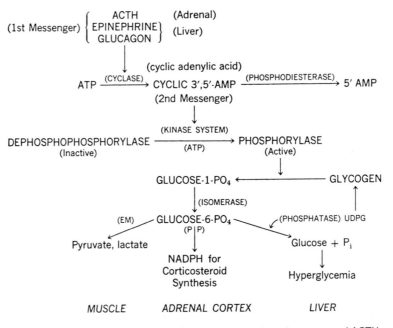

Fig. 5-7. The mechanism of phosphorylase activation by epinephrine, glucagon, and ACTH; and inhibition by insulin.

concentrations in the cells of the body. Protein kinases are not activated when cAMP concentrations are decreased by insulin.

These same events take place in adipocytes. Insulin inhibits "hormone sensitive lipase" and lipolysis is inhibited. In the absence of insulin and glucose, "hormone sensitive lipase" is activiated and lipolysis begins. In summary, cAMP increases during lipolysis and decreases during lipogenesis.

Amino acid uptake and protein synthesis in cells are stimulated while protein degradation is inhibited by insulin. Protein synthesis centers around transcription and translation. An increase in mRNA has been demonstrated in insulin-stimulated cells; however, the exact molecular mechanisms are unknown.

INSULIN DEFICIENCY (DIABETES MELLITUS)

Diabetes mellitus refers to a heterogenous group of metabolic disorders characterized by hyperglycemia and glycosuria. Other related events such as ketoacidosis, loss of minerals, nitrogen, and body weight may occur. All of these events eventually lead to coma and death if treatment is not instituted (Fig. 5-8).

Two major categories of diabetes mellitus are recognized in man: insulin-dependent diabetes mellitus (type 1; juvenile-onset) and non-insulin-dependent diabetes mellitus (type 2; maturity-onset). Patients with insulin-dependent diabetes mellitus have an absolute insulin deficiency, while individuals with non-insulin-dependent diabetes mellitus often have below normal or above normal plasma insulin levels in the fasting state, and may have an impaired insulin response to a glucose load.

Diabetes mellitus is frequently encountered in older dogs (> 7 years) and female dogs are three times as likely to be affected as male dogs. This disorder is less frequently reported in cats and other domestic species.

The majority of dogs with diabetes mellitus have clinical signs which resemble insulin-dependent diabetes mellitus of humans. Human and canine diabetes are characterized by sudden onset and marked insulin deficiency. Affected individuals are prone to ketoacidosis, and require insulin therapy to sustain life.

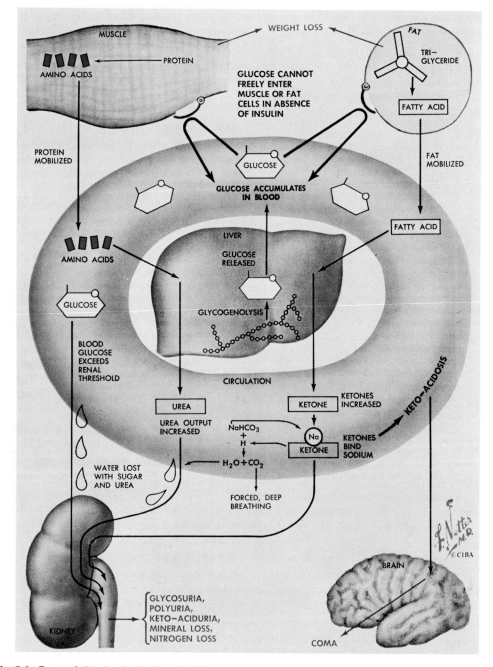

Fig. 5-8. Events following lack of insulin. (From Netter, F.: The Ciba Collection of Medical Illustrations, 4, Endocrine System and Metabolic Diseases. 1963. Also Clinical Symposia, 1963. Ciba.)

While most cases of insulin-dependent diabetes mellitus in humans occur early in life, most cases of canine diabetes are diagnosed in older animals.

A small number of canine patients will have normal or above normal fasting insulin levels in the blood, yet there is no insulin response to a glucose load. Those with fasting insulin levels above normal are usually obese. These dogs display the typical signs of diabetes mellitus, require insulin therapy to sustain life, and are prone to ketoacidosis. Therefore, they may be differentiated from human patients with non-insulin-dependent diabetes mellitus, who frequently do not have or have minimal symptoms of ketoacidosis.

Facets of Diabetes Mellitus

Some of the derangements that occur are listed below:

Hyperglycemia
Glycosuria
Diuresis
Decreased carbohydrate utilization
Increased fat and protein catabolism
Weight loss and polyphagia
Body weight loss
Loss of resistance to infections
Bilateral cataracts
Coma and death

Although there is some temporal relationship between the above-mentioned facets, it must be borne in mind that several of these processes are occurring simultaneously and the order listed is not necessarily maintained during the course of the disease.

Hyperglycemia, Glycosuria, Diuresis

A deficiency of insulin renders the animal cells unable to use the available glucose, because *glucose cannot move across the cell membrane of the majority of cells.* Since utilization of glucose is depressed, the blood glucose level begins to rise above the normal value of approximately 100 mg/dl of blood until it reaches the renal threshold for glucose which is 160 to 180 mg/dl in the dog. At this point glucose begins to appear in the urine, since *the tubules are unable to completely reabsorb this increasing amount of glucose.* The blood glucose level continues to rise until a level of 300 to 400 mg/dl may be present and the dog may be losing 3 to 4 g of glucose per kg of body weight per day through the urine. Carbohydrate intake in the diet affects the levels of glucose in the blood. The fasted animal has a less dramatic rise in blood glucose than the carbohydrate-fed animal. The loss of glucose in the urine exerts an osmotic attraction for water thereby causing an excretion of large amounts of urine and bringing about dehydration. The polyuria continues causing an intense thirst so the animal consumes large amounts of water (polydipsia).

Decreased Carbohydrate Utilization

Most tissues of the body are unable to take up and metabolize the usual amount of glucose in the absence of insulin. *Nerve cells and red blood cells are among a number of cells that do not require insulin for glucose utilization* (Fig 5-5); consequently their rate of uptake is not affected by the diabetic state. Skeletal and cardiac muscle are able to use some glucose in the absence of insulin, but the amount is reduced. In general, though, the utilization of glucose is reduced and this can be shown by a reduced glucose tolerance curve, a decreased respiratory quotient, and the fact that the fasting animal still exhibits hyperglycemia and glycosuria. The decreased utilization of carbohydrate causes catabolism of fat and protein stores of the body.

Increased Fat and Protein Catabolism

Fat catabolism is increased in the diabetic animal, since another major source of energy must be mobilized to offset decreased utilization of glucose. With increased fat catabolism the concentration of ketone bodies such as acetoacetic and beta hydroxybutyric acids increases in the blood. Ketogenesis is considered a normal part of fat metabolism, but there is a limit to the amount of ketone bodies that can be used for energy; consequently the excess ketone substances accumulate in the blood and may even appear in the urine. These give the characteristic ketone odor to the urine and breath of the diabetic animal.

Even though fat catabolism occurs elsewhere in the body, fatty metamorphosis of the liver leads to hepatomegaly. Liver failure may occur leading to icterus and elevated liver enzymes, (e.g., aspartate aminotransferase) in the serum.

The ketone bodies are released as acids and must be buffered by the blood. Some are excreted as salts; consequently there is a loss of sodium and potassium from the body. If the severity is intense and duration is prolonged, then *the acid-base balance is taxed*. Vomiting is also common. At the same time, polyuria is causing loss of electrolytes. Consequently the depletion of salt and dehydration of the body may lead to *acidosis and dehydration so severe that coma will ensue*. In the treatment of the diabetic animal the degree of ketosis is often the most urgent factor to consider.

Protein catabolism occurs simultaneously with fat catabolism. The body stores of protein, such as those in the muscle, are mobilized as a source of energy. The liberated amino acids are converted to glucose or fatty acids. Only a portion of the glucose can be used; consequently there is additional loss through the urine and body weight continues to decrease. The deaminization of amino acids liberates nitrogen to cause a rise in nonprotein nitrogen levels in the blood and urine.

In long-standing cases of canine diabetes mellitus, capillary microangiopathy, including thickening of the basment membrane, may occur. Less often, the arterioles and venules are affected. Canine microangiopathy is less frequent than in man, since the time factor is reduced. These vascular effects are usually in the kidneys, retina, and skin.

Diabetes mellitus in domestic animals does not retard tissue repair or healing as much as in the human; instead, slow healing in the dog more often accompanies excess corticosteroids as in Cushing's disease.

Weight Loss, Polyphagia

Depletion of the stores of carbohydrate, fat, and protein results in severe loss of body weight. Even with a voracious appetite, the animal continues to lose weight, since many energy-yielding substances are being lost in the urine.

Coma and Death

Many factors lead to coma, but perhaps dehydration, acidosis, and ketonemia are of utmost importance. Frequently the animal is found in a state of coma and must be treated immediately. Neutralization of the ketone substances and hydration must occur quickly in order to prevent death.

Causes of Diabetes Mellitus

Studies of human diabetes mellitus have shown a definite familial hereditary predisposition to the condition. This predisposition, although hereditary, can possibly be manifested in several ways: an inherent gluconeogenic state such as hyperproduction of ACTH could lead to chronic hyperglycemia and finally islet cell exhaustion; a familial tendency toward high sugar diets could bring about the same chain of events leading to exhaustion of the islet cells; an abnormal nitrogen metabolism might produce an alloxan-like substance which is toxic to B cells; another possibility is that the enzyme insulinase may be present in abnormally high levels thereby lowering prematurely the level of insulin. Others have suggested insulin inhibitors as being prevalent in the diabetic animal. Cattle recovered from foot-and-mouth disease have a high incidence of diabetes mellitus as do humans and mice which experience related viruses. Not enough work has been done in domestic animals to be able to classify the conditions as to cause.

In the dog, diabetes mellitus is often a sequela to chronic pancreatitis, an infection of the acinar cells which may involve the islets. Although the pancreatitis may be controlled, permanent damage to the islet cells may remain. In chronic diabetes mellitus, *the dog often develops cataracts*. The mechanism underlying this relationship is unknown. Because the retinopathy occurs in dogs with long-standing diabetes, cataract removal may not be indicated.

Glucagon must be considered a possible cause of diabetes mellitus. In man, some diabetic patients have elevated levels of glucagon which could come from the pancreatic A cells or an enteric source. The ensuing hyperglycemia may lead to B cell exhaustion.

The B cells of most species are so susceptible to injected growth hormone that one wonders if overproduction of endogenous somatotropin could be a cause of diabetes mellitus.

Experimental Diabetes Mellitus

Much of the early work on insulin and the metabolic role of insulin was performed on pancreatectomized animals. These studies were confounded, especially in long-term studies, due to the fact that the pancreas is a diffuse organ in mammals. Therefore, it is difficult to remove all of the endocrine cells. Chemical techniques may be used to eliminate the undesirable consequences of surgery, including trauma, pain, stress, and loss of exocrine tissue. Alloxan and streptozotocin are the drugs that selectively destroy B cells and thus induce experimental diabetes mellitus. A major disadvantage with these chemical techniques is that all of these agents induce side effects, which include liver and kidney injuries and bone marrow depression. Streptozotocin is less toxic than alloxan and may be useful clinically to treat tumors of B cells, called insulinomas. This approach is still experimental because it is difficult to overcome the drug toxicity problems.

Insulin Therapy

Insulin formulations are usually made from porcine and bovine insulin extracts. These formulations can be divided into three categories, according to promptness, and duration of action following subcutaneous injection. They are classified as fast-, intermediate-, and long-acting types. The ranges of durations of action for these types of insulin in the human diabetic are 6 to 14, 18 to 24, and 36 hours, respectively. If diabetes mellitus is diagnosed in dogs or cats before severe ketoacidosis develops, treatment with isophane (NPH) insulin, an intermediate-acting preparation, or protamine zinc insulin, a long-acting preparation is recommended. Isophane insulin has been widely used by veterinarians and its use is based on the contention that the duration of action is 24 hours when administered to dogs and cats. It is now clear that isophane insulin is only effective in most dogs and cats for about 12 hours, rather than 24 hours. Since the duration of action is shorter than previously thought, most dogs and cats need two rather than one daily injection of isophane insulin for adequate control of blood levels of glucose.

The use of protamine zinc insulin is increasing. Although it was once thought that the duration of action was 36 hours, it is now apparent that the duration of action of protamine zinc insulin in a dog or cat is only about 24 hours. Most diabetic dogs and cats can be adequately maintained with a single daily injection of protamine zinc insulin. The insulin dosage must be adjusted after blood glucose levels are taken at 12 and 24 hours postinjection. In addition, the diabetic dog or cat should be fed twice a day. Diabetic animal patients can often be maintained for several years, but this regimen is time-consuming.

If severe ketoacidosis occurs, the animals will become dehydrated and comatose. When these signs develop, appropriate emergency treatment is required. Treatment with intravenous fluids plus a fast-acting crystalline insulin will usually stabilize the patient.

Sulfonylureas which increase insulin release from the B cells are used in human medicine to treat non-insulin-dependent diabetics. Diabetic dogs and cats usually have an absolute deficiency of insulin, consequently these oral hypoglycemic agents are not useful. Tolbutamide, the prototype of the sulfonylureas, is hepatotoxic to the dog.

Hyperinsulinism (Hypoglycemia)

An excess of insulin from injection or hyperproduction by the B cells may induce hypoglycemia. The nervous system in particular is affected and the following signs develop: incoordination, muscular weakness, tremors, and finally unconsciousness and convulsions. *The nervous system is primarily dependent on glucose for energy, hence the dysfunction.*

The dog occasionally has a tumor of the islet cells bringing on hyperinsulinism and hypolgycemia. The appearance of hypoglycemic signs after an overdosage of insulin is dependent upon objective signs in the domestic animal. This is in contrast to the human subject in whom subjective symptoms such as tingling of the limbs, dizziness, and muscular weakness can be detected by the patient and the falling blood glucose level alleviated by the oral ingestion of sugar.

When the rate of fall in blood glucose is rapid, the early signs of hyperinsulinism are those elicited by a compensating release of epinephrine, these early signs include tachycardia, weakness, hunger, and sweating. Epinephrine favors glycogenolysis in the liver. This degree of hypoglycemia stimulates ACTH release, thereby bringing this glucose elevating scheme into play. Thus a physiological balance (reciprocal relationship) exists between insulin and epinephrine bringing about a steady blood glucose level—the liver being the storehouse for glycogen.

Excess insulin may bring on coma or convulsion in the dog, young ruminants, and man but not the bird or mature ruminants. The goat requries large doses of insulin and low blood glucose (10 to 20 mg/dl for 5 to 8 hours) in order to induce apathy and sluggishness. Parenteral glucose infusion would be the treatment of choice following insulin overdosage.

Hyperinsulinism in older dogs is usually due to an adenoma (30 to 45%) or carcinoma (55 to 70%) of the islets. Diagnosis depends on persistent hypoglycemia, glucose tolerance tests, determinations of levels of insulin in serum or plasma, or exploratory laparotomy. Adenomas are usually well-circumscribed and may be surgically removed with fair success.

GLUCAGON

Shortly after the discovery of insulin, it became evident that the administration of crude extracts of the pancreas into experimental animals produced inconsistent hypoglycemia. It was hypothesized that a hyperglycemic factor, which counteracted the insulin-induced hypoglycemia, was present in these extracts. This factor, named glucagon, was isolated and characterized thirty years after the discovery of insulin.

Glucagon is synthesized as an 18,000 dalton prohormone and stored in granules in the A cells of the pancreatic islets. The prohormone is cleaved to form the active molecule, a simple peptide with 29 amino acids and a molecular weight of 3500, prior to release from the granule (Fig. 5-9).

Glucagon release is stimulated during hypolgycemia and inhibited during hyperglycemia. Insulin and somatostatin also inhibit glucagon release. Amino acids stimulate both glucagon and insulin release. Gastrointestinal peptides such as cholecystokinin, gastrin and gastric inhibitory polypeptide, and catabolic hormones such as catecholamines, growth hormone, and glucocorticoids stimulate release of glucagon.

The major metabolic effect of glucagon is to stimulate hepatic glycogenolysis. Glucagon acts in hepatic cells by activating adenylate cyclase and a cAMP dependent protein kinase. During glycogenolysis phosphorylase is activated while glycogen synthase is inhibited. The activation of phosphorylase promotes the degradation of hepatic glycogen to glucose which then enters the bloodstream. Gluconeogenesis in the liver is also stimulated by glucagon. During gluconeogenesis, amino acids from skeletal muscle and non-glucose compounds, such as lactate and glycerol, are converted to glucose.

In summary, insulin is an anabolic hormone whereas glucagon is a catabolic hormone. Although other catabolic hormones play a role in maintaining blood glucose, these two hormones are paramount to glucose homeostasis. They function to maintain a fairly stable concentration of glucose in the blood which adequately meets the metabolic requirements during periods of activity. During the postprandial period, insulin lowers blood glucose by facilitating glucose storage and utilization. During periods of

NH$_2$

NH$_2$ NH$_2$ NH$_2$

His-Ser-Glu-Gly-Thr-Phe-Thr-Ser-Asp-Tyr-Ser-Lys-Tyr-Leu-Asp-Ser-Arg-Arg-Ala-Glu-Asp-Phe-Val-Glu-Try-Leu-Met-Asp-Thr

Fig. 5-9. Amino acid sequence of glucagon.

high metabolic demand, glucagon acts to increase blood glucose through hepatic glycogenolysis and gluconeogenesis.

SOMATOSTATIN

Somatostatin, a tetradecapeptide with a molecular weight of 1638, was isolated initially from the hypothalamus. Growth hormone release is inhibited by somatostatin; hence, it was called somatotrophin release inhibiting factor (SRIF). Since the discovery of somatostatin in pituitary extracts, this peptide has been isolated from many other tissues, including the pancreas. In the pancreas, somatostatin is synthesized in D cells. The main action of somatostatin is to inhibit the release of insulin, glucagon, and gastrointestinal peptides. The low levels of somatostatin in the blood and the ubiquitous distribution have led many investigators to conclude that the action of somatostatin is paracrine in nature. Somatostatin is synthesized as a peptide with 28 amino acids, which are then cleaved to 14 amino acids. The hormone with 28 amino acids is more potent than the tetradecapeptide form in decreasing insulin release. Somatostatin reduces glucose absorption from the gut by inhibiting the release of gastrointestinal peptides.

PANCREATIC POLYPEPTIDE

Pancreatic polypeptide is a peptide hormone containing 36 amino acids which is synthesized by F cells in the islets. The specific function of this peptide is not clear, however, inhibition of food intake has been postulated as a possible function of this peptide. Pancreatic polypeptide increases in the bloodstream after meals, especially those high in protein.

REFERENCES

1. Anderson, N. V., and Low, D. G. (1965): Diseases of the canine pancreas: a comparative summary of 103 cases. J. Am. Anim. Hosp. Assoc. *1*:189.
2. Asplin, C. M., Paquette, T. L., and Palmer, J. P. (1981): In vivo inhibition of glucagon secretion by paracrine β cell activity in man. J. Clin. Invest. *68*:314.
3. Belinger, R. E., and Siegel, E. T. (1972): Double antibody radioimmunoassay of insulin in canine serum. Am. J. Vet. Res. *33*:2149.
4. Berkow, J. W., and Ricketts, R. L. (1965): Spontaneous diabetes mellitus in dogs. J. Am. Vet. Med. Assoc. *146*:1101.
5. Black, H. E., Rosenblum, Y., and Capen, C. C. (1979): Chemically induced (streptozotocin-alloxan) diabetes mellitus in the dog: biochemical and ultrastructural studies. Am. J. Pathol. *98*:295.
6. Bloodworth, J. M. B., Jr., and Molitor, D. L. (1965): Ultrastructural aspects of human and canine diabetic retinopathy. Invest. Ophthalmol. *4*:1037.
7. Bloom, F. (1937): Diabetes mellitus in a cat. N. Engl. J. Med. *217*:395.
8. Blum. T. W., Wilson, R. B., and Kronfeld, D. S. (1973): Plasma insulin concentrations in parturient cows. J. Dairy Sci. *56*:459.
9. Bromer, W. W., Sinn, L. G., and Behrens, O. K. (1957): The amino acid sequence of glucagon. J. Am. Chem. Soc. *79*:2807.
10. Calabresi, P., and Parks, R. E., Jr. (1985): Antiproliferative agents and drugs used for immunosuppression. *In*: The Pharmacological Basis of Therapeutics, 7th Ed., A. G. Gilman, et al. (eds) New York, MacMillan, p. 1247.
11. Call, J. L., Mitchell, G. E., Jr., Ely, D. G., et al. (1972): Amino-acids, volatile fatty-acids, and glucose in plasma of insulin treated sheep. J. Anim. Sci. *34*:767.
12. Capen, C. C., and Martin, S. L. (1969): Hyperinsulinism in dogs with neoplasia of the pancreatic islets, a clincial, pathologic, and ultrastructural study. Pathol. Vet. *6*:309.
13. Caywood, D. D., Wilson, J. W., Hardy, R. M., et al. (1979): Pancreatic islet cell adenocarcinoma: clinical and diagnostic features of six cases. J. Am. Vet. Med. Assoc. *174*:715.
14. Cotton, R. B., Cornelius, L. M., and Theran, P. (1971): Diabetes mellitus in the dog: a clinicopathologic study. J. Am. Vet. Med. Assoc. *159*:863.
15. Craighead, J. E. (1972): Workshop on viral infection and diabetes mellitus in man. J. Infect. Dis. *125*:568.
16. Czech, M. P. (1977): Molecular basis of insulin action. Ann. Rev. Biochem. *46*:359.
17. de Lahunta, A., Ross, G., Loomis, W., et al. (1971): Clinical pathological conference (pancreatitis, diabetes mellitus, and myocardial degeneration in a dog). Cornell Vet. *61*:716.
18. Dileepan, K. N., and Wagle, S. R. (1985): Somatostatin: A metabolic regulator. Life Sci. *37*:2335.
19. Elahi, D., Raizes, G. S., Andres, S., et al. (1982): Interaction of arginine and gastric inhibitory polypeptide on insulin release in man. Am. J. Physiol. *242*:E343.
20. Frank, B. H., and Chance, R. E. (1983): Two routes for producing human insulin utilizing recombinant DNA technology. Munch. Med. Wochen. *125*:14.
21. Gepts, W., and Toussaint, D. (1967): Spontaneous diabetes in dogs and cats: A pathological study. Diabetologia *3*:259.
22. Gerich, J. E., Charles, M. A., and Grodsky, G. M. (1976): Regulation of pancreatic insulin and glucagon secretion. Ann. Rev. Physiol. *38*:353.
23. Gerich, J. E., Lorenzi, M., Bier, D. M., et al. (1975): Prevention of human diabetic ketoacidosis by somatostatin: Evidence for an essential role of glucagon.

N. Engl. J. Med. *292*:985.

24. Gershwin, L. J. (1975): Familial canine diabetes mellitus. J. Am. Vet. Med. Assoc. *167*:479.

25. Hedeskov, C. J. (1980) Mechanism of glucose-induced insulin secretion. Physiol. Rev. *60*:442.

26. Hedo, J. A., Villanueva, M. L., and Marco, J. (1979): Influence of plasma free fatty acids on pancreatic polypeptide secretion in man. J. Clin. Endocrinol. Metab. *49*:73.

27. Hougen, T. J., B. E. Hopkins and T. W. Smith (1978): Insulin effects on monovalent cation transport on Na-K-ATPase activity. Am. J. Physiol. *234*:C59.

28. Jeffrey, J. R. (1969): Diabetes mellitus secondary to chronic pancreatitis in a pony. J. Am. Vet. Med. Assoc. *153*:1168.

29. Johnson. R. K. (1977): Insulinoma in the dog. Vet. Clin. North Am. *7*:629.

30. Jones, K. L., Bell, R. L., Oyler, J. M., et al. (1970): Hyperglycemic effects of sodium butyrate in normal and pancreatectomized sheep. Am. J. Vet. Res. *31*:81.

31. Lacy, P. E. (1975): Endocrine secretory mechanism. Am. J. Pathol. *79*:170.

32. Lapras, M., Beurlet, J., Guillaume, J., et al. (1973): Hypoglycemic convulsions, simulating epilepsy. Report on a bitch with a secreting insulinoma in the pancreas. Rev. Med. Vet. *124*:169.

33. Larrson, L. -I., Golterman, N., DeMagistris, L., et al. (1979): Somatostatin cell processes as pathways for paracrine secretion. Science *205*:1393.

34. Ling, G. V., Lowenstine, L. J., Pulley, L. T. et al. (1977): Diabetes mellitus in dogs: A review of initial evaluation, immediate and longterm management and outcome. J. Am. Vet. Med. Assoc. *170*:521.

35. Manns, J. G., and Boda, J. M. (1965): Control of insulin secretion in sheep: the effect of volatile fatty acids and glucose. Physiologist *8*:227.

36. Manns, J. G., and Martin, C. L. (1972): Plasma insulin, glucagon, and nonesterified fatty-acid in dogs with diabetes mellitus. Am. J. Vet. Res. *33*:981.

37. Mattheeuws, D., Rottiers, R., Kaneko, J. J., et al. (1984): Diabetes mellitus in dogs: Relationship of obesity to glucose tolerance and insulin response. Am J. Vet. Res. *45*:98.

38. Maugh, T. H. (1975): Diabetes (II): Model systems indicate viruses a cause. Science *188*:436.

39. Maugh, T. H. (1975): Diabetes (III): New hormones promise more effective therapy. Science *188*:920.

40. McIntyre, N., Holdsworth, C. D., and Turner, D.S. (1964): New interpretation of oral glucose tolerance. Lancet *2*:20.

41. Meier, H. (1961): Comparative aspects of spontaneous diabetes mellitus in animals. Am. J. Med. *31*:868.

42. Meyer, D. J. (1977): Temporary remission of hypoglycemia in a dog with insulinoma after treatment with streptozotocin. Am. J. Vet. Res. *38*:1201.

43. Miller, R. E. (1981): Pancreatic neuroendocrinology: Peripheral neural mechanisms in the regulation of the islets of Langerhans. Endocrine Rev. *2*:471.

44. Mutt. V. (1980): Cholecystokinin: Isolation, structure, and function. *In*: Gastrointestinal Hormones, G. B. Jerzy Class (ed.). New York, Raven Press, p. 169.

45. Nakaki, T., Nakadate, T., Ishsi, K., et al. (1981): Postsynaptic alpha-2 adrenergic receptors in isolated rat islets of Langerhans: Inhibition of insulin release and cyclic 3':5' -adenosine monophosphate accumulation. J. Pharmacol. Exp. Ther. *216*:607.

46. Orci, L. (1982): Macro- and micro-domains in the endocrine pancreas. Diabetes *31*:538.

47. Pipleers, D., Veld, P., Maes, E., et al. (1982): Glucose-induced insulin release depends on functional cooperation between islet cells. Proc. Natl. Acad. Sci. *79*:7322.

48. Sanger, F. (1960): Chemistry of insulin. Br. Med. Bull. *16*:183.

49. Schaer, M. (1973): Diabetes mellitus in the cat. J. Am. Anim. Hosp. Assoc. *9*:548.

50. Schaer, M., Scott, R., Wilkins, R., Kay, W., Calvert, C., and Wolland, M. (1974): Hyperosmolar syndrome in the non-ketoacidotic diabetic dog. J. Am. Anim. Hosp. Assoc. *10*:357.

51. Schall, W. D. (1985): Pancreatic disorders. *In*: Handbook of Small Animal Therapeutics, L. E. Davis (ed), New York, Churchill-Livingston, 1985. p. 485.

52. Shimazu, T., and Ishikawa, K. (1981): Modulation by the hypothalamus of glucagon and insulin secretion in rabbits: Studies with electrical and chemical stimulation. Endocrinology *108*:605.

53. Szecowka, J., Lins, P. E., and Efendic, S. (1982): Effects of cholecystokinin, gastric inhibitory peptide, and secretin on insulin and glucagon secretion in rats. Endocrinology *110*:1268.

54. Tannenbaum, G. S., Ling, N., and Brazeau, P. (1982): Somatostatin-14 on pituitary and pancreatic hormone release. Endocrinology *111*:101.

55. Trenkle, A. (1972): Radioimmunoassay of plasma hormones: review of plasma insulin in ruminants. J. Dairy Sci. *55*:1200.

56. Unger, R. H., and Orci, L. (1981): Glucagon and the A cell. N. Engl. J. Med. *304*:1518.

57. Valverde, I., Vandermeers, A., Anjaneyulu, R., and Malaisse, W. J. (1979): Calmodulin activation of adenylate cyclase in pancreatic islets. Science *206*:225.

58. Wilson, J. W., and Hulse, D. A. (1974): Surgical correction of islet cell adenocarcinoma in a dog. J. Am. Vet. Med. Assoc. *164*:603.

59. Witzel, D. A., and Littledike, E. T. (1973): Suppression of insulin secretion during induced hypocalcemia. Endocrinology *93*:761.

60. Wollheim, C. B., and Sharp. G. W. G. (1981): Regulation of insulin release by calcium. Physiol. Rev. *61*:914.

61. Zarrow, M. X., Yochim, J. M., and McCarthy, J. L. (1964): Experimental Endocrinology. New York. Academic Press, Inc.

The Adrenal Gland

W. H. HSU and M. H. CRUMP

6

THE adrenal glands are paired endocrine organs located within the abdominal cavity. The hormones secreted by the adrenal glands regulate a number of metabolic processes which enable animals to function in a constantly changing environment. Each gland has two distinct functional and anatomic parts. The outer part or adrenal cortex is derived from mesodermal tissue and contains those cells which synthesize the steroid hormones called corticosteroids. The inner part or adrenal medulla is derived from ectodermal tissue from the neural crest and contains the chromaffin cells which synthesize catecholamines.

The corticosteroids from the adrenal cortex regulate the concentrations of Na^+ and K^+ in plasma in conjunction with the proper water volume to maintain cell hydration. Corticosteroids and catecholamines participate in the regulation of metabolic processes and the maintenance of proper nutrition for all cells, especially neural tissues. In general, corticosteroid hormones are involved in adaptive changes which take place over minutes, hours or days, while catecholamines regulate and induce fast responses in seconds in major organ systems, such as the cardiovascular and neuromuscular systems. A functional adrenal cortex, or the administration of steroid hormones to individuals which have dysfunction of the adrenal cortex, is requisite for life, whereas the hormones secreted by the adrenal medulla are not essential for life.

The most common dysfunctions of the adrenal gland are hyposecretion of the adrenal cortex, hypoadrenocorticism or Addison's disease, and hypersecretion of the adrenal cortex, hyperadrenocorticism or Cushing's disease. The most common clinical problem associated with the adrenal medulla in veterinary medicine is a tumor of the chromaffin cells called pheochromocytoma.

ANATOMY

The adrenal glands, literally "the glands next to the kidneys," are located within the abdominal cavity in close apposition to the kidneys. All domestic animals have paired glands with the exception of birds, which have clusters of intermixed cortical and medullary tissue in close proximity to the kidneys. The adrenal glands are highly irrigated organs with a rich network of capillaries which supply blood to the adrenal cortex and medulla. Blood carrying adrenal hormones leaves the gland via veins which enter the abdominal vena cava.

The adrenal cortex constitutes about 90% of the gland mass and can be characterized and divided from the outer to the inner part into three distinct zones: zona glomerulosa, zona fasciculata and zona reticularis (Fig. 6-1). More than 50 different steroids are synthesized and released from the adrenal cortex. These steroids fall into three classes: glucocorticoids, which received this name because of their effect on glucose homeostasis; mineralocorticoids, because of their effect on Na^+ and K^+ homeostasis; and sex steroid hormones, particularly androgens. Mineralocorticoids, in general, are synthesized in the zona glomerulosa with the exception of deoxycorticosterone. Deoxycorticosterone, which is a mineralocorticoid, is synthesized in both the zona fasciculata and zona reticularis. Glucocorticoids and sex steroids are synthesized in both the zona fasciculata and zona reticularis. Endogenous corticosteroids, such as cortisol and corticosterone, have predominantly glucocorticoid activity, while deoxycorticosterone and aldosterone have a predominant mineralocorticoid activity. Many corticosteroids have functions with overlap. A comparison of the relative potencies of several important endogenous corticosteroids is listed in Table 6-1. Cortisol is the most potent of the glucocorticoids secreted by the adrenal cortex, while aldosterone is the most potent mineralocorticoid.

Adrenocorticotropic hormone (ACTH), a peptide hormone of the adenohypophysis, has a trophic or nutritive effect on the adrenal cortex and also stimulates the synthesis of corticosteroids. A short-term deficiency of ACTH results in atrophy of the zonae fasciculata and reticularis of the adrenal cortex. The zona glomerulosa is necessary for the regeneration of cells in the zonae reticularis and fasciculata, in the event these cells die. An administration of ACTH will cause an increase in the growth of the zonae fasciculata and reticularis when there are still residual cells in the zona glomerulosa. Long-term pituitary hypofunction may eventually result in atrophy of the zona glomerulosa and mineralocorticoid deficiency.

The adrenal medulla is composed of ectodermal cells which comprise 10% of the total adrenal gland mass. The chromaffin cells synthesize and store norepinephrine and epinephrine in cytosolic granules. On the basis of the characteristics of the cytosolic granules, two types of cells have been described histologically in the adrenal medulla: (1) epinephrine-secreting cells which have large, less dense granules, and (2) norepinephrine secreting cells which have small, dense granules. These medullary or chromaffin cells are a part of the endocrine system and also an important branch of the sympathetic nervous system. The chromaffin cells, as part of the endocrine system, release the catecholamines, norepinephrine and epinephrine, which enter the circulatory system and are carried to cells throughout the body. As a part of the sympathetic nervous system, the chromaffin cells are innervated by cholinergic preganglionic nerve fibers from the central nervous system (retic-

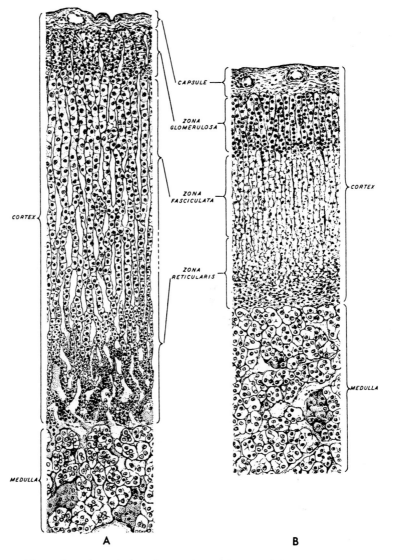

Fig. 6-1. Comparable sections through the adrenal glands of normal (*A*) and hypophysectomized (*B*) rats. Since the functional capacity of the adrenal cortex is conditioned by the release of ACTH, hypophysectomy results in tremendous shrinkage of the fascicular zone of the cortex. The medulla and glomerular zone are not influenced by hypophysectomy. Both sections are drawn to scale. (Turner, C. D, and Bognara, J. T. General Endocrinology. 6th ed., 1976. Courtesy W. B. Saunders Co.)

Table 6-1   Comparison of the Relative Potencies of Endogenous Corticosteroids

Corticosteroid	Relative Glucocorticoid Potency	Relative Mineralocorticoid Potency
Cortisol	1	1
Cortisone	0.8	0.8
Corticosterone	0.3	15
Deoxycorticosterone	0	100
Aldosterone	0.3	3000

ular formation of the medulla oblongata, pons, and hypothalamic centers). The preganglionic sympathetic fibers release acetylcholine which depolarizes the medullary cells and sympathetic nerve endings thereby causing the release of catecholamines. Thus, the medullary cells resemble postganglionic sympathetic neurons without fibers.

ADRENAL CORTEX

Chemistry and Biosynthesis of Corticosteroids

The adrenocorticoid hormones are steroid molecules which contain the cyclopentanoperhydrophenanthrene ring structure as depicted in Figure 6-2. The steroid molecule is formed by four rings called, A, B, C and D. The number of carbon atoms and their location in the molecular structure are depicted for cholesterol in Figure 6-2. The following nomenclature is internationally accepted for corticosteroids: double bonds in the structure are indicated by the Greek letter Δ, followed by a superscript number which indicates the specific carbon atom associated with the double bond. The carbon atom with the lower number is used to indicate the double bond (e.g., Δ^4 instead of Δ^5 for aldosterone, corticosterone, and cortisol in Fig. 6-2). The steroid molecule is a planar molecule because of the angles of the bonds between carbons. When the molecule is in a horizontal plane, the chemical groups attached to the molecule may extend either above (β) or below (α) the plane of the molecule. Chemical groups in position β, extending above the plane of the molecule, are represented as being attached to the carbon in the ring by a solid line, while those groups in position α are represented by a dashed line attached to the carbon (e.g., 11β-hydroxy and 17α-hydroxy in Fig. 6-2). Keto groups have double bonds and are identified by a number indicating the carbon atom to which they are attached (e.g., 3-keto).

Cholesterol, a compound with 27 carbon atoms, is the parent structure for all adrenal corticosteroids. Cholesterol may be synthe-

sized *de novo* in the body from acetate or absorbed from the gastrointestinal tract. Since cholesterol is not water-soluble, it is transported to adrenocortical cells by low-density lipoproteins in the plasma. Cholesterol passively diffuses across the plasma membrane along with the low-density lipoproteins into the cells of the adrenal cortex and either enters a biosynthetic pathway to generate corticosteroid hormones or is stored as a cholesterol ester in the cytosol. The adrenocortical cells have enzyme systems within the smooth endoplasmic reticulum and mitochondria which participate in complex biosynthetic pathways until the specific hormones are synthesized. The biosynthetic pathways of the adrenocortical hormones and other steroid hormones are illustrated in Figure 6-2.

Synthetic corticosteroids are man-made compounds from structural modifications of cortisol. Pharmacology textbooks should be consulted for more detailed information on their nomenclature and structure.

Transport, Metabolism and Elimination of Corticosteroids

Corticosteroids enter the bloodstream as non-polar molecules and circulate as free molecules or are bound extensively to plasma proteins. Only free corticosteroids are biologically active and are absorbed into cells, where they initiate their specific effects. Although all corticosteroids bind reversibly to the plasma proteins, only the binding of cortisol has been extensively studied. More than 90% of plasma cortisol is bound to two plasma proteins, albumin and transcortin. Albumin has a low affinity, but relatively high binding capacity for cortisol. Transcortin, also called corticosteroid-binding globulin, has a high affinity but low total binding capacity for cortisol. Since corticosteroids compete with each other for binding sites on transcortin, most of the cortisol in the plasma is bound to transcortin when corticosteroid concentrations are normal or below normal. Water-soluble cortisol metabolites and aldosterone have lower affinities for transcortin. When the secretion of corticosteroids is increased (e.g., in hyper-

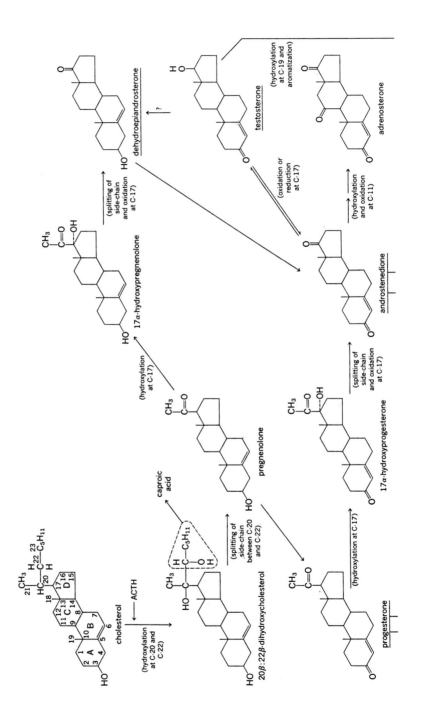

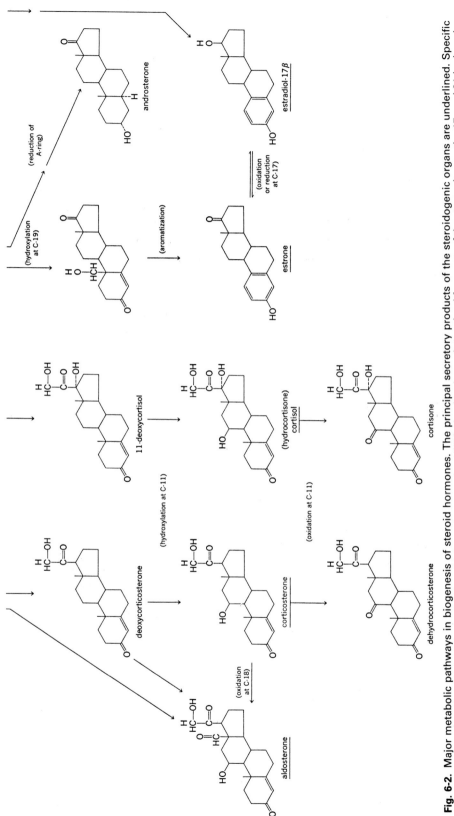

Fig. 6-2. Major metabolic pathways in biogenesis of steroid hormones. The principal secretory products of the steroidogenic organs are underlined. Specific enzymes have been characterized, and mitochondrial or microsomal participation has been determined for many of the steps shown. the 17- and 21-hydroxylations appear to require mitochondria; the 11-hydroxylation, microsomes. Also, various cofactors have been specified for many of the steps. For example, reduced nicotinamide adenine dinucleotide phosphate (NADPH) and molecular O_2 are required for the various hydroxylations and for the side chain splitting (desmolase enzyme activity.) In addition, certain ions are known to be required for the conversion of corticosterone to aldosterone by the zona glomerulosa cells of the adrenal cortex. Most of the products of catabolism of the major steroid hormones are not shown. (Gorbman A., et al.: Comparative Endocrinology, 1983 Courtesy John Wiley and Sons, Inc.)

adrenocorticism), the concentrations of free and albumin-bound steroids increase with little change in the concentration of corticosteroids bound to transcortin. Deficiency in plasma protein may lead to a shortage of transcortin, whereas hyperestrogenism (e.g., pregnancy) causes elevated transcortin levels. These changes in transcortin affect only the concentration of bound but not that of unbound or free corticosteroids.

The half-life of plasma cortisol is less than 2 hours. This is longer than the half-life of catecholamines and peptide hormones. The metabolic degradation of free adrenocortical hormones takes place mainly in the hepatic cells and to a small degree in the kidneys. As the first step, enzymes within hepatic cells reduce the 3-keto group to a 3-hydroxyl group. The next step is conjugation of the 3-hydroxyl group on the molecule to either glucuronide or sulfate. These conjugated molecules are now water-soluble and are excreted in the urine (75%) or the feces (25%).

Molecular Acitivity of Steroids

Considerable progress has been made to understand how steroid hormones act within the cell. There are at least six steps basic to steroid hormone action. These would apply to the corticosteroids as well as to the sex steroids. These steps are also illustrated in Figure 6-3.

1. Entry of the steroid hormones into the target cells. Steroid hormones are lipid-soluble and diffuse through cell membranes to the cytoplasm without depending upon a transport system.

2. Binding to a specific receptor in target cells. Target cells have inactive cytoplasmic receptors with a high affinity for particular steroids which become active sites after binding. The steroid-receptor complex undergoes a time-, temperature-, or calcium-dependent activation that affects the conformational characteristics and possibly the size of the complex.

3. Translocation to the nucleus. The steroid-receptor complex migrates into the nu-

cleus where it attaches to a particular site on the chromosome.

4. Binding of steroid-receptor complex to nuclear acceptor site. Once bound, certain components of the genome are then activated or derepressed so that new mRNA can be formed.

5. Formation of new proteins. Some of the mRNA migrates to cytosolic ribosomes in the cytosol to stimulate the synthesis of hormone-induced proteins (Fig. 6-3). The new protein mediates the hormonal action.

6. Inactivation may occur by metabolism of the steroid. The end compound may be recycled.

Glucocorticoids

Cortisol (hydrocortisone) and corticosterone are the principal glucocorticoids of the adrenal cortex. Cortisol predominates in man, horse, pig, sheep, dog and cat, but corticosterone predominates in the rabbit, mouse, and rat. The ruminant is intermediate, since it secretes sizable amounts of both. Cortisone is secreted in small amounts by adrenal glands of mammals.

The ratio of cortisol to corticosterone in adrenal venous blood of mammals is as follows: bovine, 1:1; sheep, 15–20:1; dogs, 2:1 to 5:1; humans and cats, 5:1 to 10:1; rats and rabbits, 0.05:1. Cortisol is the major secretory product in newborn calves and corticosterone does not appear in calves until 10 days after birth. Adrenal effluent blood of calves receiving ACTH infusion has a plasma cortisol concentration 4- to 5-times more than corticosterone. Cortisol is the major corticosteroid of sheep. The levels of cortisol in animals are summarized in Table 6-2.

Control of Glucocorticoid Secretion

The output of glucocorticoids by the adrenal cortex is minimal in the absence of ACTH stimulation from the adenohypophysis (Fig. 6-4). ACTH stimulates the synthesis of the glucocorticoids, cortisol and corticosterone, and the mineralocorticoids, deoxycorticosterone and aldosterone. However, the secretion of aldosterone is also under non-pituitary con-

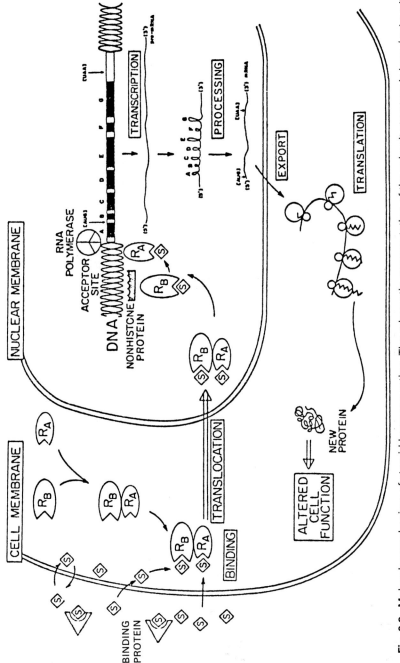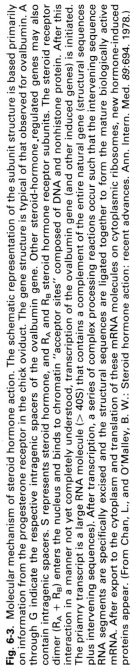

Fig. 6-3. Molecular mechanism of steroid hormone action. The schematic representation of the subunit structure is based primarily on information from the progesterone receptor in the chick oviduct. The gene structure is typical of that observed for ovalbumin. A through G indicate the respective intragenic spacers of the ovalbumin gene. Other steroid-hormone regulated genes may also contain intragenic spacers. S represents steroid hormone, and R_A and R_B steroid hormone receptor subunits. The steroid receptor dimer ($R_A + R_B$) enters the nucleus and binds to chromatin "acceptor sites" composed of DNA and nonhistone protein. After this interaction in a manner not yet completely understood, transcription of the ovalbumin gene (and other induced genes) is initiated. The priamry transcript is a large RNA molecule (> 40S) that contains a complement of the entire natural gene (structural sequences plus intervening sequences). After transcription, a series of complex processing reactions occur such that the intervening sequence RNA segments are specifically excised and the structural sequences are ligated together to form the mature biologically active mRNA. After export to the cytoplasm and translation of these mRNA molecules on cytoplasmic ribosomes, new hormone-induced proteins appear. (From Chan, L., and O'Malley, B. W.: Steroid hormone action: recent advances. Ann. Intern. Med. *89*:694. 1978.)

Table 6-2   Plasma Cortisol and Corticosterone of Domestic Species

Species	Plasma Cortisol (ng/ml)			Method	Reference
	Range	Mean	SD* or SEM[†]		
Dog	6.0–28.5	17.8	1.32[†]	RIA	Chen et al.
	< 3.0–77.5	19.4	3.0*	RIA	Johnston & Mather
	9.4–37.0	23.2	6.9*	RIA	Becker et al.
Cat	< 3.0–82.8	17.0	2.8*	RIA	Johnston & Mather
Sheep					
Nonpregnant		6.0	1*		Linder
Pregnant		7.0	2*		Linder
Goat	8.0–19.0	12.0			Linder
Cattle	0.1–16.1	4.9	0.2*	CPB	Seren
Hereford bulls					
at 21°C	16.4–20.5	18.4	0.9*	Fluorometric	Rhynes & Ewing
at 35°C	10.3–15.8	11.2	0.75*	Fluorometric	Rhynes & Ewing
(corticosterone)					
at 21°C	2.7–3.9	3.0	0.2*	Fluorometric	Rhynes & Ewing
at 35°C	2.2–3.4	2.8	0.15*	Fluorometric	Rhynes & Ewing
Cows					
Suckled		9.4	0.09[†]	CPB	Wagner & Oxenreider
Milked		6.8	0.05[†]	CPB	Wagner & Oxenreider
Nonlactating		4.5	0.04[†]	CPB	Wagner & Oxenreider
Pregnant		26.0	3.0*		Linder
Mare		13.7	4.0[†]	RIA	Bottoms et al.
(corticosterone)		2.2	0.4[†]	RIA	
Swine		8.1	2.9[†]	RIA	Bottoms et al.
(corticosterone)		2.4	0.8[†]	RIA	

* Standard deviation.
[†] Standard error of the mean.

trol, which will be discussed later. ACTH activates cholesterol esterase to stimulate the formation of free cholesterol from cholesterol ester that is bound to low density lipoprotein. The effects of ACTH on steroid synthesis are mediated by the cyclic nucleotides, cAMP and cGMP. High concentrations of ACTH activate adenylate cyclase which converts ATP to cAMP. Protein kinases, activated by the cAMP, in turn activate the enzyme, cholesterol esterase. This activated enzyme acts on cholesterol ester to form free cholesterol. Lower concentrations of ACTH promote calcium-dependent activation of guanylate cyclase to increase the formation of cGMP. The cells contain cGMP-dependent kinases which are required to stimulate the synthesis of a labile protein for steroidogenesis. It is not known whether this labile protein participates in the activation of cholesterol esterase.

In addition to the effects on the synthesis of corticosteroids, ACTH is required for the growth and maintenance of the adrenal gland. The trophic effects of ACTH on the adrenal cortex appear to be mediated by cAMP.

The hypothalamic-adenohypophyseal control of corticosteroid synthesis and the regulation of the release of corticotropin releasing hormone (CRH) and ACTH are illustrated in Figure 6-4, and the interrelationship of these hormones is also discussed in Chapter 2. As depicted in the figure, there are many factors affecting the release of ACTH from the pituitary gland, but the central coordinator is CRH (Fig. 6-4). This hormone is released from the hypothalamus and carried by the portal system to the adenohypophysis, where it stimulates the release of ACTH.

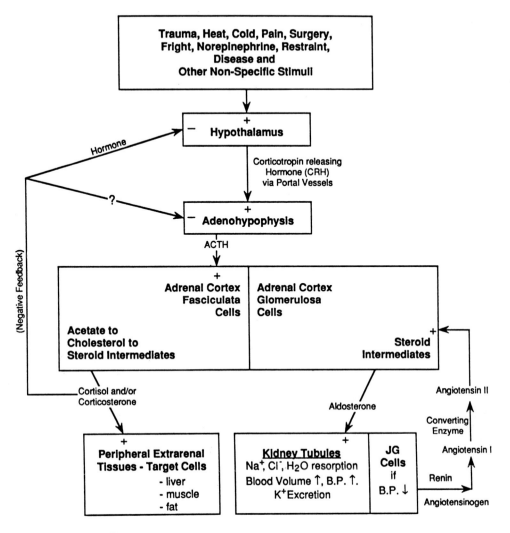

Fig. 6-4. Control of steroid secretion in the adrenal cortex.

Effects of Glucocorticoids

Cortisol affects a wide range of activities in the body, including metabolism of carbohydrates, proteins, and fats and inflammatory processes. Glucocorticoids also reduce the number of certain leukocytes such as lymphocytes and eosinophils in the circulation, decrease growth, and inhibit wound healing. Cortisol and corticosterone have some effects on electrolyte and water metabolism. These varied functions are indicative of many receptors in the cells from many different target tissues.

In addition to the effects of external factors (stressors) and negative feedback control on ACTH output, a third modulator is *diurnal* changes. In pigs and mares glucocorticoid output is highest in the morning (4 to 10 AM), having risen during sleep, and lowest in the afternoon and early evening. A rise in ACTH precedes the glucocorticoid rise by 1 to 2 hours. This is probably reversed in nocturnal species. The cat and dog do not have a morning rise in glucocorticoids.

CARBOHYDRATE METABOLISM. Cortisol increases gluconeogenesis, inhibits peripheral glucose utilization, and increases tissue stores of glycogen, especially in the liver by increasing the production of glycogen synthase. Hyperglycemia could lead to glucosuria but may temporarily alleviate the hypoglycemia in the ketotic dairy cow.

PROTEIN METABOLISM. Cortisol causes catabolism of muscle proteins leading to negative nitrogen balance and an increase in urinary elimination of nitrogn and uric acid. Anabolism of proteins is inhibited by cortisol and growth ceases in young animals.

Cortisol causes the blood level of amino acids to rise due to the increased breakdown of muscle protein, often leading to muscle wasting and weakness. The transport of amino acids across all extrahepatic cell membranes decreases, but hepatic transport increases under the influence of cortisol. This mobilization of amino acids along with (1) conversion of amino acids to glucose (gluconeogenesis), (2) increased formation of plasma and liver protein by the liver, and (3) increased deamination by the liver characterizes the effects of cortisol. Most of these may simply depend on altered membrane permeability to amino acids in the liver.

FAT METABOLISM. The influence of glucocorticoids on fat metabolism is not well understood. The induced gluconeogenesis does favor catabolism of fats, as well as shifting of the body stores of fats, and prolonged hypersecretion often leads to a pendulous abdomen. This mobilization of fat stores causes an increased circulating level of fatty acids, thereby favoring their use for energy. In addition, the glucocorticoids facilitate the effects on adipokinetic hormones such as catecholamines, glucagon, and growth hormone in eliciting lipolysis.

ENDOCRINE SYSTEM. When plasma levels of glucocorticoids are high for several weeks or longer, the excess hormones may suppress the production of ACTH by the anterior pituitary and/or the release of CRH. Atrophy of the adrenal cortex follows. When ACTH is given in excess, the adrenal cortex hypertrophies.

MUSCULOSKELETAL SYSTEM. Hyperadrenocorticism, a condition which develops from adrenal hypersecretion or prolonged therapy with glucocorticoids, may cause muscular weakness resulting from loss of muscle protein associated with an increase in gluconeogenesis. Muscular weakness is also observed in cases of hypoadrenocorticism, but in this case, the muscular weakness is thought to be due to systemic hypotension.

Prolonged administration of high doses of glucocorticoids increases renal excretion of calcium and phosphorus while there is a concomitant decrease in gastrointestinal absorption of these two elements. Losses of calcium and phosphorus induce osteoporosis and lead to bone fractures.

HEMOPOIETIC SYSTEM. Administration of glucocorticoids may cause eosinopenia, monocytopenia, lymphocytopenia, and neutrophilia. Prolonged therapy may cause involution of lymph nodes, thymus, and spleen. A decrease in the number of circulating lymphocytes, monocytes, and eosinophils may result from redistribution of these cells to other body compartments. After the administration of glucocorticoids, the thymus-derived lymphocytes (T cells) decrease proportionately more than the lymphocytes derived from the bone marrow cells (B cells). The neutrophilia, induced by glucocorticoids, is the result of an increase in the number of neutrophils entering the bloodstream from bone marrow and from a diminished rate of removal from the circulation. The overall functional activity of these neutrophils, however, is decreased.

Glucocorticoids tend to increase the number of red blood cells (polycythemia). This effect is attributed to a retardation of erythrophagocytosis.

SUSCEPTIBILITY TO INFECTION, ANTI-INFLAMMATORY AND IMMUNOSUPPRESSIVE EFFECTS. Glucocorticoids suppress protein synthesis of connective tissue in response to injury, whether chemical, thermal, mechanical, anaphylactic, or derived from infections. These steroids only inhibit the early stages of the inflammatory response including: edema, fibrin deposition, capillary dilatation, migration of leukocytes into the inflamed area, and phagocytic activity of leukocytes, but also the later stages of the inflammatory response, such as capillary and fibroblast proliferation, deposition of collagen, and scar formation. Glucocorticoids reduce the movement of neutrophils and monocyte-macrophages toward the inflammatory site, yet do not impair the phagocytic activity of these macrophages or reduce their ability to digest microorganisms.

Glucocorticoids are thought to stabilize the phospholipid components of the cell and organelle membranes, thereby maintaining cellular integrity. The membrane-stabilizing effect of glucocorticoids may be due to the inhibition of phospholipase A_2, an enzyme which increases the releases of arachidonic acid from phosphatidyl-inositol, a membrane phospholipid. Arachidonic acid is the precursor of prostaglandins, leukotrienes and related compounds called autacoids which play important roles in chemotaxis and inflammation. Glucocorticoids also protect cells from lysosomal proteolytic enzymes which may be released from the lysosomes of the injured adjacent cells.

Glucocorticoids inhibit the neutrophilic synthesis of plasminogen activator, an enzyme that converts plasminogen to plasmin (fibrinolysin). Plasmin is thought to facilitate the recruitment and movement of leukocytes into areas of inflammation by hydrolyzing fibrin and other proteins. The ability of glucocorticoids to inhibit the recruitment of leukocytes may be their most important action as anti-inflammatory agents.

The use of glucocorticoids as therapeutic agents is associated with immunosuppression and with a modest fall in antibody titers; however, the immunosuppressive activity of glucocorticoids is usually not detrimental and in fact glucocorticoids are used therapeutically to prevent cell-mediated immune reactions or delayed hypersensitivity (e.g., graft rejection). Lymphocytes, previously sensitized to a particular antigen, bind the antigen in tissues where the inflammatory response is occurring. These activated lymphocytes produce soluble factors called lymphokines that control the cellular response to infection. The macrophage migration inhibitory factor, a lymphokine, causes macrophages to accumulate in the inflammatory area by inhibiting their movement away from the inflammatory site. Therapeutic levels of glucocorticoids usually do not alter the production of migration inhibitory factor by T cells, but the effect of this factor on macrophages is blocked by glucocorticoids, thus the macrophages do not accumulate locally.

CARDIOVASCULAR SYSTEM. Glucocorticoid-deficient animals have a reduced cardiac output, limited cardiac reserve, hypotension, and impaired delivery of oxygen and nutrients to peripheral tissues. Capillary permeability is usually increased, and glucocorticoid-deficient animals are hyporesponsive to the vasopressor effect of catecholamines.

Administration of glucocorticoids, especially in large doses, decreases capillary permeability, increases vasomotor response of the small blood vessels, and increases cardiac output. Synthetic glucocorticoids are used in the treatment of circulatory shock due to endotoxins, hemorrhage, or trauma. In addition, the membrane-stabilizing effect of glucocorticoids may prevent the release of lysosomal enzymes and autacoids, such as histamine and bradykinins. However, the benefit of using massive doses of glucocorticoids as therapeutic agents is still controversial and thus, there are no definite guidelines.

PARTURITION. Depending on the species, glucocorticoids can cause luteolysis and induce uterine contractions. This will be discussed in Chapter 18.

BEHAVIORAL CHANGES. Behavioral changes such as a feeling of well-being and appetite improvement are frequently manifested following glucocorticoid therapy. They occur despite such terminal conditions as cancer. Depressive states associated with other diseases may warrant such therapy provided corticoid therapy per se is not contraindicated. Occasionally the dog or cat may react to corticoid therapy with depression or even viciousness (dog).

OTHER EFFECTS. The glucocorticoids may increase the secretion of pepsin and hydrochloric acid. These hormones also exert an androgenic action which appears in both sexes following prolonged therapy. Hyaluronidase activity may be inhibited. Convulsive thresholds apparently are lowered.

Stress and Disease

A discussion of the endocrinology of the adrenal cortex would be incomplete without mentioning stress and disease. Adrenalectomized animals are limited in their ability to withstand "stresses" such as extremes of muscular activity or temperature, infections, trauma (including surgery), fright, or lack of food and water. The administration of glucocorticoids to adrenalectomized animals enhances the animal's ability to withstand stress. Domestic animals certainly experience stressors of this nature in their day-to-day existence.

Plasma levels of glucocorticoids rise after exposure to several or any of the stresses. These stresses cause an increase in ACTH release, which in turn causes the adrenal cortex to increase the secretion of glucocorticoids. Continued high levels of glucocorticoids by any cause will suppress inflammatory reactions. In some cases, this might be of value, but in others it would not be of value to the animal, since it would permit infections to spread. Dissemination of infection may be offset by the simultaneous administration of antibiotics.

Cattle shipped for long distances are often stressed by extreme temperature changes, fatigue, lack of food and water, and fright. These stresses cause massive release of ACTH which leads to an increase in the plasma concentration of glucocorticoids. As a result, the defense mechanisms of these animals are depressed and, therefore, they are more susceptible to infection.

Mineralocorticoids (Aldosterone)

Aldosterone is a mineralocorticoid synthesized and released from cells in the zona glomerulosa of the adrenal cortex. The affinity of aldosterone for plasma proteins is relatively low; approximately one third of plasma aldosterone is unbound, one-half is loosely associated with albumin, and the remainder is bound to transcortin. The half-life of aldoste-

rone in plasma is approximately 15 minutes.

The action of aldosterone may be described as enhancing Na^+ and water uptake, and K^+ and H^+ excretion. Aldosterone acts on epithelial cells in the collecting tubules of the kidneys, salivary ducts, sweat glands, stomach, and colon to absorb Na^+. The K^+ and H^+ are excreted at the luminal membrane, in exchange for Na^+.

Aldosterone, like all of the other steroid molecules, diffuses passively across cell membranes and binds to a specific receptor-protein in the cytosol. This aldosterone-receptor complex is then translocated to the nucleus where it stimulates mRNA transcription and synthesis, resulting eventually in protein synthesis by the ribosomes in the cytosol. Because of the time required for protein synthesis, the action of aldosterone after uptake by the cells is not evident until 15 to 30 minutes later.

The synthesis and release of aldosterone is regulated by 2 major systems: (1) the renin-angiotensin-aldosterone system, and (2) the hypothalamic-pituitary-adrenal cortex system (Fig. 6-4).

The Renin-Angiotensin-Aldosterone System

Renin, a potent indirect stimulus for the production of aldosterone, is a proteolytic enzyme, which is synthesized and stored in the juxtaglomerular cells surrounding the afferent arterioles of the kidney glomeruli. The concentration of renin in the blood is the major regulator of the renin-angiotensin-aldosterone system. Renin converts angiotensinogen, an α_2 globulin in plasma, to angiotensin I, a decapeptide. Angiotensin I is converted to angiotensin II, an octapeptide, by a "converting enzyme." Angiotensin II, which has a plasma half-life of approximately one minute, interacts with receptors on the cells of the glomerular zone to initiate aldosterone synthesis. Angiotensinases in the bloodstream inactivate angiotensin II.

Angiotensin II interacts with receptors on cells in the glomerular zone to induce aldosterone synthesis. Two sites in the synthetic pathway are acted on by angiotensin II (Fig. 6-2). The first step is to increase the conversion of cholesterol to pregnenolone, a common intermediate in the synthesis of all adrenal steroids. Next, angiotensin II increases the oxidative conversion of corticosterone to aldosterone, the major physiological mineralocorticosteroid.

Four interdependent factors regulate the release of renin: the juxtaglomerular cells, the macula densa cells of the distal tubules, the sympathetic nervous system via β_1-adrenergic receptors, and plasma K^+.

The juxtaglomerular cells function as miniature pressure transducers which are responsive to pressure changes in the afferent arterioles of the glomeruli. Any slight decrease in pressure will elicit an increase in renin release. As the blood pressure increases, renin release is inhibited.

The distal tubules in the kidneys are in close apposition to the afferent arterioles. The epithelial cells lining the tubules in this area are called macula densa cells, and together with the juxtaglomerular cells are known as the juxtaglomerular apparatus. The macula densa cells, acting as chemoreceptors, monitor the Na^+ concentration in the tubules. An increase in tubular concentration of Na^+ causes the release of renin from the juxtaglomerular apparatus.

The sympathetic nervous system also stimulates the juxtaglomerular cells to release renin via β_1-adrenergic receptors. In addition, high plasma K^+ concentrations increase renin release while low plasma K^+ concentrations have no effect on renin release.

The Hypothalamic-Pituitary-Adrenal Cortex System

ACTH increases aldosterone synthesis as well as all corticosteroid hormones. High levels of ACTH are necessary to induce the synthesis of aldosterone. The effect is relatively transient since aldosterone synthesis decreases in 1-2 days even when ACTH levels are still high. The synthesis of deoxycorticosterone, however, continues as long as ACTH persists. Deoxycorticosterone is not an important mineralocorticoid in normal animals, because aldosterone is 30 times more potent than deoxycorticosterone with regard to mineralocorticoid activity (Table 6-1).

Adrenal Sex Steroids

The zona reticularis of the adrenal cortex has been recognized as a source of sex steroids in man and possibly other species. Tumors of the adrenal are known to cause masculinization or feminization in any species. Furthermore, estrogens, androgens, and progesterone are present in the extracts of normal adrenal glands. Castrated animals produce some sex steroids. With our current understanding of adrenal steroidogenesis (see Fig. 7-6), overproduction of a sex steroid could occur if the direction was shifted or if a block or defect occurred in the enzyme involved in the steroidogenic scheme.

Although estrogens and progesterone have been isolated from adrenal vein blood of several domestic animals, the full physiological significance of these steroids in normal animals has not been clarified.

Inhibitors of Corticosteroid Secretion

Three pharmacologic agents, mitotane (O, P'-DDD), metyrapone, and aminoglutethimide are inhibitors of corticosteroid secretion and thus, are potentially useful in alleviating hyperadrenocorticism and tumors of the adrenal cortex.

Mitotane, a derivative of the insecticide DDT, selectively destroys the cells of the zonae reticularis and fasciculata but the mechanism of this cytotoxic action is unknown. This compound is used in both humans and animals. Metyrapone reduces the production of cortisol and corticosterone by inhibiting the 11β-hydroxylation reaction; therefore, biosynthesis is terminated at 11-deoxycortisol and deoxycorticosterone (Fig. 6-2). Since these compounds have essentially no inhibitory influence on ACTH secretion, the treated animals have an increased release of ACTH and renal secretion of 11-deoxycorticosteroids. Metyrapone has been used in human medicine to test the capacity of the pituitary gland to respond to a decreased concentration of plasma cortisol. The use of this drug in the treatment of hyperadrenocorticism is controversial, since the excessive release of ACTH induced by the administration of metyrapone may overcome the suppressive effect of the drug on cortisol secretion.

Aminoglutethimide inhibits the conversion of cholesterol to dihydroxycholesterol (Fig. 6-2), thus blocking the production of all corticosteroids. This potent drug has been used successfully in the treatment of Cushing's syndrome in humans.

Hyperfunction of the Adrenal Cortex

Hyperadrenocorticism (Cushing's syndrome, cortisol excess) results in many clinical and pathological manifestations of an elevated circulating level of the glucocorticoids. Overproduction of the mineralocorticoids has not been documented in domestic animals. Hyperadrenocorticism is one of the most common endocrine diseases of the dog. It occasionally occurs in the horse but is rare in other domestic species including cats. The classification and discussion will be concerned mainly with our knowledge of the disease in the dog.

Hyperadrenocorticism in the dog may be classified as: (1) *secondary adrenocorticism* (bilateral adrenal hyperplasia) due to adenoma of the pituitary gland with oversecretion of ACTH (80% of natural cases); (2) *primary adrenocorticism* due to adrenal cortex neoplasm (10 to 20% of natural cases); (3) *pharmacological* elevation of glucocorticoid levels by excessive and prolonged administration of glucocorticoids.

The overadministration of glucocorticoids in the dog as a means of alleviating chronic conditions such as allergies and skin conditions is increasing. Iatrogenic canine Cushing's syndrome, resulting from prolonged glucocorticoid therapy, can lead to *hypoadrenocorticism* upon discontinuation of therapy, since the adrenal cortex has been rendered dysfunctional by the therapy. Secondary (pituitary-dependent) hyperadrenocorticism is due to ACTH but not CRH.

Hyperadrenocorticism is a slowly developing, insidious disease affecting many organ systems. A complete discussion of the diagnosis, management, and therapy of the condition may be obtained in textbooks on veterinary clinical medicine.

Clinical Signs

Hyperadrenocorticism from any cause results in elevation of urine and plasma concentrations of cortisol and corticosterone. Because there is some overlap with normal values, other clinical signs need to be considered in a diagnosis. The clinical signs of hyperadrenocorticism are mainly manifestations of excess glucocorticoids.

The clinical signs vary but usually include the following:

Polydipsia and polyuria
Polyphagia
Pendulous abdomen
Bilateral alopecia
Hyperpigmentation of skin
Skin atrophy; thinness with visible vessels
Hepatomegaly (fatty liver)
Muscle weakness and atrophy
Lethargy
Persistent anestrus or atrophied testes
Calcinosis cutis
Heat intolerance
Hypertrophy of the clitoris
CNS dysfunction and convulsions

Treatment

The spontaneous hyperadrenocorticism may be controlled pharmacologically, surgically or by a combination of these two approaches. In the absence of treatment, death is usually expected within a year from the time of diagnosis. The most economical and safest form of treatment for pituitary dependent hyperadrenocorticism is a pharmacologic approach using the drug, mitotane. For radiographically demonstrable adrenocortical carcinomas, surgical ablation followed by treatment with mitotane to control metastasis, is preferred. Mitotane is also recommended for the treatment of primary hyperadrenocorticism with no visible tumors by abdominal radiography.

Hypofunction of the Adrenal Cortex

Hypoadrenocorticism is recognized and diagnosed primarily in the middle-aged dogs (3–

5 years old), less often in the cat, and infrequently in other domestic species. The incidence is 3–4 times greater in female dogs than in male dogs. Adrenocortical insufficiency is insidious and progressive, often reaching acute manifestations. This disease is not only due to a shortage of the glucocorticoids, but usually includes a deficiency of the *mineralocorticoids*. Since the mineralocorticoids are life-sustaining, the management of this disease is important.

Hypoadrenocorticism in the dog may be classified as either primary or secondary hypoadrenocorticism.

Primary hypoadrenocorticism

1. *Bilateral idiopathic adrenocortical atrophy*. Deficiency of all glucocorticoids, mineralocorticoids, and adrenal sex steroids. Etiology unknown but often relegated to autoimmune reaction. At least 75% of cases belong to this type.
2. *Destruction of both adrenal cortices* by infectious diseases, infarctions, or tumors.
3. *Extensive bilateral adrenal cortical hemorrhage.*
4. *Pharmacologic inhibition of the adrenal cortex* by excessive administration of synthetic glucocorticoids.

Secondary hypoadrenocorticism

1. *ACTH deficiency* leading only to glucocorticoid deficiency. Rare.

Adrenal cortical insufficiency (Addison's disease) may be chronic with vomiting, muscular weakness, anorexia, depression, diarrhea, and dehydration which may eventually lead to an addisonian crisis. In the acute condition or addisonian crisis, cardiovascular weakness may lead to circulatory collapse, severe depression, unconsciousness, coma, and death. Therapy should be initiated immediately before laboratory analyses are completed.

Cows in late pregnancy may suffer from toxemia possibly due to secondary adrenal cortex hypofunction. The administration of ACTH and/or glucocorticoids will alleviate clinical signs.

Although some of the signs of glucocorticoid deficiency exist, it is the mineralocorticoid deficiency that must be corrected. First, attention must be directed toward the correction of the Na^+ and K^+ imbalance. Kidney dysfunction causes elevated levels of blood urea, hyperkalemia, and hyponatremia. A decrease in serum Na^+ and, to a lesser extent, the slight elevation of K^+ aid in the diagnosis. The ECG changes, spiking of the T wave and flattening of the P wave, are diagnostic. The determination of the plasma concentration of cortisol is one of the best diagnostic tests.

In contrast to canine hyperadrenocorticism, where only one hormone (cortisol) is in excess, all three groups are deficient in hypoadrenocorticism.

Treatment of the acute addisonian crisis must include the correcton of the severe dehydration, mineral imbalance, and circulatory collapse. This can be accomplished when the analysis of blood electrolytes can be accompanied by intravenous fluid therapy to reverse the condition. During the addisonian crisis, therapy must include intravenous injections of glucocorticoids plus intramuscular or subcutaneous injections of deoxycorticosterone acetate (DOCA). Thereafter, maintenance doses of DOCA and glucocorticoid therapy can be given.

Therapy must be continued to sustain life. Fortunately, the use of long-acting DOCA or implants along with the oral administration of a glucocorticoid is an effective therapy. Considerable care must be expended to attain the proper therapeutic dose. A high Na^+ diet is beneficial. Some clinicians prefer oral fludrocortisone, a synthetic corticosteroid with potent glucocorticoid and mineralocorticoid activity.

Therapeutic Uses of Glucocorticoids

Glucocorticoids, particularly synthetic corticoids, are frequently used in veterinary medicine. There are five basic indications for their use: (1) replacement in the hypoadrenocortical state, (2) anti-inflammation, (3) immunosuppression, (4) treatment of shock, and (5) reduction of cerebrospinal edema. A veterinary clinical textbook should be consulted for detailed information on the uses of glucocorticoids.

When prescribing glucocorticoids, one

should remember that the administration of glucocorticoids, especially for prolonged periods of time, will inhibit ACTH production by the pituitary gland, which in turn, may cause atrophy and further potentiate hyposecretion of the adrenal cortex. This condition is called iatrogenic secondary hypoadrenocorticism.

ADRENAL MEDULLA

Biosynthesis of Catecholamines

The catecholamines, including dopamine, norepinephrine and epinephrine, are a group of compounds which contain the catechol nucleus, a benzene molecule with adjacent hydroxyl groups and an amine group. Catecholamines are synthesized from the amino acids phenylalanine or tyrosine in the chromaffin cells of the adrenal medulla and in adrenergic and dopaminergic neurons (Fig. 6-5). Phenylalanine is converted to tyrosine by phenylalanine hydroxylase, an enzyme widely distributed in the body. Tyrosine is absorbed directly from the blood by the chromaffin cells of the adrenal medulla and hydrolyzed to dopa, the rate limiting step in the synthetic pathway. Dopa is then decarboxylated to form dopamine in the cytosol of the cells. After being taken up into the granules of chromaffin cells, dopamine is converted to norepinephrine by dopamine β-hydroxylase. The granules in some adrenomedullary cells contain phenylethanolamine-N-methyl transferase which catalyzes the conversion of norepinephrine to epinephrine (Fig. 6-5). Glucocorticoids in the blood bathing the medullary cells may induce the synthesis of phenylethanolamine-N-methyl transferase. Therefore, the glucocorticoids, through their action on this enzyme, may enhance the synthesis of epinephrine. The catecholamines are stored inside granules in the adrenomedullary cells and in adrenergic neurons throughout the body. The medullary granules also contain ATP, calcium, and chromagranin, a granule protein.

Release and Fate of Catecholamines

Acetylcholine, which is released from the preganglionic fibers, stimulates chromaffin cells in the adrenal medulla and sympathetic nerve endings causing depolarization of the plasma membrane and a concomitant influx of Ca^{++} into the cells. Calcium and energy in the form of ATP are required for the release of catecholamines from the chromaffin cells. The membranes of the catecholamine-containing granules fuse with the plasma membranes of the chromaffin cells and the contents of the granules are expelled from the cell by exocytosis.

The ratio of norepinephrine to epinephrine released from the adrenal medulla varies among species. Equal amounts of epinephrine and norepinephrine are released in the cat. Dogs and horses release mainly epinephrine, while other domestic species release mainly norepinephrine. The sympathetic emergency discharge of catecholamines may occur under a variety of conditions. Stimuli such as cold, apnea, and hypoglycemia cause the release of massive amounts of norepinephrine and epinephrine and elicit strong sympathetic responses. Behavioral changes also increase the selective release of catecholamines from the adrenal medulla. Conditioned behavioral responses are followed by the release of more norepinephrine than epinephrine, whereas unconditioned responses or unexpected changes cause the release of more epinephrine than norepinephrine.

The half-life of catecholamines in blood is approximately 2 minutes in most species. The metabolic transformation of circulating catecholamines by the enzyme catechol-O-methyl transferase takes place in the cytosol of cells in the brain, liver, and kidneys. Monoamine oxidase, a mitochondrial enzyme in adrenomedullary cells and adrenergic neurons, has a major role in the regulation of catecholamines in these cells. These transformed catecholamines, which are biologically inactive, are water soluble and are excreted in the urine.

The nerve endings of the sympathetic nervous system have an amine transport system

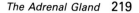

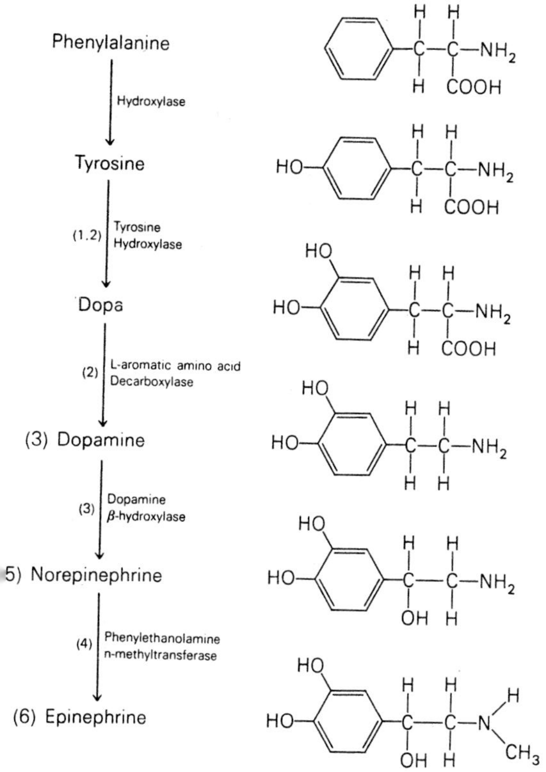

Phenylalanine

↓ Hydroxylase

Tyrosine

(1,2) Tyrosine Hydroxylase

↓

Dopa

(2) L-aromatic amino acid Decarboxylase

(3) Dopamine

(3) Dopamine β-hydroxylase

5) Norepinephrine

(4) Phenylethanolamine n-methyltransferase

↓

(6) Epinephrine

Fig. 6-5. Structure and biosynthesis of epinephrine and norepinephrine: (1) = the rate-limiting step; (2) = occurs within axoplasm; (3) = occurs within amine storage granule; (4) = occurs primarily within cytoplasm of adrenal medullary chromaffin cells; (5) = stored primarily within amine storage granule of adrenergic neurons (6) = stored within amine storage granule of chromaffin cells. (From Adams, H. R.: *In* Veterinary Pharmacology and Therapeutics, 4th ed. Ames, The Iowa State University Press, 1977.)

which actively takes up norepinephrine from the extracellular fluid. Norepinephrine is incorporated into the storage granules and recycled. Approximately 50% of norepinephrine in the extracellular space is removed by this uptake mechanism. Cytosolic enzymes, such as monoamine oxidase, transform any catecholamines which are not in the granules.

Classification of Catecholamine Receptors

The concept of different receptors was proposed in an effort to explain the many inconsistencies and contradictions in the action of catecholamines.

Adrenergic Receptors

According to the result of pharmacologic studies there are two types of adrenergic receptors — α and β. Alpha-receptors generally mediate the stimulatory effects of epinephrine and norepinephrine on smooth muscle, while β-receptors generally mediate the inhibitory effects of these catecholamines on smooth muscle, except for cardiac muscle where β-receptors mediate an increase in force and rate of myocardial contraction. Adrenergic receptors also mediate the effects of epinephrine and norepinephrine on hormone release. In this respect, α-receptors generally mediate the inhibitory effects and β-receptors generally mediate stimulatory effects. A number of agonists (activators) and antagonists (blockers) for α and β-receptors are listed in Table 6-3.

According to the current theory, the α- and β-receptors can be further classified into α_1, α_2, β_1, and β_2 (Table 6-3). As illustrated in Figure 6-6, α_1-receptors are located at post-

Table 6-3 Representative Agonists and Antagonists for Adrenergic and Dopamine Receptors

α-Adrenergic Agonists
1. $\alpha_1 + \alpha_2$: norepinephrine, epinephrine
2. α_1: phenylephrine, methoxamine
3. α_2: clonidine, xylazine

α-Adrenergic Antagonists
1. $\alpha_1 + \alpha_2$: phentolamine, tolazoline
2. α_1: phenoxybenzamine, prazosin
3. α_2: yohimbine, idazoxan

β-Adrenergic Agonists
1. $\beta_1 + \beta_2$: isoproterenol, epinephrine
2. β_1: norepinephrine, dopamine, dobutamine
3. β_2: metaproterenol, albuterol

β-Adrenergic Antagonists
1. $\beta_1 + \beta_2$: propranolol, nadolol
2. β_1: metoprolol, atenolol
3. β_2: butoxamine, ICI 118551

Dopamine Agonists
1. $D_1 + D_2$: dopamine
2. D_1: SK&F 38393
3. D_2: apomorphine, LY 141865

Dopamine Antagonists
1. $D_1 + D_2$: butaclamol
2. D_1: SCH 23390
3. D_2: haloperidol, domperidone

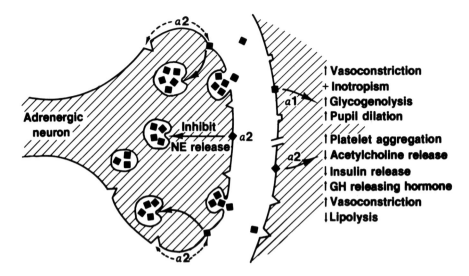

Fig. 6-6. Schematic representation of the synapse of a sympathetic (adrenergic) nerve ending showing the anatomical location of presynaptic and postsynaptic α-receptors and some of the effects mediated by them.

synaptic sites, and mediate effects such as vasoconstriction, positive inotropic responses, glycogenolysis, and pupil dilation, which is due to contraction of the dilator muscle of the iris. There are two kinds of α_2-receptors, presynaptic and postsynaptic. Activation of presynaptic α_2-receptors decreases the release of norepinephrine from the sympathetic nerve endings. The presynaptic α-receptors serve a feedback, autoregulatory role by participating in the inhibition of norepinephrine release, when the concentration of norepinephrine in the synaptic cleft is high. Activation of the postsynaptic α_2-receptors increases vasoconstriction and the release of growth hormone releasing hormone, but decreases the release of a number of neurotransmitters (e.g., acetylcholine) and hormones (e.g., insulin and vasopressin). Activation of these receptors also decreases lipolysis and increases platelet aggregation in several species.

With regard to the subtypes of β-receptors, β_1-receptors are located at postsynaptic sites, and mediate effects such as cardiac activation, intestinal relaxation, and lipolysis. The β_2-receptors are located both presynaptically and postsynaptically. The activation of presynaptic β_2-receptors increases norepinephrine re-

lease, while activation of postsynaptic β_2-receptors increases uterine relaxation, bronchodilation, and glycogenolysis. In the regulation of norepinephrine release, the presynaptic α_2-receptors predominate over the presynaptic β_2-receptors.

Specific agonists and antagonists for adrenergic receptors are listed in Table 6-3.

Dopamine Receptors

Dopamine receptors mediate the actions of dopamine on vascular smooth muscle, endocrine glands, and on the central and peripheral nervous systems. Based on their interaction with adenylate cyclase, dopamine receptors can be classified into two classes, D_1 and D_2. Stimulation of D_1-receptors activates adenylate cyclase to increase cAMP formation, while stimulation of D_2-receptors inhibits adenylate cyclase. In general, vasodilation and release of parathyroid hormone have been clearly associated with activation of D_1-receptors, whereas inhibition of the release of norepinephrine from the sympathetic nerve endings, inhibition of the secretion of aldosterone, prolactin, and renin, and inhibition of emesis appear to result from activation of D_2-receptors. In addition, activation of both types of receptors seems to be necessary for normal motor behavior.

Specific agonists and antagonists for dopamine receptors are listed in Table 6-3.

Regulation of Adrenergic Receptors

Adrenergic receptors are dynamic molecules while under constant changes. These changes include alterations in the number of receptors, changes in the receptor affinity for catecholamines, and variations in the physiologic response of the target tissue. These changes are classified as either homologous or heterologous regulation.

Homologous regulation of adrenergic receptors refers to changes in the number of and affinity for the adrenergic receptors by the corresponding agonist. Prolonged exposure of adrenergic receptors to agonists (Table 6-3) causes a decrease in the number of receptors and is referred to as "down regulation." The mechanism for this phenomenon is unknown. Conversely, a decrease in the concentration of adrenergic agonists will result in an increase in the number of receptors and this is called "up regulation." The physiologic response of target tissues changes as the number of receptors changes; a decrease in receptor numbers is reflected by a diminution of the response, while an increase in receptor numbers magnifies the response of the target tissue.

The affinity of the agonist for the receptor is another factor affecting the regulation of the adrenergic receptor. Receptors which regulate adenylate cyclase, such as α_2- and β-receptors, have a decreased affinity for adrenergic agonists during prolonged exposure to the agonist.

Adrenergic receptors may also be regulated by substances other than adrenergic agonists. This regulation is called heterologous regulation. For example, thyroid hormones increase the number of β_1-adrenergic receptors in the myocardium, therefore, they enhance the stimulatory effect of catecholamines on the heart. The exact molecular interactions involved in these receptor alterations are unknown.

Physiologic and Pharmacologic Effects of Catecholamines

The catecholamines in general have profound effects on metabolism and smooth muscles. The important actions of norepinephrine and epinephrine are summarized in Table 6-4.

Cardiovascular System

Catecholamines increase the force and rate of myocardial contraction. Force of contraction is increased by activation of β_1- and α_1-receptors, while heart rate is increased by activation of β_1-receptors. Norepinephrine increases vasoconstriction by activation of α_1- and α_2-receptors.

Blood vessels in the various tissues of the body respond to epinephrine differently (see Table 6-4). Small doses of epinephrine may dilate blood vessels in certain tissues, such as skeletal muscles and liver by activating β_2-receptors, while higher concentrations of epinephrine constrict blood vessels by activating α_1- and α_2-receptors. However, epinephrine, regardless of dose, causes consistent vasoconstriction in the renal and mesenteric arteries, indicating that α-receptors predominate over β_2-receptors in these arteries.

Respiratory System

Epinephrine initially causes a brief period of apnea when given intravenously to animals. The apnea is probably due to a reflex inhibition of the respiratory center in the medulla oblongata by the baroreceptor mechanism (because of the pressor effect of epinephrine) and in part due to a direct inhibition of the respiratory center.

Epinephrine can increase respiration by peripheral actions, particularly the relaxation of bronchial muscles. Bronchodilation is mediated by β_2-adrenergic receptors. Epinephrine and norepinephrine increase the contraction of the pulmonary blood vessels to relieve congestion within the bronchioles. This effect is mediated by α-receptors.

Smooth Muscles

Epinephrine and norepinephrine are largely stimulatory to smooth muscle of the vascu-

Table 6-4   Responses of Effector Organs to Norepinephrine and Epinephrine

Effector Organs	Type of Adrenergic Receptor[1]	Responses[2]
Eye		
Radial muscle, iris	α_1	Contraction (mydriasis) ++
Ciliary muscle	β	Relaxation for far vision +
Heart		
S-A node	β_1	Increase in heart rate ++
Atria	β_1	Increase in contractility and conduction velocity ++
A-V node	β_1	Increase in automaticity and conduction velocity +
His-Purkinje system	β_1	Increase in automaticity and conduction velocity +++
Ventricles	β_1	Increase in contractility, conduction velocity, automaticity, and rate of idioventricular pacemakers +++
Arterioles		
Coronary	$\alpha; \beta_2$	Constriction +; dilatation[3] ++
Skin and mucosa	α	Constriction +++
Skeletal muscle	$\alpha; \beta_2$	Constriction ++; dilatation[3,4]
Cerebral	α	Constriction (slight)
Pulmonary	$\alpha; \beta_2$	Constriction +; dilatation[3]
Abdominal viscera	$\alpha; \beta_2$	Constriction +++; dilatation[4] +
Renal	$\alpha_1; \beta_2$	Constriction +++; dilatation[4] +
Veins (Systemic)	$\alpha_1; \beta_2$	Constriction ++; dilatation ++
Lung		
Tracheal and bronchial muscle	β_2	Relaxation +
Bronchial glands	$\alpha_1; \beta_2$	Decreased secretion; increased secretion
Stomach		
Motility and tone	$\alpha_2; \beta_2$	Decrease (usually)[5] +
Sphincters	α	Contraction (usually) +
Secretion	$\alpha_2; \beta$	Inhibition
Intestine		
Motility	$\alpha_1; \beta_1$	Decrease[5] +
Sphincters	α	Contraction (usually) +
Secretion	α_2	Inhibition
Gallbladder and Ducts	β_2	Relaxation +
Kidney	β_1	Renin secretion ++
Urinary Bladder		
Detrusor	β	Relaxation (usually) +
Trigone and sphincter	β	Contraction ++
Ureter		
Motility and tone	α	Increase
Uterus	$\alpha; \beta_2$	Pregnant: contraction; relaxation (β_2)[7] Nonpregnant: relaxation (β_2)[7]
Sex Organs, Male	α	Ejaculation +++
Skin		
Pilomotor muscles	α	Contraction ++
Sweat glands	α	Localized secretion[6] +
Spleen Capsule	$\alpha; \beta_2$	Contraction +++; relaxation +
Skeletal Muscle	β_2	Increased contractility; glycogenolysis; K^+ uptake
Liver	$\alpha_1; \beta_2$	Glycogenolysis and gluconeogenesis[7] +++

Table 6-4   Cont.

Effector Organs	Type of Adrenergic Receptor[1]	Responses[2]
Pancreas		
Acini	α	Decreased secretion +
Islets (β cells)	α_2	Decreased release +++
	β_2	Increased release +
Fat Cells	β_1	Lipolysis[7] +++
	α_2	Antilipolysis +
Salivary Glands	α_1	Potassium and water secretion +
	β	Amylase secretion +
Pineal Gland	β	Melatonin synthesis
Posterior Pituitary	β_1	Incrased antidiuretic hormone release +
	α_2	Decreased antidiuretic hormone release +

[1] Where a designation of subtype is not provided, the nature of the subtype has not been determined unequivocally.
[2] Responses are designated as weak + to strong +++ to provide an approximate indication of the degree of adrenergic activity in the control of the various organs and functions listed.
[3] Dilatation predominates *in situ* due to metabolic autoregulatory phenomena.
[4] Over the range of concentration of physiologically released, circulating epinephrine, β-receptor response (vasodilatation) predominates in blood vessels of skeletal muscle and liver; α-receptor response (vasoconstriction) in blood vessels of other abdominal viscera. The renal and mesenteric vessels also contain specific dopaminergic receptors, activation of these receptors causes dilatation.
[5] It has been proposed that adrenergic fibers terminate at the inhibitory β-receptors on smooth muscle fibers, and at the inhibitory α_2-receptors on parasympathetic cholinergic (excitatory) ganglion cells of Auerbach's plexus.
[6] Paws and some other sites ("adrenergic sweating").
[7] There is significant variation among species in the type of receptor that mediates certain metabolic responses.
(Modified from Goodman and Gilman: The Pharmacological Basis of Therapeutics 7th ed., 1985).

lar system and inhibitory to the non-sphincter smooth muscle of the visceral system. These effects are summarized in Table 6-4. The stimulatory effects are usually mediated by α-receptors, whereas the inhibitory effects are usually mediated by β-receptors.

The responses of uterine smooth muscles to catecholamines vary with the dose given, species, phase of the sexual cycle, and stage of gestation. In general, stimulation of β-receptors causes relaxation while stimulation of α-receptors causes uterine smooth muscle to contract.

Catecholamines inhibit gastrointestinal smooth muscle via two mechanisms: (1) a direct inhibition of smooth muscle, which is mediated by β_1-receptors, and (2) an inhibition of acetylcholine release in Auerbach's (myenteric) plexus which is mediated by the α_2- receptors in the preganglionic parasympathetic fibers (Fig. 6-7).

Norepinephrine stimulates erection of the hair, which is part of the "fight or flight" response of most species. This effect is mediated by α-receptors.

Metabolism

Glycogenolysis in the liver and muscle is stimulated by norepinephrine and epinephrine. The action they induce is mediated by β_2-receptors and to a lesser degree by α_1-receptors (Table 6-3). β_2-Adrenergic receptors are activated by epinephrine, which leads to an increase in intracellular cAMP. Cyclic AMP stimulates protein kinases to activate phosphorylase. Activated phosphorylase degrades glycogen to glucose-6-phosphate. The stimulation of α_1-adrenergic receptors by epi-

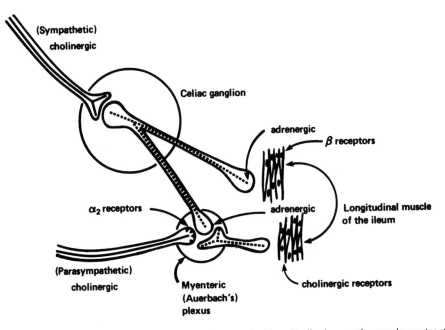

Fig. 6-7. Schematic representation of the autonomic control of longitudinal smooth muscle contraction in the ileum. Acetylcholine released from the preganglionic fibers stimulates the release of acetylcholine and norepinephrine in the ganglionic fibers of the parasympathetic and sympathetic nervous systems, respectively. Acetylcholine released from the postganglionic fibers increases contraction of longitudinal smooth muscle. Norepinephrine inhibits longitudinal smooth muscle via two mechanisms: (1) a direct inhibition of the muscle layer that is mediated by β-receptors, and (2) an inhibition of acetylcholine release from Auerbach's plexus that is mediated by α_2-adrenergic receptors in the preganglionic parasympathetic fibers.

nephrine and norepinephrine in the liver increases cytosolic Ca^{++}, by mobilizing this ion from the intracellular storage sites. This α_1-effect, for instance, increases glycogenolysis in the canine liver.

Norepinephrine and epinephrine also affect insulin and glucagon release. Activation of β_2-adrenergic receptors of the pancreatic islets increases the release of insulin and glucagon, while activation of α_2-adrenergic receptors decreases insulin release (see Chapter 5).

The effect of epinephrine and norepinephrine on the mobilization of free fatty acids from adipose tissue is mediated by β_1-receptors. In the presence of β_1-adrenergic blockers, catecholamines decrease lipolysis, which is mediated by α_2-receptors.

Catecholamines potentiate the stimulatory effect of thyroid hormones on the metabolic rate of animals. In addition, the concentration of plasma K^+ is regulated, to a degree, by the

catecholamines. Epinephrine induces a transient hyperkalemia, a β_2-adrenergic effect, mainly due to release of K^+ from the liver.

Central Nervous System

Both epinephrine and norepinephrine are found throughout the CNS. Their actions range from depression to excitation. Their mechanisms of action within the CNS are not completely understood, but the current concept is that α_1-receptors mediate CNS excitation, while α_2-receptors mediate CNS depression.

Mechanism of Action

Although the mechanism of action of catecholamines is not fully understood, certain cellular events have been identified. Activation of α_1- and α_2-receptors leads to an increase in the concentration of cytosolic Ca^{++}. However, the sources of Ca^{++} appear to be different; activation of α_1-receptors increases the release of Ca^{++} from intracellular storage sites while activation of α_2-receptors increases the influx of Ca^{++} from the extracellular fluid. In addition, α_2-adrenergic activity is associated with the inhibition of adenylate cyclase in some cells, such as adipocytes, platelets, and adrenergic nerve endings. An increase in adenylate cyclase activity is associated with activation of both β_1- and β_2-receptors. Furthermore, an increase in adenylate cyclase activity is associated with activation of D_1-receptors, while a decrease in adenylate cyclase activity is associated with activation of D_2-receptors.

Hyperfunction of the Adrenal Medulla (Pheochromocytomas)

Pheochromocytomas, which in Greek means "dusky-colored tumors," are red-brown in color and are functional neuroendocrine tumors that arise from chromaffin cells of the adrenal medulla and in other parts of the body. The occurrence of these tumors has been reported only for some of the domestic species. They occur in 0.5% of the canine population. Pheochromocytomas occasionally occur in horses, but have not been described in cats. Most pheochromocytomas are thought to be benign, but these tumors can secrete large quantities of catecholamines. However, the clinical signs of hypersecretion of catecholamines are usually vague. The diagnosis of a pheochromocytoma in animals is difficult, because the measurements of arterial blood pressure and catecholamine metabolites in the urine, which are essential for the diagnosis of these tumors, are rarely done in veterinary medicine. In fact, accurate diagnosis of a pheochromocytoma is usually only made during the post-mortem examination. Pheochromocytomas may also produce peptide hormones, such as ACTH and calcitonin. If a pheochromocytoma is diagnosed, surgical excision is the only satisfactory treatment. Beta-adrenergic blockers such as

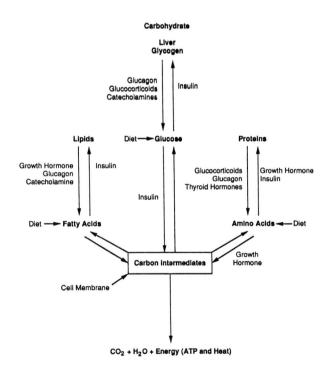

Fig. 6-8. Schematic of the hormonal regulation of carbohydrate, lipid and protein metabolism.

propranolol can be administered before and/ or during surgery to control the catechol-amine-induced tachyrhythmias.

HORMONAL REGULATION OF ENERGY METABOLISM

This section is included in this chapter as an attempt to provide a simplified overview of the complex relationship between hormones and intermediary metabolism. Metabolic ho-meostasis in animals is mainly regulated by the following six hormones: catecholamines, glu-cagon, insulin, glucocorticoids, growth hor-mone, and thyroid hormones (T_3 and T_4). The anabolic and catabolic effects of these hormones on carbohydrate, fat and protein metabolism will be discussed with respect to the metabolism of the liver, skeletal muscle, adipose and nervous tissues. A variety of dif-ferent conditions such as age, feeding or fast-ing, exercise, cold ambient temperatures, and pregnancy impose different demands on the nutritional and metabolic requirements of ani-mals. This synopsis will focus only on the general concepts of the endocrine regulation of energy metabolism (Fig. 6-8).

Fats make up approximately 80% of stored energy in the body. Protein in muscle tissue contributes approximately 20% while glyco-gen and glucose make up approximately 0.5% of the stored energy. Fat is the most efficient storage from of energy. Each gram of fat will generate 9.6 kcal as compared with 4.1 kcal of energy for a gram of either carbohydrate or protein. When the daily energy turnover of an animal is considered, carbohydrates, in the form of glucose, supply approximately one half of the required energy.

The main purpose of hormones in the regu-lation of metabolism is to bridge the gap be-tween the digestive and interdigestive periods to insure a constant supply of energy at all times and in every condition.

Carbohydrate Metabolism

The pancreatic hormones, insulin and glu-cagon, are the most important regulators of blood glucose (see Chapter 5). Insulin lowers blood glucose and inhibits glycogenolysis, while glucagon raises blood glucose and stim-ulates hepatic glycogenolysis. In addition, catecholamines stimulate glycogenolysis and thus, by increasing the plasma levels of glu-cose, make energy available to the cells. These hormones bring about rapid changes in the plasma levels of glucose and in this regard, their participation may be summarized by classifying insulin as an anabolic hormone and glucagon and catecholamines as catabolic hormones.

Glucocorticoids and thyroid hormones are catabolic in that they increase glycogenolysis and hyperglycemia, while growth hormone slows glucose entry into cells. The action of these hormones is slow when compared to glu-cagon and the catecholamines.

Fat Metabolism

Insulin stimulates lipogenesis while glu-cagon, growth hormone and catecholamines stimulate lipolysis in adipose tissue. Gluco-corticoids inhibit lipogenesis. In general, as glycogenolysis increases, lipolysis increases. When glucose concentrations are inadequate or low, ketone bodies from faulty fat metab-olism increase in the bloodstream and pro-duce metabolic acidosis.

Protein Metabolism

The endocrine effect on protein synthesis may be summarized by stating that insulin stimulates protein synthesis while inhibiting protein breakdown and gluconeogenesis. Growth hormone stimulates protein synthesis and gluconeogenesis. Growth hormone in-creases gluconeogenesis by increasing the uti-lization of plasma amino acids.

The cellular actions regulated by hor-mones are schematically summarized in Figure 6-9.

In summary, hormones modulate the me-tabolism of carbohydrates, fats and proteins by shifting energy from storage sites to supply available energy and vice versa so that the daily energy and nutrient requirements are met.

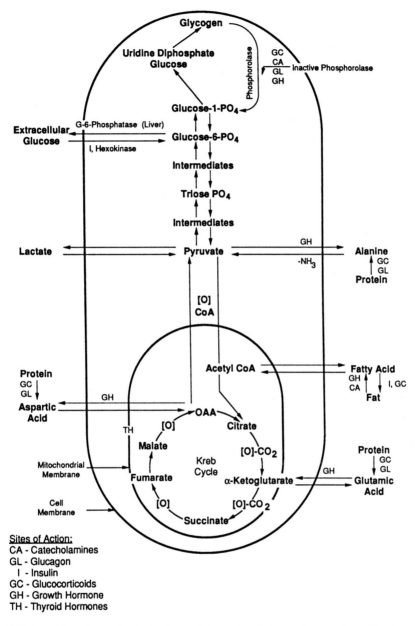

Fig. 6-9. Cellular metabolism of carbohydrates, fats and proteins and some sites of hormone action.

REFERENCES

1. Adams, H. R., and Parker, J. L. (1979): Pharmacologic management of circulatory shock: cardiovascular drugs and corticosteroids. J. Am. Vet. Med. Assoc. 175:86.
2. Adams, H. R. (1984): New perspectives in cardiopulmonary therapeutics: Receptor selective adrenergic drugs. J. Am. Vet. Med. Assoc. 185:966.
3. Ahlquist, R. P. (1948): A study of the adrenotropic receptors. Am. J. Physiol. 153:586.
4. Ariens, E. J., and Simonis, A. M. (1983): Physiological and pharmacological aspects of adrenergic receptor classification. Biochem. Pharmacol. 32: 1539.
5. Ask, J. A., and Stene-Larsen, G. (1984): Functional α_1-adrenoceptors in the rat heart during β-receptor blockade. Acta Physiol. Scand. 120:7.
6. Balfour, W. E., Comline, R. S., and Short, R. V. (1959): Changes in the secretion of 20 α-hydroxypregn-4-en-3-one by the adrenal gland of young calves. Nature 183:467.

7. Balow, J. E., and Rosenthal, A. S. (1973): Glucocorticoid suppression of macrophage migration inhibitory factor. J. Exp. Med. *137*:1031.

8. Becker, M. J., Helland, D., and Becker, D. N. (1976): Serum cortisol (hydrocortisone) values in normal dogs as determined by radioimmunoassay. Am. J. Vet. Res. *37*:1101.

9. Baylink, D. J. (1983): Glucocorticoid-induced osteoporosis. N. Engl. J. Med. *309*:306.

10. Berthelsen, S., and Pettinger, W. A. (1977): A functional basis for classification of α-adrenergic receptors. Life Sci. *21*:595.

11. Bishop, C. R., Athens, J. W., Boggs, D. R., et al. (1968): Leukokinetic studies. XIII. A nonsteady-state kinetic evaluation of the mechanism of cortisone-induced granulocytosis. J. Clin. Invest. *47*: 249.

12. Blaschko, H. (1959): Development of current concepts of catecholamine formation. Pharmacol. Rev. *11*:307.

13. Bonneau, N., and Reed, J. H. (1971): Adrenocortical insufficiency in a dog. Can. Vet. J. *12*:100.

14. Bottoms, G. D., Roesel, O. F., Rausch, F. D., et al. (1972): Circadian variation in plasma cortisol and corticosterone in pigs and mares. Am. J. Vet. Res. *33*:785.

15. Braun, R. K., Bergman, E. N., and Albert, T. F. (1970): Effects of various synthetic glucocorticoids on milk production and blood glucose and ketone body concentrations in normal ketotic cows. J. Am. Vet. Med. Assoc. *157*(7):941.

16. Brezonck, E. M., and McQueen, R. D. (1970): Adrenocortical function during aging in the dog. Am. J. Vet. Res. *31*:1269.

17. Brodde, O. -E. (1986): Molecular pharmacology of β-adrenoceptors. J. Cardiovasc. Pharmacol. *8*:S16.

18. Burton, R. M., and Westphal, U. (1972): Steroid hormone binding proteins in blood plasma. Metabolism *21*:253.

19. Bush, I. E. (1953): Species differences and other factors influencing adrenal cortical secretion. Colloq. Endocrin., Ciba Found. *7*:210.

20. Campbell, J. R., and Watts, C. (1973): Assessment of adrenal function in dogs. Br. Vet. J. *129*:134.

21. Capen, C. C., and Koestner, A. (1967): Functional chromophobe adenomas of the canine adenohypophysis. Pathol. Vet. *4*:326.

22. Capen, C. C., Martin, S. L., and Koestener, A. (1967): Neoplasms in the adenohypophysis of dogs. Pathol. Vet. *4*:301.

23. Chan, L., and O'Malley, B. W. (1978): Steroid hormone action: recent advances. Ann. Intern. Med. *89*:694.

24. Chen, C. L., Kumar, S. A., Williard, M. D., et al. (1978): Serum hydrocortisone (cortisol) values in normal and adrenopathic dogs as determined by radioimmunoassay. Am. J. Vet. Res. *39*(1):179.

25. Critchley, J. A. J. H., Fllis, P., and Unger, A. (1980): The reflex release of adrenaline and noradrenaline from the adrenal glands of cats and dogs. J. Physiol. *298*:71.

26. Cupps, T. R., and Fauci, A. S. (1982): Corticosteroid-mediated immunoregulation in man. Immunol. Rev. *65*:133.

27. Davis, J. O., and Freeman, R. H. (1976): Mechanism regulating renin release. Physiol. Rev. *56*:1.

28. Delmage, D. A. (1972): Three cases of alopecia in the dog related to adrenocortical dysfunction. J. Small Anim. Pract. *13*:265.

29. Dunlop, D., and Shanks, R. (1968): Selective blockade of adrenoceptive β-receptors in the heart. Br. J. Pharmacol. *32*:201.

30. Eberhart, R. J., and Patt, J. A. Jr. (1971): Plasma cortisol concentrations in newborn calves. Am. J. Vet. Res. *32*:1291.

31. Edelman, I. S., and Marver, D. (1980): Mediating events in the action of aldosterone. J. Steroid. Chem. *12*:219.

32. Eiler, H., Goble, D., and Oliver, J. (1979): Adrenal gland function in the horse: Effects of Cosyntropine (synthetic) and corticotropin (natural) stimulation. Am. J. Vet. Res. *40*:724.

33. Enright, J. B., Goggin, J. E., Frye, F. L., et al. (1970): Effects of corticosteroids on rabies virus infections in various animal species. J. Am. Vet. Med. Assoc. *156*:765.

34. Euler, U. S. Von (1960): Twenty years of noradrenaline. Pharmacol. Rev. *18*:29.

35. Farr, M. J., and Olsen, R. G. (1978): Suppression of the cell-mediated immune system of the horse by systemic corticosteroid administration. J. Eq. Med. Surg. *2*:129.

36. Fauci, A. S., Dale, D. C., and Balow, J. E. (1976): Glucocorticosteroid therapy: Mechanisms of action and clinical considerations. Ann. Intern. Med. *84*: 304.

37. Feldman, E. C. (1981): Effect of functional adrenocortical tumors on plasma cortisol and corticotropin concentrations in dogs. J. Am. Vet. Med. Assoc. *178*:823.

38. Feldman, E. C. (1984): Hypoadrenocorticism. Vet. Clin. North Am. Vet. Pract. *14*:751.

39. Ferguson, J. L., Roesel, O. F., and Bottoms, G. D. (1978): Dexamethasone treatment during hemorrhagic shock: Blood pressure, tissue perfusion, and plasma enzymes. Am. J. Vet. Res. *39*:817.

40. Franklin, R. T. (1984): The use of glucocorticoids in treating cerebral edema. Comp. Cont. Educ. Pract. Vet. *6*:442.

41. Fuller, R. W. (1973): Control of epinephrine synthesis and secretion. Fed. Proc. *32*:1772.

42. Ganjam, V. K., and Estergreen, V. L. Jr. (1970): Cortisol and corticosterone in bovine plasma and the effect of ACTH. J. Dairy Sci. *53*:480.

43. Gann, D. S., Dallman, M. F., and Engleland, W. C. (1981): Reflex control and modulation of ACTH and corticosteroids. Int. Rev. Physiol. *24*:157.

44. Granelli-Piperano, A., Vassali, J. D., and Reich, E. (1977): Secretion of plasminogen activator by human polymorphonuclear leuckocytes. Modulation of glucocorticoids and other effects. J. Exp. Med. *146*:1693.

45. Gwazdavkas, F. C., Thatcher, W. W., and Wilcox, C. J. (1972): Adrenocorticotropin alteration of bovine peripheral plasma concentrations of cortisol, corticosterone and progesterone. J. Dairy Sci. *55*: 1165.

46. Hall, S. S. (1972): Iatrogenic hyperadrenocorticism due to prolonged Azium therapy. Southwestern Vet. *26*:62.

47. Hardee, G. E., Lai, J. W., Semrad, S. D., et al. (1983): Catecholamines in equine and bovine plasmas. J. Vet. Pharmacol. Ther. *5*:279.
48. Hinshaw, L. B., Beller, B. K., Archer, L. T. et al. (1979): Recovery from lethal *E. coli* shock in dogs. Surg. Gynecol. Obstet. *149*:545.
49. Hirata, F., Schiffmann, E., Venkatasubamanian, K., et al. (1980): A phospholipase A_2 inhibitory protein in rabbit neutrophils induced by glucocorticoids. Proc. Natl. Acad. Sci. *77*:2533.
50. Hoffman, B. B., and Lefkowitz, R. J. (1980): Alpha-adrenergic receptor subtypes. N. Engl. J. Med. *302*:1391.
51. Hoffsis, G. F., Murdick, P. W., Tharp, V. L., et al. (1970): Plasma concentrations of cortisol and corticosterone in the normal horse. Am. J. Vet. Res. *31*:1379.
52. Horton, R. (1973): Aldosterone: review of its physiology and diagnostic aspects of primary aldosteronism. Metabolism *22*:1525.
53. Insel, P. A. (1984): Identification and regulation of adrenergic receptors in target cells. Am. J. Physiol. *247*:E53.
54. Johnston, S. D., and Mather, E. C. (1978): Canine plasma cortisol measured by RIA. Am. J. Vet. Res. *39*:1766.
55. Johnston, S. D., and Mather, E. C. (1979): Feline plasma cortisol (hydrocortisone) measured by radioimmunoassay. Am. J. Vet. Res. *40*:190.
56. Kaiser, C., and Jain, T. (1985): Dopamine receptors: Functions, subtypes and emerging concepts. Med. Res. Quarterly *5*:145.
57. Keeton, K. S., Schechter, R. D., and Schalm, O. W. (1972): Adrenocortical insufficiency in dogs. Mod. Vet. Pract. *53*:25.
58. Kelly, D. F., Siegel, E. T., and Berg, P. (1971): The adrenal gland in dogs with hyperadrenocorticalism. A pathologic study. Vet. Pathol. *8*:385.
59. Lands, A. M., Arnold, A., McAuliff, J. P., et al. (1967): Differentiation of receptor systems activated by sympathomimetic amines. Nature *214*:597.
60. Langer, S. Z. (1974): Presynaptic regulation of catecholamine release. Biochem. Pharmacol. *23*:1793.
61. Lavelle, R. B. (1976): The treatment of Cushing's disease in the dog. Vet. Rec. *98*:406.
62. Lefer, A. M., (1975): Corticosteroids and circulatory function. *In:* Handbook of Physiology, Vol. 6, H. Blaschko, *et. al.* (eds) Washington D. C., American Physiological Society, p. 191.
63. Linder, H. R. (1959): Blood cortisol in the sheep: normal concentration and changes in ketosis of pregnancy. Nature *184*(Suppl. 21):1645.
64. Linder, H. R. (1967): Comparative aspects of cortisol transport: Lack of firm binding to plasma proteins in domestic ruminants. J. Endocrinol. *28*:301.
65. Ling, G. V., Stabenfeldt, G. H., Comer, K. M., Gribble, D. H., and Schechter, R. D. (1979): Canine hyperadrenocorticism: pretreatment clinical and laboratory evaluation of 117 cases. J. Am. Vet. Med. Assoc. *174*:1211.
66. Lorenz, M. D., Scott, D. W., and Pulley, L. T. (1973): Medical treatment of canine hyperadrenocorticoidism with o,p'DDD. Cornell Vet. *63*:646.
67. Lubberink, A. A. M. E., Rijnberk, A., der Kinderen, P. J., and Thijsen, J. H. H. (1971): Hyper-

68. Macadam, W. R., and Eberhart, R. J. (1972): Diurnal variation in plasma corticosteroid concentration in dairy cattle. J. Dairy Sci. *55*:1792.
69. Mandel, S. (1982): Steroid myopathy. Postgrad. Med. *72*:207.
70. Marple, D. N., Judge, M. D., and Aberle, E. D. (1972): Pituitary and adrenocortical function of stress susceptible swine. J. Anim. Sci. *35*:995.
71. Martin, S. L., Murdick, P. W., and Capen, C. C. (1971): Laboratory evaluation of adrenocortical function in dogs. *In* Current Veterinary Therapy IV, edited by R. W. Kirk. Philadelphia, W. B. Saunders Co.
72. Marver, D, (1980): Aldosterone action in target epithelia. Vitam. Horm. *38*:57.
73. Meijer, J. C., de Bruijne, J. J., Rijnberk, A., et al. (1978): Biochemical characterization of pituitary-dependent hyperadrenocorticism in the dog. J. Endocrinol. *77*:111.
74. Meijer, J. C., Mulder, G. H., Rijnberk, A., et al. (1978): Hypothalamic corticotrophin releasing factor activity in dogs with pituitary-dependent hyperadrenocorticism. J. Endocrinol. *79*:209.
75. Moore, J. N., Steiss, J., Nicholson, W. E., and Orth, D. N. (1979): A case of pituitary adrenocorticotropin-dependent Cushing's syndrome in the horse. Endocrinology *104*:576.
76. Mulnix, J. A. (1971): Hypoadrenocorticism in the dog. J. Am. Anim. Hosp. Assn. *7*:220.
77. Mulnix, J. A. (1975): Adrenal cortical disease in dogs. Vet. Scope *19*:12.
78. Mulnix, J. A., van den Brom, E. W., Lubberink, A. A. M. E., et al. (1976): Gamma camera imaging of bilateral adrenocortical hyperplasia and adrenal tumors in the dog. Am. J. Vet. Res. *37*:1467.
79. Nara, P. L., Krahowka, S., and Powers, T. E. (1979): Effects of prednisolone on the development of immune responses to canine distemper virus in Beagle pups. Am. J. Vet. Res. *40*:1742.
80. O'Malley, B. (1974): Steroid hormone receptors. Session IX. Fifty-sixth Annual Meeting of the Endocrine Soc. Endocrinology *94*:21.
81. Osbaldiston, G. W., and Johnson, J. H. (1972): Effect of ACTH and selected glucocorticoids on circulating blood cells in horses. J. Am. Vet. Med. Assoc. *161*:53.
82. Paape, M. J., Desjardins, C., Schultze, W. D., et al. (1972): Corticosteroid concentrations in jugular and mammary vein blood plasma of cows after overmilking. Am. J. Vet. Res. *33*:1753.
83. Parrillo, J. E., and Fauci, A. S. (1979): Mechanism of glucocorticoid action on immune processes. Ann. Rev. Pharmacol. Toxicol. *19*:179.
84. Paterson, J. Y. F. (1964): The distribution and turnover of cortisol in sheep. J. Endocrinol. *28*:183.
85. Perchellet, J., and Sharma, R. K. (1979): Mediating role of calcium and guanosine 3', 5-monophosphate in adrenocorticotropin induced steroidogenesis by adrenal cells. Science *23*:1259.
86. Rae, P. A., Gutmann, N. S., Tsao, J., et al. (1979): Mutations in cyclic AMP-dependent protein kinase and corticotropin (ACTH)-sensitive adenylate cyclase affect adrenal steroidogenesis. Proc. Natl.

function of the adrenal cortex: a review. Aust. Vet. J. *47*:504.

Acad. Sci. *76*:1896.

87. Reid, I. A., Morris, B. J., and Ganong, W. F. (1978): The renin-angiotensin system. Ann. Rev. Physiol. *40*:377.

88. Rhynes, W. E., and Ewing, L. L. (1983): Plasma corticosteroids in Hereford bulls exposed to high ambient temperature. J. Anim. Sci. *36*:369.

89. Richkind, M., and Edquist, L. E. (1973): Peripheral plasma levels of corticosteroids in normal beagles and greyhounds measured by a rapid competitive protein binding technique. Acta Vet. Scand. *14*: 745.

90. Rijnberk, A., der Kinderen, P. J., and Thijssen, J. H. H. (1968): Investigations on the adrenocortical function of normal dogs. J. Endocrinol. *41*:387.

91. Rijnberk, A., der Kinderen, P. J., and Thijssen, J. H. H. (1968): Spontaneous hyperadrenocorticism in the dog. J. Endocrinol. *41*:397.

92. Ross, J. N. (1979): Comprehensive patient management in shock. J. Am. Vet. Med. Assoc. *175*(1):92.

93. Santen, R. J. (1980): Adrenal of male dog secretes androgens and estrogens. Am. J. Physiol. *239*:E109.

94. Schechter R. D., Stabenfeldt, G. H., Gribble, D. H., et al. (1973): Treatment of Cushing's syndrome in the dog with an adrenocorticolytic agent (o,p'.DDD). J. Am. Vet. Med. Assoc. *162*:629.

95. Scott, D. W., and Greene, C. E. (1974): Iatrogenic secondary adrenocortical insufficiency in dogs. J. Am. Anim. Hosp. Assn, *10*:555.

96. Sebranek, J. G., Marple, D. N., Cassens, R. G., et al. (1973): Adrenal response to ACTH in the pig. J. Anim. Sci. *36*:41.

97. Seren, E. (1973): ACTH and glucocorticoids in cattle. Folia Vet. Lat. *3*:584.

98. Shaw, K. E., and Nichols, R. E. (1962): The influence of age upon the circulating 17-hydroxy-corticosteroids of cattle subjected to blood sampling and exogenous adrenocorticotrophic hormone and hydrocortisone. Am. J. Vet. Res. *23*:1217.

99. Short, R. V. (1959): The secretion of sex hormones by the adrenal gland. Biochem. Soc. Symp. *59*:84.

100. Siegel, E. T., Kelly, D. F., and Berg, P. (1970): Cushing's syndrome in the dog. J. Am. Vet. Med. Assoc. *157*:2081.

101. Stark, K. (1977) Regulation of noradrenaline release by presynaptic receptor systems. Rev. Physiol. Biochem. Pharmacol. *77*:1.

102. Steinberg, D. (1966): Catecholamine stimulation of fat mobilization and its metabolic consequences. Pharmacol. Rev. *18*:217.

103. Swift, G. A., and Brown, R. H. (1976): Surgical treatment of Cushing's syndrome in the cat. Vet. Rec. *99*:374.

104. Temple, T. E., and Liddle, G. W. (1970): Inhibitors of adrenal steroid synthesis. Ann. Rev. Pharmacol. *10*:199.

105. Thompson, E. B., and Lippman, M. E. (1974): Mechanism of action of glucocorticoids. Metabolism *23*:159.

106. Thurley, D. C. (1972): Prenatal growth of the adrenal gland in sheep. N. Z. Vet. J. *20*:177.

107. Tumisto, J., and Mannisto, P. (1985): Neurotransmitter regulations of anterior pituitary hormones. Pharmacol. Rev. *37*: 249.

108. Twedt, D. C., and Wheeler, S. L. (1984): Pheochromocytoma in the dog. Vet. Clin. North. Am. *14*:767.

109. Unger, A., and Phillps, J. H. (1983): Regulation of the adrenal medulla. Physiol. Rev. *63*:687.

110. Unger, R. H., Dobbs, R. E. and Orci, L. (1978): Insulin, glucagon, and somatostatin secretion in the regulation of metabolism. Ann. Rev. Physiol. *40*:307.

111. Wagner, W. C., and Oxenreider, S. L. (1972): Adrenal function in the cow. Diurnal changes and the effects of lactation and neurohypophyseal hormones. J. Anim. Sci. *34*:630.

112. Westley, H. J., and Kelley, K. W,. (1984): Physiological concentrations of cortisol suppress cell-mediated immune events in the domestic pig. Proc. Soc. Exp. Biol. Med. *177*:156.

113. Whipp, S. C., Beary, M. E., Usenik, E. A., et al. (1967): Secretory rates of aldosterone in sodium-depleted calves. Am. J. Vet. Res. *28*:1343.

114. Whipp, S. C., Wood, R. L., and Lyon, N. C. (1970): Diurnal variation in concentrations of hydrocortisone in plasma of swine. Am. J. Vet. Res. *31*:2105.

115. Williams, G. H., and Dluhy, R. G. (1972): Aldosterone biosynthesis. Am. J. Med. *53*:595.

116. Wurtman, R. J., Pohorecky, L. A., and Baliga, B. S. (1972): Adrenocorticol control of the biosynthesis of epinephrine and proteins in the adrenal medulla. Pharmacol. Rev. *24*:411.

117. Yovich, J. V., Horney, F. D., and Hardee, G. E. (1984): Pheochromocytoma in the horse and measurement of norepinephrine levels in horses. Can. Vet. J. *25*: 21.

The Biology of Sex

M. H. PINEDA

7

Sex may be defined as the total morphological, physiological, and psychological differences that distinguish male and female. Chromosomal and phenotypic sex are recognized.

SEXUALITY

REPRODUCTION is essential to continuity of the species in all living organisms. The lower forms of life are more or less fixed in their habitat and reproduction by mitotic cellular division is advantageous, since seeking and recognizing a suitable mate are unnecessary. This form of reproduction is found in mammalian somatic cells and in the proliferative stages of gametogenesis, the formation of sex cells. The principal disadvantage of mitosis is the uniformity of the genotype of daughter cells. Except for occasional mutants, every progeny originated during mitosis is identical to its progenitor.

Evolution of Sex

In mammals, reproduction depends upon the union of anisogametes produced by dimorphic individuals designated as male and female. The evolution of sexuality is an adaptation to specialized function in multicellular organisms. Division of genetic materials between male and female provides for specialization of social function, as well as reproductive function. The most important evolutionary advantage gained by sexual reproduction is the increase in genetic variability afforded by meiotic division to form haploid gametes. Variability is produced by chiasma formation, random segregation, and recombination of chromosomal genes.

Although sexual reproduction is advantageous in terms of adaptation, the union of anisogametes from dimorphic parents is subject to temporal and spatial hazards. If gametes were released independently by the two sexes, this type of reproduction would likely lead to extinction. Thus, even in the lowest bisexual species, there are stimuli which tend to synchronize male and female partners to release their gametes at nearly the same time and in close proximity. These adversities were further complicated as land-dwelling species evolved and the gametes could no longer be released directly into an aqueous environment. Fertilization became an internal process, and

231

gestation evolved. A further hazard in sexual reproduction is that the progeny must pass through critical stages of development.

Chromosomal Sex

Chromosomal sex is determined by a single pair of sex chromosomes. The sex having similar sex chromosomes is the homozygous sex. The heterozygous sex has dissimilar sex chromosomes. Among domestic animals, the female is the homogametic sex and is designated XX. The mammalian male is the heterogametic sex and is designated XY. In poultry, hens are heterogametic and are designated ZW. Roosters are homogametic and are designated ZZ.

Chromosomal sex can be ascertained by examining interphase nuclei of somatic cells. The nuclei of somatic cells containing two X chromosomes contain a characteristic chromatin mass, the Barr body. Nuclei containing Barr bodies are chromatin-positive. Normal males are chromatin-negative. The number of bodies is one less than the total number of X chromosomes in diploid cells.

Gene expression in one of the X chromosomes of the XX somatic cells of the female appears to be inactivated or repressed early in fetal development in the eutherian mammals. This results in a ratio sex chromosome: autosomes similar to that of the XY cells of the male, compensating for the X sex chromosomal difference in the 2X females and 1X males. For a given individual, the inactivation of the X chromosome from either progenitor, paternal X or maternal X, may be of random occurrence. However, once it occurs, it remains fixed in the heredity of the somatic cells of that individual. During oogenesis, the inactivated X chromosome becomes active again while the oocyte undergoes meiosis so that each oocyte will contain an active X chromosome.

Anomalous sex chromosomal complements result from nondisjunction of the sex chromosomes during meiosis (Fig. 7-1). Best-documented among these are the XXY nuclei of Klinefelter's syndrome (seminiferous tubule dysgenesis) and the XO nuclei of Turner's syndrome (ovarian agenesis) in man. An XXY chromosomal constitution associated with testicular hypoplasia and azoospermia has been reported in the bull, horse, pig, ram, and cat. An XO syndrome associated with inactive ovaries has also been reported in the mare. Patients with Klinefelter's disease are chromatin-positive, and those with Turner's syndrome are chromatin-negative. Thus, chromatin-positiveness does not always indicate the XX chromosome complement of normal females.

Table 7-1 shows the diploid number of chromosomes of domestic species. Chromosome number plays an important role in maintaining genetic purity in nature. Interspecific mammalian hybrids, usually produced for commercial purposes, are possible. The mule and its reciprocal hybrid, the hinny, are examples. However, such hybrid progeny are usually sterile. The sterility of mules is due to chromosomal incompatibility. Mules of both sexes occasionally produce gametes, but most germ cells degenerate early in gametogenesis probably because of a block in meiosis due to incompatibility between the paternal (donkey, 62 chromosomes) and maternal (horse, 64 chromosomes) chromosomes. The mule and the hinny both have 63 chromosomes with unevenly matched pairs. Lack of pairing of homologous chromosomes in the few gametes produced by mules would not allow normal fertilization and development of their own gametes. However, mules undergo estrous cycles and are capable of gestation to term of transferred equine embryos.

Characteristic club-shaped nuclear appendages termed drumsticks occur in a small proportion of segmented neutrophils of genetic females. Drumsticks are equivalent to the sex chromatin mass in the nuclei of other somatic cells and occur with a frequency of less than 1 in 500 polymorphonuclear neutrophils of genetic males.

Recent technical advances in chromosomal analysis have contributed to the value of sex chromatin determination and the understanding of sexual abnormalities resulting from chromosomal aberrations. Cytogenetics, the science dealing with karyotype, has become a

		OOCYTE		
		Normal	Non–disjunctive	
		x	xx	o
S P E R M Normal	x	xx (=normal female)	xxx	xo
	y	xy (=normal male)	xxy	yo
Nondisjunctive	xy	xxy		
	o	xo		

Fig. 7-1. Diagram showing how normal and abnormal sex-chromosome constitutions can arise at fertilization. An O sperm or oocyte is one which carries neither an X nor a Y chromosome. Nondisjunctive gametes arise through faulty sharing out (nondisjunctive) of the sex chromsomes; YO individuals are probably not viable; XXX individuals in man, are sterile females.

Table 7-1 Numbers of Chromosomes

Animal	Diploid No.
Cat	38
Pig	38
Sheep	54
Cattle	60
Goat	60
Horse	64
Donkey	62
Dog	78
Chicken	
Rooster	78
Hen	77

Adapted from Pakes, S. P. and Griesemer, R. A.: J. Am. Vet. Med. Assoc. *146*:139, 1965, and Ohno, S.: Annu. Rev. Genet. *3*:495, 1969.

routine procedure in many pathology laboratories to aid in the diagnosis of developmental abnormalities.

Phenotypic Sex

Both male and female potentialities exist in every embryo. Most individuals differentiate in accord with their chromosomal sex, but all degrees of expression of the genetic sex occur. Furthmore, individuals may differentiate toward the sex contrary to chromosomal sex, resulting in intersexuality. Complete sex reversals are known in some species. Genetic sex is unalterably fixed at fertilization, but phenotypic sex differentiation is influenced by a number of factors such as evocators, hormones, temperature extremes, and probably other agents.

Ova from normal females carry the X chromosome, while 50% of spermatozoa carry an X, and 50% carry a Y chromosome. Theoretically, 50% of zygotes should be males, and 50% should be females (Fig. 7-2).

Sex ratio is expressed as the percentage of males or as the *number of males per 100 females.* Primary sex ratio is the ratio at conception. This is a theoretical value, but sex ratio can

be determined early in embryonal development by sex chromatin techniques. Secondary sex ratio is the proportion of males at birth, and tertiary sex ratio is the ratio at puberty. Secondary sex ratios of a number of species are displayed in Table 7-2.

The perfection of sex control on a practical scale by artificial insemination or transfer of sexed embryos would be a great asset to genetic progress in the livestock industry. Females could be ranked according to their genetic worth for highly heritable economic traits. A small percentage of the most desirable females could be bred to selectively produce male progeny for use as seminal donors. The next most valuable females could be bred to produce female replacements, and the remainder of females could produce males or females, depending on economic demand. Sex ratios have been reported to be modified by genetic selection, frequency of ejaculation, and parity of the dam. Separation of X and Y spermatozoa would be the simplest method to achieve this end. Successful attempts at separating male-

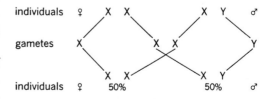

Fig. 7-2. Theoretical sex ratio at fertilization.

*Table 7-2   Secondary Sex Ratios Commonly Observed in Some
Mammals and Domestic Chickens*

Species	Number Observed	% Males (High Ratio)	Number Observed	% Males (Low Ratio)
Dog	1,400	55.4	6,878	52.4
Pig	2,357	52.8	16,233	48.8
Cattle	4,900	51.8	982	48.6
Horse	25,560	49.9	135,826	49.1
Sheep	50,685	49.5	8,965	49.2
Domestic Chicken	20,037	48.6	2,501	46.8

Data modified from various sources, especially from Lawrence, P. S.: Q. Rev. Biol. *16*:35, 1941 and from Nalbandov, A. V.: Reproductive Physiology, 2nd ed. San Francisco, W. H. Freeman and Co., 1964.

and female-determining spermatozoa have been reported, but these results are not yet repeatable.

Since the Y chromosome contains less material than the X chromosome, the Y-bearing spermatozoon has less mass. Centrifugation, sedimentation, and electrophoresis have been used to separate the two types of sperm cells. The X spermatozoa migrate to the anode, whereas Y spermatozoa are attracted to the cathode. Separation of spermatozoa on the basis of nuclear mass or membrane potential has not been reliably achieved on a practical scale. An additional route of further investigation lies in the distinct antigenic properties of the X- and Y-bearing spermatozoa, which would allow sex control by immunologic technics. The use of immunologic methods to detect the H-Y antigen, a gene product of the Y chromosome, is another approach being investigated to separate X- and Y-bearing spermatozoa. Production of offsprings from oocytes fertilized *in vitro* has been obtained in some species and the *in vitro* fertilization of oocytes with either X- or Y-bearing spermatozoa would then allow for the generation of sexed embryos for transfer.

Female monozygotic mice have been produced by removing, with microsurgery, the male pronucleus from a fertilized oocyte. Diploidy is achieved by inducing the haploid female pronucleus to replicate its chromosomes by culturing in a medium containing cytochal-asin B. The removal of the female pronucleus would generate lethal YY individuals.

DEVELOPMENT OF MALE AND FEMALE REPRODUCTIVE ORGANS

Sexual differentiation, like the differentiation of other systems, proceeds in consecutive steps (Fig. 7-3). Chromosomal sex is determined at fertilization; the establishment of gonadal sex is followed by the differentiation of the müllerian or wolffian duct system into the female or male accessory genitalia. The final step is the establishment of the psychic sex with the characteristic male or female sexual behavior.

Although the genetic sex of the conceptus is unalterably determined by its sex chromosome complement, each embryo is potentially capable of developing the genitalia of either sex, since the primitive gonad has all the cellular elements to give origin to a testicle or an ovary. The differentiation of sexual characteristics depends upon the quantitative relationship between male- and female-determining genes and their interaction with the internal environment.

Genes associated with female characteristics are believed to be located on the X chromosome. Homologous (XX) chromosomes appear to be necessary for the differentiation of the normal ovary. In Turner's syndrome (XO), diagnosed in man, rat, cat, pig, sheep, and mare, the adult gonad is an elongated mass of connective tissue. Genes for male

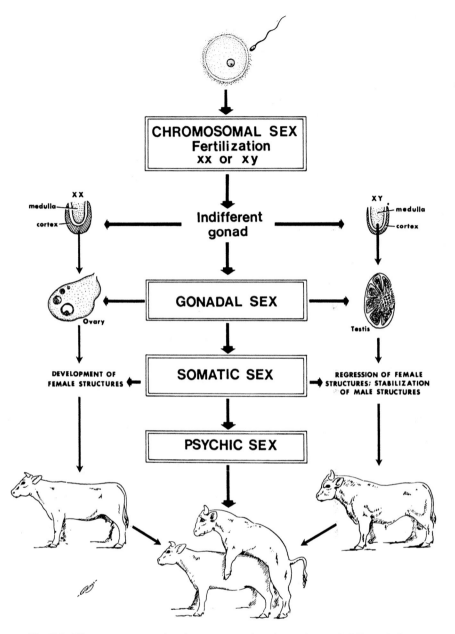

Fig. 7-3. Diagram representing four consecutive steps of sexual differentiation.

development are located on autosomes and on the Y chromosome. The presence of a Y chromosome, irrespective of the number of X chromosomes, or some form of chromosomal X-Y interaction, including the expression of the H-Y antigen, is responsible for the differentiation of the testes. In man, individuals with 45,XO syndrome are females, whereas those with 46,XY; 47,XXY; 48,XXXY; and 49,XXXXY are all males. Normally the female, being homozygous for the X chromosome, has an abundance of female-determining genes and develops as a female. Conversely in the normal male, genes for masculinity on the autosomes and Y chromosome predominate over the female determiners on the single

X chromosome, and male characteristics differentiate. The Y chromosome bears factors which determine the morphological differentiation of the testis, but its presence does not guarantee normal testicular development and functioning either in the fetus or in the adult.

The mammalian embryo has an inherent tendency to develop as a female; castration of male embryos at early stages of embryogenesis consistently results in their development as females.

Evidences accumulated in the last few years indicate that maleness and testicular differentiation in mammals is dependent upon both the Y chromosome and other associated and interacting factors. It is now known that XY cells contain genes, which code for the production of a discrete proteic factor called the H-Y (histocompatibility-Y) antigen. The H-Y antigen has been detected on preimplantation embryos and is thought to be a major sex determiner. The presence of the H-Y antigen and its interaction with cells of the undifferentiated, developing gonad would signal for the formation of the testis. Thus, the undifferentiated gonad becomes a testis when the Y chromosome is present in the heterogametic XY male and the H-Y antigen is fully expressed. When the Y chromosome is absent or if the Y chromosome is present but the H-Y antigen is not expressed, the undifferentiated gonad will become an ovary. The endogenous H-Y antigen is not recognized as foreign by the immune system of mammals. In the avian species, however, the H-Y antigen is present in the female, which is the heterogametic sex. It appears that antibodies against the H-Y antigen are generated by the immune system of the female bird, which would neutralize the H-Y antigen, preventing its male determining activity.

Despite the male-determining role of the Y chromosome in mammals, a gene on the X chromosome appears to be necessary for testosterone secretion. Moreover, male or hermaphroditic development has been observed in cocker spaniel dogs, gilts, goats, mice, and men with the XX karyotype. The cause of sex reversal in XX males has not been determined, but the abnormal translocation of genes from the Y to X chromosome or the inheritance of the condition as an autosomal, dominant or recessive, trait has been implicated. In the species mentioned, XX males were positive for H-Y antigen.

The finding of mares with an XY karyotype has also been reported. These mares were infertile and had underdeveloped gonads and uteri, resembling those of females with an XO karyotype. The case of a fertile mare with an XY constitution and low blood levels of H-Y antigen has also been reported.[51]

Gonadogenesis begins with the formation of the genital ridges in close association with the mesonephros (Fig. 7-4). Primordial germ cells migrate from the yolk sac endoderm to the genital ridges. The gonads at this stage are still sexually bipotent and consist of an inner medulla and an outer cortex. Primordial germ cells invade the medulla to form primary sex cords. At this time, gonadal differentiation occurs, and bipotentiality no longer exists. When genes for masculinity of an XY individual prevail, the medulla persists, cortical development is inhibited, and a testis develops. When genes for femaleness predominate in the XX embryo, the medulla is inhibited, and the cortex develops. In this case, the persisting primordial germ cells in the epithelium invade the cortex as the secondary sex cords, and an ovary develops. Thus, spermatozoa are derived from progenitors in the primary sex cords, and cells in the secondary sex cords are the ancestors of oocytes.

During the indifferent (or bisexual) stage, the gonad is potentially capable of either testis or ovary formation. Furthermore, discrete primordia for development of complete accessory sex structures of either sex are present. Table 7-3 shows the homologous structures that differentiate from the indifferent rudiments.

Following gonadal differentiation, the accessory genitalia develop under the influence of the gonad. When a testis has formed, the female (müllerian) duct system regresses to vestigial rudiments and the male (wolffian) elements develop under the influence of mor-

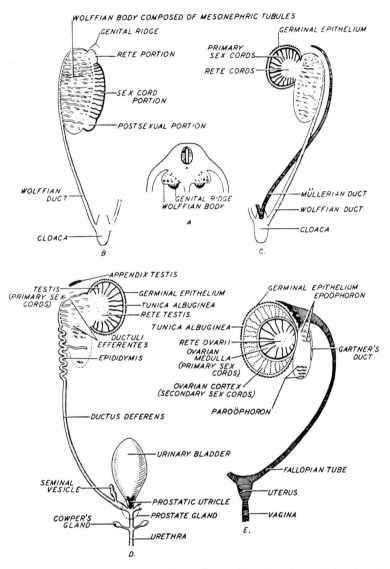

Fig. 7-4. Embryogenesis of the genital system in amniotes. *A*, section through the dorsal region of an early embryo, showing the wolffian bodies (mesonephric kidneys) and the genital ridges on their medio-lateral surfaces. *B*, The wolffian body and genital ridge in sagittal section. With respect to the fate of its parts, the genital ridge is divisible into three general regions. The wolffian (mesonephric) ducts drain the kidneys, but genital ducts as such are not present. *C*, The indifferent (ambisexual) stage. The rete cords have become enclosed by the primary sex cords. The müllerian ducts appear and temporarily coexist with the wolffian ducts in both genetic males and females. *D*, Differentiation of the male genitalia. *E*, Differentiation of the female genitalia.

The primary sex cords are shown in solid black, whereas the secondary sex cords are represented by large stipples. The müllerian ducts and their derivatives are heavily cross-hatched; the wolffian ducts are relatively unshaded. (From Turner, C. D.: General Endocrinology. 3rd ed., Philadelphia, W. B. Saunders Co., 1960.)

Table 7-3   Homologies of Male and Female Reproductive Systems

Indifferent	Male	Female
	INTERNAL GENITALIA	
Gonad	Testis	Ovary
	Rete testis	Rete ovarii*
Mesonephric tubules	Vas efferens	Epoophoron*
	Paradidymis*	Paroophoron*
	Vas aberrans*	
Mesonephric duct	Epididymis	Duct part of epoophoron*
	Vas deferens	(Gartner's duct)
	Ejaculatory duct	
	Seminal vesicle	
	Appendix of the epididymis*	
Müllerian duct	Appendage of testis*	Appendage of the ovary*
		(hydatid)
		Fimbria of oviduct
		Oviduct
	Prostatic utricle* (uterus masculinus)	Uterus
		Vagina [all or part?]
Urogenital sinus	Prostatic, membranous, and carvernous urethra	Urethra
		Vestibule
		Vagina [in part?]
	Bulbourethral glands	Vestibular glands
	(Cowper's glands)	(Bartholin's glands)
	Prostate	Paraurethral glands
	EXTERNAL GENITALIA	
Genital tubercle	Glans penis	Glans clitoris
	Corpus penis	Corpus clitoridis
Urethral folds	Raphe of scrotum and penis	Labia minora
Labioscrotal swellings	Scrotum	Labia majora

From Nalbandov, A. V.: Reproductive Physiology, 2nd ed. San Francisco, W. H. Freeman and Co., 1964.
*Rudimentary.

phogenic agents secreted by the newly formed testes: androgens and the müllerian inhibiting hormone (MIH). The androgens, mainly testosterone, secreted by the fetal testes or their metabolites, stimulate the growth and development of the wolffian system and the external genitalia of the fetus. The onset of testosterone synthesis by the fetal testes corresponds closely with the differentiation of the Leydig cells. The müllerian inhibiting hormone, secreted by the Sertoli cells of the fetal testes blocks the development of the müllerian system. MIH is a macromolecular, glyco- proteic hormone now demonstrated to be produced by the fetal testes of several species. The inhibitory activity of MIH on the müllerian system of the male fetus is limited to a short, sensitive period early in fetal development. In the calf, this sensitive period for the activity of MIH extends to day 62 of gestation. When an ovary has formed, the absence of the testicular morphogenic agents permits the müllerian system to develop, and the wolffian duct and tubules regress to vestigial rudiments. Ablation of the fetal male gonad prior to differentiation of the wolffian system causes differentiation of the müllerian system in individuals with XY constitution. The urogenital sinus, genital tubercle, and genital folds normally differentiate in accord with the wolffian or müllerian duct system (Table 7-3).

A series of major developmental changes begin to occur in the testes during the fetal period. These changes continue after birth in the late postnatal period until puberty is reached and the full expression of the male reproductive function has been established. During the early fetal period, the germ cells of the developing testes undergo mitotic proliferation and differentiate into Sertoli and fetal Leydig cells. The fetal Leydig cells secrete androgens, which influence the differentiation of the male reproductive system. In the late fetal and early postnatal periods, the germ cells cease to divide and the Leydig cells undergo regressive changes while the Sertoli cells proliferate. As puberty approaches, the Leydig cells resume their secretory activity and differentiate into the adult type. The Sertoli cells also undergo further differentiation and morphogenic changes which would lead to the establishment of a blood-testis barrier. In the prepubertal period, the germinal cells resume their mitotic activity and differentiate into spermatogonia, as spermatogenesis progresses.

The testes are in the abdominal cavity during the embryonal and fetal stages. In most mammals the testes descend, at variable periods prior to or after birth, to the scrotum. In some species, the testes are in the scrotum only during periods of sexual activity and ascend during sexual quiescence. In birds and a few mammals the testes are permanently intra-abdominal. The extra-abdominal location of the testes in domestic mammals is indispensable for normal spermatogenesis.

Development of the reproductive system is a complex series of events involving a number of developmental actions and interactions subject to error at three states. (1) The distribution of sex chromosomes during meiotic or mitotic divisions may result in sex chromosome aneuploidy in gametes. Moreover, fragments of sex chromosomes or autosomes bearing sex-influencing genes may be abnormally distributed as a result of partial or complete deletion or translocation in chiasma formation. (2) Gonadal morphogenesis may be disturbed because of abnormal corticomedullary relationships. (3) Secondary and accessory genital structures may develop abnormally under the influence of an irregular endocrine environment or as a result of teratogenic factors.

The classic example of intersexuality in veterinary medicine is the freemartin heifer. The freemartin is a genetic female which has been modified in the male direction by masculinizing factors from a heterozygous male twin. Factors from the male twin enter the blood vascular system of the female co-twin when anastomosis of placental blood vessels has occurred. Placental fusion with vascular anastomosis is said to occur in about 92% of bovine twins. Since the testicular morphogenic agents from the male twin exert their influence before the development of the ovary and müllerian system in the female twin, the sexual apparatus of the freemartin is stimulated to develop male structures. All degrees of masculinization are observed, presumably due to variable amounts of male morphogenic substance, likely MIH, reaching the reproductive system of the female co-twin. The gonads resemble testes to a greater or lesser degree, the müllerian duct system is inhibited, and wolffian ducts remain and are differentiated in varying degrees. Postnatal treatment of freemartin heifers with estrogens induces mammary growth, while postnatal treatment with androgens stimulates clitoral development with little effect on the other reproductive organs. The finding that some freemartins are chimeric (XY/XX) gave impetus to the cellular theory of freemartinism. XY cells from the male co-twin concurrently with the H-Y antigen instruct the developing female system to masculinize. Singleton freemartins with 60, XX/60, XY chimeric karyotype have been reported. These probably result from the early death and absorption of the male twin. Similar intersexes have been reported in sheep, pigs, and goats.

A large percentage of bulls born co-twin with freemartin heifers have impaired testicular steroidogenesis and reduced reproductive capability including low sperm output or azoospermia, and a high incidence of abnormal spermatozoa in their ejaculates. The finding of XX spermatogonia and primary spermatocytes in the testes of some bulls born co-twin with freemartin heifers suggests that XX germinal cells from the female co-twin may alter spermatogenesis in these chimeric bulls.

Female pseudohermaphrodites have essentially normal internal genitalia but intermediate external genitalia. The external genitals may vary from a nearly normal vulva with an enlarged clitoris to a nearly normal penis, usually with hypospadias. The male pseudohermaphrodite, with abdominal or subcutaneous testes and intermediate external genitalia, is more common among domestic species than the female pseudohermaphrodite.

True hermaphrodites have both ovarian and testicular tissues with an intermediate external genitalia. Hermaphroditic goats result from homozygosity of an autosomal recessive gene which causes XX zygotes to develop both male and female sex structures.

SEXUAL BEHAVIOR

Sexual behavior includes mating behavior, maternal behavior, and social mannerisms. This discussion will be limited to mating behavior and social mannerisms related to mating behavior.

Mating behavior has two components. The first is sex drive, or libido. The second includes all phases of copulation, including postural adjustments, intromission, ejaculation, orgasm, and postcopulatory behavior.

Internal Factors

There is generally a close relationship between ovarian function and sexual behavior in subprimate female mammals. Sexual receptivity is largely limited to periods of maximal development of ovarian follicles and the secretion of estrogens. Sexual receptivity is the ultimate criterion of estrus. However, receptive behavior sometimes occurs at other stages in the ovarian cycle and occasionally during pregnancy. Prepubertal gonadectomy usually prevents mating behavior. Ovariectomy of sexually mature females immediately abolishes mating behavior, in contrast to a gradual loss of mating behavior following orchiectomy.

Adequate doses of estrogen administered to ovariectomized adult animals restore manifestations of estrus, including mating behavior. In several species, and particularly in the bitch, treatment with estrogens followed by progesterone is needed to induce estrous behavior in ovariectomized animals. The first pubertal cycle of ewes and heifers and the first ovulatory cycle of the breeding season of ewes is usually not accompanied by normal mating behavior, presumably because progesterone from a corpus luteum of a preceding cycle is absent.

Exogenous gonadotropins may initiate mating behavior in pubertal or adult females by stimulating the secretion of ovarian steroids. In some species, estrogens restore mating behavior in hypophysectomized females, confirming that estrogens are the primary regulators of female mating behavior.

The consequences of gonadectomy in the adult male are generally less dramatic than in the female, especially when castration is performed in sexually experienced males. Prepubertal orchiectomy prevents normal mating patterns. Adult castration is followed by a gradual diminution of copulatory responses and sex drive, in that order. In castrated males, behavioral response to erogenous stimuli and copulatory responses, in that order, are restored by treatment with androgens.

The role of androgens in male sexual behavior is twofold. During fetal life of males, or within a few days after birth, androgens organize neural centers which will mediate male mating behavior. In pubertal males, androgens activate these centers.

Experimental masculinization of the developing female brain has been achieved in several species, including dogs, by the administration of androgens during the critical period of development. Behaviorally, masculinized females are incapable of displaying female sexual behavior, even in response to the administration of ovarian hormones. On the other hand, orchiectomy or the administration of antiandrogens during the critical period renders males psychological females. These feminized males display lordosis in response to mounting.

In contrast to the ability of androgens to organize neural centers for the mediation of male mating behavior, injections of estrogen in females during the period when the neural centers are organized inhibit female behavior. Thus, the absence of androgen, rather than the presence of estrogen, during the period of differentiation induces female mating patterns.

It appears that the neural centers mediating estrous behavior are located in the hypothalamus or in the mamillary bodies. Centers for male sexual behavior are less defined, but certain cortical and hypothalamic lesions cause decreased sexual activity. Lesions in the region of the amygdala of male cats apparently destroy a sex-inhibiting center, resulting in hypersexuality. Castration abolishes this hypersexuality, and testosterone restores it in the castrate.

Mating behavior is dependent upon functional levels of other hormonal factors, as well. The thyroidal secretion influences behavioral response to sexual steroids. Thyroidal activity also modifies the rate of secretion of gonadal steroids. The adrenal glands are capable of secreting androgens and estrogens, and their activity must be considered when evaluating the effects of gonadectomy.

Mating behavior varies with genotype. Sex drive, like many other measures of reproductive function, is subject to heterosis, or hybrid vigor. Homozygous twin bulls showed great similarities of the sexual pattern within pairs of twins and great differences between pairs. Beef bulls generally exhibit much less sex drive and require more sexual preparation than dairy bulls. These factors all indicate a genetic basis for male sexual behavior.

External Factors

The effects of season and nutrition are the most profound of the environmental factors which influence mating behavior. Seasonal effects are discussed in the chapter on patterns of reproduction. Light and temperature influence mating behavior through neural pathways which modify the function of the pituitary and by altering the sensitivity of the somal substrate to endocrine stimulation.

Mating activity often occurs at that portion of the year which assures an adequate supply of feed for the offspring. Nutritional deficiency, especially inadequate caloric intake, delays the onset of puberty in both males and females. Conversely, high-energy diets hasten puberty. After puberty, females are more sensitive to dietary insufficiencies than males, because of the increased demands of pregnancy and lactation.

Species differ in their response to confinement and domestication. Reproduction fails in several wild species when confined in zoos, whereas domestication with attendant provision of shelter and food has nearly obliterated seasonal reproductive activity in cattle and swine. The history of domesticated species is thus a record of the ability to adapt physiologically to a life of confinement.

Social interactions in groups of prepubertal companions are a necessary learning experience in the formation of sexual behavior. In several species and notably among subhuman primates, behavioral deficiencies develop in males reared in isolation. Males reared in isolation display arousal to the same degree as normal males, but copulatory responses are incoordinated, and intromission is rarely achieved. These behavioral deficiencies are not corrected by injections of testosterone. Deficiencies in copulatory behavior have been observed in bulls, dogs, and stallions. However, deficient males can be taught the proper copulatory patterns through patient training. The effect of rearing females in isolation is less pronounced and puberty is hastened in gilts having contact with a boar.

When groups of rams are joined with ewes, mature rams dominate the yearling rams. Dominance also occurs within both yearling and mature groups of rams. Rams joined with ewes prior to the first (silent) ovulation of the breeding season hasten the onset of estrus. Vasectomized teasers are less effective, possibly due to a loss of libido as a function of time following surgery; loss of libido has also been observed in vasectomized dogs and men.

Chemical communication between animals is well-documented, especially among the lower phyla. Sex communicants are among the compounds known as pheromones. Chemical communication is implicated as the prime mode of communication in most animal phyla. Pheromones affect behavioral centers and may alter function of the anterior pituitary by influencing the release of hypothalamic releasing or inhibitory hormones. Reproductive behavior in most species of domestic animals indicates that pheromones, acting through olfaction and taste, influence sex behavior patterns. Sex pheromones elicit one or both of two responses, attraction and mating behavior.

Anosmic rams display normal sex drive and copulatory behavior, but their ability to discriminate between estrous ewes and ewes not in estrus is impaired. Anosmic rams approach ewes at random and must rely on the precopulatory behavior of estrous ewes to discern receptive females. Rams with unimpaired olfactory capacity are capable of detecting those ewes which are more apt to accept their precopulatory advances.

Estrous bitches attract males over a considerable distance. The anal glands, vaginal secretion, and urine have been postulated as sources of sex pheromones. Saliva, urine, and preputial washings of the boar attract sows in estrus and boars exert an estrous-synchronizing effect on gilts. Steroidal compounds have been isolated from the saliva, urine, and spermatic venous blood of boars and implicated as pheromones for the sow. Valeric acid in the urine of the female cat may play an important role in facilitating mating behavior in the male cat.

In addition to olfactory and gustatory stimuli, visual, tactile, and auditory stimuli arouse mating behavior. Animals which have one of these senses impaired compensate by increased reliance on the remaining senses.

The homosexual behavior of female cattle helps range bulls to identify estrous females. Allowing bulls to observe seminal collection procedures stimulates their responsiveness at artificial insemination centers. Similarly, dogs become excited when they observe other dogs mating.

The males of most species use tactile stimuli to identify estrous females. Licking and rubbing of the female external genitalia are almost universal among domestic species. Stallions often nibble the mare's neck or withers to test receptivity, and the auditory response may in turn stimulate the horse. Rams test receptivity in ewes by thumping the ewe's chest with the foreleg. Bulls and rams are often seen to rest the head and chin on the female's rump prior to mounting. Temperature and tactile receptors on the penis are important to intromission.

Mating experience is an important factor in sexual behavior. Experienced males usually achieve copulation in less time than inexperienced males. Males trained to serve the artificial vagina learn to rely heavily on tactile stimuli. Learning of copulatory patterns decreases the dependence of neural sex centers for endocrine stimuli. Experienced stallions may maintain sex drive for more than 500 days following orchiectomy.

GAMETOGENESIS

Gametogenesis refers to the formation of the male and female gametes, the spermatozoon and the oocyte, respectively.

Spermatogenesis

Spermatogenesis is a complex process of cell division and differentiation conducive to the formation of spermatozoa. Spermatozoa are formed in the seminiferous tubules of the testes by a series of cell divisions followed by a metamorphosis which produces a highly differentiated and potentially motile cell, the spermatozoon. The seminiferous tubules form a complex system that constitutes about 90% of the testicular mass in the adult. Spermatogenesis can be divided into two phases, spermatocytogenesis and spermiogenesis. Spermatocytogenesis is the proliferative phase in which primitive germ cells are multiplied by a series of mitotic divisions followed by the meiotic divisions, which produce the haploid state. Spermiogenesis is the differentiative phase in which the nucleus and cytoplasm undergo morphologic changes to form the sperm cell.

Spermatocytogenesis begins with the mitotic division of spermatogonia on the basement membrane and proceeds toward the lumen. Spermatogonia are activated to form active, type A spermatogonia. There may be several generations of type A spermatogonia, depending on the species. Most of the type A spermatogonia divide to form intermediate spermatogonia; certain of the type A cells are retained as resting-type A spermatogonia. In this way, the type A cells provide daughter cells for the formation of spermatozoa but are not normally depleted in the process. Intermediate spermatogonia divide to form type B spermatogonia, which undergo the last of the mitotic divisions to form primary spermatocytes. Spermatocytogenesis is concluded by the meiotic divisions which produce secondary spermatocytes, then spermatids. (Fig. 7-5).

The formation of spermatids marks the end of spermatocytogenesis and the beginning of spermiogenesis. Spermiogenesis, or spermateliosis, begins in the seminiferous tubules and is completed in the epididymis as the animal approaches puberty. Spermiogenesis has been intensively studied, since normal or abnormal morphological forms develop during this phase. A series of complex structural reorganizations occurs during spermiogenesis (Fig. 7-6).

Although reproductive behavior and spermatogenesis of most domestic males are relatively independent of cyclic variations, very definite cyclic activity is seen in seminiferous tubules. In the postpubertal male, the cells of the germinal epithelium are organized in cellular associations that are about the same stage of development. They evolve synchronously from the basement membrane of the seminiferous tubule to its lumen. These cellular associations succeed one another at a point in the seminiferous tubule over time and are called stages in the cycle of the seminiferous epithelium (Fig. 7-7). One cycle of the seminiferous epithelium includes the series of changes in the cells at a specific location in the tubule between two successive appearances of the same cellular association. Each successive cell layer in a given stage, or cellular association, is derived from a cell which has completed the changes of one cycle of the seminiferous epithelium. Thus, each cycle of the seminiferous epithelium constitutes a generation interval.

The spermatogenic cycle consists of several cycles of the seminiferous epithelium and includes all events from activation of the resting spermatogonium to the release of spermatozoa generated from it. In Figure 7-7, the spermatogenic cycle is depicted as consisting of 4½ cycles of the seminiferous epithelium. The linear movement of cells is confined to progression between the basement membrane and lumen of the tubule during the spermatogenic cycle and does not occur along the long axis of the tubule.

Various investigators have classified the cellular associations in the cycle of the seminiferous epithelium into more or less distinct stages. Since the criteria for classification are arbitrary, and the starting points in the cycle have not been uniform in these studies, the number of stages and their relation to the classifications of other authors are variable.

The duration of the cycle of the seminiferous epithelium and the duration of the spermatogenic cycle vary among species but are constant for a given species (Table 7-4). The durations of the cycle of the seminiferous epithelium have been accurately determined. For practical purposes, the duration of spermatogenesis can be calculated by multiplying the duration of the cycle of the seminiferous epithelium by 4, since spermatogenesis extends over approximately 4 (3.9 to 4.7, according to criteria for classification and species) consecutive cycles.

Although Sertoli cells are the only nongerminal cells in the seminiferous epithelium, they are fundamental to normal spermatogenesis. Plasma membranes form tight junc-

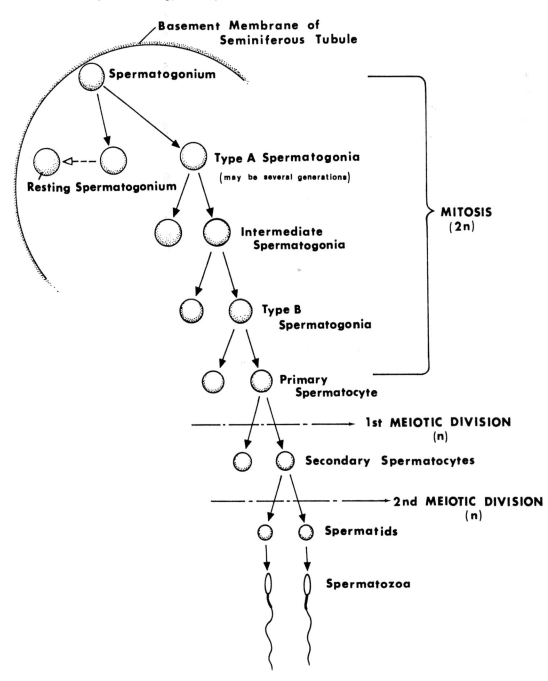

Basement Membrane of Seminiferous Tubule

Spermatogonium

Type A Spermatogonia
(may be several generations)

Resting Spermatogonium

Intermediate Spermatogonia

Type B Spermatogonia

Primary Spermatocyte

MITOSIS (2n)

1st MEIOTIC DIVISION (n)

Secondary Spermatocytes

2nd MEIOTIC DIVISION (n)

Spermatids

Spermatozoa

Fig. 7-5. Diagrammatic representation of spermatogenesis.

tions between adjacent Sertoli cells which divide the seminiferous epithelium into compartments. These compartments constitute part of a blood-testis barrier. Recent evidence indicates that these compartments provide a special testosterone-enriched microenvironment necessary for meiosis and spermiogenesis (Fig. 7-8). The morphological transformation of spermatids during spermiogenesis occurs with the spermatids embedded within

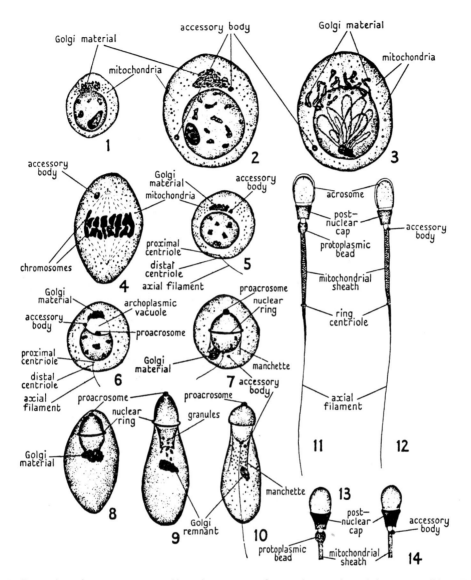

Fig. 7-6. Formation of a spermatozoon. Note the process of spermiogenesis and the responsible cellular inclusions. 1. Spermatogonium. 2. Primary spermatocyte. 3. Primary spermatocyte—early prophase. 4. Primary spermatocyte—early anaphase. 5. Young spermatid. 6–8. Spermatids. 9, 10. Late spermatids. 11. Spermatozoon. 12. Spermatozoon, showing accessory body; the protoplasmic bead is not shown. 13. Spermatozoon. 14. Spermatozoon, showing accessory body; the protoplasmic bead is not shown. (Gresson, R. A. R., and Zlotnik, I.: Q. J. Microbiol. Sci. *89*:219, 1948.)

cytoplasmic pockets of individual Sertoli cells. The Sertoli cells support the spermatogenic epithelium, have endocrine activity, and participate in spermiogenesis by phagocytosis of the residual bodies shed by the maturing spermatids. The release of spermatozoa from the cytoplasmic pockets of the Sertoli cell,

spermiation, involves marked swelling of the Sertoli cell.

The vascular supply to the germinal epithelium is outside the basement membrane of the seminiferous tubule. The Sertoli cells serve to convey nutrients and metabolites between the spermatogenic cells and the peritubular

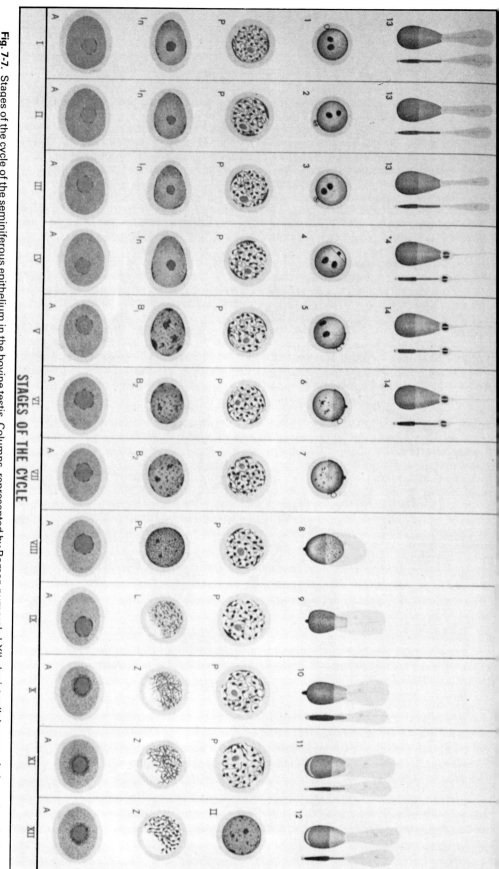

Fig. 7-7. Stages of the cycle of the seminiferous epithelium in the bovine testis. Columns, represented by Roman numerals I-XII, depict cellular associations at each of the 12 stages. Fourteen steps of spermiogenesis were identified and illustrated by spermatids (numbered 1-14) in the upper two rows with the lateral profile of the elongated spermatids (steps 10-14 of spermiogenesis) included. The types of germ cells observed in sequence are: A, type A spermatogonia; I$_n$, intermediate spermatogonia; B$_1$, type B$_1$ spermatogonia; B$_2$, type B$_2$ spermatogonia; PL, preleptotene primary spermatocytes; L, leptotene primary spermatocytes; Z, zygotene primary spermatocytes; P, pachytene primary spermatocytes; and II, secondary spermatocytes. (From Berndtson, W. E., and Desjardins, C.: The cycle of the seminiferous epithelium and spermatogenesis in the bovine testis. Am. J. Anat. *140*:167, 1974.)

STAGES OF THE CYCLE

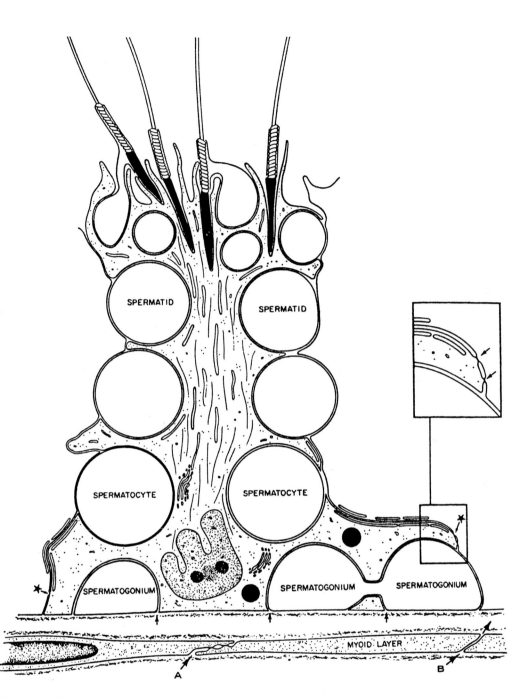

Fig. 7-8. A diagram depicting localization of the blood-testis barrier and compartmentalization of the germinal epithelium by tight junction between adjacent Sertoli cells. Note the germ cells and their relationship to a columnar Sertoli cell. The primary barrier to substances penetrating from the interstitium is the myoid layer. The majority of cell junctions in this layer are closed by a tight apposition of membranes (A). Over a small fraction of the tubule surface, the myoid junctions exhibit a 200 Å wide interspace and are therefore open (B). Material gaining access to the base of the epithelium by passing through open junctions in the myoid layer is free to enter the intercellular gap between spermatogonia and Sertoli cells. Deeper penetration is prevented by occluding junctions (stars) on the Sertoli-Sertoli boundaries. These tight junctions constitute a second and more effective component of the blood-testis barrier. In effect, Sertoli cells and their tight junctions delimit a *basal* compartment in the germinal epithelium, containing the spermatogonia and early preleptotene spermatocytes, and an *adluminal* compartment, containing the spermatocytes and spermatids. Substances traversing open junctions in the myoid cell layer have direct access to cells in the basal compartment, but to reach the cells in the adluminal compartment, substances must pass through the Sertoli cells. (From Dym, M., and Fawcett, D. W.: The blood-testis barrier in the rat and the physiological compartmentation of the seminiferous epithelium. Biol. Reprod. *3*:308, 1970.)

Table 7-4 Duration of the Cycle of the Seminiferous Epithelium and of Spermatogenesis in Some Mammals

Species	Durations, Days	
	Cycle	Spermatogenesis
Ram	10.4	49
Bull	13.5	54*
Boar	8.6	34.4
Dog	13.6	54.4*
Coyote	13.6	54.4*
Stallion	12.2	48.8*
Rabbit	10.3, 10.7, 10.9	51.8, 42–47, 48
Rat (Sprague-Dawley)	12.9	51.6
Rat (Wistar)	13	52
Monkey (Macaca mulatta)	10.5	42*
Monkey (Macaca fascularis)	9.3	37.2*
Man	16	64

Adapted from Clermont, Y.: Physiol. Rev., *52*:198, 1972. Data for the dog and coyote from Foote, R. H., et al.: Anat. Rec., *173*:341, 1972, and from Kennelly, J. J.; J. Reprod. Fertil., *31*:163, 1972. Data for the stallion from Swierstra, E. E., et al.: J. Reprod. Fertil., *40*:113, 1974.

*Duration of spermatogenesis calculated by multiplying duration of the cycle by 4.

capillaries. In line with their role in sustaining maturing germinal elements during spermatogenesis, Sertoli cells undergo a cyclic transformation which is coextensive with the cycle of the seminiferous epithelium. The Sertoli cell cycle may, in fact, be the most important coordinating factor in the spermatogenic cycle. The long-held view that the number of Sertoli cells is established before or during puberty and remains stable in the adult male may no longer be tenable. Evidences accumulated in the last few years indicate that there are seasonal variations in the number and volume of Sertoli cells in the stallion. Sertoli cell numbers increase during the breeding season and decrease during the winter months of the year. Age-related changes in the numbers of Sertoli cells have been observed in the human testes and similar changes may occur in other species, as well.

Ooogenesis

Oogonia are produced by mitotic proliferation of primordial germ cells. It is not clear in all species whether all oogonia are the direct descendants of germ cells in the secondary sex cords, or whether some of them arise by transition of peritoneal cells covering the ovary (referred to as "germinal epithelium").

Oogonia multiply by mitosis until the final generation of oogonia enter prophase of the first meiotic division, at which point they are primary oocytes. In the domestic mammals, with the exception of the bitch and the female cat, the queen, oogonia develop into primary oocytes before or shortly after birth (Fig. 7-9). In the bitch and queen, oogenesis extends after birth. In the bitch, primary oocytes are present in the ovarian follicles by approximately 50 to 60 days of age. The primary oocyte consists of the ooplasm, or vitellus, and a large spherical nucleus, sometimes called the germinal vesicle. During the first meiotic prophase, primary oocytes are surrounded by a flattened layer of follicular epithelium to form primary follicles.

The nucleus of the primary oocyte enters the dictyate, or resting, stage of the first meiotic prophase. The dictyate stage is specific to meiotic prophase in the female, since there is not a corresponding stage in spermatocytogenesis. The nucleus of the primary oocyte remains in the dictyate stage during growth

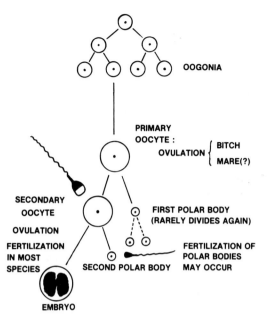

Fig. 7-9. Diagrammatic representation of oogenesis.

of the oocyte and follicle, and does not complete the first meiotic division until the follicle reaches maturity at the preovulatory stage. Resumption of meiosis beyond the dictyate stage in the mammalian oocyte depends upon the ovulatory surge of luteinizing hormone.

The granulosa cells form a diffusion barrier between the blood and the oocyte so that the ovarian follicle provides the oocyte with an appropriate environment for oocyte nourishment and maturation. This includes the maintenance of an intrafollicular temperature, particularly at the preovulatory stage, which is about 2° to 3°C lower than the systemic temperature in the female rabbit and woman. The primordial follicle consists of a primary oocyte surrounded by a single layer of follicular cells which will proliferate and develop into the membrana granulosa. Follicles containing more than one oocyte occur rarely in adult domestic animals. However, follicles with mutliple oocytes are seen in the fetal ovaries and in ovaries of newborn queens and bitches. At first, the follicular cells are in intimate contact with the vitelline membrane, or cellular membrane of the oocyte. As the

follicle grows, a complex glycoproteic layer, which will form the zona pellucida, is deposited in isolated patches between the vitelline membrane and the inner layer of granulosa cells, or corona radiata. These patches of zona material gradually coalesce to form a continuous structure around the oocyte. As the follicle matures, the zona thickens by incorporating zona material produced by the follicular cells and possibly by the oocyte. There are species differences in the process of zona formation, but in general, it follows the general pattern indicated above. Processes from the corona cells and oocyte plasma membrane maintain contact between the granulosa and the oocyte. These cellular extensions probably serve to nourish the oocyte. Contact between the oocyte and the granulosa cells may prevent maturation of the oocyte beyond the dictyate stage through some factor produced by the granulosa cells. A small peptide factor called oocyte maturation inhibitor (OMI) is presumed to maintain the oocyte in the dictyate stage of meiosis. OMI appears to be produced by the granulosa cells of the follicle (Fig. 7-10). OMI is present in the developing follicles and its concentration in the follicular fluid declines as the follicles mature. So far as is now known, OMI is absent in the follicular fluid of ovulatory follicles. The ovulatory surge of LH presumably blocks the transfer of OMI from the cumulus cells to the oocyte allowing meiosis to resume at the time of ovulation (Fig. 7-10). Oocytes isolated from preovulatory follicles resume meiosis spontaneously *in vitro*. Oocytes in developing follicles remain at the dictyate stage when cultured *in vitro*, unless they have been exposed to gonadotropins *in vivo* or gonadotropins are added to the culture medium.

As the follicle grows, lacunae are formed between the follicular cells. These lacunae coalesce to form an antrum which fills with the liquor folliculi. At this stage the primary oocyte is surrounded by a mass of granulosa cells which projects into the antrum. Many of the follicular cells in this mass, the cumulus oophorus, will be expelled with the oocyte at ovulation. During follicular growth, cells of

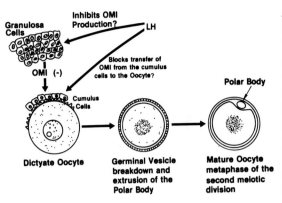

Fig. 7-10. Postulated control of meiotic maturation of mammalian oocytes. (*Adapted from*: Tsafriri, A., et al.: J. Reprod. Fertil. *64*:541, 1982.)

the surrounding connective tissue differentiate as theca interna and theca externa.

At the termination of follicular growth, the oocyte resumes the meiotic, or maturation, divisions. During the first division, the oocyte nucleus migrates toward the plasma membrane, the nuclear membrane and nucleoli disappear, and the chromosomes undergo the first meiotic division. Half of the chromatin and a small amount of cytoplasm are extruded as the first polar body.

In most domestic species, the first meiotic division is completed a few hours before ovulation, and the cell is then a secondary oocyte. (Fig. 7-9) In the bitch, however, the first maturation division and abstriction of the first polar body occur after ovulation (Fig. 7-9). Abstriction of the first polar body may be delayed for a few days following ovulation, and this delay probably accounts for the prolonged period of viability of tubal oocytes (up to 7 days) observed in this species.

The mare is a special case; in some mares the oocyte is ovulated at the dictyate stage, as in the bitch, and the abstriction of the first polar body occurs in the oviduct. In other mares, the first meiotic division is completed shortly before ovulation and the oocyte is ovulated as a secondary oocyte.

Except for the bitch and some mares, the secondary oocyte enters the second meiotic division and is usually in metaphase II at ovulation. The tubal oocyte normally completes the second maturation division when a spermatozoon penetrates the zona pellucida to "activate" the oocyte (Fig. 7-11). When the oocyte is activated, the second maturation division is completed with the formation of the second polar body. At this time, the germ cell is momentarily an ootid. The first polar body occasionally undergoes division to form two polar bodies.

The fate of unfertilized oocytes has been studied in several species. In most laboratory and domesticated animals, fertilized and unfertilized oocytes reach the uterus in 3 to 6 days after ovulation. The unfertilized oocytes of most species undergo degeneration and fragmentation in the uterus. In the mare, only fertilized oocytes pass through the oviduct and enter the uterus, whereas unfertilized oocytes are retained and degeneration and fragmentation of the unfertilized oocyte occur in the oviduct.

FERTILIZATION

Fertilization can be defined as a multiple step phenomenon initiated by the interaction, binding, and subsequent fusion of the male and female gametes. This process culminates in the formation of a single cell of a new individual, conventionally called the zygote, which has biparental nuclear heredity. From the embryological and genetic points of view, the essential aspect of fertilization is the association of the maternal (from the oocyte) and the paternal (from the spermatozoon) genomes.

Gametic Encounter

Spermatozoa unite with oocytes in the ampulla of the oviduct where fertilization occurs in domestic species. Testicular spermatozoa of most species are immotile, and movement into the epididymis is entirely passive. The forces involved include the pressure of spermatozoa and fluids in the seminiferous tubules, ciliary movements in the efferent ductuli and epididymis, absorption of seminal fluid from the epididymis and epididymal contractions. In the epididymis, sperms are moved passively toward the epididymal tail. Ejaculated sperms are motile.

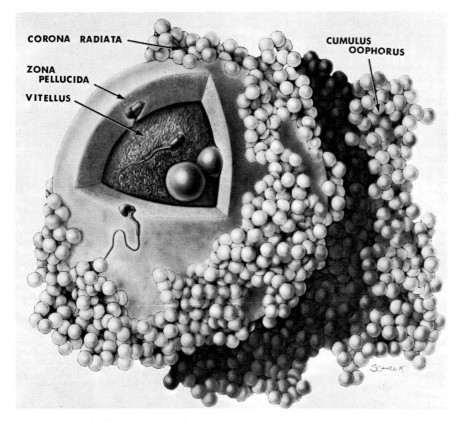

CORONA RADIATA

ZONA PELLUCIDA

VITELLUS

CUMULUS OOPHORUS

Fig. 7-11. Drawing of the layers surrounding the rabbit ovum. (From Gould, K. G.: Fed. Proc. *32*:2071, 1973.)

Ejaculation is the result of a series of muscular contractions along the male excurrent tract. The neural impulse is initiated by thermal and pressure receptors which are located primarily in the glans penis. The afferent pathway is via the internal pudic nerve to the lumbosacral section of the cord. The efferent impulse is via nerves of the hypogastric plexus.

During mating or artificial insemination, the estrogen-sensitized uterus responds with muscular contractions due to the reflexogenic release of oxytocin in response to genital stimulation. At least for a short time after mating or insemination, uterine contractions are far more important than spermatozoan motility in spermatozoal transport. However, spermatozoan motility does enhance the probability of a sperm-oocyte collision.

Ovulated oocytes normally enter the fimbria of the ipsilateral oviduct, which is in close contact with the ovary during estrus. The proper transport of fertilized eggs in the oviducts is essential to assure their arrival in the uterus at the proper time. Premature or delayed arrival results in embryonal death. Transport in the oviducts depends upon ciliary movements, segmental and peristaltic contractions of the oviduct, and probably the flow of oviductal secretions.

Oocytes are capable of fertilization and development 12 to 24 hours following ovulation in most species. In the bitch, the oocyte may be viable and fertilizable for several days after ovulation. Fertility is highest in the ampulla, decreases significantly in the isthmus, and is lost in the uterus.

Ejaculated spermatozoa of several mammalian species must be exposed to the female reproductive tract for a variable period of time before attaining the capacity to fertilize oocytes. This process of preparing a spermatozoon for the *in vivo* fertilization is termed capacitation. The secretions of the uterus and oviducts participate in the capacitation process, and the follicular fluid released at ovulation may also contribute to capacitation.

A need for the capacitation of ejaculated spermatozoa has been demonstrated for the bull, boar, cat and several species of laboratory rodents. The evidence for the necessity of capacitation in the ram, stallion, dog, and man is equivocal. It is generally believed that capacitation involves release or activation of enzymes, possibly associated with loosening or detachment of the acrosome, which enhance spermatozoal penetration of the cumulus and zona pellucida.

Capacitation can be reversed in previously capacitated spermatozoa by incubating them in seminal plasma. Thus, capacitation would involve the destruction or removal of a macromolecular decapacitation factor in seminal plasma. Spermatozoa collected from the proximal part of the vas deferens in cats or from the epididymal tail in rabbits can fertilize oocytes *in vitro* without a period of *in vivo* capacitation. Even though spermatozoal viability may not always be optimal when deposited in a foreign female tract, *in vivo* interspecies spermatozoal capacitation is possible. Furthermore, seminal plasma from the bull, boar, stallion, dog, and tomcat contain decapacitating activity for rabbit spermatozoa, suggesting that the decapacitation factor is not species-specific. The presence or absence of decapacitation factor in the seminal plasma of a given species may indicate the requirement for capacitation to occur in that species (Table 7-5). Spermatozoa from several species have been "capacitated" *in vitro* by incubation with enzymes or by inactivation in chemically defined media. *In vivo*, capacitation may represent a selective process to prevent fertilization by weak or abnormal sperms, since the cells must survive several hours in the female tract. Capacitation is more effective during the estrous phase of the ovarian cycle than during the progestational phase, and the efficiency of capacitation

Table 7-5 Need for Capacitation of Ejaculated Spermatozoa

Species	Capacitation Required	Decapacitation Factor
Ram	Probably	?
Bull	Yes	Yes
Boar	Yes	Yes
Stallion	Probably	Yes
Dog	Probably	Yes
Cat	Yes	Yes
Man	Probably	Yes

seems to be related to optimal levels of estrogens and gonadotropins, since it may be modified by exogenous hormones.

In the oviduct, encounters between spermatozoa and oocytes depend upon the number of oocytes, concentration and motility of spermatozoa, and slight movements of the oocytes. Thus, the transport of a population of spermatozoa, which have the capability to fertilize the oocyte, from the site of seminal deposition in the female genitals to the ampullary region of the oviducts is essential for successful fertilization.

Tubal oocytes of some mammals are surrounded by granulosa cells (corona radiata and cumulus oophorous) for several hours. Enzymes in sperm heads are released, exposed, or activated to attack and penetrate successive oocyte investments. The cumulus of most domestic species disintegrates within a few hours after ovulation. Hyaluronidase from spermatozoa may in some species enhance penetration of the cumulus (Figs. 7-12A and 7-13A, B). Acrosomal enzymes exposed during the acrosomal reaction disperse the cumulus and corona radiata (Fig. 7-12B). Proteolytic activity is essential to penetration of the zona pellucida, which appears to be the most difficult of the oocyte envelopes for the spermatozoa to penetrate. Active dispersal factors, such as neuraminidase and trypsin-like enzymes, such as acrosin, in addition to hyaluronidase, are present in the acrosome. During passage through the zona pellucida, the spermatozoon loses its plasma membrane and gradually loses its

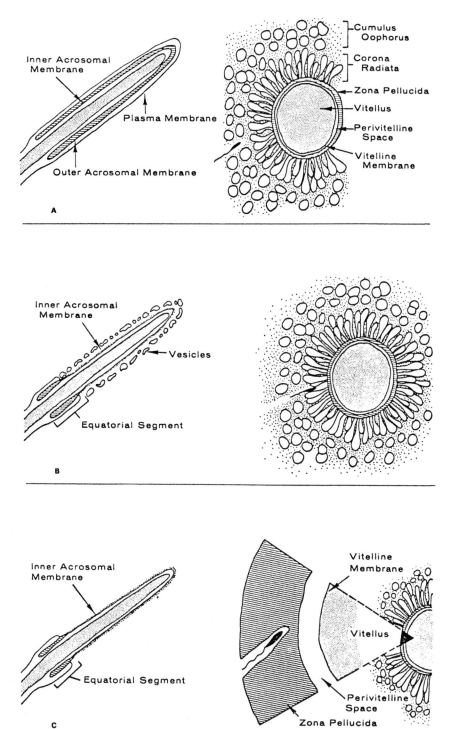

Fig. 7-12. Penetration of sperm. A, Status of capacitated sperm (left) as it penetrates cumulus (right). B, Acrosome reaction of sperm (left) as it penetrates corona (right). C, Status of reacted sperm (left) as it penetrates zona (right). (From McRorie, R. A., and Williams, W. L. Reproduced, with permission, from the Ann. Rev. of Biochem., *43*:778, 779. © 1974 by Annual Reviews, Inc.)

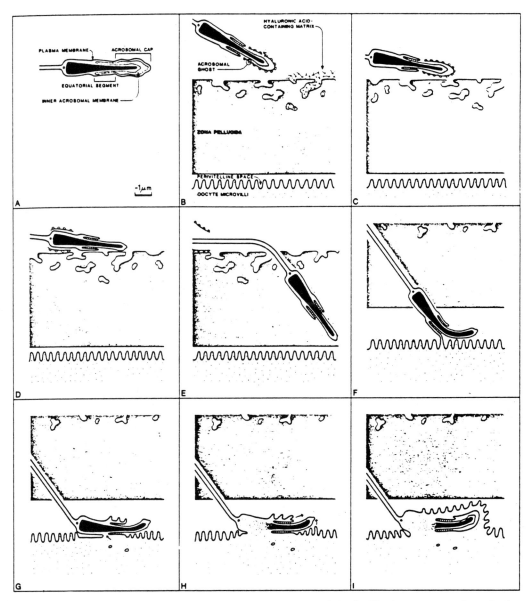

Fig. 7-13. Schematic diagram showing ultrastructural aspects of the fertilization sequence in eutherian mammals. A. An unreacted mammalian sperm head is shown; the acrosome consists of a cap and equatorial segment. The site of initiation of the acrosome reaction is not known, but it is probably the cumulus/corona radiata or zona pellucida surface. B. A sperm that has started a normal acrosome reaction is shown; the plasma membrane and outer acrosomal membrane have vesiculated, and the soluble acrosomal vesicle contents (AVC) can escape. The acrosomal ghost is formed. A granule/filament matrix containing hyaluronic acid is present in the cumulus/corona radiata and outer region of the zona pellucida (only a small portion of this matrix is shown). In some species, this matrix is also abundant in the perivitelline space. C. The sperm has attached to the zona pellucida surface by its acrosomal ghost (vesicle plus insoluble AVC.) D. The sperm then swims through a split in the anterior aspect of the ghost. E. The sperm enters the zona pellucida at an angle; the equatorial segment remains intact, and the ghost is left on the zona surface. A narrow slit forms in the zona. F, G. The sperm enters the perivitelline space, where oocyte microvilli fuse with the plasma membrane overlying the equatorial segment. H. Ooplasm flows into the sperm, and the posterior aspect of the nucleus begins decondensing. I. The perforatorium enters the oocyte last, probably in a phagocytic vesicle. In stages G and H, the sperm head bends. The equatorial segment is drawn into the oocyte while the anterior and posterior regions deflect upward toward the zona pellucida. These diagrams are approximately to scale.

outer acrosomal membrane (Fig. 7-13C to E). Cells reaching the vitelline (plasma) membrane are divested of the acrosome (Fig. 7-12C). Upon entrance of the spermatozoa into the perivitelline space, microvilli from the oocyte plasma membrane fuse with the plasma membrane at the equatorial segment of the spermatozoon (Fig. 7-13F, G). Cytoplasmic materials from the oocyte mix with that of the spermatozoon (Fig. 7-13H). The interaction of spermatozoal components with the oocyte cytoplasm is essential for the formation of the male pronucleus (Fig. 7-13I).

Oocytes of higher mammals normally undergo monospermic fertilization. The zona pellucida of most mammals allows a single spermatozoon to reach the plasma membrane. The zona pellucida is an effective barrier to prevent the fertilization of an oocyte by spermatozoa from a different species. Enzymatic digestion of the zona pellucida allows for interspecies fertilization *in vitro*. In the rabbit and a few other mammals, several spermatozoa (supplementary sperm) penetrate the zona to reach the perivitelline space, but only a single spermatozoon normally penetrates the vitellus. Thus, monospermic fertilization safeguards the constancy of the DNA content for the species. Among domestic animals, the primary block to polyspermy is a reaction in the zona pellucida. The reaction is secondary to changes in the vitelline cortex and the release of agents which alter the zona pellucida. Aging of mammalian eggs decreases the efficiency of the block to polyspermy.

Fertilization is associated with three major events: (1) the continuation of meiosis in the oocyte; (2) sperm penetration and the development of the parental pronuclei; and (3) the early stages of mitosis. A detailed description of the events of fertilization is beyond the scope of this chapter. The reader is urged to refer to the references listed in this chapter.

Experimental evidences accumulated over the past few years clearly indicate that cytoplasmic inheritance of mitochondrial DNA is an important component of eukaryotic inheritance. Mitochondria in all metazoan animals so far studied possess double-stranded DNA, which is distinguishable from nuclear DNA. The mitochondrial DNA is greatly amplified during oogenesis and mammalian oocytes are rich in mitochondria and mitochondrial DNA. It is estimated that an oocyte contains approximately 92,000 mitochondria. However, the number of mitochondria in the midpiece is low in the mammalian spermatozoa, about 72 mitochondria in the bull spermatozoon. Mitochondrial DNA is maternally inherited, that is the offsprings, regardless of their homo- or heterozygosity, including reciprocal crosses of horses and donkeys, will have the mitochondrial DNA of the mother. The maternal inheritance of mitochondrial DNA has been explained on the basis of the small number of mitochondria contributed to the oocyte by the fertilizing spermatozoon. The midpiece containing the spermatozoal mitochondria enters the oocyte at fertilization in several mammalian species. Thus, it is not possible to rule out a role of the paternal mitochondria on maternal mitochondrial replication during embryonic development. Maternal inheritance of the mitochondrial DNA may simply be the result of an overwhelming preponderance of maternal mitochondria in the oocyte.

Unequal amplification and segmentation of mitochondrial DNA during oogenesis and possibly polymorphism resulting from maternal and paternal mitochondrial interactions at fertilization, and subsequently during embryonic development, may influence the survivability of the embryo to term. A further understanding of cytoplasmic inheritance might allow for the improvement of production traits in livestock animals and resistance to diseases of importance to the veterinary profession.

Extraordinary Fertilization

Polyspermy (more than one sperm cell entering the ooplasm to form multiple male pronuclei) is pathological in mammals. Multiple pronuclei may also result from monospermic fertilization of binucleate eggs. Two female pronuclei may develop from binucleate primary oocytes or as a result of failure to abstrict the polar body at one of the maturation divisions. These multinucleate ova, like polyspermic ova, are destined to developmental failure, since the pronuclei fuse and polyploidy results. Few polyploid embryos survive to birth.

A single nucleus undergoes cleavage without syngamy in parthenogenesis, gynogenesis, and androgenesis. The oocyte nucleus is activated in the absence of fertilization to cause parthenogenesis. In gynogenesis the oocyte is activated by a spermatozoon which takes no further part in development. In androgenesis the oocyte nucleus fails to participate. The resulting embryos, like polyploid embryos, generally fail to develop to birth.

Development of the embryo is further discussed in Chapter 19.

REFERENCES

Sexuality

1. Bruere, A. N., Marshall, R. B., and Ward, D. P. J. (1969): Testicular hypoplasia and XXY sex chromosome complement in two rams: The ovine counterpart of Klinefelter's syndrome in man. J. Reprod. Fertil. *19*:103.
2. Buoen, L. C., Eilts, B. E., Rushmer, A., et al. (1983): Sterility associated with an XO karyotype in a Belgian mare. J. Am. Vet. Med. Assoc. *182*:1120.
3. Centerwall, W. R., and Benirschke, K. (1975): An animal model for the XXY Klinefelter's syndrome in man: tortoiseshell and calico male cats. Am. J. Vet. Res. *36*:1275.
4. Dunn, H. O., Lein, D. H., and Mc Entee, K. (1980): Testicular hypoplasia in a Hereford bull with 61, XXY karyotype: the bovine counterpart of human Klinefelter's Syndrome. Cornell Vet. *70*:137.
5. Epstein, C. J. (1983): Sex chromosome expression in embryonic development. Differentiation *23* (Suppl.): S31.
6. Garner, D. L., Glenhill, B. L., Pinkel, D., et al. (1983): Quantification of the X- and Y- chromosome-bearing spermatozoa of domestic animals by flow cytometry. Biol. Reprod. *28*:312.
7. Gartler, S. M., and Riggs, A. D. (1983): Mammalian X-chromosome inactivation. Ann. Rev. Genet. *17*: 155.
8. Gondos, B. (1980): Development and differentiation of the testis and male reproductive tract. *In* Testicular Development, Structure, and Function, edited by A. Steinberger and E. Steinberger, New York, Raven Press, p. 3.
9. Goodall, H., and Roberts, A. M. (1976): Differences in motility of human X- and Y-bearing spermatozoa. J. Reprod. Fertil. *48*:433.
10. Hare, W. C. D., and Betteridge, K. J. (1978): Relationship of embryo sexing to other methods of prenatal sex determination in farm animals: A review. Theriogenology *9*:27.
11. Hare, W. C. D., McFeely, R. A., and Kelly, D. F. (1974): Familial 78 XX male pseudohermaphroditism in three dogs. J. Reprod. Fertil. *36*:207.
12. Hernández-Jauregui, P., and Márquez, H. (1977): Fine structure of mule testes: Light and electron microscopy study. Am. J. Vet. Res. *38*:443.
13. Hunter, R. H. F., Baker, T. G., and Cook, B. (1982): Morphology, histology and steroid hormones of the gonads in intersex pigs. J. Reprod. Fertil. *64*:217.
14. Jost, A., and Magre, S. (1984): Testicular development phases and dual hormonal control of sexual organogenesis. *In* Sexual Differentiation: Basic and Clinical Aspects, edited by M. Serio et al., New York, Raven Press, p. 1.
15. Markert, C. L., and Petters, R. M. (1977): Homozygous mouse embryos produced by microsurgery. J. Exp. Zool. *201*:295.
16. McFeely, R. A. (1975): A review of cytogenetics in equine reproduction. J. Reprod. Fertil., (Suppl.) *23*:371.
17. Miyake, Y-I. (1973): Cytogenetical studies on swine intersexes. Jpn. J. Vet. Res. *21*:41.
18. Moruzzi, J. F. (1979): Selecting a mammalian species for the separation of X- and Y-chromosome-bearing spermatozoa. J. Reprod. Fertil. *57*:319.
19. Nalbandov, A. V. (1964): The biology of sex, Ch. 1 *In* Reproductive Physiology, 2nd ed. San Francisco, W. H. Freeman & Co., p. 3.
20. Napier, K. M., and Mullaney, P. D. (1974): Sex ratio in sheep. J. Reprod. Fertil. *39*:391.
21. Ohno, S. (1969): Evolution of sex chromosomes in mammals. Ann. Rev. Genet. *3*:495.
22. Picard, J.-Y., and Josso, N. (1984): Purification of testicular anti-Müllerian hormone allowing direct visualization of the pure glycoprotein and determination of yield and purification factor. Mol. Cell Endocrinol. *34*:23.
23. Quinlivan, W. L. G., Preciado, K., Long, T. L., et al (1982): Separation of human X and Y spermatozoa by albumin gradients and sephadex chromatography. Fertil. Steril. *37*:104.
24. Selden, J. R., Wachtel, S. S., Koo, G. C., et al. (1978): Genetic basis of XX male syndrome and XX true hermaphroditism: Evidence in the dog. Science *201*:644.
25. Short, R. V. (1975): The contribution of the mule to scientific thought. J. Reprod. Fertil., (Suppl.) *23*: 359.
26. Trujillo, J. M., Ohno, S., Jardine, F. H., et al. (1969): Spermatogenesis in a male hinny: Histological and cytological studies. J. Hered. *60*:79.
27. Vendeberg, J. L. (1983): Developmental aspects of X chromosome inactivation in eutherian and methaterian mammals. J. Exp. Zool. *228*:271.
28. Vigier B., Picard, J.-Y., and Josso, N. (1982): A monoclonal antibody against bovine anti-Müllerian hormone. Endocrinology *110*:131.
29. Vigier, B., Tran, D., Du Mesnil du Buisson, F., et al. (1983): Use of monoclonal antibody techniques to study the ontogeny of bovine anti-Müllerian hormone. J. Reprod. Fertil. *69*:207.
30. Wachtel, S. S. (1984): H-Y antigen in the study of sex determination and control of sex ratio. Theriogenology *21*:18.
31. White, K. L., Lindner, G. M., Anderson, G. B., et al. (1982): Survival after transfer of "sexed" mouse

embryos exposed to H-Y antisera. Theriogenology *18*:655.

32. Winter, H., and Pfeffer, A. (1977): Pathogenic classification of intersex. Vet. Rec. *100*:307.

Development of Male and Female Reproductive Organs

33. Allen, W. E., Daker, M. G., and Hancock, J. L. (1981): Three intersexual dogs. Vet. Rec. *109*:468.
34. Basrur, P. K., and Kanagawa, H. (1971): Sex anomalies in pigs. J. Reprod. Fertil. *26*:369.
35. Bruere, A. N., Fielden, E. D., and Hutchings, H. (1968): XX/XY mosaicism in lymphocyte cultures from a pig with freemartin characteristics. N. Z. Vet. J. *16*:31.
36. Donahoe, P. K., Ito, Y., Price, J. M., et al. (1977): Müllerian inhibiting substance activity in bovine fetal, newborn and prepubertal testes. Biol. Reprod. *16*:238.
37. Dunn, H. O., McEntee, K., Hall, C. E., et al. (1979): Cytogenetic and reproductive studies of bulls born cotwin with freemartins. J. Reprod. Fertil. *57*:21.
38. Gladue, B. A., Green, R., and Hellman, R. E. (1984): Neuroendocrine response to estrogen and sexual orientation. Science *225*:1496.
39. Gluhovschi, N., Bistricenau, M., Suciu, A., et al. (1970): A case of intersexuality in the horse with type 2A + XXXY chromosome formula. Br. Vet. J. *126*:522.
40. Greene, W. A., Mogil, L. G., Lein, D. H., et al. (1979): Growth and reproductive development in freemartins hormonally treated from 1 to 79 weeks of age. Cornell Vet. *69*:248.
41. Hare, W. C. D., McFeely, R. A., and Kelly, D. F. (1974): Familial 78 XX male pseudohermaphroditism in three dogs. J. Reprod. Fertil. *36*:207.
42. Hughes, J. P., and Trommershausen-Smith, A. (1977): Infertility in the horse associated with chromosomal abnormalities. Aust. Vet. J. *53*:253.
43. Josso, J. (1973): *In vitro* synthesis of Müllerian-inhibiting hormone by seminiferous tubules isolated from the calf fetal testis. Endocrinology *93*:829.
44. Josso, N., Forest, M. G., and Picard, J-Y. (1975): Müllerian-inhibiting activity of calf fetal testes: Relationship to testosterone and protein synthesis. Biol. Reprod. *13*:163.
45. Jost, A., Vigier, B., and Prepin, J. (1972): Freemartins in cattle: The first steps of sexual organogenesis. J. Reprod. Fertil. *29*:349.
46. Meck, J. M. (1984): The genetics of the H-Y antigen system and its role in sex determination. Perspect. Biol. Med. *27*:561.
47. Mittwoch, U., Delhanty, D. A., and Beck, F. (1969): Growth of differentiating testes and ovaries. Nature *224*:1323.
48. Nalbandov, A. V. (1964): Reproductive Physiology, 2nd ed. San Francisco, W. H. Freeman & Co., p. 5.
49. Ohno, S., Nagai, Y., Ciccarese, S., et al. (1979): Testis-organizing H-Y antigen and the primary sex-determining mechanism of mammals. Recent Progr. Horm. Res. *35*:449.
50. Saba, N., Cunningham, N. F., and Millar, P. G. (1975): Plasma progesterone, androstenedione and testosterone concentrations in freemartin heifers. J. Reprod. Fertil. *45*:37.
51. Sharp, A. J., Wachtel, S. S., and Benirschke, K. (1980): H-Y antigen in a fertile XY female horse. J. Reprod. Fertil. *58*:157.
52. Shore, L. S., Shemesh, M., and Mileguir, F. (1984): Foetal testicular steroidogenesis and responsiveness to LH in freemartins and their male co-twins. Int. J. Androl. *7*:87.
53. Turner, C. D. (1960): The Biology of Sex and Reproduction, Ch. 8. *In* General Endocrinology, 3rd ed. Philadelphia. W. B. Saunders Co., p. 272.
54. Vigier, B., Tran, D., Legeai, L., et al. (1984): Origin of anti-mullerian hormone in bovine freemartin fetuses. J. Reprod. Fertil. *70*:473.
55. Wai-Sum, O., and Baker, T. G. (1978): Germinal and somatic cell interrelationships in gonadal sex differentiation. Ann. Biol. Anim. Biochim. Biophys. *18*:351.
56. Wachtel, S. S., Hall, J. L., and Cahill, L. T. (1981): H-Y antigen in primary sex determination. *In* Bioregulators of Reproduction, 1st ed., edited by G. Jagiello and H. J. Vogel, New York, Academic Press, p. 9.
57. Wijeratne, W. V. S., Munro, I. B., and Wilkes, P. R. (1977): Heifer sterility associated with single-birth freemartinism. Vet. Rec. *100*:333.

Sexual Behavior

58. Aronson, L. R., and Cooper, M. L. (1974): Olfactory deprivation and mating behavior in sexually experienced male cats. Behav. Biol. *11*:459.
59. Wartenberg, H. (1983): Morphological aspects of gonadal differentiation. Structural aspects of gonadal differentiation in mammals and birds. Differentiation *23* (Suppl.):S64.
60. Bland, K. P. (1979): Tom-cat odour and other pheromones in feline reproduction. Vet. Sci. Comm. *3*: 125.
61. Bronson, F. H. (1971): Rodent pheromones. Biol. Reprod. *4*:344.
62. Brooks, P. H., and Cole, D. J. A. (1970): The effect of the presence of a boar on the attainment of puberty in gilts. J. Reprod. Fertil. *23*:435.
63. Bruce, H. M. (1960): A block of pregnancy in the mouse caused by proximity of strange males. J. Reprod. Fertil. *1*:96.
64. Doty, R. L., and Dunbar, I. (1974): Attraction of Beagles to conspecific urine, vaginal and anal sac secretion odors. Physiol. Behav. *12*:825.
65. Doty, R. L., and Mare, C. J. (1974): Color, odor, consistency and secretion rate of anal sac secretions from male, female, and early androgenized female Beagles. Am. J. Vet. Res. *35*:669.
66. Edgar, D. G., and Bilkey, D. A. (1964): The influence of rams on the onset of the breeding season in ewes. Proc. N. Z. Soc. Anim. Prod. *23*:79.
67. Gower, D. B. (1972): 16-unsaturated C_{19} steroids. A review of their chemistry, biochemistry and possible physiological role. J. Steroid Biochem. *3*:45.
68. Hopkins, S. G., Schubert, T. A., and Hart, B. L. (1976): Castration of adult male dogs: Effects on roaming, aggression, urine marking, and mounting. J. Am. Vet. Med. Assoc. *168*:1108.
69. Levine , S. (1966): Sex differences in the brain. Sci.

Am. *214*:84.

70. Lindsay, D. R. (1965): The importance of olfactory stimuli in the mating behavior of the ram. Anim. Behav. *13*:75.

71. Signoret, J. P. (1974): Rôle des différentes informations sensorielles dans l'attraction de la femelle en oestrus par le mâle chez les porcins. Ann. Biol. Anim. Biochim. Biophys. *14*:747.

72. Tischner, M., Kosiniak, K., and Bielański, W. (1974): Analysis of the pattern of ejaculation in stallions. J. Reprod. Fertil. *41*:329.

73. Wheeler, J. W. (1976): Insect and mammalian pheromones, Lloydia *39*:53.

74. Whitten, W. K., Bronson, F. H., and Greenstein, J. A. (1968): Estrus-inducing pheromone of male mice: Transport by movement of air. Science *161*: 584.

75. Young, W. C., Goy, R. W., and Phoenix, C. H. (1964): Hormones and sex behavior. Science *143*: 212.

Gametogenesis

76. Amann, R. P., and Schanbacher, B. D. (1983): Physiology of male reproduction. J. Anim. Sci. *57*, Suppl. 2:380.

77. Andersen, A. C., and Simpson, M. E. (1973): The Ovary and Reproductive Cycle of the Dog (Beagle). Los Altos, California, Geron X, Inc., p. 48.

78. Bellvé, A. R., and Feig, L. A. (1984): Cell proliferation in the mammalian testis: Biology of the seminiferous growth factor (SGF). Rec. Progr. Horm. Res. *40*:531.

79. Berndtson, W. E. (1977): Methods for quantifying mammalian spermatogenesis: A review. J. Anim. Sci. *44*:818.

80. Berndtson, W. E., and Desjardins, C. (1974): The cycle of the seminiferous epithelium and spermatogenesis in the bovine testes. Am. J. Anat. *140*:167.

81. Burgoyne, P. S. (1978): The role of sex chromosomes in mammalian germ cell differentiation. Ann. Biol. Anim. Biochim. Biophys. *18*:317.

82. Clermont, Y. (1972): Kinetics of spermatogenesis in mammals: Seminiferous epithelium cycle and spermatogonial renewal. Physiol. Rev. *52*:198.

83. Dym, M., and Cavicchia, J. C. (1978): Functional morphology of the testis. Biol. Reprod. *18*:1.

84. Fawcett, D. W. (1975): The mammalian spermatozoan. Dev. Biol. *44*:394.

85. Flechon, J.-E., Pavlok, A., and Kopecný, J. (1984): Dynamics of zona pellucida formation by the mouse oocyte. An autoradiographic study. Cell. Biol. *51*: 403.

86. Flood, P. F., Jong, A., and Betteridge, K. J. (1979): The location of eggs retained in the oviducts of mares. J. Reprod. Fertil. *57*:291.

87. Fulka, J., Jr., and Okolski, A. (1981): Culture of horse oocytes in vitro. J. Reprod. Fertil. *61*:213.

88. Foote, R. H., Swiestra, E. E., and Hunt, W. L. (1972): Spermatogenesis in the dog. Anat. Rec. *173*:341.

89. Grinsted, J., Kjer, J. J., Blendstrup, K., et al. (1985): Is low temperature of the follicular fluid prior to ovulation necessary for normal oocyte development? Fertil. Steril. *43*:34.

90. Hochereau de Reviers, M. T., and Courot, M. (1978): Sertoli cells and development of seminiferous epithelium. Ann. Biol. Anim. Biochim. Biophys. *18*:573.

91. Ibach, B., Weissbadi, L., and Hilscher, B. (1976): Stages of the cycle of the seminiferous epithelium in the dog. Andrologia *8*:297.

92. Johnson, L., and Nguyen, H. B. (1986): Annual cycle of the Sertoli cell population in adult stallions. J. Reprod. Fertil. *76*:311.

93. Johnson, L., and Thompson, D. L., Jr. (1983): Age-related and seasonal variation in the Sertoli cell population, daily sperm production and serum concentrations of follicle-stimulating hormone, luteinizing hormone and testosterone in stallions. Biol. Reprod. *29*:777.

94. Johnson, L., Amann, R. P., and Pickett, B. W. (1978): Scanning electron and light microscopy of the equine seminiferous tubule. Fertil. Steril. *29*: 208.

95. Johnson, L., Zane, R. S., Petty, C. S., et al. (1984): Quantification of the human Sertoli cell population: its distribution, relation to germ cell number, and age-related decline. Biol. Reprod. *31*:785.

96. Hyttel, P., Callesen, H., and Greve, T. (1986): Ultrastructural features of preovulatory oocyte maturation in superovulated cattle. J. Reprod. Fertil. *76*:645.

97. Kennelly, J. J. (1972): Coyote reproduction. I. The duration of the spermatogenic cycle and epididymal sperm transport. J. Reprod. Fertil. *31*:163.

98. Kruip, T. A. M., Cran, D. G., Van Beneden, T. H., et al. (1983): Structural changes in bovine oocytes during final maturation in vivo. Gamete Res. *8*:29.

99. Lok, D., Weenk, D., and De Rooij, D. G. (1982): Morphology, proliferation, and differentiation of undifferentiated spermatogonia in the chinese hamster and the ram. Anat. Rec. *203*:83.

100. Mather, J. P., Gunsalus, G. L., Musto, N. A., et al. (1983): The hormonal and cellular control of Sertoli cell secretion. J. Steroid Biochem. *19*:41.

101. Mauléon, P. (1967): Cinétique de l'ovogenèse chez les mammifères. Arch. d'Anat. Microsc. Morphol. Exp. *56*:125.

102. Mauléon, P., and Mariana, J. C. (1977): Oogenesis and folliculogenesis. *In* Reproduction in Domestic Animals, 3rd ed., edited by H. H. Cole and P. T. Cupps. New York, Academic Press, Inc, p. 175.

103. Motlik, J., and Fulka, J. (1976): Breakdown of the germinal vesicle in pig oocytes in vivo and in vitro. J. Exp. Zool. *198*:155.

104. Oakberg, E. F. (1978): Differential spermatogonial stem-cell survival and mutation frequency. Mutat. Res. *50*:327.

105. Ohuma, H., and Ohnamiu, Y. (1975): Retention of tubal eggs in mares. J. Reprod. Fertil., Suppl. *23*: 507.

106. Osman, D. I., and Plöen, L. (1979): Fine structure of the modified Sertoli cells in the terminal segment of the seminiferous tubules of the bull, ram and goat. Anim. Reprod. Sci. *2*:343.

107. Pedersen, H., and Seidel, G., Jr. (1972): Micropapillae: A local modification of the cell surface observed in rabbit oocytes and adjacent follicle cells.

J. Ultrastruct. Res. *39:*540.

108. Ross, M. H. (1976): The Sertoli cell junctional specialization during spermiogenesis and at spermiation. Anat. Rec. *186:*79.

109. Ross, G. T., and Lipsett, M. B. (1978): Homologies of structure and function in mammalian testes and ovaries. Int. J. Androl. Suppl. *2:*39.

110. Setchell, B. P., and Waites, G. M. H. (1975): The blood-testis barrier. *In* Handbook of Physiology, Section 7: Endocrinology, Vol. V. Male Reproductive System. edited by D. W. Hamilton and R. O. Greep. Washington, American Physiological Society, pp. 143.

111. Shehata, R. (1974): Polyovular graafian follicles in a newborn kitten with a study of polyovuly in the cat. Acta Anat. *89:*21.

112. Staigmiller, R. B., and Moor, R. M. (1984): Effect of follicle cells on the maturation and development competence of ovine oocytes matured outside the follicle. Gamete Res. *9:*221.

113. Steffenhagen, W. P., Pineda, M. H., and Ginther, O. J. (1972): Retention of unfertilized ova in uterine tubes of mares. Am. J. Vet. Res. *33:*2391.

114. Steinberger, A. (1979): Inhibin production by Sertoli cells in culture. J. Reprod. Fertil. *26:*31.

115. Steinberger, A., Heindel, J. J., Lindsay, J. N., et al. (1975): Isolation and culture of FSH responsive sertoli cells. Endocr. Res. Commun. *2:*261.

116. Swierstra, E. E. (1968): Cytology and duration of the cycle of the seminiferous epithelium of the boar; duration of the spermatozoan transit through the epididymis. Anat. Rec. *161:*171.

117. Swierstra, E. E., Gebauer, M. R., and Pickett, B. W. (1974): Reproductive physiology of the stallion. I. Spermatogenesis and testis composition. J. Reprod. Fertil. *40:*113.

118. Tesoriero, J. V. (1984): Comparative cytochemistry of the developing ovarian follicles of the dog, rabbit, and mouse: origin of the zona pellucida. Gamete Res. *10:*301.

119. Thibault, C., Gerard, M., and Menezo, Y. (1975): Preovulatory and ovulatory mechanisms in oocyte maturation. J. Reprod. Fertil. *45:*605.

120. Thompson, R. S., and Zamboni, L. (1975): Anomalous patterns of mammalian oocyte maturation and fertilization. Am. J. Anat. *142:*233.

121. Tsafriri, A., and Channing, C. (1975): An inhibitory influence of granulosa cells and follicular fluid upon porcine oocyte meiosis in vitro. Endocrinology *96:*922.

122. Tsafriri, A., Debel, N., and Bar-Ami, S. (1982): The role of oocyte maturation inhibitor in follicular regulation of oocyte maturation. J. Reprod. Fertil. *64:*541.

123. Tsutsumi, Y., Suzuki, H., Takeda, T., et al. (1979): Evidence of the origin of the gelatinous masses in the oviducts of mares. J. Reprod. Fertil. *57:*287.

124. Vanha-Pertula, T. (1978): Spermatogenesis and hydrolytic enzymes. A review. Ann. Biol. Anim. Biochim. Biophys. *18:*633.

125. Van den Wiel, D. F. M., Bar-Ami, S., Tsafriri, A., et al. (1983): Oocyte maturation inhibitor, inhibin and steroid concentrations in porcine follicular fluid at various stages of the oestrous cycle. J. Reprod. Fertil. *68:*247.

126. Van Niekerk, C. H., and Gerneke, W. H. (1966): Persistence and parthenogenic cleavage of tubal ova in the mare. Onderstepoort. J. Vet. Res. *31:*195.

127. Webel, S. K., Franklin, V., Harland, B., et al. (1977): Fertility, ovulation and maturation of eggs in mares injected with hCG. J. Reprod. Fertil. *51:*337.

128. Zamboni, L. (1970): Ultrastructure of mammalian oocytes and ova. Biol. Reprod. *2:*44.

129. Zamboni, L. (1974): Fine morphology of the follicle wall and follicle cell-oocyte association. Biol. Reprod. *10:*125.

Fertilization

130. Anderson, G. B. (1977): Fertilization, early development, and embryo transfer. *In* Reproduction in Domestic Animals, 3rd ed., edited by H. H. Cole and P. T. Cupps. New York, Academic Press, Inc., p. 286.

131. Bahr, G. F., and Engler, W. F. (1970): Considerations of volume, mass, DNA, and arrangement of mitochondria in the midpiece of bull spermatozoa. Exp. Cell Res. *60:*338.

132. Bedford, J. M. (1970): Sperm capacitation and fertilization in mammals. Biol. Reprod. Suppl. *2:*128.

133. Bedford, J. M. (1983): Significance of the need for sperm capacitation before fertilization in eutherian mammals. Biol. Reprod. *28:*108.

134. Bell, B. R., McDaniel, B. T., and Robinson, O. W. (1985): Effects of cytoplasmic inheritance on production traits of dairy cattle. J. Dairy Sci. *68:*2038.

135. Berruti, G. (1981): Multiple forms of bovine acrosin: purification and characterization. Comp. Biochem. Physiol. *69B:*323.

136. Bowen, R. (1977): Fertilization in vitro of feline ova by spermatozoa from the ductus deferens. Biol. Reprod. *17:*144.

137. Brackett, B. G. (1973): Mammalian fertilization *in vitro*. Fed. Proc. *32:*2065.

138. Brackett, B. G. (1981): Applications of in vitro fertilization. *In* New Technologies in Animal Breeding edited by B. G. Brackett et al., New York, Academic Press, p. 141.

139. Brackett, B. G., Hall, J. L., and Oh, Y-K (1978): In vitro fertilizing ability of testicular, epididymal, and ejaculated rabbit spermatozoa. Fertil. Steril. *29:*571.

140. Corselli, J., and Talbot, P. (1986): An in vitro technique to study penetration of hamster oocyte-cumulus complexes by using physiological numbers of sperm. Gamete Res. *13:*293.

141. Dale, B., and Monroy, A. (1981): How is polyspermy prevented? Gamete Res. *4:*151.

142. Dukelow, W. R. (1971): Bioassay techniques related to sperm capacitation. Acta Endocrinol. *66:*503.

143. Esbenshade, K. L., and Clegg, E. D. (1980): Acrosome reaction of sperm incubated in the uterus of gilts. Am. J. Vet. Res. *41:*1137.

144. Francisco, J. F., Brown, G. G., and Simpson, M. V. (1979): Further studies in types A and B rat mtDNAs: cleavage maps and evidence for cytoplasmic inheritance in mammals. Plasmid *2:*426.

145. Gould, K. G. (1973): Application of *in vitro* fertilization. Fed. Proc. *32:*2069.

146. Grivell, L. A. (1983): Mitochondrial DNA. Sci. Am. *248*:78.

147. Hamner, C. E., Jennings, L. L., and Sojka, N. J. (1970): Cat (Felis catus L.) spermatozoa require capacitation. J. Reprod. Fertil. *23*:477.

148. Harper, M. J. K. (1970): Cytological observations on sperm penetration of rabbit eggs. J. Exp. Zool. *174*:141.

149. Herz, Z., Northey, D., Lawyer, M., et al. (1985): Acrosome reaction of bovine spermatozoa in vivo: sites and effects of stages of the estrous cycle. Biol. Reprod. *32*:1163.

150. Holst, P. A., and Phemister, R. D. (1974): Onset of diestrus in Beagle bitch: definition and significance. Am. J. Vet. Res. *35*:401.

151. Hunter, R. H. F. (1977): Physiological factors influencing ovulation, fertilization, early embryonic development and establishment of pregnancy in pigs. Br. Vet. J. *133*:461.

152. Hunter, R. H. F., and Dziuk, P. J. (1968): Sperm penetration of pig eggs in relation to timing of ovulation and insemination. J. Reprod. Fertil. *15*:199.

153. Hunter, R. H. F., and Hall, J. P. (1974): Capacitation of boar spermatozoa: Synergism between uterine and tubal environments. J. Exp. Zool. *188*:203.

154. Hutchinson, C. A., III, Nebold, J. E., Potter, S. S., et al. (1974): Maternal inheritance of mammalian mitochondrial DNA. Nature *251*:536.

155. Iritani, A., and Niwa, K. (1977): Capacitation of bull spermatozoa and fertilization in vitro of cattle follicular oocytes matured in culture. J. Reprod. Fertil. *50*:119.

156. Leman, A. D., and Dziuk, P. J. (1971): Fertilization and development of pig follicular oocytes. J. Reprod. Fertil. *26*:387.

157. Longo, F. J. (1973): Fertilization: A comparative ultrastructural review. Biol. Reprod. *9*:149.

158. Mahi, C. A., and Yanagimachi, R. (1978): Capacitation, acrosome reaction, and egg penetration by canine spermatozoa in a simple defined medium. Gamete Res. *1*:101.

159. Mahi, C. A., and Yanagimachi, R. (1976): Maturation and sperm penetration of canine ovarian oocytes in vitro. J. Exp. Zool. *196*:189.

160. Mattner, P. E. (1963): Capacitation of ram sperm and penetration of the ovine egg. Nature *199*:772.

161. McLaren, A. (1974): Fertilization, implantation and cleavage. In Reproduction in Farm Animals, 3rd ed., edited by E. S. E. Hafez, Philadelphia, Lea & Febiger, p. 143.

162. McRorie, R. A., and Williams, W. L. (1974): Biochemistry of mammalian fertilization. Ann. Rev. Biochem. *43*:777.

163. Metz, C. B. (1972): Effects of antibodies on gametes and fertilization. Biol. Reprod. *6*:358.

164. Michaels, G. S., Hauswirth, W. W., and Laipis, P. J. (1982): Mitochondrial DNA copy number in bovine oocytes and somatic cells. Develop. Biol. *94*:246.

165. Moore, H. D. M., and Bedford, J. M. (1978): Ultrastructure of the equatorial segment of hamster spermatozoa during penetration of oocytes. J. Ultra-

struct. Res. *62*:110.

166. Moore, H. D. M., and Bedford, J. M. (1983): The interaction of mammalian gametes in the female. In: Mechanism and Control of Animal Fertilization, edited by J. F. Hartmann, New York, Academic Press, p. 453.

167. Morton, D. B. (1975): Acrosomal enzymes: Immunochemical localization of acrosin and hyaluronidase in ram spermatozoa. J. Reprod. Fertil. *45*: 375.

168. Oh, Y. K., and Brackett, B. G. (1975): Ultrastructure of rabbit ova recovered from ovarian follicles and inseminated in vitro. Fertil. Steril. *26*:665.

169. Overstreet, J. W., and Bedford, J. M. (1975): The penetrability of rabbit ova treated with enzymes or anti-progesterone antibody: A probe into the nature of a mammalian fertilizin. J. Reprod. Fertil. *44*:273.

170. Phillips, D. M. (1977): Surface of the equatorial segment of the mammalian acrosome. Biol. Reprod. *16*:128.

171. Plöen, L. (1971): A scheme of rabbit spermateleosis based upon electron microscopical observations. Z. Zellforsch. *115*:553.

172. Rogers, B. J. (1978): Mammalian sperm capacitation and fertilization in vitro: a critique of methodology. Gamete Res. *1*:165.

173. Saling, P. M., and Bedford, J. M. (1981): Absence of species specificity for mammalian sperm capacitation in vivo. J. Reprod. Fertil. *63*:119.

174. Singhas, C. A., and Oliphant, G. (1978): Ultrastructural observations of the time sequence of induction of acrosomal membrane alterations by ovarian follicular fluid. Fertil. Steril. *29*:194.

175. Srivastava, P. N., Munnell, J. F., Yang, C. H., et al. (1974): Sequential release of acrosomal membranes and acrosomal enzymes of ram spermatozoa. J. Reprod. Fertil. *36*:363.

176. Srivastava, P. N., Zaneveld, L. J. D., and Williams, W. L. (1970): Mammalian sperm acrosomal neuraminidases. Biochem. Biophys. Res. Commun. *39*: 575.

177. Talbot, P. (1985): Sperm penetration through oocyte investments in mammals. Am. J. Anat. *174*:331.

178. Thompson, R. S., and Zamboni, L. (1975): Anomalous patterns of mammalian oocyte maturation and fertilization. Am. J. Anat. *142*:233.

179. Vander Vliet, W. L., and Hafez, E. S. E. (1974): Survival and aging of spermatozoa: A review. Am. J. Obstet. Gynecol. *118*:1006.

180. Wagner, R. P. (1972): The role of maternal effects in animal breeding: II. Mitochondria and animal inheritance. J. Anim. Sci., *35*:1280.

181. Wassarman, P. M. (1983): Oogenesis: synthetic events in the developing mammalian egg. In Mechanism and Control of Animal Fertilization, edited by J. F. Hartmann, New York, Academic Press, p. 1.

182. Williams, W. L., Abney, T. O., Chernoff, H. N., et al. (1967): Biochemistry and physiology of decapacitation factor. J. Reprod. Fertil., Suppl. *2*:11.

Male Reproduction

M. H. PINEDA

8

The male gonads or testes are the primary organs of reproduction in the male. Both male and female gonads fulfill two functions: gametogenesis and steroidogenesis and share, in the adult animal, compartmentalization homologies: the Sertoli cells in the seminiferous tubules and the granulosa cells in the ovary form diffusion barriers between the germinal cells and the blood. These compartmentalizations provide a microenvironment for normal gametogenesis.

REGULATION OF GONADAL ACTIVITIES

Both gametogenic and steroidogenic testicular functions are regulated by the gonadotropins. Most of our knowledge of pituitary regulation of gonadal function is based upon the effects of hypophysectomy and replacement therapy. Unfortunately, hypophysectomy removes not only gonadotropins but also other pituitary tropins.

Hypophysectomy is a difficult surgical procedure in most species, and our knowledge of the effects of hypophysectomy is based upon data from a limited number of species. Moreover, it has not been possible to prepare gonadotropins free of contaminating pituitary hormone activities for use in replacement studies. Added to these are the problems of inadequate knowledge of the biological life, secretion, and metabolic clearance rates of a hormone for a given species. All of these factors influence the physiologic levels in the blood and in target tissues. Little is known on the activity of hormonal metabolites, and species specificity of gonadotropins. Hormone-specific antibodies have been used to study the sites of pituitary hormone production, circulating levels of pituitary hormones, and the binding of hormones to receptors in target tissues. Selective depletion of single pituitary hormones without disturbing the independent activities of other pituitary hormones may be achieved by monospecific, active, or passive immunization.

Control of Spermatogenesis

In general, the seminiferous tubules do not respond to gonadotropins in juvenile male mammals as they do in adult males, indicating an effect of somatic age independent of gonadotropins. Other factors, as yet unknown, must act upon the germinal cells to make them sensitive to gonadotropin stimulation.

There is no question, however, that the pituitary gland is essential to the function of seminiferous tubules. Normal spermatogenesis requires the synergistic activities of ICSH (LH), FSH, prolactin, androgens, and probably other hormones, as well (Fig. 8-1). Their respective roles in the spermatogenic process are not fully established, and the precise mechanisms and hormonal requirements for quantitative maintenance of normal spermatogenesis are unknown. The unavailability of pure LH and FSH complicates the separation of their roles in spermatogenesis. Experimental evidence suggests that ICSH stimulates both steroidogenic and gametogenic testicular functions. The stimulatory activity of ICSH on spermatogenesis appears to be indirect and exerted through the action of testosterone secreted by the Leydig cells. FSH is involved in spermiogenesis and spermiation by its activity on the Sertoli cells. The functional activity of the Sertoli cells shows cyclic variation in accordance to the complex requirements of spermatogenesis.

It is becoming evident that the activity of gonadotropic hormones on the testicular, gametogenic and steroidogenic cells is under the interactive control of intratesticular factors. These will be discussed in corresponding sections in this chapter.

Noxious Agents

In general, the sensitivity of germinal cells of the seminiferous epithelium to harmful agents increases as differentiation proceeds to the spermatid stage. One of the earliest changes due to harmful agents causing degeneration of the seminiferous epithelium is the appearance in the semen of spermatids and multinucleated cells from the luminal layers of the spermatogenic epithelium.

Degeneration due to irradiation is an exception to this rule, because irradiation produces its greatest destructive effect on dividing cells, and spermatogonia are more sensitive than spermatocytes. On the other hand, the most serious effects of irradiation, its nuclear effects, may be on the genetic apparatus. These effects would include mutations, translocations, and deletions. Spermatids are sensitive to the mutagenic effects of X-irradiation, spermatozoa are somewhat less sensitive, and spermatogonia are the least sensitive.

The interval between testicular damage and the appearance of changes in seminal quality depends on the cell types affected, the duration of spermatogenesis, and epididymal migration time in that species. Total epididymal migration time has been estimated to be 8 to 11 days in the bull, 13 days in the ram, 9 to 14 days in the boar, 3 to 7 days in the stallion, 14 days in the coyote, and 10 days in the rabbit. However, the transit time from the head to the body of the epididymis varies from 2 to 5 days for most of the species. This suggests that the time available for spermatozoal maturation in these two active areas of the epididymis is less than 5 days. If epididymal sperm are damaged, the semen is affected soon after application of the noxious agent. If the effect is on spermatogonia, the damage will not be apparent in the semen for several weeks after the damage is done.

In addition, the type of change in seminal quality is related to the type of damage produced, i.e., death of cells causes decreased numbers of sperm; abnormal spermateliosis results in morphological defects, and damage to the spermatozoal genetic apparatus results in embryonal and fetal death or teratogeny.

Sertoli cells are resistant to nearly all factors that harm germinal cells and are often the only tubular cells remaining after prolonged testicular insult. It remains possible, however, that damage to Sertoli cells is responsible for at least some of the apparent damage to germinal cells. For example, the sloughing of spermatids and formation of multinucleated cells may actually result from damage to Sertoli cells, even though their morphological integrity is undisturbed.

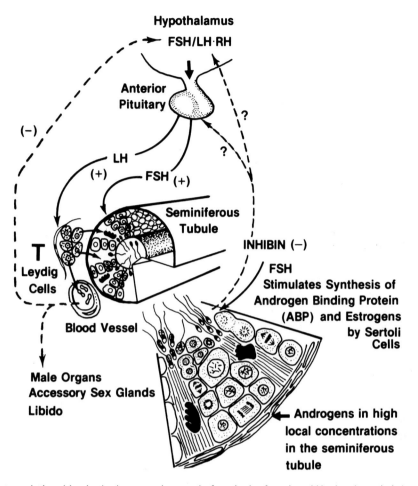

Fig. 8-1. Inter-relationships in the hormonal control of testicular function: LH stimulates (+) the secretion of testosterone by the Leydig cells, while FSH stimulates (+) the germinal epithelium and Sertoli cells. Testosterone (T) produced by the Leydig cells enters the systemic circulation, to reach and stimulate the androgen dependent organs of the male, and feedback negatively (−) on the hypothalamus decreasing release of GnRH (FSH/LH-RH). High local concentrations of testosterone stimulates the germinal epithelium. FSH stimulates the synthesis of androgen binding protein (ABP) and probably estrogens by the Sertoli cells. Inhibin secreted by the Sertoli cells suppresses plasma levels of FSH.

Seasonal Variations

Females of domestic mammals show reproductive periodicity (see Chapter 9), but males of these species show much less seasonal variation in testicular function. In general, the quality and fertility of ejaculates tend to be optimal during the reproductive season for the female of the species. Interestingly, male rats, as they gain sexual experience "learn" to discharge pituitary gonadotropins in anticipation to copulation. Similar situations occur in males from other species, such as bulls which which are trained and conditioned to regular and frequent ejaculations in artificial insemination centers. The presence of the female does not seem to be a requirement to evoke the response. For some species, seminal quality and male fertility tend to decline during the hot summer months, but it is not clear whether this is attributable to the effects of season on hypothalamo-hypophyseal pathways or to a direct effect of temperature on the testis and epididymis.

Scrotal Position

In a few species of mammals and in poultry, the testes function within the abdominal cavity. Normal, adult males of domestic mammals have scrotal testes, and the scrotal position is essential to normal gametogenic function. Males with bilateral cryptorchidism are sterile.

Experimentally, spermatogenesis is impaired when heat is applied to the scrotum or when the scrotum is insulated against heat loss. Degeneration is proportional to the degree and duration of temperature elevation.

Intrascrotal deposits of fat are also detrimental to spermatogenesis, probably because they act as insulators. There may be a genetic predisposition for the deposition of fat in the scrotum.

The scrotum, the cremaster muscles, and the spermatic vasculature constitute an efficient thermoregulatory mechanism (Fig. 8-2). The tunica dartos and cremaster muscles regulate scrotal surface area and the position of the testes with respect to the abdominal wall, and the spermatic artery and pampiniform plexus provide a heat-exchange mechanism.

Scrotal surface area and the position of the testes regulate heat loss. In hot weather, the tunica dartos and cremaster muscles are fully relaxed to allow maximum heat loss. In cold weather, these muscles contract to reduce heat loss. Arterial blood is cooled as it passes among the vessels of the pampiniform plexus and courses on the surface of the testicle before passing into the testis. Venous blood is warmed by heat exchange with the artery.

Normal spermatogenesis also depends on general homeothermy. Febrile states causing increased testicular temperature may result in disturbed spermatogenesis. Testicular hypoxia probably plays a role in heat damage and other spermatogenic disturbances.

Spermatogenesis seems to be more resistant to cooling than to heat, and the tunica dartos and cremaster muscles contract to protect the testes from the effects of cold. Low environmental temperatures ($-15°$ to $-20°C$) during winter months do not seem to interfere with testicular development, sperm production, or semen quality in boars. Within a herd, bulls that suffer scrotal frostbite as a result of exposure to severe blizzard conditions produced semen of inferior quality when compared to bulls that were not affected with scrotal necrosis.

Nutrition

Specific deficiencies in the intake and utilization of nutrients can adversely influence reproductive efficiency. Malnutrition constitutes a greater stress to spermatogenesis in prepuberal males than in postpuberal males. A markedly deficient caloric intake in prepuberal males causes hypoplasia of the testes and accessory sex glands and delays puberty.

There is evidence that energy-deficient diets adversely affect gonadotropin secretion. Mature males underfed to the point of inanition (loss of 25 to 35% of body weight) show decline in libido, suffer damage to the seminiferous epithelium, and have low volume of ejaculate and poor seminal quality.

Germinal and Leydig cells are both affected by hypovitaminosis A, resulting in poor seminal quality, testicular atrophy, hypoplasia of the accessory sex glands, and delayed puberty.

Hypovitaminosis E causes testicular damage in rats, but there is no evidence that vitamin E deficiency plays a significant role in infertility among domestic animals. Prolonged vitamin E deficiency in the ration of dairy cows and bulls produced some cases of cardiac failure but was without a measurable effect on reproduction. Very young ruminants require dietary sources of the water-soluble vitamins, but animals with functional rumens and normal ruminal flora get adequate amounts of these vitamins from the activities of the microflora.

Mineral deficiencies and the feeding of excessive amounts of phytoestrogens, goitrogens, and nitrates are associated with impaired reproductive performance in males. Although optimal nutrition after a period of deprivation appears to reverse the degenerative reproductive changes, total recovery can be prolonged.

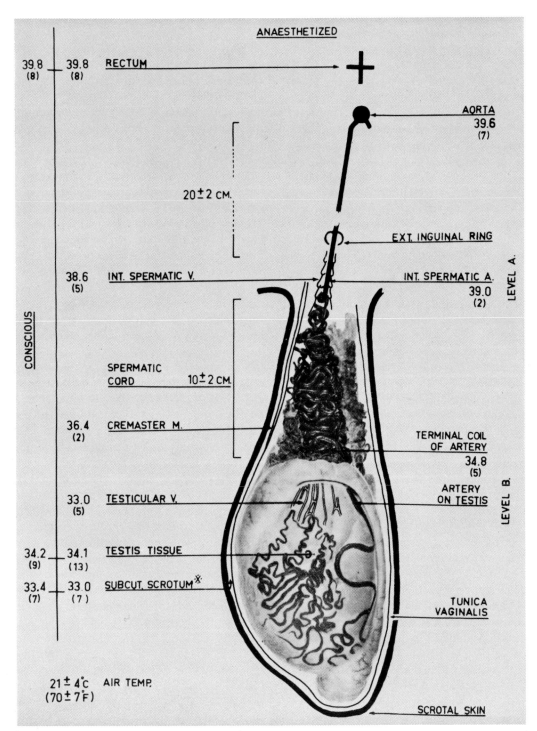

Fig. 8-2. Sites of measurements and comparisons of the temperatures recorded from conscious and anesthetized rams. Lateral aspect. The internal spermatic artery has been filled with neoprene and the cast has been exposed by removal of the pampiniform plexus and the tunica albuginea over the artery on the testis. Figures in parentheses give the number of measurements from which the average was obtained.

*Subcutaneous scrotum measurements were made beneath the posterior skin and not the anterior as shown here for the purposes of illustration only. (Waites, G. M. H., and Moule, E.R.: J. Reprod. Fertil. 2:217, 1961.)

Exogenous sex steroids may affect testicular function directly or by altering the secretion of pituitary gonadotropins. Small doses of testosterone may impair spermatogenesis by suppressing gonadotropin secretion. Prolonged treatment with large doses, while suppressing the pituitary, can maintain the seminiferous epithelium, allowing spermatogenesis to proceed. In some species, steroidal suppression of the testis has been followed by a "rebound phenomenon" after withdrawal of the steroid. Testicular rebound is presumably due to released gonadotropin secretion following withdrawal of the exogenous steroid. Testosterone injected into intact bulls severely depressed semen quality by 11 weeks (approximately the time required for the spermatogenesis and epididymal migration) after the injections were stopped, suggesting that the greatest effect was on spermatogonia. Seminal quality returned to pretreatment levels between 12 and 37 weeks after testosterone withdrawal.

Estrogens administered to 2- to 3-month old calves retard development of the seminiferous tubules and inhibit development of accessory glands. Progestins are also potent inhibitors of spermatogenesis. The pituitary-suppressing activities of sex steroids make them useful as contraceptives.

Steroidogenic Function

The fetal testes synthesize androstenedione and testosterone before and during differentiation of the accessory reproductive organs and regression of the müllerian system. The tubular genitalia, accessory sex glands, and secondary sexual characters develop and function under the influence of testicular androgens.

Secondary sexual characters can be classified as special or general and are not directly concerned with the reproductive process, although they may be important to identification and mating behavior. Special sex characters are organs or appendages which serve for adornment, attraction, or combat, and these characters often differ qualitatively between sexes. Sex plumage of birds is an outstanding example of a special secondary sex character. In some species, including deer and elk, antlers are limited to males. General sex characters, unlike special sex characters, differ quantitatively between the sexes. Muscular and skeletal development are the most notable examples of general sexual characters. (Fig. 8-3).

The extratesticular role of androgens in maintaining male secondary sex characteristics is well established. Androgens also support spermatogenesis. The germinal epithelium has a higher testosterone requirement for normal function than other androgen-dependent tissues. In fact, the close association of the Leydig cells with the seminiferous tubules (Figs. 8-1 and 8-4) probably provides high local concentrations of testosterone to the tubules. Intratesticular changes in testosterone concentration may act as a regulatory mechanism on capillary permeability and flow, altering the secretion of testosterone by the Leydig cells. This regulatory mechanism may be exerted directly on the Leydig cells or indirectly, on the Sertoli cells. A small peptide, GnRH-like factor, gonadocrinin, probably produced by the Sertoli cell appears to act locally at the interstitial-tubular system to serve as an intratesticular regulator of testosterone secretion (Fig. 8-4). The Sertoli cells also produced an androgen-binding protein (ABP), which serves as a protein carrier for testosterone. This ABP protein apparently maintains a high concentration of testosterone within the tubular compartments of the mammalian testis. The concentration of testosterone in the testicular artery leaving the pampiniform plexus is consistently higher in the monkey, rat, ram, and bull than the concentration of testosterone in systemic blood. This suggests a transfer of steroids from testicular venous blood to the testicular artery in the pampiniform plexus. The venous-arterial transfer of steroids may function to enrich the supply of testosterone and other steroids to the testes and epididymides.

The interstitial cells of the testis produce androgens, including testosterone, in response to ICSH (LH) stimulus, in synergy with FSH

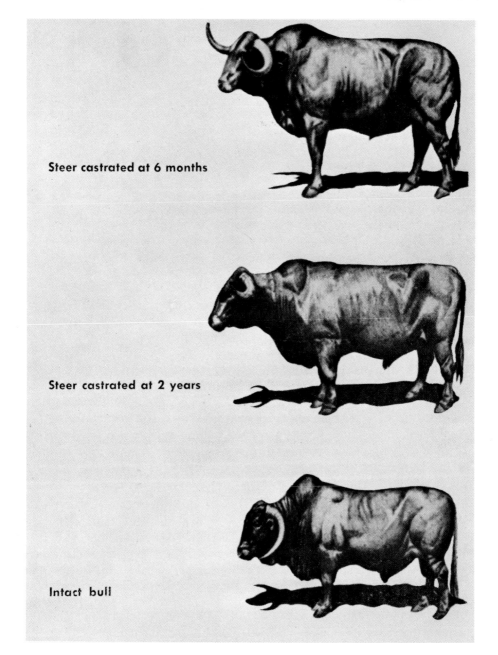

Steer castrated at 6 months

Steer castrated at 2 years

Intact bull

Fig. 8-3. Influence of sex hormones on hair, muscular development, and skeletal growth. All three animals are 12 years old. (Bonsma, J. C.: Wortham Lectures in Animal Science. College Station, Texas, Texas A & M University Press, 1965.)

and probably with prolactin. The interaction of ICSH with receptors in the Leydig cells activates the adenyl cyclase system, including protein kinase activation and RNA synthesis, resulting in an increased pregnenolone production from cholesterol by the mitochondria in the Leydig cells. Intracellular enzymatic side-chain cleavage of pregnenolone occurs in

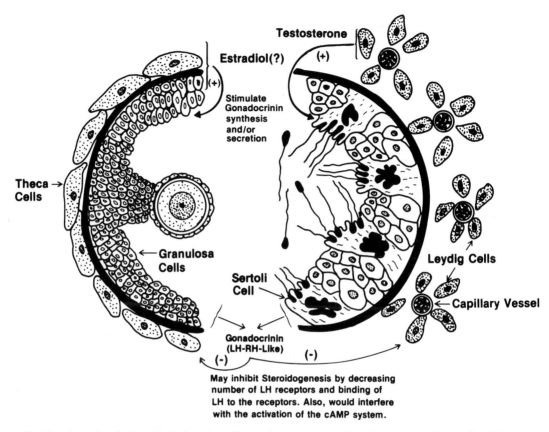

Fig. 8-4. Postulated physiologic function of gonadocrinin on the Sertoli and granulosa cells. (*Adapted from* different sources, including R. M. Sharp, J. Reprod. Fertil. *64*:517, 1982.)

the mitochondrion and leads to the production and finally, release of testosterone by the Leydig cells (Fig. 8-5). For some species, there are evidences indicating that testosterone produced by the Leydig cells is uptaken in a paracrine fashion by the Sertoli cell, which under the influence of FSH, converts it to estradiol (Fig. 8-5). The estradiol produced by the Sertoli cells may in turn have a regulatory activity in the production of testosterone by the Leydig cells, since specific receptors for estradiol have been demonstrated in the Leydig cells of some species. The adrenal cortex also secretes androgens, but the amounts normally secreted must be small, since in animals with intact adrenals, orchiectomy has a profound inhibitory influence on accessory sex organs and secondary sex characters.

Puberty, the onset of reproductive capac-

ity, is the result of complex interactions of the hypothalamus, the anterior pituitary gland, the gonads, conditioning of the target organs or "aging" of the somatic substrate, and environmental factors such as nutrition. Function of the Leydig cells precedes the formation of spermatozoa, suggesting that androgens condition the seminiferous tubules to gonadotropic stimulation.

Sexual maturity is the state of full reproductive capacity. The interval between puberty and sexual maturity is adolescence. Several seminal characteristics have been shown to change quantitatively toward mature patterns during adolescence. Indicative of increasing 17β-hydroxy-steroid dehydrogenase activity in the testes, as the animal approaches puberty, changes in the androstenedione/testosterone ratios with advancing

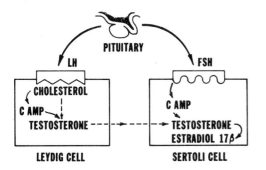

Fig. 8-5. Paracrine interactions between Leydig and Sertoli cells.

age have been found in the testes of bulls, rams, stallions, rhesus monkeys, men, and rats.

Blood levels of testosterone are shown in Table 8-1. The concentration of steroids and other hormones per unit volume of blood is highly variable among individuals and over time in the same individuals. Hormonal levels in the blood are not only dependent upon secretion, release, and metabolic clearance rates but also upon the age of the animal, season of the year, time of day, frequency of sampling, conditions of sampling (sexually stimulated versus nonstimulated; conscious versus anes-

Table 8-1   Levels of Testosterone (ng/ml) in the Systemic Blood*

Species	Testosterone (mean ± standard error of the mean)
Boar	4.00 ± 0.50
Bull·	6.70 ± 0.20
Stallion	2.10 ± 0.10
Ram	5.22 ± 0.66
Goat	6.22 ± 0.70
Dog	2.20 ± 0.70
Cat	6.33 ± 0.35

*Adapted from Andresen, Ø.: J. Reprod. Fertil. *48*: 51, 1976; Swanson, L. V., et al.: J. Anim. Sci. *33*:823, 1971; Ganjam, V. K., and Kenney, R. M.: J. Reprod. Fertil. *52*:67, 1975; Schanbacher, B. D., and Ford, J. J.: Endocrinology *99*:752, 1976; Zlotnik, G.: J. Reprod. Fertil. *32*:287, 1973; DePalatis, L., et al.: J. Reprod. Fertil. *52*:201, 1978; Taha, M. B., and Noakes, D. E.: J. Small Anim. Pract. *23*:351, 1982; Johnstone, I. P., et al.: Anim. Reprod. Sci. 7:*363*, 1984.

thetized), and the sensitivity and specificity of the assay system.

The weight, fructose content, and citric acid content of the vesicular glands generally reflect the endocrine activity of the testes.

The classic methods of studying the effects of testicular hormones are castration and replacement therapy. Interpretation of the results of these methods must include several important considerations. The changes occurring after orchiectomy may reflect the residual effects of extragonadal influences which are synergized or antagonized by testicular steroids. The effects of replacement therapy may be primary or secondary to effects on other systems. Testicular steroids may exert permissive effects on target organs which allow the effects of a second factor to be expressed.

Male sex steroids have both androgenic and anabolic activities. The androgenic activity stimulates growth and function of accessory reproductive organs and the development of special sex characters, which constitutes the basis for bioassay of these hormones. The anabolic activity stimulates constructive metabolism and the development of general sex characters (Figs. 8-6 and 8-7).

Body Size and Shape

Larger body size with more massive development of component parts in males is nearly universal among animals. Bulls, in which mature body weight is frequently double the weight of mature females of the same breed, are extraordinary examples (Fig. 8-7). Gonadal steroids influence ossification of the epiphyses in both sexes.

Steroids with androgenic activity have myotropic activity. Massive muscular development in the male can be related to copulatory postural requirements and aggressive social mannerisms related to mating behavior.

Complex interrelationships exist between fat compartments and sexual function. Excessive fat deposition has been related to lowered reproductive function in both sexes. Excessive fat deposits in the neck of the scrotum appear to lower seminal quality, probably by insu-

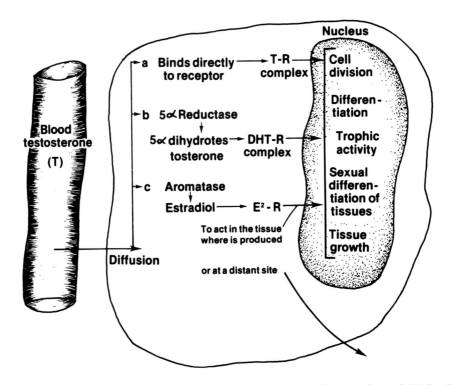

Fig. 8-6. Major pathways of metabolism of testosterone in target cells. (Adapted from: C. W. Bardin, and J. F. Catterall: Science *211*:1285, 1981.)

lating against normal heat loss. Effects on the steroidogenic function are unknown. Fat depots may sequester the fat-soluble steroid hormones.

Other Characteristics

Greater longevity among the females of several species is known, but it is not always clear whether the difference is a direct effect of gonadal steroids. Male sex steroids influence hair pigmentation and growth in mammals and feather pigmentation and growth in poultry. The hair coat of highly masculine males tends to be darker, especially in certain body regions, than the coat of castrates or females. Hair fibers of males are coarser than those of females or castrates.

Testis-Pituitary Relationships

The pituitary gland has several sexual dichotomies. The female generally has a larger gland than the male. Sex differences in the relative percentages of acidophils, basophils, and chromophobes, as well as differences in the staining qualities of the chromophilic granules have been reported. Sex differences in total gonadotropic potency and the relative activities of FSH and LH are common, but considerable species variation exists as to which sex has the greater potencies. The preoptic area of the female hypothalamus contains a center which regulates the ovulatory surge of LH. This center is not functional in males.

Leydig cell function declines as the male ages. The mechanisms acting to induce a hypofunctional activity of the Leydig cells in the aged animal remain undetermined. In some species, such as in rodents, total gonadotropic output declines with age, while it increases in other species, such as in humans. Age-related, intracellular changes in the Leydig cells may

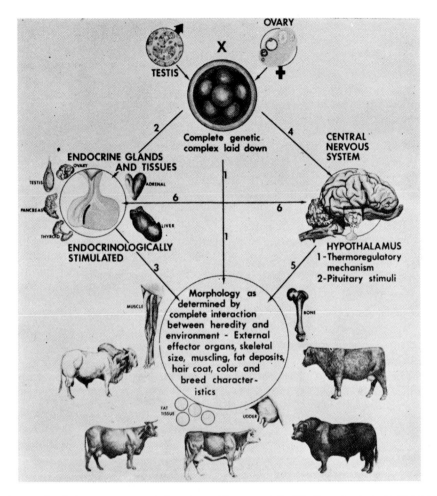

Fig. 8-7. Interaction between genes and phenotype. (Bonsma, J. C.: Wortham Lectures in Animal Science. College Station, Texas, Texas A & M University Press, 1965.)

influence the response of these cells to local intratesticular factors and to pituitary control of their secretory activity.

Following castration, the male hypophysis enlarges more than the female gland, abolishing the sex difference in size. Vacuolated "signet ring" basophils form in the pituitary glands of both sexes in some species following castration, and the percentage of basophils and gonadotropic activity increase. Estrogens are generally more effective than androgens in preventing castrational changes in the pituitary of either sex.

Testosterone inhibits the secretion of pitui-

tary gonadotropins by a negative feedback mechanism. The relative pituitary-depressing and androgenic activities, like the relative anabolic and androgenic activities, vary among the androgenic steroids. Thus, some androgens suppress pituitary gonadotropin secretion to a greater extent than they stimulate spermatogenesis, accessory sex organs, and secondary sex characters.

The existence of inhibin, a nonsteroidal pituitary inhibitor of gonadal origin, was first postulated by McCullagh in 1932.[95] Recent studies suggest that inhibin is produced by the Sertoli cells and is present in testicular fluid, seminal plasma, and the ovarian follicular fluid. Inhibin selectively suppresses plasma levels of FSH without altering LH levels in castrated animals. In intact animals, inhibin appears to participate in the control of FSH secretion by the pituitary gland through a negative feedback action.

Testis-Adrenal Relationships

Adrenal cortices normally produce androgens, and adrenal androgen secretion may be greatly increased in a variety of pathological conditions, including adrenal hyperplasia or neoplasia, nymphomania in cattle, and adrenal virilism in women.

Special Sex Characters

In some species and in certain breeds within species, some body characters are qualitatively different according to sex and are thus special sex characters. These include dichromism of the pelage (hair coat), horns in ungulates, vocalization, and behavior at urination.

The production of pheromones (see Chapter 7) is, in some cases, a secondary sex character, since some pheromones are sex-specific and dependent on gonadal steroids. The Bruce and Whitten factors are pheromones produced by male rodents, which affect the reproductive cycle in females. Androgenic ($C_{19} - \Delta^{16}$) steroids synthesized by the testes of the boar are released into the systemic circulation during sexual excitement. These steroids are metabolized to 5α-androsterone type of steroids in the salivary glands and are released in the saliva of the boar. These steroids induce a pheromonal response in the female pig in estrus, which results in the mating stance. These $C_{19} - \Delta^{16}$ steroids are also stored in the fat of the male and are responsible for the boar taint, the unpleasant, urine-like odor of cooked pork meat. Orchiectomy abolishes the activities of both substances. Other chemical communicants are concerned with sexual behavior and identification of appropriate sex partners, and gonadectomy alters their activities. Moreover, castration has been reported to alter the development of olfactory perception.

Testis-Accessory Sexual Organ Relationships

The male accessory sex organs include the efferent ducts, epididymides, vasa deferentia and their ampullae, vesicular glands, prostate, bulbourethral glands, urethra, urethral glands, prepuce, preputial glands, penis, and scrotum. The effects of castration on these organs vary with the age and stage of development at which orchiectomy is performed. In general, prepuberal castration prevents normal development, and postpuberal castration leads to atrophy. In adults, function is a more accurate index of androgenic activity than size of the sexual accessory organs. The accessory sexual organs of males castrated as adults may retain their precastration size because the stroma is maintained while function is severely impaired.

In addition to stimulating growth of the penis, androgens stimulate cleavage of the preputial lamellae to form the preputial cavity. Preputial adhesions in prepuberal bulls may be mistaken for a pathological process when electroejaculation is used to stimulate protrusion of the penis. The development of the penile spines in the cat is directly related to androgen levels.

Hypertrophic or hyperplastic enlargement of the prostate is a common ailment in intact, aged male dogs. Castration often corrects the condition.

Seminal fructose levels decline rapidly following castration, and injections of testosterone restore the function of the vesicular glands. There appears to be a progressive loss of sensitivity of the vesicular glands to androgen stimulation following orchiectomy, and estrogens may synergize with testosterone or act to sensitize the vesicular glands to the stimulatory effect of testosterone.

Factors Affecting Leydig Cell Function

As would be expected, the steroidogenic function of the testis parallels the gametogenic activity in seasonal breeders. As a result, the accessory glands and special sex characters undergo corresponding changes in these species.

In contrast to the severe damaging effect of the intra-abdominal or other ectopic position of the testes on the germinal epithelium and spermatogenesis, the Leydig cells of artificially cryptorchid testes are functional for a time, as evidenced by the size of accessory sex glands, male aggressiveness, and libido. There are indications, however, that accessory glandular function is affected. Cryptorchid testes weigh less, are less capable than scrotal testes to respond to gonadotropic stimulation, and may not secrete androgens normally. The endocrine activity of the Sertoli cells is also affected by cryptorchidism. In some species, high blood levels of FSH have been associated with crytorchidism, suggesting that inhibin secretion is impaired.

Restriction of dietary intake, resulting in energy deficiency, causes atrophy and functional depression of the accessory sex glands. Energy restriction in rams reduces the testicular blood flow and uptake of oxygen and glucose, as well as the daily output of testosterone. Exposure to severe cold ($-5°C$) causes atrophy of the accessory sex glands similar to that from restriction of dietary energy. Low temperatures may reduce the flow of blood to the testis and thus cause a depression in androgen secretion.

The results of experiments to evaluate the effects of exogenous testosterone on Leydig cell function must be viewed in the knowledge that doses equal to or greater than physiological levels may suppress Leydig cell function yet maintain androgen-dependent organs. Leydig cell tumors are the most common testicular tumors in dogs and bulls.

Testicular Estrogens

Estrogens have been isolated from the testes of stallions, bulls, boars, dogs, and man. The level of estrogenic activity in testicular venous blood from stallions is 20 times greater than the level in peripheral blood. Levels of estrogens in the blood of the spermatic vein are higher than those in the peripheral blood of several species, including the canine. Estrogens, like androgens, are transferred from the testicular vein to the testicular artery. In several species, levels of estrogens in the blood of the testicular artery are consistently higher than the levels of estrogens in systemic blood. In bulls, about 12% of the estrogens in testicular venous blood are transferred to the testicular artery.

The mechanisms involved in the transfer of steroids from the testicular vein to the artery in the pampiniform plexus and its physiological role remain to be determined. The ability of the testes to synthesize estrogens implies the presence of enzymes necessary for aromatization of the A ring and removal of the C-19 methyl group of the steroid molecule. Sertoli cells contain the necessary enzymes for the conversion, under the control of FSH, of testosterone to estrogens in general and estradiol in particular.

The urine of stallions and male mules is one of the richest sources of estrogens, and the daily output of urinary estrogen in the stallion exceeds that of the nongravid mare by a factor of 100 to 200. In spite of this, the stallion is one of the most impressively masculine of all males. Estrone is the major urinary estrogen in the stallion; there are relatively small levels of estradiol and no detectable levels of estriol. Estrone is also the major estrogen in the urine of male mules. The testes of the stallion have a low 17β-(testosterone) dehydrogenase activity and very high 19-(androstenedione) hydroxylase and aromatizing activities, compared to other species. As a consequence, most of the androstenedione, which serves as a precursor for both testosterone and estrone, is converted to estrone.

The ejaculate of the bull, stallion, and particularly the boar contains relatively high concentrations of estrogens. It has not been conclusively established whether the estrogens in the semen are contributed by the testes, the accessory sex glands, or by both. Spermatozoa released from the Sertoli cells at spermiation may act as estrogen carriers.

Generally, Sertoli cell tumors in dogs are feminizing, and some tumors contain high levels of estrogenic activity. Canine Sertoli cell tumors produce estrone and estradiol-17β.

Sertoli cells are the most probable source of testicular estrogens. Since the estrogens are more potent than androgens in inhibiting pituitary gonadotropin secretion, estrogens in the male may play an important role in regulating the pituitary-gonadal axis.

THE EXCURRENT TRACT

The excurrent tract includes the rete testis, the efferent ducts, the epididymis, the vas deferens, and the urethra. Semen is composed of spermatozoa and other cellular elements, and fluids contributed by a number of organs, including the accessory sex glands (Fig. 8-8). The relative contribution of the organs participating in the formation of semen varies between species and even between ejaculates from the same animal. The rete testis is a network of straight tubules connecting the convoluted seminiferous tubules with the efferent ducts. The convoluted seminiferous tubules are the sperm-producing tubules; the straight tubules do not have germinal epithelium but a simple, cuboidal epithelium. The rete testis tubules are mostly intratesticular, but they become extratesticular after penetrating the tunica albuginea to join the efferent ducts. The union of the rete tubules with

the efferent ducts is extratesticular in the stallion and ram, and probably is also extratesticular in other domestic species. The number of efferent ducts (ductuli efferentes) for the domestic species is shown in Table 8-2.

The simple cuboidal epithelium of the rete tubules becomes columnar, containing both ciliated and nonciliated cells at the union with the efferent ducts. The efferent ducts lie under the head of the epididymis and converge to form the epididymal tubule. The epididymal tubule is a single, highly convoluted tubule which may be as long as 50 meters in the bull and 70 meters in the stallion. Anatomically, the epididymis is divided into: head (caput), body (corpus), and tail (cauda). However, the anatomical division of the epididymis does not correspond with its histological and functional characteristics.

The term *spermateliosis*, or *spermiogenesis*, is usually applied only to that phase of spermatogenesis in which spermatids are transformed into spermatozoa before spermiation, the release of spermatozoa into the lumen of the seminiferous tubules. Spermatozoa do, however, undergo additional physicochemical changes between the rete testis and cauda epididymis which are associated with phys-

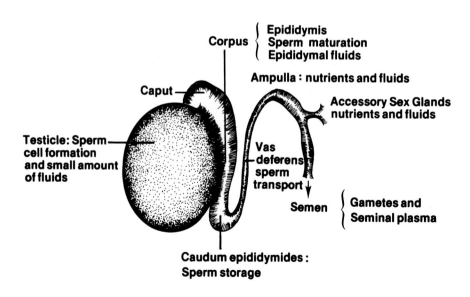

Fig. 8-8. Organs participating in the formation of semen.

Table 8-2 Number of Ductuli Efferentes in Domestic Species

Species	Range	Relative Frequency* of Blind-ending Ductuli
Boar	14–16	—
Bull	13–16	Common
Cat	14–17	—
Dog	13–15	—
Goat	18–19	Common
Ram	17–20	Common
Stallion	14–17	Common

*Spermiostasis in the head of the epididymis is common in the goat, ram and bull, and may be associated with the number of blind-ending ductuli. (*Adapted From*: N. A. Hemeida et a.: Am. J. Vet. Res., *39*:1892, 1978.)

iologic changes in the cells. These changes are described as maturation and are needed for fertilization.

The nonmotile spermatozoa released into the seminiferous tubules are propelled through the rete testis into the epididymis by the contracting activity of the testicular capsule and the seminiferous tubules, and by the flow of testicular fluids (Fig. 8-9). During migration through the epididymis, spermatozoa develop the capacity for motility and fertility, while their resistance to thermal stress is decreased. Spermatozoa acquire the progressive, forward motility typical of mature sperm as they pass through the epididymides. The metabolic pattern of testicular spermatozoa differs from epididymal and ejaculated cells, indicating enzymatic changes within the cells, a change in metabolic substrate, or both.

Seminal fluid is absorbed in the efferent ducts and caput epididymis, causing sperm concentration to fluctuate throughout the epididymis. The absorptive capacity of the epididymis may be related to the fact that it develops from the mesonephros. The specific gravity of sperm cells in the cauda is greater than that of sperm cells in the caput. Changes

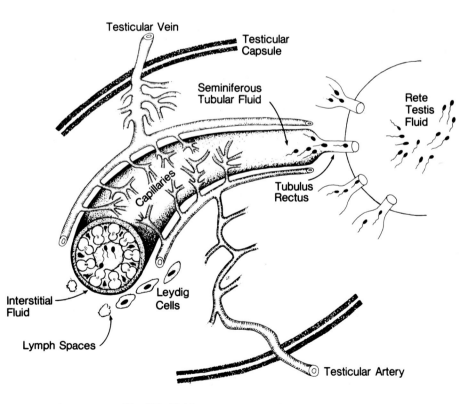

Fig. 8-9. Fluid compartments of the testis.

in the fluid environment of spermatozoa in the epididymis include changes in the concentration of electrolytes, especially sodium, potassium and chloride, and of amino acids and proteins, phospholipids, and enzymes.

Sodium and potassium are reciprocally related in the spermatozoa and seminal plasma of several species. Potassium is concentrated in the cells, whereas the sodium concentration is high in seminal plasma.

Testicular and ejaculated spermatozoa from the boar, bull, and ram show qualitative changes in phospholipid and fatty acids during epididymal passage and ejaculation. Epididymal spermatozoa of these species contain more total lipid than ejaculated cells. These changes in cellular lipids suggest that certain lipids are implicated in maturation, perhaps by serving as metabolic substrates for spermatozoa during their passage through the epididymis.

Testicular spermatozoa are more resistant to cold shock than epididymal spermatozoa and resistance to thermal stress decreases from the head to the tail of the epididymis. Ejaculated spermatozoa have even less thermal resistance, and spermatozoa from second ejaculates survive freezing or cold shock better than those from the first ejaculate. Changes in cellular lipids may be associated with changes in susceptibility of the cells to thermal shock, probably as a result of changes in membrane permeability.

As spermatids differentiate into spermatozoa, most of the cytoplasm enters into the formation of the midpiece and tail or is passed off through the posterior regions of the cell. Some of this cytoplasm persists at the base of the head, moves down the midpiece, and is eventually lost from most spermatozoa during epididymal passage; the residual bead of cytoplasm is called the cytoplasmic or kinoplasmic droplet.

No physiological role has been defined for the cytoplasmic droplet, although the rods and granules in the droplet have been postulated to constitute an endogenous source of energy for spermatozoa in the proximal epididymis. These droplets are rich in hydrolase enzymes

and their disappearance in the distal epididymis and ejaculate may thus be related to observed differences in metabolism of cells from various segments of the excurrent ducts. Large numbers of droplets in ejaculated spermatozoa indicate a disturbance in maturation or suggest frequent ejaculations.

Spermatogenesis proceeds throughout the year in most domestic males, even though females may be out of season. This fact raises the question of the disposition of unejaculated spermatozoa during periods of sexual rest. In some rodents, spermiophages from the basal layer of cells lining the epididymis phagocytize spermatozoa in cases of obstructive azoospermia. However, in vasectomized animals or animals with obstruction of the vas deferens, spermatozoa accumulate in the epididymis, causing dilation and rupture of the epididymal tubule. There is a constant flow of semen from bulls and rams with fistulated vas deferens which suggests the unejaculated spermatozoa are constantly eliminated through the vas deferens into the urethra. It is generally believed that the daily produced but unejaculated spermatozoa are released into the urethra and washed out during micturition since variable, but considerable numbers of spermatozoa are found in the urine of sexually rested animals and men. However, spermatozoa have been found in the urine withdrawn with a catheter from the urinary bladder of rams or by cystocentesis from the bladder of dogs and cats before ejaculation indicating that spermatozoa had flowed into the bladder during sexual rest. A series of old, but largely ignored, and new evidence clearly indicates that the pathway of least resistance in nonejaculatory situations is for the flow of fluid and spermatozoa into the bladder, probably due to a relative higher resistance to the outflow presented by the penile urethra. Thus, retrograde flow of spermatozoa into the bladder during periods of sexual rest may provide a mechanism for the disposal of the daily produced but unejaculated spermatozoa. Furthermore, recent studies have demonstrated that there is retrograde flow of spermatozoa into the urinary bladder during electroejaculation in the bull,[128] ram,[148] and cat,[129] and as a consequence there are considerable losses of spermatozoa in the urine. Retrograde flow of spermatozoa into the bladder may not be limited to ejaculation induced by electrical stimulation since dogs and cats in which semen was collected with an artificial vagina had significant numbers of spermatozoa in the bladder. The percentage of retrograde flow, estimated by dividing the total number of spermatozoa in the urine by the total number of spermatozoa displaced during ejaculation (total number of spermatozoa in the urine plus total number of spermatozoa in the ejaculate) varies considerably among species, between and within animals, and with seminal collections. The percentage of retrograde flow may reach values as high as 50% or even exceed 90%. A retrograde flow of 100% should be termed retrograde ejaculation, since the ejaculate would be devoid of spermatozoa. Retrograde ejaculation is a pathologic condition that appears to be more frequent in men than in domestic animals. It appears that the retrograde flow of spermatozoa into the bladder is also a component of the ejaculatory process when semen is collected by artificial means and probably occurs at the beginning of the seminal emission (Fig. 8-10).

In addition to its roles in sperm transport and maturation, the epididymis functions to store viable spermatozoa. Spermatozoa accumulate in the tail of the epididymis, which acts as a reservoir. Ejaculated spermatozoa in man, cat, dog, stallion, and probably in other species originate mainly from their site of storage in the cauda epididymides and to a lesser degree from the vasa deferentia. A large reservoir of mature spermatozoa in the tail of the epididymis is important for species, such as the ram, that copulate frequently. The location of the tail of the epididymis in the most distal, cooler part of the scrotum may be related to the storage function. While stored in the tail of the epididymis, spermatozoa from several species are immotile and do not acquire motility until exposed to the accessory sex gland secretions during ejaculation. Epididymal spermatozoa, however, can be rendered motile experimentally by incubation in

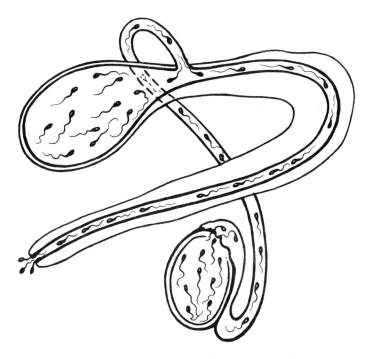

Fig. 8-10. Apparent pathways of spermatozoal displacement during ejaculation.

their own epididymal fluid (Table 8-3) or in appropriate, chemically defined solutions. The existence of "immobilin," a high molecular weight epididymal glycoprotein, has been postulated. Immobilin would inhibit spermatozoal motility by creating a viscoelastic epididymal environment for the spermatozoa stored in the tail of the epididymis.

Epididymal dysfunction has been related to altered seminal quality, including increased morphological defects and akinesia.

Morphological defects of sperm have also been related to degeneration of the epididymal epithelium. Bulls, rams, and dogs with microscopic focal interstitial epididymitis frequently have lowered seminal quality, including an abnormally high percentage of spermatozoa displaying morphological defects.

Epididymal function depends on androgen stimulation. In some species, such as rodents and monkeys, the need for androgens to maintain the structural and functional integrity of the epididymis is higher than that of other accessory sex glands. This may be true for other species, as well.

During emission, spermatozoa and testicular and epididymal fluids are conveyed by peristaltic contractions of the muscular walls of the excurrent ducts into the pelvic urethra. Near the pelvic urethra of some species, an increase in the glandular elements of the deferent ducts forms the ampullae of the vasa. The glands of the ampullae are similar to those of the vesicular glands (which also are embryologic tributaries of the wolffian duct), and their secretion provides the first notable carbohydrate substrate to semen. No distinct ampulla is formed in the boar or the tomcat.

The urethra receives ducts of a number of glandular tributaries, of which the accessory glands are prominent. Urethral glands have not been extensively studied in domestic mammals, but urethral glands are not found in the bull.

Emission of contributions from the excurrent ducts and various accessory glands occurs in sequential fashion in the stallion, boar, and dog. In the bull and ram, emission is nearly instantaneous, with a mixing of con-

Table 8-3   Motility of Spermatozoa Incubated In Their Own Epididymal Fluid*

Spermatozoa From	Species		
	Boar	Bull	Ram
Testis	−	−	−
Epididymis			
caput	−	−	−
corpus	−	+	+
cauda	−	++	+++

*Adapted From: J. L. Dacheux and M. Paquignon: Reprod. Nutr. Develop. *20*:1085, 1980.

tributions from various portions of the tract. However, presperm, sperm-rich, and postsperm fractions of bull ejaculates have been collected with an electroejaculator and during collection with the artificial vagina.

THE ACCESSORY SEX GLANDS

The accessory glands include the vesicular glands, the prostate, and the bulbourethral (Cowper's) glands. The occurrence and development of these structures vary widely among species (Fig. 8-11). Unlike mammals, birds such as the chicken and turkey do not have accessory sex glands, but secretory cells in the epithelium of the excurrent ducts add products to the semen.

Normal development and function of the accessory sex glands are controlled by testosterone, and the synergistic action of estrogens may also be required. In some species testosterone must be converted to dihydrotestosterone to be physiologically active on the accessory glands.

The accessory glands contribute most of the volume to the ejaculate. Motility and metabolic activity of sperm are stimulated as the accessory gland secretions are added to the contributions from the testes and epididymides during ejaculation. Sperm-coating antigens are also secretory products of the accessory sex glands. A great deal of study has been devoted to the effects of accessory glandular constituents on the physiology of sperm *in vitro*, but remarkably little is known about the role of normal or abnormal acces-

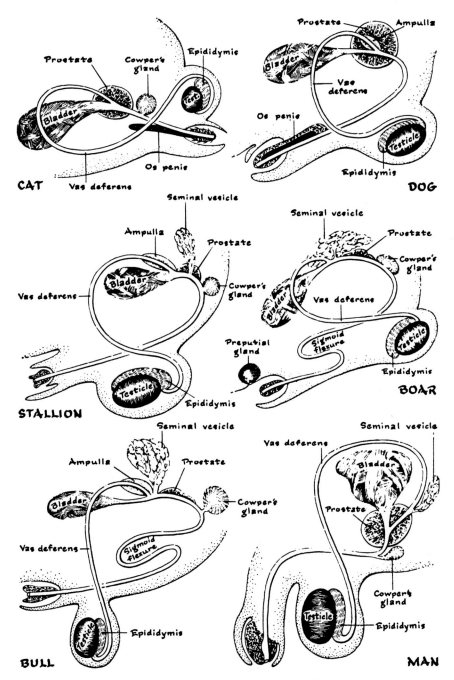

Fig. 8-11. Reproductive systems of the male cat, the dog, the stallion, the boar, the bull, and man. Compare the relative sizes of the various accessory glands and note that all these species have the prostate; that the dog and the cat have no seminal vesicles; that the dog has no Cowper's gland; that the cat, the boar, and man have no ampullar swelling; that the bull and the boar have the sigmoid flexure of the penis; that the dog and the cat have the os penis; that only the boar has the preputial pouch. (From Nalbandov, A. V.: Reproductive Physiology, 2nd ed. San Francisco, W. H. Freeman and Co., 1964.)

sory glandular secretions in the function of spermatozoa while in the female tract.

Artificial insemination of caput and corpus epididymal and even testicular spermatozoa results in fertilized oocytes, but the fertility of these cells is less than that of mature spermatozoa (Fig. 8-12).

Epididymal rabbit sperm and spermatozoa from the vas deferens in cats are capable of fertilizing oocytes *in vitro*, without capacitation. Ejaculated spermatozoa, however, require capacitation in many species.

The vesicular and prostate glands have been removed from boars and rats without impairing fertility, and the breeding efficiency of bulls in natural service has been acceptable following seminal vesiculectomy. The seminal vesicles are not, as their name implies, places of sperm storage. Vesicular glands are a preferable designation and more accurately describes their function. Sixty to 90% of the volume of fluid in normal ejaculates comes from the accessory glands, and the vesicular glands when present contribute a major portion. Vesicular glands are absent in the dog and tomcat (Table 8-4).

The bovine and porcine prostates are composed of the body, which overlies the origin of

Table 8-4   Accessory Glands in Domestic Species

Species	Vesicular Glands	Prostate	Cowper's
Bovine	+	+	+
Ovine	+	+	+
Equine	+	+	+
Porcine	+	+	+
Canine	−	+	−
Feline	−	+	+

the pelvic urethra, and the disseminate prostate, which surrounds the pelvic urethra. The ram's prostate consists of two lateral lobes which are connected by an isthmus dorsal to the origin of the pelvic urethra. The prostate gland of the dog, being the only accessory gland present, is well developed, contributes a large volume of fluid to the ejaculate, and is mostly delivered as the postsperm fraction of the ejaculate.

The bulbourethral glands of most species of domestic mammals are relatively small, compact, round bodies located above the urethra near the pelvic outlet. The bulbourethral glands of the boar are large and cylindrical.

THE PENIS AND PREPUCE

With the exception of the dog, vaginal intromission of the penis requires erection. The penis of the dog contains a bone, the os penis, which facilitates vaginal entry without full erection. Erection is accomplished by synergy of two mechanisms. The cavernous bodies of the penis become engorged through expansion of the arterioles, while the corresponding venules, which have strategically placed valves, contract. Secondly, the ischiocavernosus and bulbospongiosus muscles contract to compress the dorsal vein of the penis against the ischial arch. Structural abnormalities in the blood vessels of the penis may cause impotency in bulls, boars, and other species due to a deficient penile erection or the inability to sustain an erection until ejaculation has occurred. A pressure, greatly exceeding arterial pressure, develops in the corpus cavernosum penis during erection, reaching a peak

Percentage of Fertility

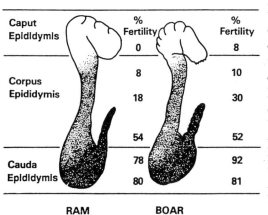

		% Fertility		% Fertility
Caput Epididymis		0		8
Corpus Epididymis		8		10
		18		30
		54		52
Cauda Epididymis		78		92
		80		81
	RAM		BOAR	

Fig. 8-12. Fertility of spermatozoa from different regions of the epididymis in the ram and boar. (Adapted from: J. L. Dacheux and M. Paquignon: Reprod. Nutr. Develop. *20*:1085, 1980.)

pressure at ejaculation. For the bull, the pressure in the corpus cavernosum reaches a mean of more than 14,000 mm of Hg during ejaculation. Pressures of this magnitude help to explain the development of hematomas of the penis, a common clinical entity in bulls.

The extent to which the cavernous bodies expand to enlarge the penis during erection depends upon the development and composition of the tunics of connective tissue which surround and send trabeculae into the spongy tissues. Ruminants and boars have fibroelastic penes which enlarge slightly during erection, and protrusion of the penis is primarily achieved by straightening of the sigmoid flexure due to relaxation of the retractor penis muscle. The body of the dog's penis has considerable fibrous tissue, whereas the connective tissues of the glans are weakly developed and consist of a large proportion of elastic fibers and smooth muscle. Erection involves primarily the glans penis. Enlargement of the bulbus glandis and contraction of vestibular muscles after intromission "lock" the dog's penis in the bitch's vagina. The stallion has no sigmoid flexure and protrusion results by enlargement of the highly vascular penis, which is invested with elastic fibers and smooth muscle. The pressure in the corpus cavernosum of the stallion seldom reaches pressures higher than 1,500 mm of Hg during ejaculation.

The glans penis of the cat has cornified spines which function to stimulate the ovulatory response in this reflexogenously ovulating species. The canine glans penis has a long collum glandis and a prominent bulbus glandis. A distinct corona glandis appears just behind the urethral process in the erect canine penis.

The bull's penis is surrounded by lamellae important in the support and protrusion of the penis, which appears to be peculiarly susceptible to deviations during erection and protrusion. Spiral deviation of the bull's penis occurs commonly within the vagina during normal ejaculation. The architecture of the lamellae suggests that the penis is structurally adapted to perform the spiral deviation.

In the clinical condition known as "corkscrew penis," service is prevented because spiraling occurs before intromission.

Except for the cat, the penes of most domestic animals are suspended by the prepuce from the ventral abdomen. The dog's prepuce is loose, allowing the glans penis to be directed posteriorly when the bulbus glandis engages the vulva. The penis of the cat is directed backward and downward from the ischial arch.

The penis is not free in the preputial cavity at the time of birth in most domestic animals. At birth, the epithelial surfaces of the penis and sheath are adhered as the balanopreputial fold. The fold is split into parietal and visceral layers by a cytolytic process which forms vesicles that coalesce to form the preputial cavity. Separation of the parietal and visceral layers is influenced by androgens.

The balanopreputial fold is continuous in the boar. In dogs and bulls, the fold is discontinuous ventral to the urethra, leaving a band of fibrous tissue between the ends of the solid primary fold (Fig. 8-13). This band forms the frenulum in the dog and may persist in the bull to cause severe deviation of the penis or to prevent complete protrusion.

BIOLOGY OF SPERMATOZOA

The spermatozoon is a highly specialized cell which has evolved to perform the sole

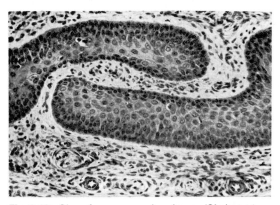

Fig. 8-13. Glans from a pup, showing an 'S'-shaped mesodermal primordium of the frenulum interrupting the balanopreputial fold ventral to the urethra. Trichrome stain; × 350. (From Bharadwaj, M. B., and Calhoun, M. L.: Am. J. Vet. Res. *22*:767, 1961.)

function of fertilizing an oocyte. The head is specialized to penetrate the oocyte to deliver its genetic payload. The tail contains the metabolic machinery to produce energy and provides the propelling mechanism for motility. Figure 8-14 is a diagrammatic representation of a bovine spermatozoon.

The head, which is usually flattened, is primarily a nucleus covered anteriorly by the acrosome (galea capitis, or head cap) composed of an outer and inner acrosomal membrane, connected by bridges, which apparently maintain the spacing and parallel arrangement and posteriorly, by the postnuclear membrane. Between the nucleus and the acrosome lies the perinuclear substance. The perforatium or apical body is part of the perinuclear substance and may play a role in fertilization (Chapter 7). The ultrastructure of the head of a bull's spermatozoon is illustrated in Figure 8-15. The shape of the head varies greatly among species. During spermateliosis the spermatid nucleus gradually takes the shape characteristic of the species, as the chromatin condenses.

The tail consists of the middle piece, principal piece, and terminal piece. A delicate neck joins the middle piece and head. The metabolic apparatus, a sheath of mitochondria, surrounds the flagellar filament in the middle piece. When compared to the mammalian oocyte, the number of mitochondria in the middle piece is small. Spermatozoal mitochondria, as the oocyte mitochondria, contain DNA, but the contribution of spermatozoal mitochondrial DNA to the oocyte during fertilization appears to be negligible, since the mitochondrial DNA is maternally inherited in the offspring (see Chapter 7). The flagellar fibrils extend the length of the tail. Figures 8-16 and 8-17 illustrate the ultrastructure of the tail.

Our meager knowledge of the physiology of spermatozoa in the female genital tract limits the usefulness of measurements of seminal characteristics *in vitro*. This is particularly true of measures of metabolic activity. One of the first decisive discoveries of the influence of the female environment on spermatozoal

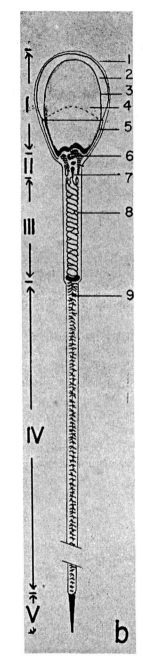

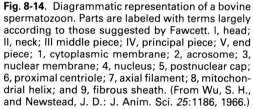

Fig. 8-14. Diagrammatic representation of a bovine spermatozoon. Parts are labeled with terms largely according to those suggested by Fawcett. I, head; II, neck; III middle piece; IV, principal piece; V, end piece; 1, cytoplasmic membrane; 2, acrosome; 3, nuclear membrane; 4, nucleus; 5, postnuclear cap; 6, proximal centriole; 7, axial filament; 8, mitochondrial helix; and 9, fibrous sheath. (From Wu, S. H., and Newstead, J. D.: J. Anim. Sci. *25*:1186, 1966.)

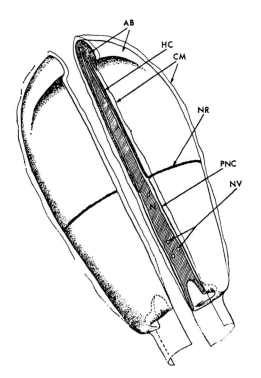

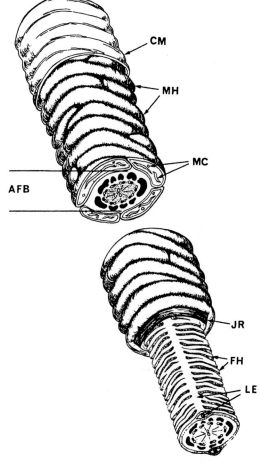

Fig. 8-15. Graphic illustration summarizing the ultrastructural features of the bovine sperm head. Apical body (AB); head cap (HC); cell membrane (CM); nuclear ring (NR); nucleus (N); postnuclear cap (PNC); nuclear vacuoles (NV). (From Saacke, R. G., and Almquist, J. O.: Am. J. Anat. *115*:144, 1964.)

Fig. 8-16. Graphic illustration summarizing ultrastructural features of the middle piece and anterior portion of the principal piece of tail of sperm. The cell membrane has been partially removed and the flagellum cut to show internal structure. Cell membrane (CM); mitochondrial helix (MH); mitochondrial cristae (MC); Jensen's ring (JR); fibrous helix (FH); longitudinal element (LE); axial fiber bundle (AFB), consisting of the nine outer coarse fibers, the nine inner fibers or doublets and the central pair of fibers. (From Saacke, R. G., and Almquist, J. O.: Am. J. Anat. *115*:165, 1964.)

function was the phenomenon of spermatozoal capacitation (Chapter 7).

Substantial concentrations of glycerylphosphorylcholine, primarily an epididymal contribution, are found in the semen of rams, bulls, stallions, goats, rabbits, and man. Spermatozoa are incapable of metabolizing this abundant seminal substrate *in vitro*, but glycerylphosphorylcholine diesterase activity has been found in the uterine washings of the ewe, cow, sow, rat, and mouse. The products of uterine hydrolysis, glycerol and phosphoglycerol, could serve as energy sources by entering the glycolytic pathway. Uterine glycerylphosphorylcholine diesterase activity is regulated by ovarian steroids and is greatest when estrogen levels are high. Secretions of the female reproductive tract have been reported to stimulate the metabolic activity of bull, boar, rabbit, and rooster spermatozoa.

An overwhelming abundance of spermatozoa are deposited in the female tract during natural service and the apparent requirement for a minimum number of motile sperm in the artificial insemination dose results in the presence of large numbers of cells in the female tract following insemination. Among domestic mammals, the survival of sperm in the female gential tract is usually limited to a few days at or

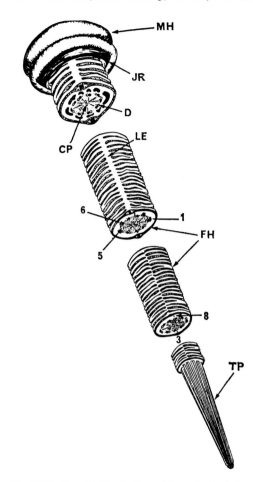

Fig. 8-17. Graphic illustration of the principal piece and terminal piece of tail of sperm. The cell membrane has been removed and the principal piece has been cut at various locations to show internal structure. Mitochondrial helix (MH); Jensen's ring (JR); central pair of fibers (CP); doublet (D); longitudinal element (LE); fibrous helix (FH); terminal piece (TP). (From Saacke, R. G., and Almquist, J. O.: Am. J. Anat. *115*:169, 1964.)

near the time of ovulation. The dog is a notable exception, since motile, fertile spermatozoa are present in large numbers for 4 to 6 days after copulation, and some motile cells are present as long as 11 days after mating. Removal of spermatozoa is accomplished by mechanical evacuation, leukocytic phagocytosis, and cytolysis.

THE SEMEN

The efficient production of meat, milk, and other animal products depends first and fore-most upon successful reproduction. The maximal utilization of superior genetic material in the gametes of companion, sporting, and work animals is of primary concern to the breeders of these animals, as well. At the present stage of technology in animal reproduction, the greatest selection pressure is exerted against the male gametes. The male is immensely more capable of yielding a harvest of germ cells than is the female, and spermatozoa from single sires are used to fertilize oocytes in as many dams as possible. From this point of view, submaximal fertility in individual males is of relatively greater consequence than submaximal fertility in individual females. The development of superovulation and embryo recovery and transfer techniques facilitates the utilization of superior genes in females. Thus, the role of the female's fertility is becoming important to increase reproductive rates in species such as the bovine and equine, which have characteristically low reproductive rates.

Evaluation of Seminal Quality

Lagerlöf[229] reviewed the history of the evaluation of seminal quality and histological investigations of the testes associated with infertility. An evaluation of seminal quality is an important consideration in assessing fertility levels and for diagnosing male reproductive disorders. Histological examinations of tissues from the male reproductive tract are essential to the understanding of seminal physiology and pathology, but they are of distinctly limited value in clinical veterinary medicine until biopsy techniques for obtaining meaningful samples of tissue have been perfected.

There are some distinct limitations to relating seminal quality to fertility, and these limitations must be appreciated. The seminal ejaculate is a composite of contributions from the testes, excurrent ducts, and accessory sex glands. The seminal sample reflects the function of each portion of the reproductive tract and its interactions with all other portions. Since the secretion of accessory glandular fluid is reasonably concurrent with ejaculation, the accessory gland contributions are a fairly accurate reflection of current functional status. The epididymal and testicular contributions, on the other hand, reflect past events in these portions of the tract.

Physical and Chemical Properties of Semen

The composition of semen varies among species, individuals of the same species, and ejaculates of the same individual. Seminal samples may be modified by disease, frequency of ejaculation (including masturbation), nutrition and other management factors, season, age, amount of sexual preparation, method of collection, magnitude of retrograde flow, procedures of handling the ejaculate during and after collection, analytic techniques and variation among technicians, pharmacological agents, and normal physiologic variation. Each potential source of variation should be recognized and accounted for in the interpretation of analyses of seminal quality. Many of these sources of variation can be controlled. Collection, handling, and analytic techniques should be standardized, and analytic procedures should be as objective and as repeatable as possible.

No single measurement of seminal quality has been found to be a reliable criterion for predicting fertility. Correlations of fertility with measures of quality in semen used for artificial insemination have the distinct advantage that individual ejaculates are used to inseminate relatively large numbers of females. Correlation coefficients based on the results of artificial insemination are usually biased, however, by the large number of spermatozoa inseminated and by the use of semen which has been selected for high quality. Seminal characteristics are better correlated to fertility when the samples are drawn from an unselected population. Many biological correlations are not straight-line relationships over the range of all possible values for the independent variable (Fig. 8-18). The coefficient of correlation between seminal characteristic and fertility will depend upon the range of values of the characteristic

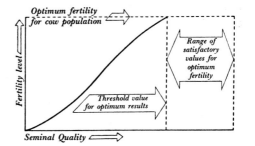

Fig. 8-18. Increasing fertility with increasing values of bull semen characteristics until threshold for optimum fertility is reached. (From Salisbury, G. W., and VanDemark, N. L.: Physiology of Reproduction and Artificial Insemination of Cattle. San Francisco, W. H. Freeman & Co., 1961.)

in the seminal samples used to determine the relationship.

In addition to the possibility of bias in the seminal samples used in computing relationships between seminal quality and fertility, there is the possibility of bias in the female population. The more females inseminated by single ejaculates, the less will be the bias in this direction. A further advantage of computing the relationship of seminal quality to fertility in artificial insemination programs is that male mating behavior is eliminated as a variable. Moreover, the inseminating dose, within the limits of processing error and technician error, is the same for all inseminations.

It is nearly impossible to obtain reliable coefficients of correlation that apply to natural mating. Single females are inseminated by single ejaculates containing large yet variable numbers of spermatozoa. Furthermore, there is no way to separate the contributing secretions from the female's tract to accurately measure the seminal characteristics of that ejaculate. Seminal quality must be characterized before or after the breeding period, and the number of females exposed per unit time is quite restrictive.

An examination of seminal quality should incorporate as many useful measurements of seminal characteristics as possible within the limits of practicality. The procedures will be modified by the purpose of the evaluation. Routine seminal analyses at an artificial insemination center usually include volume, sperm concentration, and percentage and rate of motility as minimal procedures. Examinations of seminal quality for research purposes usually include these plus a variety of additional measures of physical, chemical, and metabolic characteristics. In evaluating sires for potential breeding soundness, the results of the seminal analysis must always be interpreted in terms of the intended use of the sire and after a thorough physical examination. Valuable sires, especially those destined for service in artificial insemination, should be examined for venereal diseases or other infectious diseases that may be transmitted through insemination. Attempts to diagnose specific infertilities may include hormone assays, microscopic examination of tissues obtained by testicular biopsy, chemical analysis of semen to assess testicular and accessory sex glandular function, special studies of sperm morphology and ultrastructure, *in vitro* fertilization, and heterospermic inseminations.

A thorough discussion of the properties of semen is beyond the scope of this chapter. Table 8-5 gives published values of seminal characteristics, and reference should be made to reviews and original papers listed in the references under the headings of *Biology of Spermatozoa, Evaluation of Seminal Quality,* and *Physical and Chemical Properties of Semen.*

MATING

Copulatory behavior is composed of several elements which vary among species and individuals, but the pattern is remarkably similar. The male mounts the female from the rear and *clasps* his forelegs about her laterolumbar region (Fig. 8-19A). Rapid movement of the forelegs along the female's sides is termed *palpation.* Palpation is frequently accompanied by rapid, piston-like movements of the pelvis, called *pelvic thrusts* (Fig. 8-19B). If intromission is not achieved and the male dismounts, the mount is termed *incomplete copulation* or *attempt.* When intromission is achieved, with or without ejaculation, the mount is called a *complete copulation* (Fig. 8-19 C and D). Copulatory

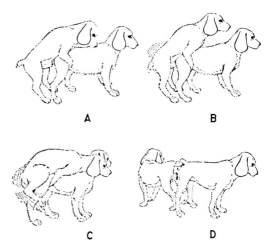

Fig. 8-19. Different stages in mating behavior of the male dog (drawn from motion picture prints): A, mounting and clasping; B, pelvic thrusting; C, intense ejaculatory reaction; D, copulatory lock. (From Hart, B. J.: J. Comp. Physiol. Psychol. *64*: 390, 1967.)

behavior of the male goat is depicted in Figure 8-20 A-F. Copulation with ejaculation is followed by a *refractory period,* during which mating behavior in the male is not aroused by any sexual stimuli. The refractory period may be shortened by intensifying the sexual stimulus. When the refractory period is excessively prolonged, the male is said to be *satiated.* Satiation is followed by a *recovery period* of quiescent mating behavior.

Frequency of copulation varies with the species and among the domestic species, varies with a number of factors such as breed, health, ratio of males to females, and dimensions of the breeding area. Rams and tom cats may copulate several times in an hour. Some rams have been observed to copulate over 50 times in 24 hours. Bulls are also frequent copulators, especially after a period of sexual rest. Stallions and boars may copulate 3 to 4 times in a day but are satiated after fewer ejaculations than the ram or bull. Dogs, probably because of the prolonged ejaculation with vaginal locking, and boars because of the prolonged ejaculation and large volume of ejaculate, are capable of only a few ejaculations in a 24-hour period.

Table 8-5 **Composition of Semen (Values are mg/dl of semen unless otherwise indicated.)**

Constituent or Property	Bull	Ram	Stallion	Boar	Dog	Cat
1. Volume of ejaculate, ml	4.0(2.0–10.0)	1.0(0.7–2.0)	70(30–300)	250(150–500)	6.0(2.0–16.0)	0.06(0.03–0.09)
2. Spermatozoa, millions/ml	1000(300–2000)	3000 (2000–5000)	120(30–800)	100(25–300)	65(10–200)	—
3. Total number of spermatozoa in ejaculate (millions)	4,000 (2,000–12,000)	3,000 (2,000–11,000)	8,400 (3,600–13,000)	25,000 (15,000–50,000)	390(60–3,000)	61(22–117)
4. Spermatozoa, size,* μm	65; 9 × 4 × 1 13; 44	—	58; 7 × 4 × 2 10; 42	57; 8 × 4 × 1 11; 38	60; 7 × 4 × 1 10; 34	—
5. Specific gravity	1.034(1.015–1.053)	—	—	—	1.011	—
6. Freezing point depression °C	0.61(0.54–0.73)	0.64(0.55–0.70)	0.60(0.58–0.62)	0.62(0.59–0.63)	(0.58–0.60)	—
7. Conductivity, mho × 10⁻⁴	105(90–115)	63(50–80)	123(110–130)	129(125–134)	(129–138)	—
8. pH	6.9(6.4–7.8)	6.9(5.9–7.3)	7.4(7.2–7.8)	7.5(6.8–7.9)	6.4(6.1–7.0)	8.3(8.1–8.6)
9. Water, g/dl	90(87–95)	85	98	95(94–98)	98	—
10. Carbon dioxide, ml/dl	16	16	24	50	—	—
11. Sodium	230(140–280)	190(120–250)	70	650(290–850)	89(56–124)	—
12. Potassium	140(80–210)	90(50–140)	60	240(80–380)	8.2(8–8.3)	—
13. Calcium	44(35–60)	10(6–15)	20	5(2–6)	0.7(0.4–0.9)	—
14. Magnesium	9(7–12)	8(2–13)	3	11(5–15)	0.5(0.3–1.0)	—
15. Chloride	180(110–290)	86	270(90–450)	330(260–430)	630–670	—
16. Phosphorus, Total	82	142	19	357	13	—
17. Acid-soluble P	35	132	14	171		—
18. Inorganic P	9	12	17	2		
19. Lipid P	9	3	—	6		
20. Nitrogen, Total	897	875	310	615(335–765)	361(299–406)	
21. Nitrogen, nonprotein	48	57	55	22	25	
22. Ammonia	2	2	1	1		
23. Urea	4	44	3	5		
24. Uric acid	3	6	3	3		
25. Creatine	3	21	—	—		
26. Creatinine	12	—	12	0.3		
27. Ergothioneine	(O-trace)	(O-trace)	7.6	15		
28. Spermine	0	—	0	0		
29. Phosphorylcholine	Trace	0	0	0		
30. Glycerylphosphorylcholine	350(100–500)	1650(1100–2100)	(40–100)	(110–240)		
31. Fructose	530(150–900)	250	2(0–6)	13(3–50)	Trace	
32. Citric acid	720(340–1,150)	140(110–260)	26(8–53)	130(30–330)	Trace	
33. Lactic acid	30(15–40)	40	15	30		
34. Inositol	35(25–46)	12(7–14)	30(20–47)	530(380–630)		
35. Ascorbic acid	6(3–9)	5(2–8)	—	—		
36. Phosphatase, acid† U/dl	170(50–340)	High	—	—		
37. Phospatase, alk.† U/dl	400(100–3500)	—	—	—		
38. Amylase	+	—	—	—	+	
39. Cholinesterase	—	++	—	++		
40. Cytochrome	+	++	+	+		
41. β-glucuronidase	+++	++	+	0	+	
42. Hyaluronidase	+++	+	—	++	+	
43. 5-Nucleotidase	+++	+	—	—		

Adapted from different sources, including: White, I. G.: Anim. Breeding Abstr. 26:110, 1958; Boucher, J. H. et al.: Cornell Vet. 48:67, 1958; Polakoski, K. L., and Kopta, M. In: Biochemistry of Mammalian Reproduction, 1982, p. 97; Olar, T. T., et al.: Biol. Reprod. 29:114, 1983; Dooley, M. P., and Pineda, M. H.: Am. J. Vet. Res. 47:286, 1986.
*Values are, respectively: total length; length × width × thickness of head; length of mid-piece; length of tail. †U = units, one unit indicating activity necessary for liberation of 1 mg. phenol from monophenylphosphate in one hour at 37°C.

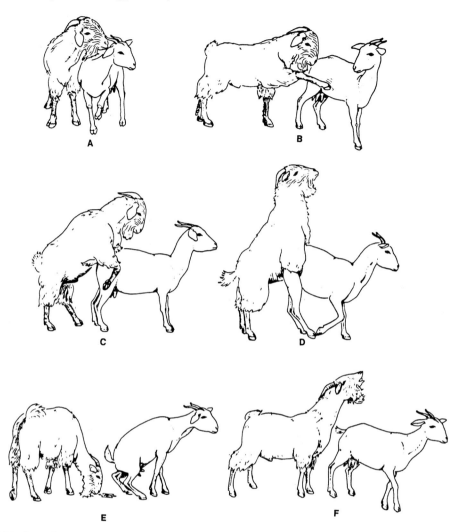

Fig. 8-20. Sexual responses of the male goat. A, Nudging the female. B, Flexing the foreleg against the female in short, choppy kicking motions. C, Mounting without intromission. D, Intromission and ejaculation as characterized by a deep penile thrust and backwards retraction of the forelegs. The upward head bounce, shown here, occurs evidently at the moment of ejaculation. E, Olfactory investigation of female urine. F, Characteristic posture of the flehmen response that occurs just after sniffing urine of an estrous or anestrous female. (Adapted from Hart, B. L., and Jones, T.O.A.C.: Effects of castration on sexual behavior of tropical male goats. Horm. Behav. *6*:251, 252, 1975.)

Sexual experience is an important factor in sexual behavior. Sexual behavior persists for variable periods after castration. Postcastration sexual behavior depends upon the species, age, and sexual experience of the male.

Ejaculation depends on the normal integrity and function of the autonomic nervous system, which coordinates seminal emission, closure of the urinary bladder sphincters, and ejaculatory displacement of seminal compon-ents through the penile urethra. The contractile activity of the urethral musculature seems to be under the control of catecholamines. The existence of adrenergic receptors in the urethra of the horse have been reported.

Copulatory patterns are influenced by the anatomy of the penis and the contributions of the accessory glands to seminal volume (Table 8-6). The duration of copulation is roughly proportional to the duration of ejacu-

Table 8-6 *Relationship Between Type of Penis, Volume of Ejaculate, Speed of Ejaculation,
and Site of Seminal Deposition*

Species	Type of Penis	Volume of Ejaculate		Type of Ejaculation	Site of Deposition
		Mean	(Range)		
Bull	Fibroelastic	4.00 ml	(1.7–10.0 ml)	Rapid	Vagina
Ram	Fibroelastic	1.00 ml	(0.7–2.0 ml)	Rapid	Vagina
Boar	Fibroelastic	250.00 ml	(150–500 ml)	Prolonged	Uterus
Stallion	Vascular	70.00 ml	(30–300 ml)	Prolonged	Uterus
Dog	Vascular (os penis)	6.00 ml	(2.0–16.0 ml)	Prolonged	Vagina
Cat	Vascular (os penis) with spines	0.06 ml	(0.03–0.09 ml)	Rapid	Vagina

lation. Copulation is rapid in the bull, billy goat, and ram, which have fibroelastic penes and ejaculate relatively small volumes of semen. The refractory period is relatively short in these species. The boar also has a fibroelastic penis, but the volume of the ejaculate is remarkably large, and copulation is prolonged. The stallion has a vascular penis and ejaculates a large volume of semen; copulation is accordingly prolonged. The dog's penis is uniquely adapted to the prolonged emission of the prostatic fluid while the bulbus glandis is engaged in the vulva. The "belling" of the glans of the stallion's penis probably plays a similar role. Copulation may be characterized by repeated intromissions in species, such as the cat and rabbit, in which LH, the ovulatory hormone, is released by a neuroendocrine reflex.

Optimal service frequency varies considerably among unselected males. Thus, it is difficult to make general recommendations. Each male should be used according to his own capabilities within the limits of the conditions under which he is used. Among the factors to be considered are:

1. PHYSICAL CONDITION. Males with physical debilities must be used in limited service. Excessively fat or thin males are considered debilitated for breeding purposes.

2. SEMINAL QUALITY AND SPERM RESERVES. Males with semen of high quality and a high daily output of sperm should be used heavily. Males with inferior seminal quality or low daily output of sperm should not be used or used in limited service. Daily sperm production (DSP) refers to the number of spermatozoa produced daily by the testes and can be expressed as the number of spermatozoa produced per gram of testis or as the total number of spermatozoa produced. DSP is estimated by quantitative histological analysis of testicular tissue. Daily sperm output (DSO) refers to the number of sperm ejaculated and collected by artificial vagina or by electroejaculation after a period of frequent collections to deplete the sperm reserves (Table 8-7). In all of the domestic species studied to date, the DSP is higher than the DSO. Several factors, including spermatozoal losses in the collection equipment, phagocytosis and epididymal absorption of spermatozoa, or overestimation of the DSP have been considered to explain the difference between the DSP and DSO. Lino[145] and co-workers first proposed that the DSP for the ram could be estimated by determining the number of spermatozoa voided in the urine during periods of sexual rest. Lino's observations were largely ignored or disputed on the assumption that the large number of spermatozoa in the urine of sexually rested rams was due to masturbation. The finding of a significant percentage of retrograde flow of spermatozoa into the bladder during electroejaculation of rams, bulls, and cats, or during ejaculation induced by digital manipulation of the penis in dogs, suggests that the determination of the total number of spermatozoa in the ejaculate and in the urine collected immediately after ejaculation would accurately estimate the total number of sper-

Table 8-7   *Daily Sperm Production and Daily Sperm Output in Four Domestic Species**

| Species | Daily Sperm (10^9) | | | |
| | Production | | Output | |
	Mean	Range	Mean	Range
Stallion	8.0	5.7–10.6	7.0	4.4–8.7
Bull	5.3	3.2–6.7	2.7	1.7–4.0
Boar	16.5	—	16.3	—
Dog	0.48	—	0.37	—

*Adapted from Gebauer, M. B., et al.: J Anim. Sci. *39*:732, 1974 (Stallion); Swierstra, E. E.: Can. J. Anim. Sci. *46*:107, 1968 (Bull); Swierstra, E. E.: Biol. Reprod. *2*:23, 1970 (Boar); Olar, T. T., et al.: *Biol. Reprod.* 29: 1114, 1983 (Dog).

matozoa displaced during the ejaculatory process. Thus, Lino's approach could be adapted to monitor the DSP of each individual animal in a variety of experimental or field situations.

Testicular diameter is a simple clinical measurement related to spermatogenic activity. Spermatogenic deficiencies which are heritable should not be perpetuated, and males with such deficiencies should not be used as sires. Fortunately, some reproductive deficiencies are self-limiting. Unfortunately, sires with such deficiencies may be outstanding in other characteristics upon which selection is based, and a sound reproductive apparatus has been historically overlooked as a criterion for selection.

3. BREEDING MANAGEMENT. The ultimate efficiency of use of a male can be obtained through artificial insemination. Males used in hand breeding programs in which estrous females are presented to the male for single or limited multiple services may be used to inseminate more females than when pasture or random mating is practiced.

The size and topography of breeding pastures limit the number of females which may be assigned to a male in pasture breeding programs. When several males are together in a breeding pasture, social dominance and fighting reduce the effectiveness of the individual sires. Males in multisire pastures should be managed to reduce this problem to a minimum by keeping them dispersed.

4. LENGTH OF BREEDING SEASON. Males may be used to inseminate more females in a prolonged breeding season, especially if the number of females is evenly distributed over the breeding period.

5. INDIVIDUAL MATING BEHAVIOR. We sorely need some easily measured criteria that are correlated to mating behavior. For example, some bulls are known to inseminate cows with a single service, then move on to seek other estrous cows; other bulls serve a single female repeatedly before serving other cows in heat. Some bulls travel over large pastures daily in search of estrous cows; some bulls wait for cows in heat to come to water or a salt lick; still other bulls prefer to group and fight. Unfortunately, the complex interactions between males and females may limit the usefulness of measures of mating behavior. For example, bulls are known to "fall in love" with certain females, and the bull may devote his undivided attention to a single cow throughout estrus, and sometimes proestrus, as well, while other cows in heat are unable to attract his service.

Recommendations for service frequency are presented for each of the domestic species in the corresponding Chapters for Reproductive Patterns.

SPERM TRANSPORT

Efficient transport of a number of viable spermatozoa from the site of deposition during insemination (Table 8-6) to the site of gametic encounter in the ampulla of the oviduct is essential to fertilization. In most mammals, the transport of spermatozoa is rapid, and they reach the oviduct shortly after insemination. The highest concentration of spermatozoa is found at the site of seminal deposition, and the number of spermatozoa decreases rapidly in the ovarian direction so that few sperm cells reach the site of gametic encounter in the oviducts.

For a short time following mating or artificial insemination, uterine contractions are more important to the transport of spermatozoa in the female tract than is spermatozoal motility. The rate of transport through the tract is too rapid to be accounted for by sperm motility. Moeller and VanDemark[329] estimated the maximum velocity of bull sperm *in vitro* as 126 cm per hour. Since the bovine reproductive tract is about 65 cm in length, the fastest spermatozoon would require about 30 minutes to reach the ampulla of the oviduct. Bull spermatozoa have been found in the ovarian portion of the oviduct within 2.5 minutes following intracervical deposition of motile cells and within 4.3 minutes following insemination of nonmotile cells. Although few spermatozoa are rapidly transported to the ampullary region of the oviducts, these may not participate in fertilization. The establishment of a population of viable, fertile spermatozoa within the oviducts is a much slower process. In the sheep, significant numbers of viable spermatozoa enter the oviducts within 6 to 8 hours after mating, remain arrested in the caudal isthmus for about 18 hours, until the time of ovulation, when they are transported to the anterior oviduct. Similar rates in the transport of a population of spermatozoa have been observed for heifers, gilts, and laboratory rodents. It is possible that the retention of spermatozoa in the isthmus is related to a more efficient spermatozoal capacitation and may serve to protect the capacitated spermatozoa from the anterior oviductal environment, since capacitated spermatozoa are relatively fragile and short-lived. Motility of the female genital tract appears to be the dominant force in transporting

sperm to the oviducts in other species, as well. Spermatozoal motility does influence transcervical migration and distribution of sperm in the female tract, however, and may be important in the penetration of the oocyte during fertilization.

The reflexogenous release of oxytocin in response to visual and tactile stimuli also plays a role in the transport of sperm in cattle, in which natural mating and artificial insemination cause milk ejection and increased uterine contractions. Motile or nonmotile bull sperm were transported from the cervix to the tubal infundibulum of excised cow tracts in 2.5 to 5 minutes when oxytocin was present in the perfusate. When oxytocin was absent from the perfusate, cells did not penetrate beyond the body of the uterus. Epinephrine inhibits the effect of oxytocin in stimulating both milk ejection and uterine motility in the cow. For this reason, cows should be handled as quietly as possible in preparation for milking or breeding. However, oxytocin secreted at the time of mating does not seem to have a significant effect on sperm transport in ewes.

Spermatozoal transport into and through the cervix was inhibited in ewes that had grazed subterranean clover with estrogenic activity. Because ewes that graze pastures containing plants with high estrogenic activity also have a high incidence of maternal dystocia (difficult birth) due to uterine inertia, the impaired transport of spermatozoa may also be due to the inhibition of myometrial activity. Foreign devices such as an intrauterine plastic spiral in one horn of the uterus in ewes prevent sperm transport in both horns, probably as a result of impairment of neurogenic stimuli to myometrial activity. Finally, uterine contractions are in the form of segmentation waves which would tend to disperse semen throughout the uterus. Seminal plasma, identified by its characteristic components or by radioactive labeling of components, is distributed rapidly throughout the uterus.

Although uterine contractions are unquestionably important for the rapid transport of spermatozoa in most species, other mechanisms of transport cannot be regarded as unimportant to the reproductive process. Natural insemination usually occurs several hours before ovulation, and the rate of transport may be less important to conception and fertilization rates than the number of cells at the fertilization site in the ampulla of the oviduct. Additional factors influencing spermatozoal transport include the motility of spermatozoa, negative intrauterine pressure, the movement of genital fluids, the propensity of spermatozoa for rheotaxis (counterflow orientation), ciliary movements in the oviduct, and volume and concentration of spermatozoa in the inseminating dose.

The cervix, the uterotubal junction and possibly the isthmus of the oviduct are especially critical areas of spermatozoal transport, and only a fraction of the cells in the preceding segment of the tract passes these critical barriers (Fig. 8-21 and 8-22). The glans penis of the boar penetrates the cervix of the sow and the cervix is fully relaxed at the height of estrus in mares. Transport through the cervix may be influenced by the flow of cervical mucus, which undergoes physical and chemical changes related to the ovarian cycle, muscular contractions of the uterus and cervix, a negative uterine pressure due to a pumping action of the abdomen, and spermatozoal motility.

Segmenting and peristaltic contractions occur in the wall of the oviduct, but the peristaltic waves progress from the ovarian toward the uterine end of the oviduct. Ciliary movements are also abovarian, but the flow of oviduct fluids may then orient the spermatozoa toward the ovary. There is some controversy concerning the selectivity of the uterotubal barrier. Motile rat spermatozoa freely penetrate the uterotubal junction in estrous or diestrous rats, but dead rat sperm and inert particles do not pass, and foreign sperm pass through only rarely. On the other hand, nonmotile and foreign spermatozoa pass the uterotubal junction, even in the presence of an intrauterine foreign body, and goat sperm are successfully transported in the reproductive tract of the ewe.

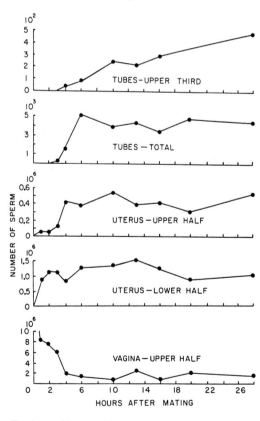

Fig. 8-21. Changes in sperm number in various sections of the genital tract of the rabbit after copulation. (Braden, A. W. H.: Aust. J. Biol. Sci. *6*:693, 1953.)

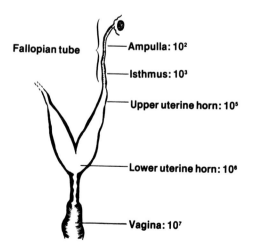

Fig. 8-22. Declining gradient in numbers of spermatozoa within the reproductive tract of the cow. (Compiled from different sources.)

REFERENCES

Control of Spermatogenesis

1. Amann, R. P. (1983): Endocrine changes associated with onset of spermatogenesis in Holstein bulls. J. Dairy Sci. *66*:2606.
2. Anderson, L. L. (1977): Development in calves and heifers after hypophysial stalk transection or hypophysectomy. Am. J. Physiol. *232*:E497.
3. Baumans, V., Dijkstra, G., and Wensing, C. J. G. (1981): Testicular descent in the dog. Zbl. Vet. Med. C. *10*:97.
4. Bellvé, A. R., and Feig, L. A. (1984): Cell proliferation in the mammalian testis: Biology of the seminiferous growth factor (SGF). Rec. Progr. Horm. Res. *40*:531.
5. Berndtson, W. E. (1977): Methods for quantifying mammalian spermatogenesis: A review. J. Anim. Sci. *44*:818.
6. Bonsma, J. C. (1940): The Influence of Climatological Factors on Cattle. Rep. Dept. Agric. So. Afr. No. 223. Bonsma, J. C. (1965). Wortham Lectures in Animal Science. College Station, Texas A & M University Press.
7. Bowler, K. (1972): The effect of repeated applications of heat on spermatogenesis in the rat: A histological study. J. Reprod. Fertil. *28*:325.
8. Bustos-Obregon, E., Courot, M., Flechon, J. E., et al. (1975): Morphological appraisal of gametogenesis. Spermatogenic process in mammals with particular reference to man. Andrologia *7*:141.
9. Courot, M., Hochereau-de-Reviers, M.-T., Monet-Kuntz, C., et al. (1979): Endocrinology of spermatogenesis in the hypophysectomized ram. J. Reprod. Fertil. *26*(Suppl.):165.
10. Dorrington, J. H., Roller, N. F., and Fritz, I. B. (1975): Effects of follicle-stimulating hormone on cultures of Sertoli cell preparations. Mol. Cell Endocrinol. *3*:57.
11. Forest, M. G. (1983): Role of androgens in fetal and pubertal development. Horm. Res. *18*:69.
12. Frankenhuis, M. T., Wensing, C. J. G., and Kremer, J. (1981): The influence of elevated testicular temperature and scrotal surgery on the number of gonocytes in the newborn pig. Int. J. Androl. *4*:105.
13. Frey, H. L., Peng, S., and Rajfer, J. (1983): Synergy of abdominal pressure and androgens in testicular descent. Biol. Reprod. *29*:1233.
14. Fritz, I. B., Louis, B. G., Tung, P. S., et al. (1978): Action of hormones on Sertoli cells during maturation. Ann. Biol. Anim. Biochim. Biophys. *18*:555.
15. Gebauer, M. R., Pickett, B. W., and Swierstra, E. E. (1974): Reproductive physiology of the stallion. III. Extra-gonadal transit time and sperm reserves. J. Anim. Sci. *39*:737.
16. Glover, T. D., and Young, D. H. (1963): Temperature and the production of spermatozoa. Fertil. Steril. *14*:441.
17. Gomez, W. R., and VanDemark, N. L. (1974): The male reproductive system. Ann. Rev. Physiol. *36*:307.
18. Hart, B. L., and Ladewig, J. (1979): Serum testosterone of neonatal male and female dogs. Biol. Reprod. 21:289.
19. Hidiroglou, M. (1979): Trace elements deficiencies and fertility in ruminants: A review. J. Dairy Sci. *62*:1195.
20. Howard, B., Jr. (1969): Fertility in the ram following exposure to elevated ambient temperature and humidity. J. Reprod. Fertil. *19*:179.
21. Kellaway, R. C., Seamark, R. F., and Ferrant, R. K. (1971): Sterilization of cattle by induced cryptorchidism. Aust. Vet. J. *47*:547.
22. Kennelly, J. J. (1972): Coyote reproduction. I. The duration of the spermatogenic cycle and epididymal sperm transport. J. Reprod. Fertil. *31*:163.
23. Kroes, R., Berkvens, J. M., Loendersloot, H. J., et al. (1971): Oestrogen-induced changes in the genital tract of the male calf. Zbl. Vet. Med, *18*:717.
24. Mather, J. P., Gunsalus, G. L., Musto, N. A., et al. (1983): The hormonal and cellular control of Sertoli cell secretion. J. Steroid Biochem. *19*:41.
25. McCarthy, M. S., Convey, E. M., and Hafs, H. D. (1979): Serum hormonal changes and testicular response to LH during puberty in bulls. Biol. Reprod. *20*:1221.
26. Meinecke, C. F. and McDonald, L. E. (1961): The effects of exogenous testosterone on spermatogenesis of bulls. Am. J. Vet. Res. *22*:209.
27. Moyle, W. R., Kuczek, T., and Bailey, C. A. (1985): Potential of a quantal response as a mechanism for oscillatory behavior: Implications of our concepts of hormonal control mechanisms. Biol. Reprod. *32*:43.
28. Ross, G. T., and Lipsett, M. B. (1978): Homologies of structure and function in mammalian testes and ovaries. Int. J. Androl. Suppl. *2*:39.
29. Sanborn, B. M., Tsai, Y. H., Steinberger, A., et al. (1978): Biochemical aspects of the interaction of androgens with Sertoli cells. Ann. Biol. Anim. Biochim. Biophys. *18*:615.
30. Schanbacher, B. D., and Ford, J. J. (1979): Photoperiodic regulation of ovine spermatogenesis: relationship to serum hormones. Biol. Reprod. *20*:719.
31. Sharpe, R. M. (1983): Local control of testicular function. Quart. J. Exp. Physiol. *68*:265.
32. Sharpe, R. M. (1984): Intratesticular factors controlling testicular function. Biol. Reprod. *30*:29.
33. Solari, A. J., and Fritz, I. B. (1978): The ultrastructure of immature Sertoli cells. Maturation-like changes during culture and the maintenance of mitotic potentiality. Biol. Reprod. *18*:329.
34. Steinberger, E. (1971): Hormonal control of mammalian spermatogenesis. Physiol. Rev. *51*:1.
35. Stone, B. A. (1981/1982): Heat induced infertility of boars: the inter-relationship between depressed sperm output and fertility and an estimation of the critical air temperature above which sperm output is impaired. Anim. Reprod. Sci. *4*:283.
36. Swierstra, E. E. (1968): Cytology and duration of the cycle of the seminiferous epithelium of the boar; duration of spermatozoa transit through the epididymis. Anat. Rec. *161*:171.
37. Swierstra, E. E. (1970): The effect of low ambient temperatures on sperm production, epididymal sperm reserves and semen characteristics of boars. Biol. Reprod. *2*:23.
38. Terner, C. (1977): Progesterone and progestins in the male reproductive system. Ann. N. Y. Acad. Sci. *286*:313.

39. Van der Molen, H. J., Van Beurden, M. O., Blankenstein, M. A., et al. (1979): The testis: Biochemical actions of trophic hormones and steroids on steroid production and spermatogenesis. J. Steroid Biochem. *11*:13.

40. Voglmayr, J. K., Setchell, B. P., and White, I. G. (1971): The effects of heat on the metabolism and ultrastructure of ram testicular spermatozoa. J. Reprod. Fertil. *24*:71.

Steroidogenic Function

41. Abdel-Raouf, M. (1960): The postnatal development of the reproductive organs in bulls with special reference to puberty. Acta Endocrinol. *34*, Suppl. 49.

42. Amann, R. P., and Ganjam, U. K. (1976): Steroid production by the bovine testis and steroid transfer across the pampiniform plexus. Biol. Reprod. *15*: 695.

43. Andresen, O.. (1976): Concentrations of fat and plasma 5α-androstenone and plasma testosterone in boars selected for rate of body weight gain and thickness of back fat during growth, sexual maturation and after mating. J. Reprod. Fertil. *48*:51.

44. Aronson, L. R., and Cooper, M. L. (1967): Penile spines of the domestic cat. Anat. Rec. *157*:71.

45. Bardin, C. W., and Catterall, J. F. (1981): Testosterone: a major determinant of extragenital sexual dimorphism. Science *211*:1285.

46. Barenton, B., Blanc, M. R., Caraty, A., et al. (1982): Effect of cryptorchidism in the ram: changes in the concentrations of testosterone and estradiol and receptors for LH and FSH in the testis, and its histology. Mol. Cell Endocrinol. *28*: 13.

47. Bartke, A., Hafiez, A. A., Bex, F. J., et al. (1978): Hormonal interactions in the regulation of androgen secretion. Biol. Reprod. *18*:44.

48. Bedrak, E., and Samuels, L. T. (1969): Steroid biosynthesis by the equine testis. Endocrinology *85*: 1186.

49. Benahmed, M., Bernier, M., Ducharme, J. R., et al. (1982): Steroidogenesis of cultured purified pig Leydig cells: secretion and effects of estrogens. Mol. Cell. Endocrinol. *28*:705.

50. Bergh, A. (1983): Paracrine regulation of Leydig cells by the seminiferous tubules. Int. J. Androl. *6*:57.

51. Berndtson, W. E., Pickett, B. W., and Nett, T. M. (1974): Reproductive physiology of the stallion. IV. Seasonal changes in the testosterone concentration of peripheral plasma. J. Reprod. Fertil. *39*:115.

52. Boyden, T. W., Pamenter, R. W., and Silvert, M. A. (1980): Testosterone secretion by the isolated canine testis after controlled infusions of hCG. J. Reprod. Fertil. *59*:25.

53. Brooks, R. I., and Pearson, A. M. (1986): Steroid hormone pathways in the pig, with special emphasis on boar odor: a review. J. Anim. Sci. *62*:632.

54. Bubenik, G. A., Brown, G. M., and Grota, L. J. (1975): Localization of immunoreactive androgen in testicular tissue. Endocrinology *96*:63.

55. Bustos-Obregon, E. (1976): Ultrastructure and function of the lamina propria of mammalian seminiferous tubules. Andrologia *8*:179.

56. Cahoreau, C., Blanc, M. R., Dacheux, J. L., et al. (1979): Inhibin activity in ram rete testis fluid: depression of plasma FSH and LH in the castrated and cryptorchid ram. J. Reprod. Fertil. Suppl. *26*: 97.

57. Carroll, E. J., Aanes, W. A., and Ball, L. (1964): Persistent penile frenulum in bulls. J. Am. Vet. Med. Assoc. *144*:747.

58. Chari, S., Duraiswami, S., and Franchimont, P. (1978): Isolation and characterization of inhibin from bull seminal plasma. Acta Endocrinol. *87*:434.

59. Claus, R., and Hoffmann, B. (1980): Oestrogens, compared to other steroids of testicular origin, in blood plasma of boars. Acta Endocrinol. *94*:404.

60. Claus, R., Schopper, D., and Hoang-Vu, C. (1985): Contribution of individual compartments of the genital tract to oestrogen and testosterone concentrations in the ejaculates of the boar. Acta Endocrinol. *109*:281.

61. Comhaire, F., Mattheeuws, D., and Vermeulen, A. (1974): Testosterone and oestradiol in dogs with testicular tumors. Acta Endocrinol. *77*:408.

62. Davies, A. G. (1981): Role of FSH in the control of testicular function. Arch. Androl. *7*:97.

63. De Palatis, L., Moore, J., and Falvo, R. E. (1978): Plasma concentrations of testosterone and LH in the male dog. J. Reprod. Fertil. *52*:201.

64. Dierschke, D. J., Walsh, S. W., Mapletoft, R. J., et al. (1975): Functional anatomy of the testicular vascular pedicle in the Rhesus monkey: Evidence for a local testosterone concentrating mechanism. Proc. Soc. Exp. Biol. Med. *148*:236.

65. Eik-Nes, K. B. (1975): Biosynthesis and secretion of testicular steroids. *In* Handbook of Physiology, Section 7, Vol. V, Male Reproductive System, edited by D. W. Hamilton and R. O. Greep. Washington, D. C., American Physiological Society, p. 95.

66. Einer-Jensen, N., and Waites, G. M. H. (1977): Testicular blood flow and a study of the testicular venous to arterial transfer of radioactive krypton and testosterone in the Rhesus monkey. J. Physiol. *267*:1.

67. Ewing, L. L., Zirkin, B. R., Cochran, R. C., et al. (1979): Testosterone secretion by rat, rabbit, guinea pig, dog, and hamster testes perfused in vitro: correlation with Leydig cell mass. Endocrinology *105*: 1135.

68. Flor-Cruz, S. V., and Lapwood, K. R. (1978): A longitudinal study of pubertal development in boars. Int. J. Androl. *1*: 317.

69. Fonda, E. S., Diehl, J. R., Barb, C. R., et al. (1981): Serum luteinizing hormone, testosterone production and cortisol concentrations after PGF2α in the boar. Prostaglandins *21*:933.

70. Franchimont, P. (1982): Intragonadal regulation of reproduction. Int J. Androl. Suppl. *5*:157.

71. Franchimont, P., Chari, S., Hagelstein, M., et al. (1975): Existence of follicle stimulating hormone inhibiting factor "inhibin" in bull seminal plasma. Nature *257*:402.

72. Frankenhuis, M. T., and Wensing, C. J. G. (1979): Induction of spermatogenesis in the naturally cryptorchid pig. Fertil. Steril. *31*:428.

73. Ganjam, V.K., and Kenney, R. M. (1975): Androgens and oestrogens in normal and cryptorchid stallions. J. Reprod. Fertil., Suppl. *23*:67.
74. Garnier, D.-H., Cotta, Y., and Tergui, M. (1978): Androgen radioimmunoassay in the ram: Results of direct plasma testosterone and dehydroepiandrosterone measurement and physiological evaluation. Ann. Biol. Anim. Biochim. Biphys. *18*:265.
75. Ginther, O. J., Mapletoft, R. J., Zimmerman, N., et al. (1974): Local increase in testosterone concentration in the testicular artery in rams. J. Anim. Sci. *38*:835.
76. Godfrey, R. W., Randel, R. D., Forrest, D. W., et al. (1985): The concentration of estradiol-17β in bovine semen. J. Anim. Sci. *60*:760.
77. Graham, J. M., and Desjardins, C. (1981): Classical conditioning: Induction of luteinizing hormone and testosterone secretion in anticipation of sexual activity. Science *210*:1039.
78. Gray, R. C., Day, B. N., Lasley, J. F., et al. (1971): Testosterone levels of boars at various ages. J. Anim. Sci. *33*:124.
79. Hafiez, A. A., Bartke, A., and Lloyd, C. W. (1972): The role of prolactin in the regulation of testis function: The synergistic effects of prolactin and luteinizing hormone on the incorporation of [I-^{14}C] acetate into testosterone and cholesterol by testes from hypophysectomized rats *in vitro*. J. Endocrinol. *53*:223.
80. Hammerstedt, R. H., and Amann, R. P. (1976): Effects of physiological levels of exogenous steroids on metabolism of testicular, cauda epididymal and ejaculated bovine sperm. Biol. Reprod. *15*:678.
81. Harris, J. M., Irvine, C. H. J., and Evans, M. J. (1983): Seasonal changes and serum levels of FSH, LH and testosterone and in semen parameters in stallions. Theriogenology *19*:311.
82. Hitzeman, J. W. (1968): Effect of the interstitial-cell-stimulating hormone on testicular enzymes during spermatogenesis. J. Exp. Zool. *169*:335.
83. Hsueh, A. J. W., and Schaeffer, J. M. (1985): Gonadotropin-releasing hormone as a paracrine hormone and neurotransmitter in extra-pituitary sites. J. Steroid Biochem. *23*:757.
84. Johnson, L., and Neaves, W. B. (1981): Age-related changes in the Leydig cell population, seminiferous tubules, and sperm production in stallions. Biol. Reprod. *24*:703.
85. Johnson, L., and Thompson, D. L., Jr. (1983): Age-related and seasonal variation in the Sertoli cell population, daily sperm production and serum concentrations of follicle-stimulating hormone, luteinizing hormone and testosterone in stallions. Biol. Reprod. *29*:777.
86. Johnstone, I. P., Bancroft, B. J., and McFarlane, J. R. (1984): Testosterone and androstenedione profiles in the blood of domestic tom cats. Anim. Reprod. Sci. *7*:363.
87. Jost, A. (1965): Gonadal hormones in the sex differentiation of the mammalian fetus. *In* Organogenesis, edited by R. L. DeHaan and H. Ursprung. New York, Holt, Rinehart and Winston, p. 611.
88. Juniewicz, P. E., and Johnson, B. H. (1981): Influence of adrenal steroids upon testosterone secretion by the boar testis. Biol. Reprod. *25*:725.
89. Katongole, C. B., Naftolin, F., and Short, R. V.

(1974): Seasonal variations in blood luteinizing hormone and testosterone levels in rams. J. Endocrinol. *60*:101.
90. Lacroix, A., and Pelletier, J. (1979): LH and testosterone release in developing bulls following LH-RH treatment. Effect of gonadectomy and chronic testosterone propionate pre-treatment. Acta Endocrinol. *91*:719.
91. Lee, V. W. K., Keogh, E. J., Burger, H. G., et al. (1976): Studies on the relationship between FSH and germ cells: Evidence for selective suppression of FSH by testicular extracts. J. Reprod. Fertil., Suppl. *24*:1.
92. Lieberman, S., Greenfield, N. J., and Wolfson, A. (1984): A heuristic proposal for understanding steroidogenic processes. Endocrinology *5*:128.
93. Lloyd, J. W., Thomas, J. A., and Mawhinney, M. G. (1975): Androgens and estrogens in the plasma and prostatic tissue of normal dogs and dogs with benign prostatic hypertrophy. Invest. Urol. *13*:220.
94. Lluarado, J. G., and Dominguez, O. V. (1963): Effect of cryptorchidism on testicular enzymes involved in androgen biosynthesis. Endocrinology *72*:292.
95. McCullagh, D. R. (1932): Dual endocrine activity of the testis. Science *76*:19.
96. Muduuli, D. S, Sanford, L. M., Palmer, W. M. et al. (1979). Secretory patterns and circadian and seasonal changes in luteinizing hormone, follicle stimulating hormone, prolactin and testosterone in the male pygmy goat. J. Anim. Sci. *49*:543.
97. Parlow, A. F., Bailey, C. M., and Foote, W. D. (1973): The unusual effect of gonadectomy on pituitary gonadotrophins in the male bovine. J. Reprod. Fertil. *33*:441.
98. Peters, H. (1976): Intrauterine gonadal development. Fertil. Steril. *27*:493.
99. Peyrat, J.-P., Meusy-Desolle, N., and Garnier, J. (1981): Changes in Leydig cells and luteinizing hormone receptors in porcine testis during postnatal development. Endocrinology *108*:625.
100. Pierrepoint, C. G., Davies, P., Millington, D., et al. (1975): Evidence that the deferential veins act as a local transport system for androgen in the rat and the dog. J. Reprod. Fertil. *43*:293.
101. Pierrepoint, C. G., Galley, J. McI., Griffiths, K., et al. (1967): Steroid metabolism of a Sertoli cell tumor of the testis of a dog with feminization and alopecia and of the normal canine testis. J. Endocrinol. *38*:61.
102. Rawlings, N. C., Hafs, H. D., and Swanson; L. V. (1972): Testicular and blood plasma androgens in Holstein bulls from birth through puberty. J. Anim. Sci. *34*:435.
103. Reiffsteck, A., Dehennin, L., and Scholler, R. (1982): Estrogens in seminal plasma of human and animal species: identification and quantitative estimation by gas chromatography-mass spectrometry associated with stable isotope dilution. J. Steroid Biochem. *17*:567.
104. Rowson, L. E. A., and Skinner, J. D. (1968): Some Effects of Orchiopexy on the Testes of Unilateral Cryptorchid Pubescent Rams. *In* Proc. VIth Int. Cong. Anim. Reprod. & AI., Paris, Vol. 1, p. 313.
105. Sanford, L. M., Simaraks, S., Palmer, W. M., et al. (1982): Circulating estrogen levels in the ram: in-

fluence of season and mating, and their relationship to testosterone levels and mating frequency. Canad. J. Anim. Sci. *62*:85.

106. Sanford, L. M., Winter, J. S. D., Palmer, W. M., et al. (1974): The profile of LH and testosterone in the ram. Endocrinology *96*:627.

107. Schanbacher, B. D., and Ford, J. J. (1976): Seasonal profiles of plasma luteinizing hormone, testosterone, and estradiol in the ram. Endocrinology *99*:752.

108. Setchell, B. P., and Main, S. J. (1975): The blood-testis barrier and steroids. *In* Hormonal Regulation of Spermatogenesis, edited by F. S. French, V. Hansson, E. M. Ritzen, and S. N. Neyfeh. New York, Plenum Press, p. 513.

109. Setchell, B. P., Laurie, M. S., Flint, A. P. F. et al. (1983): Transport of free and conjugated steroids from the boar testis in lymph, venous blood and rete testis fluid. J. Endocrinol. *96*:127.

110. Setoguti, T., Esumi, H., and Shimizu, T. (1974): Electron microscopic studies on dog testicular interstitial cells. Arch. Histol. Jpn. *37*:97.

111. Sharpe, R. M. (1982): Cellular aspects of the inhibitory actions of LH-RH on the ovary and testis. J. Reprod. Fertil. *64*:517.

112. Sharpe, R. M. (1984): Intratesticular factors controlling testicular function. Biol. Reprod. *30*:29.

113. Steinberger, A. (1979): Inhibin production by Sertoli cells in culture. J. Reprod. Fertil. *26*:31.

114. Swierstra, E. E., Gebauer, M. R., and Pickett, B. W. (1974): Reproductive physiology of the stallion. I. Spermatogenesis and testis composition. J. Reprod. Fertil. *40*:113.

115. Taha, M. B., and Noakes, D. E. (1982): The effect of age and season of the year on testicular function in the dog, as determined by histological examination of the seminiferous tubules and the estimation of peripheral plasma testosterone concentrations. J. Small Anim. Pract. *23*:351.

116. Taha, M. B., Noakes, D. E., and Allen, W. E. (1982): Hemicastration in the beagle dog; the effects on libido, peripheral plasma testosterone concentrations, seminal characteristics and testicular function. J. Small Anim. Pract. *23*:279.

117. Vincent, D. L., Kepic, T. A., Lathrop, J. C., et al. (1979): Testosterone regulation of luteinizing hormone secretion in the male dog. Int. J. Androl. *2*:241.

118. Weathersbee, P. S., and Lodge, J. R. (1976): Serum testosterone and estrogen concentrations in the Holstein-Friesian bull after successive ejaculations. Am. J. Vet. Res. *37*:465.

119. Wrobel, K.-H., Sinowatz, F., and Mademann, R. (1981): Intertubular topography in the bovine testis. Cell Tissue Res. *217*:289.

120. Zlotnik, G. (1973): Testosterone levels in intersex goats. J. Reprod. Fertil. *32*:287.

The Excurrent Tract

121. Amann, R. P. (1970): Sperm Production Rates. *In* The Testis edited by A. D. Johnson, W. R. Gomes, and N. L. Vandemark, New York, Academic Press, p. 433.

122. Amann, R. P. (1981): A critical review of methods for evaluation of spermatogenesis from seminal characteristics. J. Androl. *2*:37.

123. Amann, R. P., Hay, S. R., and Hammerstedt, R. H. (1982): Yield, characteristics, motility and cAMP content of sperm isolated from seven regions of ram epididymis. Biol. Reprod. *27*:723.

124. Amann, R. P., Johnson, L., and Pickett, B. W. (1977): Connection between the seminiferous tubules and the efferent ducts in the stallion. Am. J. Vet. Res. *38*:1571.

125. Bedford, J. M. (1978): Anatomical evidence for the epididymis as the prime mover in the evolution of the scrotum. Am. J. Anat. *152*:483.

126. Brooks, D. E. (1983): Epididymal functions and their hormonal regulation. Aust. J. Biol. Sci. *36*: 205.

127. Dacheux, J. L., and Paquignon, M. (1980): Relations between the fertilizing ability, motility and metabolism of epididymal spermatozoa. Reprod. Nutr. Develop. *20*:1085.

128. Dooley, M. P., Pineda, M. H., Hopper, J. G., et al. (1984): Retrograde Flow of Semen Caused by Electroejaculation in the Domestic Cat. Proc. 10th Int. Cong. Anim. Reprod. & AI. Univ. of Illinois, Urbana-Champaign, Vol. III, Brief Comm. 363.

129. Dooley, M. P., Pineda, M. H., Maurer, R. R., et al. (1986): Evidence for retrograde flow of spermatozoa into the urinary bladder of bulls during electroejaculation. Theriogenology *26*:101.

130. Dym, M. (1976): The mammalian rete testis—a morphological examination. Anat. Rec. *186*:493.

131. Ellis, L. C., Groesbeck, M. D., Farr, C. H., et al. (1981): Contractility of seminiferous tubules as related to sperm transport in the male. Arch. Androl. *6*:283.

132. Essenhigh, D. M., Chir, M., Adran, G. M., et al. (1969): The vesical sphincters and ejaculation in the ram. Br. J. Urol. *41*:190.

133. Frenette, M. D., Dooley, M. P., and Pineda, M. H. (1986): Effect of flushing the vasa deferentia at the time of vasectomy on the rate of clearance of spermatozoa from the ejaculates of dogs and cats. Am. J. Vet. Res. *47*:463.

134. Garbers, D. L., Wakabayashi, T., and Reed, P. W. (1970): Enzyme profile of the cytoplasmatic droplet from bovine epididymal spermatozoa. Biol. Reprod. *3*:327.

135. Hammerstedt, R. H., Hay, S. R., and Amann, R. P. (1982): Modification of ram sperm membranes during epididymal transit. Biol. Reprod. *27*:745.

136. Hemeida, N. A., Sack, W. O., and McEntee, K. (1978): Ductuli efferentes in the epididymis of boar, goat, ram, bull, and stallion. Am. J. Vet. Res. *39*: 1892.

137. Hess, R. A., Thurston, R. J., and Biellier, H. V. (1976): Morphology of the epididymal region and ductus deferens of the turkey (Meleagris gallopavo). J. Anat. *122*:241.

138. Hopwood, M. L., Faulkner, L. C., and Gassner, F. X. (1963): Effect of exhaustive ejaculation on composition of bovine semen. J. Dairy Sci. *46*:1409.

139. Hovell, G. J. R., Ardran, G. M., Essenhigh, D. M., et al. (1969): Radiological observations on electrically-induced ejaculation in the ram. J. Reprod. Fertil. *20*:383.

140. Johnson, A. L., and Pursel, V. G. (1975): Cannula-

tion of ductus deferens of the boar: A surgical technique. Am. J. Vet. Res. *36*;315.

141. Inskeep, P. B., and Hammerstedt, R. H. (1982): Changes in metabolism of ram sperm associated with epididymal transit or induced by exogenous carnitine. Biol. Reprod. *27*:735.

142. Johnson, L., Amann, R. P., and Pickett, B. W. (1980): Maturation of equine epididymal spermatozoa. Am. J. Vet. Res. *41*:1190.

143. Jones, R. (1978): Comparative biochemistry of mammalian epididymal plasma. Comp. Biochem. Physiol. *61B*:365.

144. Koefoed-Johnsen, H. H. (1964): "Sperm production in bulls. The excretion of sperm with the urine at each ejaculation frequences" (sic). In Danish, title from English summary. Ann. Report Royal Veterinary and Agricultural College, Copenhagen, A/S Carl F. R. Mortensen, p. 23.

145. Lino, B. F., Braden, A. W. H., and Turnbull, K. E. (1967): Fate of unejaculated spermatozoa. Nature *213*:594.

146. Oslund, R. M. (1928): The physiology of the male reproductive system. J. Am. Med. Assoc. *40*:829.

147. Pickett, B. W., and Komarek, R. J. (1967): Lipid and dry weight of bovine seminal plasma and spermatozoa from first and second ejaculates. J. Dairy Sci. *50*:742.

148. Pineda, M. H., Dooley, M. P., Hembrough, F. B., et al. (1987): Retrograde flow of spermatozoa into the urinary bladder of rams. Am. J. Vet. Res. *48*:562.

149. Pineda, M. H., Reimers, T. J., and Faulkner, L. C. (1976): Disappearance of spermatozoa from the ejaculates of vasectomized dogs. J. Am. Vet. Med. Assoc. *168*:502.

150. Quinn, P. J., White, I. G., and Wirrick, B. R. (1965): Studies of the distribution of the major cations in semen and male accessory secretions. J. Reprod. Fertil. *10*:379.

151. Riar, S. S., Setty, B. S., and Amiya, B. K. (1973): Studies on physiology and biochemistry of mammalian epididymis: Histology, enzyme and electrolyte composition of epididymis—a comparative study. Ind. J. Exp. Biol. *11*:365.

152. Schultz, W. H. (1935): Studies on the rat's genitourinary tract. Quantitative measurements of intravesical volume and pressure and of the urethral outflow. J. Urol. *34*:156.

153. Scott, T. W., Voglmayr, J. K., and Setchell, B. P. (1967): Lipid composition and metabolism in testicular and ejaculated ram spermatozoa. Biochem. J. *102*:456.

154. Tischner, M. (1971): Transport of unejaculated spermatozoa through the pelvic part of the urogenital tract in the ram. J. Reprod. Fertil. *24*:271.

155. Tischner, M. (1972): The role of the vasa deferentia and the urethra in the transport of semen in rams. Acta Agr. et Silv. *12*:77.

156. Usselman, M. C., and Cone, R. A. (1983): Rat sperm are mechanically immobilized in the caudal epididymis by "immobilin", a high molecular weight glycoprotein. Biol. Reprod. *29*:1241.

157. Voglmayr, J. K., Waites, G. M. H., and Setchell, B. P. (1966): Studies on spermatozoa and fluid collected directly from the testis of the conscious ram. Nature *210*:861.

The Accessory Sex Glands

158. Barnes, G. W. (1972): The antigenic nature of male accessory glands of reproduction. Biol. Reprod. *6*: 384.

159. Boesel, R. W., Klipper, R. W., and Shain, S. A. (1977): Identification of limited capacity androgen binding components in nuclear and cytoplasmic fractions of canine prostate. Endocr. Res. Commun. *4*:71.

160. Bowen, R. A. (1977): Fertilization in vitro of feline ova by spermatozoa from the ductus deferens. Biol. Reprod. *17*: 144.

161. Davies, D. C., Hall, G., Hibbitt, K. G., et al. (1975): The removal of the seminal vesicles from the boar and the effects on the semen characteristics. J. Reprod. Fertil. *43*:305.

162. Joshi, H. S., and Raeside, J. I. (1973): Synergistic effects of testosterone and oestrogens on accessory sex glands and sexual behaviour of the boar. J. Reprod. Fertil. *33*:411.

163. MacMillan, K. L., and Hafs, H. D. (1969): Reproductive tract of Holstein bulls from birth through puberty. J. Anim. Sci. *28*:233.

164. Nalbandov, A. V. (1964): Reproductive Physiology, 2nd ed. San Francisco, W. H. Freeman & Co., p. 50.

165. Rodger, J. C. (1976): Comparative aspects of the accessory sex glands and seminal biochemistry of mammals. Comp. Biochem. Physiol. *55B*:1.

166. Wales, R. G., and White, I. G. (1965): Some observations on the chemistry of dog semen. J. Reprod. Fertil. *9*:69.

167. Wilson, J. D., and Gloyna, R. E. (1970): The intranuclear metabolism of testosterone in the accessory organs of reproduction. Recent Prog. Horm. Res. *26*:309.

Penis and Prepuce

168. Ashdown, R. R. (1962): Persistence of the penile frenulum in young bulls. Vet. Rec. *74*:1464.

169. Ashdown, R. R., and Gilanpour, H. (1974): Venous drainage of the corpus cavernosum penis in impotent and normal bulls. J. Anat. *117*;159.

170. Ashdown, R. R., and Majeed, Z. Z. (1976): The shape of the free end of the bovine penis during erection and protrusion. Vet. Rec. *99*:354.

171. Ashdown, R. R., and Pearson, H. (1973): Studies on "Corkscrew Penis" in the bull. Vet. Rec. *93*:30.

172. Ashdown, R. R., and Pearson, H. (1973): Anatomical and experimental studies on eversion of the sheath and protrusion of the penis in the bull. Res. Vet. Sci. *15*:13.

173. Ashdown, R. R., Barnett, S. W., and Ardalani, G. (1981): Impotence in the boar: Angioarchitecture and venous drainage of the penis in normal boars. Vet. Rec. *109*:375.

174. Ashdown, R. R., Barnett, S. W., and Ardalani, G. (1982): Venous drainage of the ovine corpus cavernosum penis. J. Anat. *134*:621.

175. Ashdown, R. R., Barnett, S. W., and Ardalani, G. (1982): Impotence in the boar 2: clinical and anatomical studies on impotent boars. Vet. Rec. *110*:349.

176. Ashdown, R. R., David, J. S. E., and Gibbs, C.

(1979): Impotence in the bull: (1) Abnormal venous drainage of the corpus cavernosum penis. Vet. Rec. *104*:423.

177. Ashdown, R. R., Gilanpour, H., David, J. S. E., et al. (1979): Impotence in the bull: (2) Occlusion of the longitudinal canals of the corpus cavernosum penis. Vet. Rec. *104*:598.

178. Ashdown, R. R., Ricketts, S. W., and Wardley, R. C. (1968): The fibrous architecture of the integumentary coverings of the bovine penis. J. Anat. *103*: 567.

179. Beckett, S. D., Hudson, R. S., Walker, D. F., et al. (1973): Blood pressures and penile muscle activity in the stallion during coitus. Am. J. Physiol. *225*: 1072.

180. Beckett, S. D., Reynolds T. M., Walker, D. F., et al. (1974): Experimentally induced rupture of corpus cavernosum penis of the bull. Am. J. Vet. Res. *35*:765.

181. Beckett, S. D., Walker, D. F., Hudson, R. S. et al. (1975): Corpus spongiosum penis pressure and penile muscle activity in the stallion during coitus. Am. J. Vet. Res. *36*:431.

182. Beckett, S. D., Walker, D. F., Hudson, R. S., et al. (1974): Corpus cavernosum penis pressure and penile muscle activity in the bull during coitus. Am. J. Vet. Res. *35*:761.

183. Bharadwaj, M. B., and Calhoun, M. L. (1961): Mode of formation of the preputial cavity in domestic animals. Am. J. Vet. Res. *22*:764.

184. Grandage, J. (1972): The erect dog penis: A paradox of flexible rigidity. Vet. Rec. *91*:141.

185. Kainer, R. A., Faulkner, L. C., and Abdel-Raouf, M. (1969): Glands associated with the urethra of the bull. Am. J. Vet. Res. *30*:963.

186. Seidel, G. E., and Foote, R. H. (1967): Motion picture analysis of bovine ejaculation. J. Dairy Sci. *50*:970.

187. Young, S. L., Hudson, R. S., and Walker, D. F. (1977): Impotence in bulls due to vascular shunts from the corpus cavernosum penis. J. Am. Vet. Med. Assoc. *171*:643.

Biology of Spermatozoa

188. Amann, R. P. (1981): A critical review of methods for evaluation of spermatogenesis from seminal characteristics. J. Androl. *2*:37.

189. Atherton, R. W. (1979): A review of the spectrometric quantitation of spermatozoal motility. *In* The spermatozoon, edited by D. W. Fawcett and J. M. Bedford, Baltimore, Urban and Schwarzenberg, p. 421.

190. Bahr, G. F., and Engler, W. F. (1970): Considerations of volume, mass, DNA, and arrangement of mitochondria in the midpiece of bull spermatozoa. Exp. Cell Res. *60*:338.

191. Bustos-Obregon, E., and Flechon, J.-E. (1975): Comparative scanning electron microscope study of boar, bull and ram spermatozoa. Cell Tissue Res. *161*:329.

192. Doak, R. L., Hall, A., and Dale, H. E. (1967): Longevity of spermatozoa in the reproductive tract in the bitch. J. Reprod. Fertil. *13*:51.

193. Dott, H. M. (1975): Morphology of stallion spermatozoa. J. Reprod. Fertil. *23*:41.

194. Fawcett, D. W. (1970): A comparative view of sperm ultrastructure. Biol. Reprod. (Suppl.) *2*:90.

195. Fawcett, D. W. (1975): The mammalian spermatozoon. Develop. Biol. *44*:394.

196. Fawcett, D. W. (1977): What makes cilia and sperm tails beat? N. Engl. J. Med. *297*:46.

197. Fawcett, D. W., and Philips, D. M. (1969): The fine structure and development of the neck region of the mammalian spermatozoon. Anat. Rec. *165*:153.

198. Fawcett, D. W., Anderson, W. A., and Philips, D. M. (1971): Morphogenic factors influencing the shape of the sperm head. Develop. Biol. *26*:220.

199. Fiser, P. S., and Fairfull, R. W. (1983): Effect of changes in photoperiod on freezability of ram spermatozoa. Cryobiology 20:684.

200. Garner, D. L., Gledhill, B. L., Pinkel, D., et al. (1983): Quantification of the X- and Y-chromosome-bearing spermatozoa of domestic animals by flow cytometry. Biol. Reprod. *28*:312.

201. Gledhill, B. L. (1970): Enigma of spermatozoal deoxyribonucleic acid and male infertility: A review. Am. J. Vet. Res. *31*:539.

202. Jones, R. C. (1973): The plasma membrane of ram, boar and bull spermatozoa. J. Reprod. Fertil. *33*: 179.

203. Kozima, Y. (1966): Electron microscopic study of the bull spermatozoon. Jpn. J. Vet. Res. *14*:1.

204. Morstin, J., and Courot, M. (1974): Ultrastructure des spermatozoïdes de taureaux de différente fecondance. Morphologie ultrastructurale, glycoprotéines acrosomiques et membranaires, charges négatives de surface. Ann. Biol. Anim. Biochim. Biophys. *14*: 581.

205. Phillips, D. M. (1972): Comparative analysis of mammalian sperm motility. J. Cell Biol. *53*:561.

206. Plattner, H. (1971): Bull spermatozoa: A re-investigation by freeze-etching using widely different cryofixation procedures. J. Submicr. Cytol. *3*:19.

207. Revell, S. G., and Wood, P. D. P. (1978): A photographic method for the measurement of motility of bull spermatozoa. J. Reprod. Fertil. *54*:123.

208. Russell, L., Peterson, R. N., and Freund, M. (1980): On the presence of bridges linking the inner and outer acrosomal membranes of boar spermatozoa. Anat. Rec. *198*:449.

209. Saacke, R. G., and Almquist, J. O. (1964): Ultrastructure of bovine spermatozoa. I. The head of normal, ejaculated sperm. Am. J. Anat. *115*:143.

210. Sharma, O. P. (1976): Scanning electron microscopy of equine spermatozoa. J. Reprod. Fertil. *48*: 413.

211. Srisvastava, P. N., Zaneveld, L. J. D., and Williams, W. L. (1970): Mammalian sperm acrosomal neuraminidases. Biochem. Biophys. Res. Comm. *39*:575.

212. Wallace, J. C., and White, I. G. (1965): Studies of glycerylphosphorylcholine diesterase in the female reproductive tract. J. Reprod. Fertil. *9*:163.

213. Wu, S. H., and Newstead, J. D. (1966): Electron microscope study of bovine epididymal spermatozoa. J. Anim. Sci. *25*:1186.

214. Zaneveld, L. J. D., Wagner, L., Schlumberger, H. D., et al. (1974): Immunological and biochemical

studies on fractionated bull spermatozoa. J. Reprod. Fertil. *38*:411.

Evaluation of Seminal Quality

215. Almquist, J. O. (1982): Effect of long term ejaculation at high frequency on output of sperm, sexual behavior, and fertility of Holstein bulls; relation of reproductive capacity to high nutrient allowance. J. Dairy Sci. *65*:814.
216. Amann, R. P. (1981): A critical review of methods for evaluation of spermatogenesis from seminal characteristics. J. Androl. *2*:37.
217. Amann, R. P., and Schanbacher, B. D. (1983): Physiology of male reproduction. J. Anim. Sci. *57* (Suppl. 2):380.
218. Bane, A. (1961): Acrosome Abnormality Associated with Sterility in Boar. *In* Proc. IV Int. Congr. Anim. Reprod. The Hague, p. 810.
219. Boucher, J. H., Foote, R. H., and Kirk, R. W. (1958): The evaluation of semen quality in the dog and the effects of frequency of ejaculation upon semen quality, libido, and depletion of sperm reserves. Cornell Vet. *48*:67.
220. Brackett, B. G. (1981): Applications of in vitro fertilization. *In* New Technologies in Animal Breeding, edited by B. G. Brackett, G. E. Seidel, and S. N. Seidel, New York, Academic Press, p. 141.
221. Carroll, E. J., Ball, L., and Scott, J. A. (1963): Breeding soundness in bulls—a summary of 10,940 examinations. J. Am. Vet. Med. Assoc. *142*:1105.
222. Corselli, J., and Talbot, P. (1986): An in vitro technique to study penetration of hamster oocyte-cumulus complexes by using physiological numbers of sperm. Gamete Res. *13*:293.
223. Hackett, A. J., and Macpherson, J. W. (1965): Some staining procedures for spermatozoa, a review. Can. Vet. J. *6*:55.
224. Hartman, C. G. (1965): Correlations among criteria of semen quality. Fertil. Steril. *16*:632.
225. Hemsworth, P. H., and Galloway, D. B. (1979): The effect of sexual stimulation on the sperm output of the domestic boar. Anim. Reprod. Sci. *2*:387.
226. Hirao, K. (1975): A multiple regression analysis of six measurements of bovine semen characteristics for fertility. Int. J. Fertil. *20*;204.
227. Hulet, C. V., and Ercanbrack, S. K. (1962): A fertility index for rams. J. Anim. Sci. *21*;489.
228. Johnson, L., and Thompson, D. L., Jr. (1983): Age-related and seasonal variation in the Sertoli cell population, daily sperm production and serum concentrations of follicle-stimulating hormone, luteinizing hormone and testosterone in stallions. Biol. Reprod. *29*:777.
229. Lagerlöf, N. (1966): The History of Cytological and Histological Examination of Sperm and Testis. Proc. Int. Symp. on Physiology and Pathology of Spermatogenesis, Rijksuniversteit Gent, p. 5.
230. Linford, E., Glover, F. A., Bishop, C., et al. (1976): The relationship between semen evaluation methods and fertility in the bull. J. Reprod. Fertil. *47*:283.
231. Mader, D. R., and Price, E. O. (1984): The effects of sexual stimulation on the sexual performance of Hereford bulls. J. Anim. Sci. *59*:294.

232. Nunes, J. F., Corteel, J.-M., Combarnous, Y., et al. (1982): Role du plasma seminal dans la survie in vitro des spermatozoides de bouc. Reprod. Nutr. Develop. *22*:611.
233. O'Connor, M. L., Gwazdauskas, F. C., McGuilliard, M. L., et al. (1985): Effect of adrenocorticotropic hormone and associated hormonal responses on semen quality and sperm output of bulls. J. Dairy Sci. *68*:151.
234. Olar, T. T., Amann, R. P., and Pickett, B. W. (1983): Relationships among testicular size, daily production and output of spermatozoa, and extragonadal spermatozoal reserves of the dog. Biol. Reprod. *29*:1114.
235. Quinn, P. J., and White, I. G. (1966): Variation in semen cations in relation to semen quality and methods of collection. Fertil. Steril. *17*:815.
236. Saacke, R. G. (1982): Components of seminal quality. J. Anim. Sci. *55*(Suppl. 2):1.
237. Seidel, G. E., Jr., and Foote, R. H. (1969): Influence of semen collection techniques on composition of bull seminal plasma. J. Dairy Sci. *52*:1080.
238. Seidel, G. E., Jr., and Foote, R. H. (1973): Variance components of semen criteria from bulls ejaculated frequently and their use in experimental design. J. Dairy Sci. *56*:399.
239. Weisgold, A. D., and Almquist, J. O. (1979): Reproductive capacity of beef bulls. VI. Daily spermatozoal production, spermatozoal reserves and dimensions and weight of reproductive organs. J. Anim. Sci. *48*:351.

Physical and Chemical Properties of Semen

240. Amann, R P., and Hammerstedt, R. H. (1980): Validation of a system for computerized measurements of spermatozoal velocity and percentage of motile sperm. Biol. Reprod. *23*:647.
241. Atherton, R. W., (1975): An objective method for evaluating Angus and Hereford sperm motility. Int. J. Fertil. *20*: 109.
242. Bartlett, D. J. (1962): Studies on dog semen. I. Morphological characteristics. J. Reprod. Fertil. *3*: 173.
243. Bartlett, D. J. (1962): Studies on dog semen. II. Biochemical characteristics. J. Reprod. Fertil. *3*: 190.
244. Bielański, W. (1975): The evaluation of stallion semen in aspects of fertility control and its use for artificial insemination. J. Reprod. Fertil., Suppl. *23:19*.
245. Boucher, J. H., Foote, R. H., and Kirk, R. W. (1958): The evaluation of semen quality in the dog and the effects of frequency of ejaculation upon semen quality, libido, and depletion of sperm reserves. Cornell Vet. *48*:67.
246. Brotherton, J. (1975): The counting and sizing of spermatozoa from ten animal species using a Coulter counter. Andrologia *7*:169.
247. Brown-Woodman, D. D. C., and White, I. G. (1974): Aminoacid composition of semen and secretions of the male reproductive tract. Aust. J. Biol. Sci. *27*:415.
248. Casillas, E. R., Elder, C. M., and Hoskins, D. D. (1978): Adenyl cyclase activity in maturing bovine

spermatozoa. Activation by GTP and polyamines. Fed. Proc. *37*:1688.

249. Clark, J. B. K., Graham, E. F., Lewis, B. A., et al. (1967): D-mannitol, erythritol and glycerol in bovine semen. J. Reprod. Fertil. *13*:189.

250. Couture, M., Ultstein, M., Leonard, J., et al. (1976): Improved staining method for differentiating immature germ cells from white blood cells in human seminal fluid. Andrologia *8*:61.

251. Crabo, B., Gustafsson, B., Bane, A. P., et al. (1967): The concentration of sodium, potassium, calcium, inorganic phosphate, protein, and glycerylphosphorylcholine in the epididymal plasma of bull calves. J. Reprod. Fertil. *13*:589.

252. Dacheux, J. L., O'Shea, T., and Paquignon, M. (1979): Effects of osmolality, bicarbonate and buffer on the metabolism and motility of testicular epididymal and ejaculated spermatozoa of boars. J. Reprod. Fertil. *55*:287.

253. Dooley, M. P., and Pineda, M. H. (1986): Effect of method of collection on seminal characteristics of the domestic cat. Am. J. Vet. Res. *47*:286.

254. Gebauer, M. R., Pickett, B. W., and Swierstra, E. E. (1974): Reproductive physiology of the stallion. II. Daily production and output of sperm. J. Anim. Sci. *39*:732.

255. Hammerstedt, R. H., and Amann, R. P. (1976): Effects of physiological levels of exogenous steroids on metabolism of testicular, cauda epididymal and ejaculated bovine sperm. Biol. Reprod. *15*:678.

256. Harasymowycz, J., Ball, L., and Seidel, G. E., Jr. (1976): Evaluation of bovine spermatozoal morphologic features after staining or fixation. Am. J. Vet. Res. *37*:1053.

257. Hood, R. D., Witters, W. L., Foley, W. C., et al. (1967): Free amino acids in porcine spermatozoa. J. Anim. Sci. *26*:1101.

258. Hudson, M. T., Wellerson, R., Jr., and Kupferberg, A. B. (1965): Sialic acid in semen, spermatozoa and serum of mammals. J. Reprod. Fertil. *9*:189.

259. James, R. W., Heywood, R., and Street, A. E. (1979): Biochemical observations on beagle dog semen. Vet. Rec. *104*:480.

260. Johnson, L., Berndtson, W. E., and Pickett, B. W. (1976): An improved method for evaluating acrosomes of bovine spermatozoa. J. Anim. Sci. *42*:951.

261. Kamidono, S., Hamaguchi, T., Okada, H., et al. (1984): A new method for rapid spermatozoal concentration and motility: a multiple-exposure photography system using the Polaroid camera. Fertil. Steril. *41*:620.

262. King. G. J., and Macpherson, J. W. (1966): Alkaline and acid phosphatase activity, pH and osmotic pressure of boar semen. Can. J. Comp. Med. Vet. Sci. *30*:304.

263. Komarek, R. J., Pickett, B. W., Gibson, E. W., et al. (1965): Lipid of porcine spermatozoa, seminal plasma and gel. J. Reprod. Fertil. *9*:131.

264. Komarek, R. J., Pickett, B. W., Gibson, E. W., et al. (1965): Composition of lipids in stallion semen. J. Reprod. Fertil. *10*:337.

265. MacMillan, K. L., Desjardins, C., Kirton, K. T., et al. (1967): Relationship of glycerylphosphorylcholine to other constituents of bull semen. J. Dairy Sci. *50*:1310.

266. Mann, T. (1964): The Biochemistry of Semen and of the Male Reproductive Tract, 2nd ed. New York, John Wiley & Sons, Inc.

267. Mann, T. (1975): Biochemistry of stallion semen. J. Reprod. Fertil., Suppl. *23*:47.

268. Matousek, J. (1985): Biological and immunological roles of proteins in the sperm of domestic animals (Review). Anim. Reprod. Sci. *8*:1.

269. Moore, H. D. M. (1979): The net surface charge of mammalian spermatozoa as determined by isoelectric focusing. Changes following sperm maturation, ejaculation, incubation in the female tract, and after enzyme treatment. Int. J. Androl. *2*:449.

270. Pickett, B. W., and Back, D. G. (1973): Procedures for preparation, collection, evaluation, and insemination of stallion semen. Colo. State Univ., Animal Reproduction Laboratory, Ft. Collins. Information Series #2-1.

271. Pickett, B. W., Faulkner, L. C., and Sutherland, T. M. (1970): Effect of month and stallion on seminal characteristics and sexual behavior. J. Anim. Sci. *31*:713.

272. Pickett, B. W., Sullivan, J. J., and Seidel, G. E., Jr. (1975): Reproductive physiology of the stallion. V. Effect of frequency of ejaculation on seminal characteristics and spermatozoal output. J. Anim. Sci. *40*:917.

273. Pineda, M. H., Dooley, M. P., and Martin, P. A. (1984): Long-term study on the effect of electroejaculation on seminal characteristics of the domestic cat. Am. J. Vet. Res. *45*:1038.

274. Pineda, M. H., and Dooley, M. P. (1984): Effects of voltage and order of voltage application on seminal characteristics of electroejaculates of the domestic cat. Am. J. Vet. Res. *45*:1520.

275. Polakoski, K. L., and Kopta, M. (1982): Seminal Plasma. Chapter 4. *In* Biochemistry of Mammalian Reproduction, edited by L. J. D. Zaneveld and R. T. Chatterton, New York, John Wiley and Sons, Inc., pp. 97, 99-101, 103, 112.

276. Prakash, C. (1974): Séparation des spermatozoïdes mobiles des autres cellules at des débris cellulaires présents dans le sperme bovine. Ann. Biol. Anim. Biochim. Biophys. *14*:363.

277. Quinn, P. J., White, I. G., and Wirrick, B. R. (1965): Studies of the distribution of the major cations in semen and male accessory secretions. J. Reprod. Fertil. *10*:379.

278. Roussel, J. D., and Stallcup. O. T. (1967): Distribution of lactic dehydrogenase and transaminase in the genital tissues of Holstein-Friesian bulls. J. Dairy Sci. *50*:1306.

279. Saito, S., Zeitz, L., Bush, I. M., et al. (1967): Zinc content of spermatozoa from various levels of canine and rat reproductive tracts. Am. J. Physiol. *213*:749.

280. Salamon, S. (1964): The effect of frequent ejaculation in the ram on some semen characteristics. Aust. J. Agric. Res. *15*:950.

281. Scott, T. W., Voglmayr, J. K., and Setchell, B. P. (1967): Lipid composition and metabolism in testicular and ejaculated ram spermatozoa. Biochem. J. *102*:456.

282. Seidel, G. E., Jr., and Foote, R. H. (1970): Compartmental analysis of sources of the bovine ejaculate. Biol. Reprod. *2*:189.

283. Setchell, B. P. (1974): Secretions of the testis and epididymides. J. Reprod. Fertil. *37*:165.

284. Swierstra, E. E., and Rahnefeld, G. W. (1967): Semen and testis characteristics in young Yorkshire and Lacombe boars. J. Anim. Sci. *26*:49.

285. Wales, R. G., Wallace, J. C., and White, I. G. (1966): Composition of bull epididymal and testicular fluid. J. Reprod. Fertil. *12*:139.

286. Wales, R. G., and White, I. G. (1965): Some observations on the chemistry of dog semen. J. Reprod. Fertil. *9*:69.

287. White, I. G. (1958): Biochemical aspects of mammalian semen. Anim. Breeding Abstr. *26*:109.

288. White, I. G., and Lincoln, G. J. (1960): The yellow pigmentation of bull semen and its content of riboflavin, niacin, thiamine and related compounds. Biochem. J. *76*:301.

Mating

289. Aron, C. (1979): Mechanisms of control of the reproductive function by olfactory stimuli in female mammals. Physiol. Rev. *59*:229.

290. Aronson, L. R., and Cooper, M. L. (1974): Olfactory deprivation and mating behavior in sexually experienced male cats. Behav. Biol. *11*:459.

291. Beach, F. A. (1970): Coital behavior in dogs. IX. Sequelae to "coitus interruptus" in males and females. Physiol. Behav. *5*:263.

292. Beach, F. A. (1975): Hormonal modification of sexually dimorphic behavior. Psychoneuroendocrinology *1*:3.

293. Carter, C. S., and Davis, J. M. (1977): Biogenic amines, reproductive hormones and female sexual behavior: a review. Behav. Rev. *1*:213.

294. Garcia-Sacristan, A., Casanueva, C. R., Castilla, C., et al. (1984): Adrenergic receptors in the urethra and prostate of the horse. Res. Vet. Sci. *36*:57.

295. Gebauer, M. R., Pickett, B. W., and Swierstra, E. E. (1974): Reproductive physiology of the stallion. II. Daily production and output of sperm. J. Anim. Sci. *39*:732.

296. Hahn, J., Foote, R. H., and Seidel, G. E., Jr. (1969): Testicular growth and related sperm output in dairy bulls. J. Anim. Sci. *29*:41.

297. Hart, B. J. (1967): Sexual reflexes and mating behavior in the male dog. J. Comp. Physiol. Psychol. *64*:388.

298. Hart, B. L., and Kitchell, R. L. (1966): Penile erection and contraction of penile muscles in the spinal and intact dog. Am. J. Physiol. *210*:257.

299. Hart, B. L., and Jones, T. O. A. C. (1975): Effects of castration on sexual behavior of tropical male goats. Horm. Behav. *6*:247.

300. Hopkins, S. G., Schubert, T. A., and Hart, B. L. (1976): Castration of adult male dogs: Effects on roaming, aggression, urine marking, and mounting. J. Am. Vet. Med. Assoc. *168*:1108.

301. Jarman, P. (1983): Mating system and sexual dimorphism in large, terrestrial, mammalian herbivores. Biol. Rev. *58*: 485.

302. Kedia, K., and Markland, C. (1975): The effect of pharmacological agents on ejaculation. J. Urol. *114*:569.

303. Kimura, Y. (1970): On peripheral nerves controlling ejaculation. Tohoku J. Exp. Med. *105*:177.

304. Kimura, Y., Miyamoto, A., Urano, S., et al. (1982): The spinal monoaminergic systems relating to ejaculation. I. Ejaculation and dopamine. Andrologia *14*:341.

305. Knight, T. W. (1977): Methods for the indirect estimation of testes weight and sperm numbers in Merino and Romney rams. N. Z. J. Agric. Res. *20*:291.

306. Lande, R., and Arnold, S. J. (1985): Evolution of mating preference and sexual dimorphism. J. Theor. Biol. *117*:651.

307. Lino, B. F. (1972): The output of spermatozoa in rams. II. Relationship to scrotal circumference, testis weight and the number of spermatozoa in different parts of the urogential tract. Aust. J. Biol. Sci. *25*:359.

308. Lino, B. F., Braden, A. W. H., and Turnbull, K. E. (1967): Fate of unejaculated spermatozoa. Nature *213*:594.

309. MacLusky, N. J., and Naftolin, F. (1981): Sexual differentiation of the central nervous system. Science *211*:1294.

310. McMillan, K. L., and Hafs, H. D. (1968): Gonadal and extragonadal sperm numbers during reproductive development of Holstein bulls. J. Anim. Sci. *27*: 697.

311. Rosenblatt, J. S., and Aronson, L. R. (1958): The decline of sexual behavior in male cats after castration with special reference to the role of prior sexual experience. Behavior *12*:285.

312. Swierstra, E. E. (1966): Structural composition of Shorthorn bull testes and daily spermatozoa production as determined by quantitiative testicular histology. Can. J. Anim. Sci. *46*:107.

313. Swierstra, E. E. (1970): The effect of low ambient temperatures on sperm production, epididymal sperm reserves, and semen characteristics of boars. Biol. Reprod. *2*:23.

314. Tischner, M., Kosiniak, K., and Bielański, W. (1974): Analysis of the pattern of ejaculation in stallions. J. Reprod. Fertil. *41*:329.

Sperm Transport

315. Austin, C. R. (1975): Sperm fertility, viability and persistence in the female tract. J. Reprod. Fertil., Suppl. *22*:75.

316. Baker, R. D., and Degen, A. A. (1972): Transport of live and dead boar spermatozoa within the reproductive tract of gilts, J. Reprod. Fertil. *28*:369.

317. Baker, R. D., Dziuk, P. J., and Norton, H. W. (1968): Effect of volume of semen, number of sperm and drugs on transport of sperm in artificially inseminated gilts. J. Anim. Sci. *27*:88.

318. Hancock, J. L., and McGovern, P. T. (1968): The transport of sheep and goat spermatozoa in the ewe. J. Reprod. Fertil. *15*:253.

319. Hunter, R. H. F. (1975): Physiological aspects of sperm transport in the domestic pig, Sus scrofa. I. Semen deposition and cell transport. Br. Vet. J. *131*:565.

320. Hunter, R. H. F. (1975): Physiological aspects of sperm transport in the domestic pig, Sus scrofa. II. Regulation, survival and fate of cells. Br. Vet. J.

131:681.

321. Hunter, R. H. F. (1981): Sperm transport and reservoirs in the pig oviduct in relation to the time of ovulation. J. Reprod. Fertil. *63*:109.

322. Hunter, R. H. F., and Nichol, R. (1983): Transport of spermatozoa in the sheep oviduct: preovulatory sequestering of cells in the caudal isthmus. J. Exp. Zool. *228*:121.

323. Hunter, R. H. F., and Wilmut, I. (1982/ 1983): The rate of functional sperm transport into the oviducts of mated cows. Anim. Reprod. Sci. *5*:167.

324. Hunter, R. H. F., Barwise, L., and King, R. (1982): Sperm transport, storage and release in the sheep oviduct in relation to the time of ovulation. Br. Vet. J. *138*:225.

325. Larsson, B., and Larsson, K. (1985): Distribution of spermatozoa in the genital tract of artifically inseminated heifers. Acta Vet. Scand. *26*:385.

326. Lightfoot, R. J., Corker, K. P., and Neil, H. G. (1967): Failure of sperm transport in relation to ewe infertility following prolonged grazing on oestrogenic pastures. Aust. J. Agric. Res. *18*:755.

327. Lightfoot, R. J., and Restall, B. J. (1971): Effects of site of insemination, sperm motility and genital tract contractions on transport of spermatozoa in the ewe. J. Reprod. Fertil. *26*:1.

328. Mattner, P. E., and Braden, A. W. H. (1963): Spermatozoa in the genital tract of the ewe. I. Rapidity of transport. Aust. J. Biol. Sci. *16*:473.

329. Moeller, A. N., and VanDemark, N. L. (1955): *In vitro* speeds of bovine spematozoa. Fertil. Steril. *6*: 506.

330. Parker, W. G., Sullivan, J. J., and First, N. L. (1975): Sperm transport and distribution in the mare. J. Reprod. Fertil., Suppl. *23*:63.

331. Phillips, D. M. (1972): Comparative analysis of mammalian sperm motility. J. Cell Biol. *53*:561.

332. VanDemark, N, L., and Moeller, A. N. (1951): Speed of spermatozoan transport in reproductive tract of estrous cow. Am. J. Physiol. *165*:674.

Female Reproductive System

M. H. PINEDA

9

Classical physiologists, by tradition, have generally sought to ascertain principles governing the steady state. The most notable feature of the female reproductive system is the total absence of a steady state. By virtue of its ever changing functional status, the female reproductive system is clearly the prime example of a dynamic system. Its changes may be subtle, but just as small daily lengthenings of sunlight yield a season, so do subtle changes in hormonal status yield a reproductive cycle. Some events in the cycle can be traced on a day-to-day basis, but others occur at such a pace that a reading must be made every 3 hr or even more often in order to obtain a true account of the shifting functional status. Even during long periods of gestation, the physiological indicators must show a constantly unfolding pattern, else the pregnancy cannot progress. Although the underlying morphological and biochemical processes that manifest these cyclic events and the neural and endocrine mechanisms that generate the cyclicity are only partially understood, a massive volume of information is at hand.

(From R. O. Greep, Preface to Handbook of Physiology, Section 7, Am. Physiol. Soc., Wash. D.C., 1973.)

Like the mammalian male gonad, the female gonad also produces gametes and hormones that regulate and integrate the functional activity of the reproductive system. However, the homology probably ends at this point because the participation of the female in the reproductive processes is more intense and demanding of bodily energetic expenditures than those of the male of the species. Spermatozoal production is continuous for males of both monoestric and seasonally breeding species and fertile ejaculates are possible in the nonbreeding season. The reproductive processes of the female are cyclic and substantially fewer gametes are released at each ovulation, as compared to the number of gametes released by the male at each ejaculation. The reproductive participation of the male ends with deposition of semen in the genitals of the female at the time of mating. At this time, the reproductive participation of the female is only beginning, since she must contribute to the gestation, development, and survival of the offspring. To be successful, the reproductive activities of the female and male must be exquisitely coordinated. The female releases her gametes at ovulation in synchrony with behavioral changes which ensure the attraction of the male for mating. In addition, the female must provide synchronous and adequate oviductal and uterine environments for gametic encounter and fertilization; for embryonic development, attachment, gestation, and successful completion of pregnancy. On top of all of these biologically costly and debilitating demands, the pregnant female has to provide for the delivery and feeding of the newborn after parturition.

Reproduction, essential as it is for the survival of the species, is not necessary for the survival of the individual. If one considers the demands of the reproductive processes imposed upon the female of the species, it should not be surprising that the reproductive activities are often the first to be arrested when the female is confronted with debilitating, nutritional deficiencies, or with life-threatening diseases. In many ways, years of domestication and selection for specific traits, such as milk production, have imposed further burdens on the female and, as a consequence, nonpregnant cycles are increasingly common or even the norm. In the nondomesticated, wild species in which there has been no man-made selection for production traits, the nonpregnant cycle is an oddity.

The female reproductive system consists of the ovaries, oviducts (uterine tubes or fallopian tubes), uterus, cervix, vagina, and vulva. The ovary is the female gonad; the vulva and clitoris form the external genitalia, and the other organs are referred to as the internal genitalia. Students are encouraged to review the macro- and microscopic anatomy of the female reproductive system in appropriate textbooks. Figure 9-1 shows the genitalia of the mare.

ORIGIN AND DEVELOPMENT OF THE REPRODUCTIVE ORGANS

The embryologic development of the male and female reproductive organs is the same prior to sexual differentiation. Review Chapter 7, Biology of Sex. Reference is made to Table 7-3 for the homologies of the male and female reproductive systems. Failure of differentiation of these systems in whole, or in part, can lead to some of the intersexes and sterility in domestic animals.

OVARIES

The ovaries, as the testes, are paired organs that serve both a gametogenic and an endocrine function. This dual role is complementary, interdependent, and necessary for successful reproduction.

Gross Anatomy

The ovaries are formed in the embryo under the influence of the X-chromosomes (see Chapter 7). The differentiating female gonad remains permanently located in the abdominal cavity.

The shape of the ovary varies according to the species and stage of the estrous cycle, but there are some generalizations that can be made depending upon whether the female is a polytocous (litter bearing; see Fig. 9-24) or a monotocous (single bearing) species. The functional ovary of a polytocous animal (sow, bitch, or cat) has several follicles or corpora lutea which give the appearance of a cluster of grapes. The monotocous animal (cow, ewe, and mare) has an ovoid-shaped ovary, unless a follicle or corpus luteum is present; then the

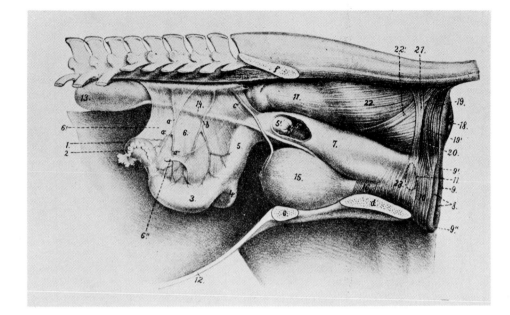

Fig. 9-1. Lateral view of genital organs and adjacent structures of mare. Removal of the other abdominal viscera has allowed the ovaries and uterus to sink down; this has, however, the advantage of showing the broad ligaments of the uterus. 1, Left ovary; 2, uterine or fallopian tube; 3, left cornu uteri; 4, right cornu uteri; 5, corpus uteri; 5′, portio vaginalis uteri, and 5″, os uteri, seen through window cut in vagina; 6, broad ligament of uterus; 6″, round ligament of uterus; 7, vagina; 8, labia vulvæ; 9, rima vulvæ; 9′, dorsal commissure, and 9″, ventral commissure, of vulva; 10, constrictor vulvæ; 11, position of vestibular bulb; 12, ventral wall of abdomen; 13, left kidney; 14, left ureter; 15, urinary bladder; 16, urethra; 17, rectum; 18, anus; 19, 19′, unpaired and paired parts of sphincter ani externus; 20, retractor ani cut at disappearance under sphincter ani externus; 21, suspensory ligament of anus; 22, longitudinal muscular layer of rectum; 22′, rectococcygeus; 23, constrictor vaginæ; a, utero-ovarian artery, with ovarian (a′) and uterine (a″) branches; b, uterine artery; c, umbilical artery; d, ischium; e, pubis; f, ilium. (After Ellenberger, in Leisering's Atlas; Sisson, and Grossman: The Anatomy of the Domestic Animals. Courtesy W. B. Saunders Co.)

ovary takes on a distorted shape depending on the size of the structure. The mare has a kidney-shaped ovary because of the ovulation fossa which is the site of all ovulations. Table 9-1 gives some pertinent data on the common domestic animals.

Figure 9-2 shows the anatomical relationship between the ovary and the oviduct in the ewe. Figure 9-3 depicts an idealized section showing the sequence of events in a mammalian ovary, including follicular growth and maturation, ovulation and release of the oocyte, and corpus luteum formation and regression. The figure is idealized and composite because it shows all the ovarian events as occurring at the same time, without distinction to the follicular and luteal phases of the cycle.

The epithelium covering the mammalian ovary is a single layer of cuboidal or low columnar cells called the *germinal epithelium*. This layer covers the entire ovary except in the mare where it is limited to the ovulation fossa. Beneath the germinal epithelium is the tunica albuginea and then the large mass of follicles.

Ovarian Follicles

The origin of the embryonic elements which eventually form the ovarian follicle is one of the most controversial and still unresolved problems in embryology. Recent studies seem to indicate that, at least for the ewe, the undifferentiated and the differentiated gonad are colonized by invasive mesonephric cells which become associated with the germinal cells of

Table 9-1 Comparative Anatomy of the Adult Ovary and Reproductive Tract*

	Animal					
	Cow[†]	Ewe[†]	Sow[†][‖]	Mare[†]	Bitch[‡]	Cat[§]
Ovary						
Shape	Almond-shaped	Almond-shaped	Berry-shaped (cluster of grapes)	Kidney-shaped; with ovulation fossa	Oval, slightly flattened	Oval, slightly flattened
Weight of one ovary (gm)	10–20	3–4	3–10	40–80	8–1	.3–1
Mature Graafian follicles						
Number	1–2	1–4	10–25	1–2	3–15	2–10
Diameter (mm)	12–19	5–10	8–12	25–70	2–4	1–2
Ovary which is the more active	Right	Right	Left	Left	—	—
Mature corpus luteum						
Shape	Spheroid or ovoid	Spheroid or ovoid	Spheroid or ovoid	Pear-shaped	Spheroid	Spheroid
Diameter (mm)	20–25	9	10–15	10–25	2–5	1.5–3
Maximum size attained (days from ovulation)	10	7–9	14	14	5–14	5–14
Regression starts (days from ovulation)	14–15	12–14	13	17	—	—
Oviduct						
Length (cm)	25	15–19	14–30	20–30	4–7	3–5
Uterus						
Type	Bipartite	Bipartite	Bicornuate	Bipartite	Bicornuate	Bicornuate
Length of horn (cm)	35–40	10–12	40–110	15–25	10–14	6–10
Length of body (cm)	2–4	1–2	5	15–20	1.4–2	1.5–2
Surface lining of endometrium	70–120 caruncles	88–96 caruncles	Slight longitudinal folds	Conspicuous longitudinal folds	Longitudinal folds	Longitudinal folds
Cervix						
Length (cm)	8–10	4–10	10–23	7–8	1.5–2	1–1.5
Outside diameter (cm)	3–4	2–3	2–3	3.5–4	.5–1.5	.4–.6
Cervical lumen						
Shape	2–5 Annular rings	Annular rings	Corkscrew-like	Conspicuous folds	Irregular	Irregular
Os Uteri						
Shape	Small & protruding	Small & protruding	Ill-defined	Clearly-defined	Slightly protruding	—
Anterior Vagina						
Length (cm)	25–30	10–14	10–23	20–35	5–10	—
Hymen	Ill-defined	Well-developed	Ill-defined	Well-developed	Ill-defined	Ill-defined
Vestibule						
Length (cm)	10–12	2.5–3	6–8	10–12	2–5	.5–1.5

*All data vary with age, breed, and parity and are only estimates.
[†]From Hafez, E. S. E.: Reproduction in Farm Animals, 5th. ed. Philadelphia, Lea & Febiger, 1987.
[‡]Data for mature beagle, from the literature and Cole, H. H., and Cupps, P. T.: Reproduction in Domestic Animals, 3rd ed. New York, Academic Press, 1977.
[§]Estimates with some data from the literature.
[‖]After Cowan, F. T., and Macpherson, J. W.: Can. J. Comp. Med. Vet. Sci. 30:107, 1966.

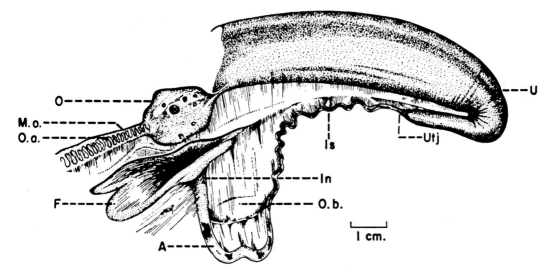

Fig. 9-2. Anatomical relationship between the ovary and the oviduct in the ewe. *A*, ampulla; *F*, fimbriae; *In*, infundibulum; *Is*, isthmus; *M.o.*, mesovarium; *O*, ovary; *O.a.*, ovarian artery; *O.b.*, ovarian bursa; *U*, uterus; *Utj*, uterotubal junction. Note the suspended loop to which the ovarian bursa is attached. The oviduct in the ewe is pigmented. (Hafez, E. S. E. (Ed.): Reproduction in Farm Animals, Lea & Febiger, 4th ed. Philadelphia 1987.)

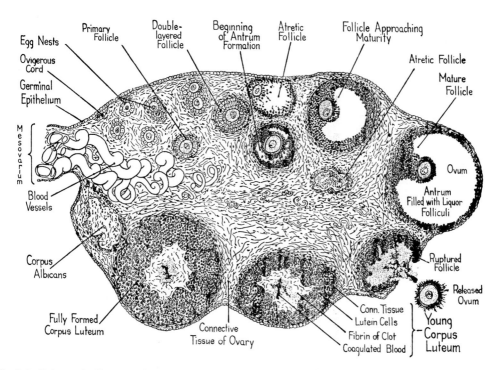

Fig. 9-3. Schematic diagram of an ovary, showing the sequence of events in origin, growth, and rupture of an ovarian (graafian) follicle and formation and retrogression of corpus luteum. Follow clockwise around ovary, starting at the mesovarium. (Patten: Human Embryology. Courtesy Blakiston Division of McGraw-Hill Book Co.)

the ovarian surface. The ovigerous cords, which are transitory, are formed in close association with the mesonephric cells (Fig. 9-3). These mesonephric cells, later participate in the organization and probably in the formation of definite ovarian structures, such as follicles. The superficial epithelium of the ovary penetrates the albuginea of the ovary and forms cords and crypts in the ovarian cortex. These cords and crypts were formerly thought to contribute to the oocyte population, and the name germinal epithelium is derived from this belief. Some invaginations of the superficial epithelium terminate in fragmented cords, forming nests of epithelial-like cells in close proximity to growing follicles. The close association of these nests of cells from the superficial epithelium to the follicle may provide a continuous source of granulosa cells to the developing follicles during postpuberal life.

From the morphologic point of view, the ovarian follicles may be classified (Fig. 9-4) in three major groups: (1) primordial or uni-

laminar follicles; (2) growing follicles, and (3) graafian follicles. It must be noted, however, that folliculogenesis, defined as the formation of a graafian or mature follicle from a pool of primordial nongrowing follicles, is a highly dynamic and rapid process that occurs at certain stages of the female cycle.

(1) *Primordial (primary) follicles* consist of an oocyte surrounded by a single layer of epithelial, flattened granulosa cells with irregularly-shaped nuclei. Thecal cells are not present at this stage of folliculogenesis. Primordial, unilaminar follicles lack a distinct vasculature. A discrete follicular capillary bed develops later in the growing follicles (Fig. 9-4). This unilaminar stage of development is reached at birth in the newborn heifer, and the ovary may contain as many as 150,000 of these follicles (Fig. 9-5). The number of primordial follicles decrease to as few as 1,000 in a cow by 15 to 20 years of age. A similar age-related decline in the number of primordial follicles present in the ovaries of newborn animals occurs in other species. The number

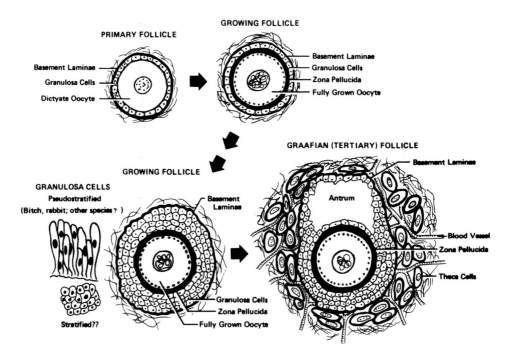

Fig. 9-4. Schematic representation of ovarian follicular growth. (Adapted from different sources, including G. F. Erickson et al.: Endocrine Reviews, *6*:371, 1985.)

FOLLICLES (No.)

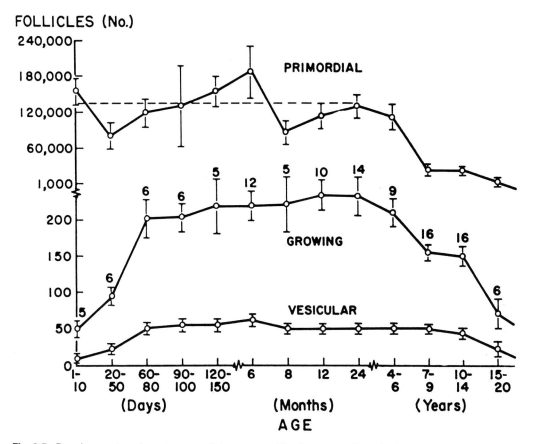

Fig. 9-5. Development and senescence of the postnatal bovine ovary. Quantitative analysis of the follicles of the postnatal bovine ovary. Primordial oocytes encompassed by a single layer of follicle cells. Broken line represents average for animals aged 0 to 24 months. Growing follicles with two or more layers of follicle cells, but without a fully-formed vesicle. Vertical bars and numerals represent the standard error and number of ovarian pairs analyzed, respectively. (After Erickson, B. H.: J. Anim. Sci. *25* (3): 1966.)

of primordial follicles that undergo folliculogenesis to reach the mature, graafian stage from puberty on is only a small fraction of the number of follicles available in the pool of primordial follicles. Most follicles will either undergo a process of regression called *atresia* at some stage of folliculogenesis, or remain as primordial follicles with no sign of growth. Primordial follicles containing more than one oocyte (polyovular) have been seen in several species (Fig. 9-6). Figures 9-6 through 9-9 show aspects of folliculogenesis in the heifer.

(2) *Growing follicles* are follicles that have left the resting stage as primordial follicles, have begun growth, but have not developed a thecal layer or antrum (cavity). In at least 2 species, the rabbit and the bitch, the granulosa cells form a pseudostratified epithelium, with all of the cellular elements reaching the basal lamina of the follicular wall. The position of the nucleus and the height of the cell gives the appearance of stratification in cross sections of growing and mature follicles. Hence, it is possible that similar arrangement and pseudostratification may be also the norm for growing and mature follicles of the other domestic species. This may be particularly true for those species that have large follicles and a thick follicular wall. Reaching the basement membrane would allow an equal and better distribution of nutrients to all of the granulosa cells. In this chapter, ref-

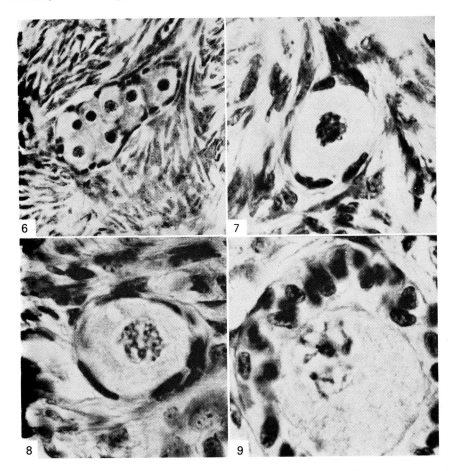

Fig. 9-6. Three primordial follicles. The one on the left contains 5 oocytes. The two oocytes to the right form solitary primordial follicles. 395 × H. E. (cow)

Fig. 9-7. Primordial follicle with oocyte and its nucleus. The chromosomes form a compact bunch which occupies only a portion of the nucleus. 990 × H. E. (cow)

Fig. 9-8. Eccentric section through an oocyte nucleus in a primordial follicle. The chromosomes are in the pachytene stage and the nucleolus is visible although weakly stained. 990 × H. E. (cow)

Fig. 9-9. Growing follicle with a "2-layered epithelium." Chromosomes are in the pachytene stage, the nucleolus is visible. 990 × H. E. (cow)
(From Rajakoski, E.: Acta Endocrinol. *34* (Suppl. 52): 1, 1960.)

erence is made to the "layer" of granulosa cells to indicate the histologic appearance of the granulosa cells in thick, cross sections of the follicle.

A growing follicle is characterized as developing 2 or more "layers" of granulosa cells surrounding the oocyte (Figs. 9-4 and 9-9 through 9-11). With continued growth, additional "layers" of granulosa cells appear to surround the oocyte. A zona pellucida sur-

rounding the oocyte may be seen at this stage (see Chapter 7). The number of growing follicles in an ovary at a given time is relatively small in the domestic species and varies with the stage of the estrous cycle. By the onset of puberty as many as 200 growing follicles may be present in the ovary of a heifer.

(3) *Graafian follicles* (vesicular follicles) are follicles in which an antrum is clearly visible (Figs. 9-10 through 9-13). The graafian follicle

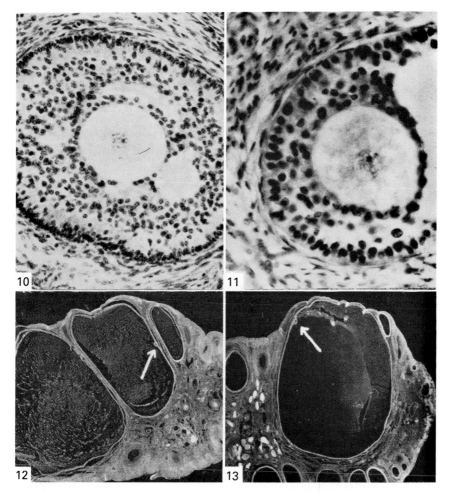

Fig. 9-10. Transitional phase between growing and graafian follicle. Note the pools of liquor folliculi in the granulosa. 200 × H. E. (cow)

Fig. 9-11. Small graafian follicle. Liquor folliculi fills the antrum, the granulosa is compact. 200 × H. E. (cow)

Fig. 9-12. Photograph of a serial section of the ovary from a heifer killed on the twentieth day of the cycle. Cumulus oophorus (arrow) in a normal follicle with a diameter of 8.3 mm. 4 ×. (cow)

Fig. 9-13. Photograph of a serial section of the ovary from a heifer killed on the twenty-first day of the cycle. Cumulus oophorus (arrow) in a normal follicle 12.5 mm in diameter. 4 ×. (cow) (After Rajakoski, E.: Acta Endocrinol. *34* (Suppl. 52): 1, 1960.)

protrudes from the surface of the ovary (Figs. 9-3 and 9-21) and as the antrum enlarges, the granulosa layer is evened out except at the cumulus oophorus where the oocyte rests in a nest of granulosa cells. The diameter of the oocyte of the cow is 80 to 120μ at this stage and is surrounded by the zona pellucida. Two layers of thecal cells, theca interna and theca externa, are now discernible and, together with the granulosa cells, form the wall of the follicle (Fig. 9-14). The theca externa, formed by myoid-type (muscle) cells and fibrocytes is the outermost layer of the follicular wall. These myoid cells have cytoplasmic features, such as parallel microfilaments containing actin and myosin, suggesting a role of

Surface

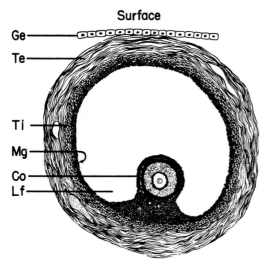

Ge
Te
Ti
Mg
Co
Lf

Fig. 9-14. Graafian follicle. *Co*, cumulus oophorus; *Ge*, germinal epithelium; *Lf*, liquor folliculi; *Mg*, membrana granulosa; *Te*, theca externa; *Ti*, theca interna. (From Hafez, E. S. E. (Ed.): Reproduction in Farm Animals, 5th ed. Philadelphia, Lea & Febiger, 1987.)

these cells in follicular contractility. The theca interna (Fig. 9-14) is formed by fibrocytes and by cells, which undergo dramatic differentiation into epithelioid cells, rich in granules and cytoplasmic organelles, as the follicle matures. Maximal differentiation of the cells of the theca interna occurs late in the process of follicular maturation, in the large antral follicles at the time of estrus. The innermost layer of the follicular wall is formed by the granulosa cells (Figs. 9-11 and 9-14), which are separated from the thecal cells and ovarian stroma throughout folliculogenesis by a well-defined basal lamina or basement membrane. This membrane becomes discontinuous near the time of follicular rupture, during ovulation. The granulosa cells maintain contact with the oocyte during folliculogenesis and in the preantral and antral stages form the cumulus oophorus. The cumulus cells maintain contact with the oocyte, even as the follicular fluid fills the antrum and eccentrically displaces the oocyte. As the follicle matures, the granulosa cells also undergo morphologic differentiation, including epithelioid changes and increased cytoplasmic

organelles, suggestive of steroidogenic function. The granulosa cells, and to a lesser degree the cells of the theca interna, show adherens- and gap-type of intercellular junctions. Gap junctions are also observed between the cells of the cumulus oophorus and the oocyte. The number of gap junctions between granulosa cells increases as folliculogenesis progresses toward the mature graafian stage of the follicle. Gap junctions between granulosa cells play an important role in the movement of small molecules, ions, and nutrients from the basement membrane toward the antrum. In addition, gap junctions may serve as channels for hormonal communication between the peripheral cells of the follicle and the oocyte.

Primordial follicles lack an independent vasculature. The capillary bed, confined to the thecal layer, develops as the thecal cells are formed around the follicle. These thecal capillaries increase in size and concentrate in the theca interna, in close proximity to the basement membrane. Blood flow through these capillaries also increases as the follicle matures.

The permeability of the follicular wall increases in the preovulatory period in some species. In general, the follicular wall appears to offer little resistance to the entry of several blood constituents into the follicle, since the composition of the follicular fluid is similar to that of the blood plasma. However, either through metabolic or secretory activities of the follicular cells, the follicular fluid has a lower concentration of gonadotropins and a higher concentration of steroid hormones than in the peripheral blood. Thus, the follicular fluid may serve the function of storing the steroid hormones produced by the follicular cells. In addition, the follicular fluid functions as a vehicle for the transport of the oocyte from the rupturing follicle at the time of ovulation through the oviduct, concurrently providing factors for spermatozoal capacitation, fertilization, and initial embryonic development.

The ovarian follicle is a structural and functional unit which produces steroid hormones (estrogens) and peptide hormones, including inhibin, oocyte maturation inhibiting factor, relaxin in some of the domestic species, and gonadocrinin, a GnRH-like hormone. Steroidogenic function of the ovarian follicle and its local and gonadotropic control will be discussed later in this chapter.

In addition, the follicle provides a chemical and physical micro-environment including lower temperature than the somatic temperature, for oocyte growth and maturation. As discussed in Chapter 7, in the primordial follicle, the oocyte is in a quiescent stage of meiosis, arrested at the diplotene stage or dictyate stage (germinal vesicle). During the preovulatory growth of the follicle, likely under the influence of LH, the oocyte undergoes in most species the meiotic maturation and becomes a secondary oocyte (Fig. 9-15). This process takes place around 12 hours prior to ovulation in most of the domestic species. The oocyte maturation inhibiting factor (OMI, see Fig. 7-10, Chapter 7) plays an important role to maintain the oocyte in the arrested, dictyate stage of meiosis. The close association of the oocyte with the cells of the cumulus oophorus and corona radiata during

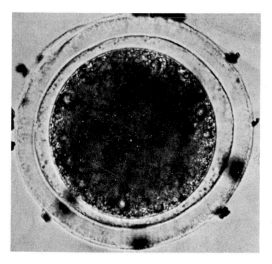

Fig. 9-15. Unfertilized ovum of cow (× 400). (From Hammond, J.: Physiology of Farm Animals. London, Butterworths Scientific Publications, 1957.) See Chapter 19 for pictures of the fertilized oocyte.

follicular maturation and the presence of numerous gap junctions among the cells of the cumulus facilitate factors secreted by follicular cells and nutrients present in the follicular fluid to reach, stimulate, nourish, and control the growth and maturation of the oocyte.

(4) *Follicular atresia.* Few of the follicles and oocytes that undergo growth and maturation at each cycle are destined to ovulate. In fact, in most species, the great majority of follicles present in the ovaries at birth will undergo degenerative changes and atresia as the animal ages. The atretic changes of the follicle may occur at any stage of follicular development. Many theories have been proposed to explain this wastage of follicles and oocytes, including the participation of androgens secreted by the ovary, yet the factors and mechanisms causing it remain largely undetermined.

Avian Ovaries

The avian ovary is an unusual organ. Domestic fowls have been selected to lay large numbers of eggs, far beyond the need for perpetuation of the species. Birds are oviparous and must provide for the nutrition of the embryo outside the body of the female. Consequently, a large amount of yolk must be provided for nutrition of the embryo in birds. In birds, only the left ovary is functional under normal conditions. The right ovary is rudimentary and ordinarily nonfunctional. This condition sets the stage for a phenomenon (sex-reversal) sometimes reported in the popular press, whereby a hen is reported to have changed sex and become a rooster. If the left ovary ceases its function due to destruction by disease, accident, or surgical removal, then the rudimentary right ovary may become an ovotestis and secrete androgens. Under this condition, the female develops secondary sex characteristics of the male including comb, plumage, spurs, and behavioral changes such as crowing and copulatory attempts. The wolffian duct system does not develop so there is no connection between the newly developed testes and the exterior.

Unequal Function of Ovaries

The two ovaries do not function equally in most domestic species, and through sequential estrous cycles one of the ovaries is more active than the other. Ewes, cows, and goats ovulate more frequently from the right than from the left ovary. In the ewe and goat 54 to 60% of the ovulations occur in the right ovary and in the cow 60 to 65% of the oocytes are released from the right ovary. The proximity of the left ovary to the rumen may be responsible for the unequal activity of the left ovary of ruminants, possibly due to extrinsic factors such as temperature fluctuations and mechanical effects caused by the rumen. However, it is not clear whether or not intrinsic factors play any role.

In the sow the left ovary is the most functional providing 55 to 60% of the oocytes. The *mare ovulates* approximately 60% of the oocytes from the left ovary.

While unilateral orchiectomy is not followed by true compensatory hypertrophy of the contralateral testis, unilateral ovariectomy in adult, cycling animals is always followed, in time, by a compensatory and functional hypertrophy of the remaining ovary. The number of follicles that ovulate from the remaining ovary increases after unilateral ovariectomy in litter-bearing species and the number of offsprings born after compensatory hypertrophy is not different from the number produced by intact females. Compensatory hypertrophy may result from more gonadotropins becoming available to the remaining ovary. Surprisingly, however, the side of ovariectomy (left versus right) does not seem to influence the compensatory response of the remaining ovary, which suggests that intrinsic rather than extrinsic factors may be responsible for the unequal ovarian function observed in domestic species.

TUBULAR GENITAL TRACT

The tubular components of the female genital tract are the oviducts, uterus, and vagina. The tubular genital tract of the female serves as the transportation route for the sperm to the oviduct where fertilization occurs. In addition, the oviduct captures the oocytes at ovulation at the fimbriated end and serves as a route for the movement of the developing embyro to the uterus, where gestation occurs. Finally at the end of gestation, the fetus is expelled through the cervix and vagina at parturition and is termed a *newborn.*

The cyclic physiological changes of the tubular genital tract will be considered in the section on the estrous cycle and in the chapters on patterns of reproduction of the six species. Table 9-1 and Figure 9-16 show the comparative anatomy of the uterus of the various species. This varies from a duplex uterus with two separate cervices in the rabbit to a rather simple uterus in the higher form of primates. The pig has a bicornuate uterus with well-developed elongated uterine horns, so that litters may be accommodated adequately. The cat and dog utilize the bicornuate uterus for somewhat equal distribution of the embryos of the litter. The cow and ewe, which usually are monotocous, utilize only one horn during pregnancy. However, there may be some utilization of the other horn by the fetal membranes for placentation. The mare's uterus approaches the form of the primate which lacks distinct uterine horns.

Oviducts (Uterine Tubes)

The oviducts, also called uterine tubes or fallopian tubes, are paired convoluted tubes that extend from the ovaries to the uterus. The ovarian end is funnel-shaped and embraces the ovary in varying degrees at ovulation depending on the species. In the rat and the mouse the ovarian end completely envelops the ovary to form a sac commonly referred to as the *bursa ovarica.* A small opening permits communication with the peritoneal cavity. In the bitch and mink the bursa has a slit large enough to permit the ovary to move through it. The infundibulum of the sow almost completely envelops the ovary. The fingered or fimbriated ends of the oviducts do not enclose the ovary in other domestic animals. In the cow and the ewe the ovarian bursa is only partially complete, whereas in the mare the

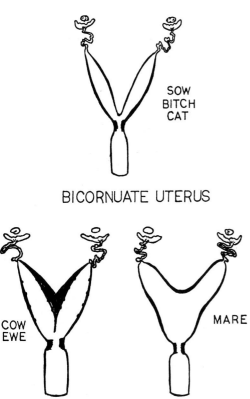

BICORNUATE UTERUS

SOW
BITCH
CAT

BIPARTITE UTERUS

COW
EWE

MARE

Fig. 9-16. Schematic anatomy of the uteri of several domestic species.

prevent the movement of bacteria from the uterus into the oviduct and peritoneal cavity. Yet it must allow semen deposited in the female genitals during copulation to pass into the oviduct. Also the embryo moves through this junction into the uterus at the proper time (Fig. 9-17). The embryo remains in the oviduct for 3 to 6 days in domestic animals. This delay is critical and necessary for embryonic development and survival.

The oviduct is a tortuous organ of small diameter in all domestic species. The lumen of the oviduct is honeycombed in appearance as seen in Figure 9-18. The muscle wall of the oviduct is well developed and responds to hormones. Estrogen priming enhances its response to oxytocin. Oxytocin appears to cause the infundibular end of the oviduct to embrace the ovary. Estrogen dominance enhances cilia activity in the upper oviduct and facilitates the transport of oocytes from the fimbria to the ampulla within 2 hours. Final stages of capacitation and fertilization occur here, and the embryos remain in this middle part of the oviduct but near the ampulla-isthmus junction for 2 to 3 days. Muscular movements probably displace the embryos the remaining distance into the uterus in one more day except in the

bursa encloses only the ovulation fossa.

The bursa consists of a thin peritoneal fold of the mesosalpinx. At the time of ovulation the fimbriated end of the oviduct embraces the ovary and captures the ova. The efficiency of ovum pickup seems to be as good in the nonbursal- as in the bursal-containing species.

The middle portion of the oviduct is called the ampulla, and the portion next to the uterus is the isthmus. There does not seem to be a well-developed valve at the junction of the oviduct and uterus. However, there is good evidence in several species that the folds of mucosa may serve as a deterrent to the movement of fluids from the oviduct into the uterus, except at the proper time. The degree of edema of the folds may control the patency of the utero-tubal junction. This junction may

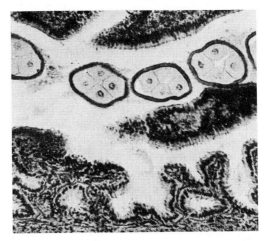

Fig. 9-17. Photograph of the four-cell stage of segmenting embryos in the oviduct of the dog. (Reproduced, by permission, from Evans and Cole: The Oestrous Cycle in the Dog. Memoirs of the University of California, 9, no. 2.)

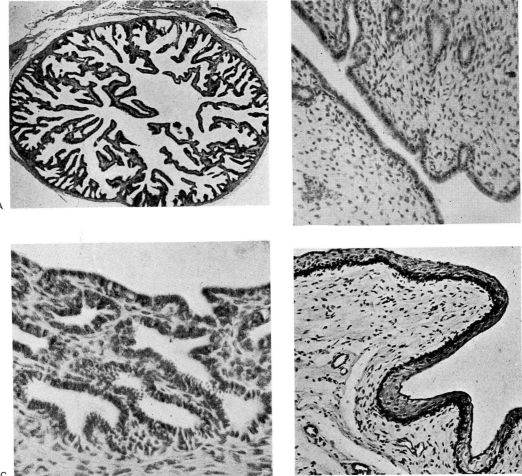

Fig. 9-18. Female duct system. *A*, oviduct. *B*, Uterus of estrous rabbit. *C*, Uterus of luteal phase rabbit. *D*, Vagina. (From McDonald, L. E., et al.: Am. J. Vet. Res. *12*(48):419, 1952.)

bitch and mare which require about 6 to 7 days for embryos to reach the uterus.

Timing of the movement of the embryos into the uterus is important for continued development. Too early or too late uterine entry will cause death of the embryo.

The epithelial lining of the lumen of the oviduct is simple columnar and ciliated. If both ends of the oviduct are ligated, fluid accumulates which is high in lactate, pyruvate, sodium, and calcium ions. Therefore, the oviduct contributes ions and fluid for transporting ova, sperm, and embryos and provides a microenvironment favorable for initial embryonic development.

Uterus

In domestic animals the uterus consists of two horns (cornua) and a body. The development of longer uterine horns is common to litter bearing species, such as the sow, bitch, and queen (Fig. 9-16). The broad ligament supports the uterus and is subject to considerable stretching, especially during pregnancy. During nonpregnancy the uterus is held in the dorsal pelvic area. In the mare and cow, the uterus can be palpated through the rectal wall. For pregnancy diagnosis, restricted rectal palpation is possible in large ewes, goats, and sows by individuals with small hands and thin arms. The uterus is a remarkable organ in that it can enlarge and extend itself to accommodate the conceptus yet retain the capacity to involute following parturition, even approaching the original size and form.

The uterus is composed of three distinct layers: (1) the serous membrane, which is an extension of the peritoneum, (2) the myometrium consisting of three muscle layers which are subject to considerable hypertrophy, and (3) the endometrium consisting of the epithelial lining of the lumen, the glands, and the connective tissue. There is a rich blood supply to the uterus which varies according to the stage of the estrous cycle and in the pregnant animal increases as gestation progresses, since the developing fetus and enlarged uterus require additional blood nutrients.

Myometrial and endometrial changes occur during every cycle under direct control of the ovarian hormones, estrogen and progesterone. These changes are similar to, but less intense than, those that occur during pregnancy. The myometrium is responsible for uterine contractions during estrus and copulation and for limited uterine activity throughout the estrous cycle. In addition, uterine activity during pregnancy enhances the spacing of fetuses in polytocous species. At the time of parturition the myometrium primed by estrogens is very sensitive to oxytocin.

The endometrial epithelium lining the uterus is simple columnar in most species. This epithelium extends into the uterine glands. Endometrial glandular development is cyclic, responding to rising levels of estrogen and progesterone during the estrous cycle and pregnancy. Figure 9-18 shows the glandular development of the uterus. The uterine epithelium contacts the fetal membranes and is the site for exchange of nutrients and waste. The type of placental attachment varies greatly with the species (see Chapter 18). Ruminants have specialized sites of attachment called cotyledonary areas. These are highly specialized localized points of contact with the fetal membranes; consequently, glandular development does not occur at these points.

The uterus serves several functions other than to be an incubator for the embryo or fetus during gestation. The uterine glands secrete "uterine milk" which serves as the nutrient medium for the free living embryo for several weeks preceding implantation. In addition to the role of the uterus as a preselector and passageway of spermatozoa deposited on the vagina or cervix to the oviduct (see Chapter 8), the uterus and associated structures perform endocrine functions in both the cycling and pregnant animal. During implantation, in conjunction with developing placental structures, the uterus acts as a barrier to the maternal, immunological rejection of the embryo or fetus. From this point of view, the spermatozoa and seminal components from the male, deposited in the female tract during mating, are the first foreign, antigenic challenges to the female immune system. The seminal plasma, however, appears to contain immunosuppressants that may protect the spermatozoa from local, uterine and oviductal, immune reactions. Once fertilization has occurred, the developing embryo which, as a new entity is immunologically dissimilar to the female, is not rejected by the mother. On the contrary, the embryo attaches to the endometrium and normally develops to term. Several theories have been proposed to explain the lack of maternal immune rejection of the embryo or fetus. These will be discussed in Chapter 18, Pregnancy and Parturition. It is noteworthy to point out here, however, that during the period of implantation and for most of gestation, the female is under the influence of progesterone, which is a hormone with powerful immunosuppressive properties.

A nonimmunologic embryonic reduction occurs in the uterus of the mare when more than one embryo is present in the uterus. The incidence of double ovulation is estimated to be about 16% for the mare, but the incidence of twin births is approximately 1%. It seems that the embryo that reaches the uterus first somehow prevents the development or interferes with the survival of the embryo reaching the uterus later. This phenomenon occurs between days 17 and 40 of the pregnant cycle.

Cervix

The cervix is the doorway to the uterus, a physiological barrier separating the external environment from the internal environment of the animal. Outside the cervix lies the vagina, which is usually contaminated with microorganisms from the external environment.

The cervix is a thick-walled sphincter-like organ. It has a thick, muscular wall capable of contracting to close the passageway or of relaxing to allow the passage of semen at estrus or of the fetus at parturition. The lumen of the cervix is tortuous and has folds that fit together. The cow, ewe, and sow have transverse ridges known as annular rings. In the sow the rings display a corkscrew appearance. The spiral twisting of the tip of the boar's penis penetrates these rings in the sow. Ring development is less apparent in the mare, but the vaginal end of the cervix is well constricted to form the *os uteri*.

The cervix has a tall columnar epithelium interspersed with goblet cells which have an important secretory function. Goblet cell secretion is a mucus which varies in amount and viscosity depending on the gonadal hormone balance. Uterine fluids move through the cervix during the flushing process occurring at estrus. During estrus the cervix is hyperemic, but the condition should not be confused with an inflammatory process. At midcycle, or during pregnancy, the cervix is blanched and constricted. Under the influence of progesterone the goblet cells secrete a thick, sticky, mucus which is so tenacious that it forms quite a definite barrier. Such mucus is sometimes referred to as the "cervical seal." The mucous seal of pregnancy should not be penetrated by an instrument such as an artificial insemination pipet. If the natural flora of the vagina are carried into the uterus, it can become infected and the fetus may die. This is one of the hazards of intrauterine insemination in dairy cattle, since estrus sometimes occurs during pregnancy in the cow (3 to 5% of all cows).

Vagina

The vagina serves as a passageway for the fetus, outwardly at parturition and inwardly for semen following copulation. In addition, the exterior limits of the vagina mark the confluence of the urinary tract with the reproductive tract.

The epithelial lining of the vagina undergoes cyclic changes under the influence of the ovarian hormones. Under the influence of estrogen, especially at estrus, the epithelium is stratified squamous, whereas during midcycle, under the influence of progesterone, the epithelium has many low cuboidal cells. The vaginal smear of the rat can be used to determine accurately the stage of the estrous cycle. In domestic animals, only the bitch has a vaginal smear that serves as an indicator of the stage of the estrous cycle. The mucous secretions in the vagina come mostly from the cervix, since most of the vagina does not have glands.

The hymen is a transverse fold of the posterior portion of the vagina which is broken at the time of the first copulation. Occasionally, especially in the heifer, the hymen forms an unusually persistent band of connective tissue that must be relieved by a minor surgical procedure.

White Shorthorns are occasionally affected by a recessive hereditary condition called "white heifer disease." The condition is recognized by abnormal development of the reproductive tract. The most common manifestations are persistent hymens or absence of the cervix or of portions of the uterus.

EXTERNAL GENITALIA

The external genitalia consists of the labia majora and minora and the clitoris. The clitoris is the embryological homologue of the penis and consists of erectile tissue. The labia are the homologues of the scrotum. The labia minora are poorly developed in domestic animals, but the labia majora are well developed. The labia majora respond to the cyclic levels of estrogen and progesterone. During proestrus and estrus, while estrogen dominates, the labia are swollen, congested, and edematous in domestic animals. These are useful signs for breeding management. Sebaceous glands surrounding the vulva and the glands of Bartholin within the vestibule secrete a lubricating mucus to enhance the copulatory process.

PUBERTY

Puberty is the age at which the male or female gonad becomes capable of releasing gametes. In the female, this would be associated with estrus and ovulation. For the female, however, puberty is customarily defined as the age at which she will display the first overt estrus or heat, because the signs of estrus are easily detectable. It must be noted that puberty in the female, as in the male (Chapter 8), is not a sudden event, but the result of a gradual process of maturation of the reproductive system, conducive to the sexual maturity of the female and competence to reproduce successfully.

Many aspects of the endocrine events occurring during the transitional period leading to puberty remain unclear or undetermined. For instance, the pituitary gland of fetal and newborn animals responds to exogenous stimulation with GnRH by secreting and releasing gonadotropins, as a postpubertal animal would. Furthermore, the gonads of prepubertal animals are capable of superovulatory responses to exogenous gonadotropin stimulation, even when given well in advance to the normal age of puberty. The quality of the superovulatory response, however, increases as the animal approaches the expected age of puberty for the species. This indicates the need for a certain degree of somatic development before spontaneous gonadotropin surges and puberty can occur. For most of the domestic species, the available evidence indicates that hypothalamic centers are sensitive, in a negative feedback fashion, to small amounts of steroid hormones, mainly estradiol, secreted by the prepubertal gonad. As the animal matures, the hypothalamus becomes less sensitive to the negative feedback of gonadal steroids and begins to respond by

secreting gonadotropin releasing factors. The pituitary gland subsequently responds by secreting gonadotropins, which in turn stimulate the gonads. Thus, puberty could be considered as a series of endocrine events which are dependent on the release from hypothalamic repression. This release occurs when a suitable stage of somatic development is attained.

The modulating activity of the brain, concurrent with the participation of other endocrine glands, such as the thyroid, pineal, and thymus, appears to be needed for the occurrence of puberty.

Some domestic species, such as the heifer and the ewe-lamb, undergo one or more "silent or quiet" estruses and ovulations before they display full estrous behavior and establish the characteristic pattern of cyclic activity of the female. Progesterone secreted by a short-lived corpus luteum, concurrent with the shift from a high to low hypothalamic sensitivity to the negative feedback of gonadal steroids, and changes in the patterns of LH secretion have a major role in the establishment of the postpubertal, estrual activity of the female.

Factors Affecting Puberty

Many factors, including interaction with the opposite sex, adequate to high levels of nutrition, favorable climate, and lack of a stressful environment, favor the onset of puberty. Other factors, such as confinement of females, probably because of pheromones, undernutrition, and adverse climate and environment, discourage the onset of puberty. Particular species and breed differences in the onset of puberty will be discussed in Chapters 11 to 17.

Breed and Genetic Influences

In general, smaller breeds experience puberty at an earlier age. Bitches of small breeds frequently experience first estrus several months earlier than bitches of large breeds. Jersey heifers have an average puberty age of 8 months, Guernseys, and Holsteins, 11 months and Ayrshires, 13 months. Perhaps the selection for genes controlling breed size was concurrent with the selection of other genetic traits such as age at puberty.

Climatic Effects

Puberty in man occurs earlier in the tropics than in the temperate zones. But good comparative data are not available in domestic animals. However, temperate climates, including the interaction of temperature, humidity, diurnal variation and daylight, favor early puberty in all animals.

Seasonal Effects

An unusual situation exists in the seasonal-breeding sheep, since age at puberty can be overridden to some extent by the occurrence of the breeding season. If the hypothalamo-pituitary-ovarian axis is sufficiently developed, then puberty can be initiated at an early date. For example, ewe lambs born early in the spring may show first estrus that fall when they are only 180 days of age. But ewe lambs born late in the spring or the early summer may not show first estrus until the breeding season in the fall of the following year when these females have reached 400 to 500 days of age.

Effect of Nutrition

A high plane of nutrition favors an earlier puberty, and a low plane of nutrition delays puberty. This is particularly true for nonseasonal-breeding animals. Considerable work has been done in this area, especially in heifers, and a more complete discussion can be found in Chapter 12. Apparently there is an interaction of nutrition, body weight gain, and age, since animals maintained under good nutrition reach puberty at an earlier age. *But poor nutrition is not able to prevent the eventual onset of puberty*, although severe delays can be caused to the extent that the age of puberty can be doubled.

Effect of Sex

The generalization that females of all species reach puberty at an earlier age than males is traditionally found in textbooks dealing with animal reproduction. However, evidence to the contrary is abundant and the statement may be incorrect. For instance, more bull calves, lambs, billy goats, dogs, and likely males from other species as well, produce ejaculates containing spermatozoa, and therefore have reached puberty, at an earlier age than the majority of females display the signs of the first overt estrus. Beagle dogs reach puberty as early as 6 months of age, whereas Beagle bitches seldom reach puberty before 10 months of age. Holstein bull calves produce ejaculates with significant numbers of spermatozoa by 8 to 9 months of age, whereas Holstein heifers usually come into estrus about 9 to 13 months of age. Comparative studies to determine age of puberty in males and females of the same species and genetic background, using animals reared and maintained under the same conditions of feeding and management, need to be performed. The easiness of detecting the behavioral signs of estrus, as opposed to the difficulties of collecting ejaculates from untrained, pubescent males, may have contributed to the belief that the age of puberty is earlier for the female of the species.

THE ESTROUS CYCLE

At puberty, the female develops a rhythmic pattern of physiologic events, which induce detectable morphologic changes in the reproductive system and behavioral changes in the animal. These physiologic and behavioral changes are cyclic and repeated over time, unless normally interrupted by pregnancy or abnormally, by a variety of pathologic conditions. Behavioral changes are easier to detect than the morphologic changes within the reproductive organs and hence, it is customary to use the period of sexual receptivity, called estrus or heat, as the central pivot for the cyclic changes. During the period of estrus or heat, the female stands and will accept the advances of the male for mating. During any other part of the cycle, the female rejects the mating advances of the male. Because there is only one period of estrus in each cycle, conventionally the sequence of events that occur between two successive estruses is termed an estrous or estrual cycle. The interestrous interval is the time elapsed from the beginning of an estrus to the beginning of the next estrus. This interestrous interval is then used as a conventional unit of measurement for the duration of the estrous cycle. The period of estrus varies, according to the species, from a few hours to several days. There is also variation in the length of estrus between individuals of the same species. It is conventional to designate the day or days of estrus as Day 0 of the cycle, regardless if the length of estrus is less than or more than one day. When needed, and particularly for species that normally have several days of estrus, each day of estrus may be designated as E1, E2, and so forth.

Ovulation occurs during estrus (in most of the domestic species) or shortly after estrus (cow). The behavioral and physiologic changes associated with ovulation, development and full functional activity of the corpus luteum, and the associated behavioral changes of the female (rejection to mating) are used to describe the estrous cycle. The first day the female refuses to mate is referred to as the first day of diestrus or day 1 of the cycle. Pertinent endocrine events and associated changes in the reproductive organs will be discussed later in this chapter.

According to the periodicity of presentation of estrous cycles, the domestic species can be classified as monoestric or polyestric. Monoestric species, such as the bitch, have only one or two cycles per year. Monoestric species typically present a prolonged period of sexual inactivity called anestrus. Polyestric species are those that, in the absence of mating or when mated with a sterile male, have several estrous cycles during the year. These can be further classified as seasonally polyestrous or seasonal breeders and continuously polyestrous or nonseasonal breeders. Seasonal breeders such as the ewe, goat, and mare present several cycles but only during a particular season of the year. Continuously polyestrous or nonseasonal breeders, such as the cow and the sow, cycle year around. This classification is somewhat arbitrary, because changes in the geographic location and the provision of favorable climatic conditions may induce

seasonally polyestrous species to become continuously polyestrous, or at the very least, extend the breeding season.

Based on ovarian changes, which can be categorized according to the role of copulation in ovulation, the activity or inactivity of the resulting corpus luteum, and the associated behavioral responses of the female, it is possible to classify species into three general types:

(1) One type is exemplified in nonseasonal breeders such as the cow and sow, or the mare and ewe during the breeding season. The infertile cycle in these species culminates in spontaneous ovulation of mature follicles. Corpora lutea automatically form and become functional for a definite period of time. In the absence of pregnancy, the corpus luteum regresses and a subsequent cycle ensues. The bitch fits in this pattern insofar as ovulation and luteal function are concerned. However, the bitch differs from the other species in this category in that the corpora lutea of the bitch remain functional for approximately the same length of time whether pregnancy occurs or not and that a long period of anestrus follows the functional demise of the corpus luteum.

(2) The rat and mouse provide an example of another type of estrous cycle in which ovulation is spontaneous, but the corpora lutea which form are not functional unless mating occurs. These estrous cycles are short (4 to 5 days) when female rats are not mated and longer (12 days) if cervical stimulation takes place.

(3) The third type of estrous cycle is one in which ovulation fails unless the male copulates with the female. The rabbit, cat, and mink are examples of this type and are commonly referred to as reflex or induced ovulators. In the rabbit successive groups of follicles mature and degenerate rhythmically and at any time there are a number of follicles capable of being ovulated if copulation occurs. The queen has periods of anestrus during the year and seasonal periods of breeding in which ovarian follicles develop and secrete estrogens to induce behavioral responses, and definite estrous stances that last for several days (see

Chapter 17). If mating does not occur, these follicles regress and subsequent periods of follicular growth and estruses recur several times during the breeding season. From this point of view, the queen could be classified as a seasonally pseudopolyestrous species. Copulation in these species stimulates afferent neural pathways via the hypothalamus causing release of luteinizing hormone which in turn promotes the ovulatory process.

Phases of the Estrous Cycle

The estrous cycle of domestic animals is traditionally classified into five somewhat arbitrary and sometimes difficult to distinguish stages called phases of the estrous cycle. These phases are called *proestrus, estrus, metestrus, diestrus, and anestrus* (Fig. 9-19).

Proestrus is the period of rapid follicular growth under gonadotropic stimulation, and the period in which the corpus luteum from the previous cycle in polyestrous species regresses. At this stage, the animal is exposed and behaviorally responds to the progressively increasing levels of estrogens secreted by the developing follicles. In most of the domestic species, proestrus is associated with progressively declining levels of progesterone

due to the regression of the corpus luteum from the preceding cycle. In the bitch, proestrus lasts for seven to nine days and is clearly identifiable by well-defined changes in the external genitalia and behavioral signs due to increasing sexual excitement. Proestrus is not clinically evident in the other domestic species and lasts only for 2 to 3 days.

Estrus is defined as the period of *sexual receptivity*, during which mating and ovulation occur in most species, and the corpus luteum begins to form.

The beginning of estrus is a gradual phenomenon. The detection of the precise time of the onset of estrus is difficult. It depends on many factors, chief of which is the change in behavior of the female (and male). Duration of estrus is usually based on the period of acceptance of the male and varies from 14 to 18 hours in the cow to 7 to 10 days in the mare and bitch. Breed, age, and environmental temperature may influence the duration of estrus. High environmental temperatures shorten the duration of estrus in sows. Copulation early in estrus will usually shorten the period of sexual receptivity. Split estrus is common in mares: estrus usually lasts 7 to 10 days, but there may be 1 to 2 days in this period when the mare is not sexually receptive. Proestrus and that portion of the estrual period prior to ovulation form part of the follicular phase of the cycle.

Metestrus is the transitional period between ovulation and the full development of the corpus luteum. During metestrus, the reproductive system switches from estrogen to progesterone dominance. Because the location of metestrus in relation to the other phases of the cycle is variable among species, the phase of metestrus is only of academic significance. For most domestic species, such as the bitch, mare, sow, ewe, and goat that ovulate before the end of estrus, or for the reflex ovulator species (queen), the period of metestrus is partially or totally included within the phase of estrus. For species that ovulate after the end of estrus (cow), the phase of metestrus forms part of the diestrual phase of the cycle.

Diestrus is the phase of the cycle during

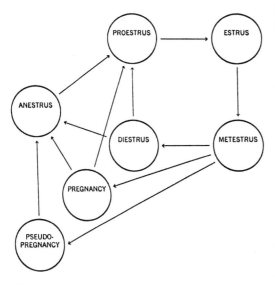

Fig. 9-19. The estrous cycle of domestic animals.

which the corpus luteum fully develops and the reproductive organs are under the dominant influence of progesterone. Metestrus and diestrus form the luteal phase of the cycle.

Even though in the nonpregnant animal diestrus is the longest phase of the cycle for all of the domestic species, lasting from 13 to 16 days, the duration of diestrus depends primarily on the occurrence or nonoccurrence of conception. The bitch is an exception, as discussed in Chapter 16.

In the nonmated animal, in those mated with sterile males, or in those in which conception did not occur, the corpus luteum regresses at the end of diestrus, and diestrus is followed by either proestrus and a subsequent cycle in the continuously polyestrous and in the seasonally polyestrous species during the breeding season, or by a period of sexual inactivity, or anestrus, in monoestric species.

Anestrus is a stage of sexual quiescence characterized by the lack of estrous behavior. Anestrus is a normal stage of the reproductive function in the prepubertal and in aged animals of all species. Anestrus is also normal for the pregnant animal of all species. In fact, pregnancy is the most common cause of anestrus in polyestrous species. After puberty, anestrus is normal in nonpregnant animals for the monoestric species, such as the bitch, for the seasonally polyestrous species during the nonbreeding season, and for the lactating female of some species.

The endocrine mechanisms involved in anestrus are not clearly defined. For some species, such as the bitch, ovarian gonadotropic stimulation is high during anestrus, as demonstrated by follicular development and estrogen secretion, however the bitch does not express estrous behavior. Silent ovulatory cycles, without behavioral signs of estrus, occur at the time of puberty in some species and at the beginning or end of the breeding season in seasonally polyestrous species.

In all domestic species, anestrus may occur as a pathological condition caused by a variety of factors, including nutritional deficiencies, environmental influences that cause endocrine imbalances, diseases of the ovaries and uterus, and infectious diseases causing early embryonic death or abortion. All of these factors result in economic losses due to reproductive failure.

Ovarian Changes During the Estrous Cycle

As described previously, the follicle in single-bearing species or several follicles in litter-bearing species, which are destined to ovulate, develop from a pool of primordial follicles and mature to the preovulatory, graafian stage under gonadotropic stimulation. One to three days before the onset of estrus, depending on the species, graafian follicles destined for ovulation begin to enlarge rapidly and become turgid. The theca interna hypertrophies, and the oocyte, with attached cumulus oophorus, moves from the embedded position in the granulosa layer toward the enlarged fluid-filled antrum of the graafian follicle (Fig. 9-14).

There is a positive correlation between anterior pituitary gonadotropin output and ovarian follicular growth and activity in most species. The follicles of most mammals enlarge very little during the luteal phase, but undergo a surge of growth 1 to 3 days before expected ovulation (Fig. 9-20).

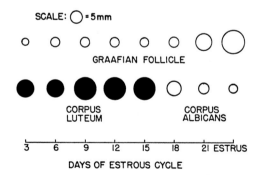

Fig. 9-20. Relative morphologic changes in the ovarian follicles during the estrous cycle of the sow. Note the rapid increase in follicular size shortly before ovulation. Also, corpora albicantia regress in size rather rapidly but are still evident at the subsequent estrus. (From Hafez, E. S. E. (Ed.): Reproduction in Farm Animals, 5th ed. Philadelphia, Lea & Febiger, 1987.)

Ovulation

There are species differences in the number of follicles that reach the preovulatory stage and in the number of days needed in each estrous cycle to reach this stage. The existence of waves of follicular growth during the estrous cycle, as opposed to the continued development of follicles, is either postulated or shown to occur for some of the domestic species. These will be discussed for each of the domestic species, in the corresponding chapter on pattern of reproduction.

Ovulation involves the breakdown of the wall of the ovarian follicle and the release of its contents, including the maturing oocyte. A transparent area appears in the follicular membrane near the apex when ovulation is impending. The point of ovulation can be seen in the resulting corpora lutea for days after ovulation in most of the species. Hemorrhagic areas develop in the vascular network of the follicle membrane, and there is extravasation of blood into the liquor folliculi near the time of ovulation. The granulosa cells lose cell-to-cell contact as the follicle approaches ovulation, probably by dissociation of the gap junctions. The oocyte and the cells of the cumulus, which at this time are projected into the follicular antrum, separate from the pedicle of the cumulus and become freed into the follicular fluid of the antrum. Cells from the granulosa layer reveal signs of luteinization due to gonadotropic, mainly LH stimulation. The connective tissue of the thecal layers dissociates during the preovulatory period, and the outer, thecal layers separate during final preovulatory changes. An avascular stigma or papilla is macroscopically recognizable on the apical surface of the follicle when ovulation is imminent. As the protrusion of the papilla progresses, the layers of the follicular wall, including the adjacent superficial epithelium of the ovary, stretch and thin until the follicular wall breaks and the follicular contents are released (Fig. 9-21).

The participation of the myoid cells of the follicular wall and the significance of follicular contractility in the process of ovulation remains a controversial issue. It has long been known that the mammalian ovarian tissues display contractile activity, probably under the control of autonomic nerves extending to the ovary and catecholamines present in the follicular wall and fluid of some species. Several lines of evidence suggest that the contraction of myoid elements in the follicular wall may be a contributing force to dissociate the thecal tissue at the stigma, and to provide the force for the mechanical rupture of the follicular wall. The oocyte appears to passively flow out of the rupturing follicle, rather than being expelled out by contraction of the follicular wall. Because ovulation is a traumatic process of rupture of tissue and subsequent hemorrhage occurs, the myoid elements may participate in the postovulatory process of tissue repair.

In the domestic species, with the exception of the mare, ovulation occurs within 24 hours following the ovulatory surge of LH. In the mare, ovulation occurs, prior to the peak of LH, while LH levels in the blood are still rising.

At the cellular level, a ripe follicle possesses the appropriate hormone receptors and metabolic components needed to respond to an ovulatory surge of LH. A model[49] based on the hypothesis that the ovulatory surge of LH induces inflammatory changes in the follicular wall has been proposed. According to this model, thecal fibroblasts are in a quiescent "stationary" phase of activity before the ovulatory surge of LH. The fibroblasts secrete a procollagenase which is bound up in the extracellular collagen matrix.

Gonadotropin stimulation rapidly increases the synthesis of cyclic AMP in the follicle and accelerates steroidogenic activity in the theca interna. The rising level of steroids, particularly estrogens, and prostaglandins in the follicle serve to transform the fibroblasts from the stationary to the proliferative state. These proliferating fibroblasts produce collagenase, which in turn initiates collagenolysis in the follicle wall. The modified proteins that are released by this degradative process induce an acute inflammatory reaction which

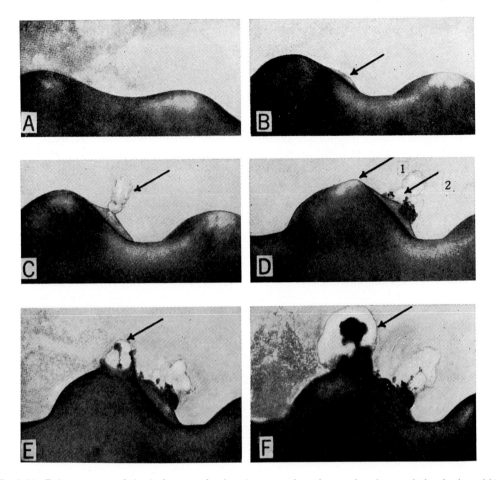

Fig. 9-21. Enlargements of single frames of a time-lapse motion picture showing ovulation in the rabbit. (From Hill, Allen, and Kramer, *Anat. Rec.*, vol. 63, 1935.) *A*, Profile view of two follicles about 1½ hours before rupture. *B*, Same follicles about ½ hour before rupture. *C*, Exudation of clear fluid in early phases of rupture. *D*, At arrow *1*, a new follicle becomes conical as the time of its rupture approaches. At arrow *2*, the exudate from the follicle shown starting to rupture in *C* has become more abundant and contains some blood (dark). *E*, The follicle indicated by arrow *1* in *D* is now beginning to rupture. The blood-tinged exudate from the follicle which started to rupture in *C*, and showed more vigorous exudation in *D* (arrow *2*), can be seen partly behind the more recently rupturing follicle. *F*, The rupture of the follicle which is indicated by the arrow in *E*. Time elapsed between the photographs shown in *E* and *F*, 8 seconds. The ovum is carried out with this final gush of fluid from the ruptured follicle. (Patten: Foundations of Embryology. Courtesy McGraw-Hill Book Co.)

results in histamine release, leukocyte migration, and further release of prostaglandins. The prostaglandins then stimulate a second phase of cyclic AMP synthesis and elevate the blood flow through the inflamed region.

There is a gross reduction in the tensile strength of the collagenous layers which encapsulate the follicle. By morphologic design, the thin region at the apex of the follicle is the area most susceptible to distention under the stress of a small, but important, intrafollicular pressure. Rupture is imminent as the degraded follicle wall begins to dissociate under this stress. By the time of rupture, the enzymatic activity has depolymerized the ground substance in the cumulus oophorus to the extent that the corona radiata is dislodged and can be expelled from the follicle.

Corpus Luteum (CL) Development

The corpus luteum (plural, corpora lutea) is a temporary endocrine organ which, for most of the domestic species, functions for only a few days in the cycling nonpregnant animal. During the diestrual phase of the cycle, the corpus luteum produces maximal amounts of progesterone. If a viable embryo is not present in the uterus by diestrus day 11 or 12 in the sow, day 12 in the ewe, day 14 in the mare, and day 16 in the cow, the corpus luteum undergoes luteolysis and regresses. Among the domestic species, the bitch and pseudopregnant queen are exceptional in that the presence of a viable embryo is not necessary for diestrual luteal maintenance (see Chapters 16 and 17).

Following ovulation there is enough hemorrhage into the follicular cavity, especially in the mare and cow, for a blood clot to develop. The blood-filled follicle now devoid of the oocyte is commonly referred to as a *corpus hemorrhagicum*. This clot of blood serves as a physical framework and a nutrient medium for the quick proliferation of the granulosa and thecal cells, which by differentiating into luteal cells, are mainly responsible for the rapid development of this endocrine organ.

The growth of the luteal cells is one of the fastest known in biology. Within 3 to 4 days the blood clot is invaded by the new luteal cells so that the blood-filled cavity loses its dark coloration.

Following ovulation, the granulosa cells remaining in the collapsed follicle and thecal cells carried from the theca interna by invading capillaries begin to hypertrophy, take on lipid material, and become the lutein or luteal cells of mature corpora lutea.

The corpus luteum is one of the most vascular organs of the body. Columns of luteal cells are separated by vessels which must nourish this new organ during its metabolic activity (steroid synthesis). The newly formed organ is termed a *corpus luteum verum* if the animal becomes pregnant and the corpus continues to function. In the cycling nonpregnant animal the newly formed organ is termed a *corpus luteum spurium*, since it is destined to regress.

The corpus luteum of an infertile cycle will also undergo regression by the end of diestrus. The retrogressive luteal changes are first microscopic and then grossly visible. The lutein cells degenerate rapidly showing cytoplasmic vacuolation and pyknotic nuclei. Progesterone production plummets sharply, even more dramatically than the anatomic changes. Corpora lutea then decrease in size along with degeneration of capillaries. Gradually the lutein cells are replaced by fibroblasts, and the other cells become enmeshed in the forming connective tissue. The degenerating avascular nonfunctional corpus is termed a *corpus luteum albicans* (white) or simply a *corpus albicans*. Slow physical degeneration occurs, usually taking 2 to 3 weeks. For several additional estrous cycles, a visible connective tissue scar remains on the ovary.

In the sow, ovarian weight increases after day 3 and reaches a peak by day 10 of the estrous cycle. This weight increase is attributed to the growth of the corpora lutea. Luteal tissue gradually changes from a dark red (hemorrhage) to a pale purple by day 15. Following day 15, corpora lutea rapidly change from pale purple to a yellowish cream and then to a white by day 18 in the nonpregnant sow. The change in color is due to the decrease in vascularity during this regressive phase. The size of corpora lutea decreases rapidly after day 18, and within 3 weeks most have regressed completely (Fig. 9-22).

Gross and histological ovarian changes in the cow and the ewe before, during, and after ovulation are somewhat different from those in the sow due to the number and location of corpora lutea within the ovary. The corpora lutea of sheep reach maximum size by day 13 and at this time are reddish-pink. Corpora lutea become pale as diestrus progresses, and after day 14 degeneration is rapid because the estrous cycle of the ewe is shorter. After ovulation in the cow, the granulosa cells hypertrophy and become filled with droplets of a yellow lipid material as the corpus luteum forms. Maximum size of the bovine corpus luteum is

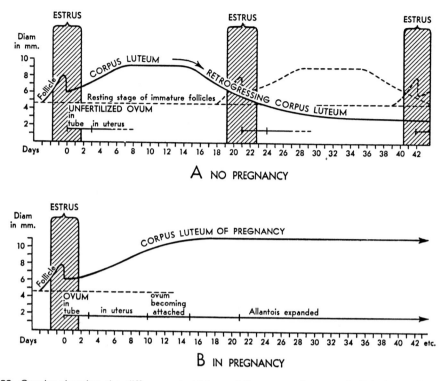

Fig. 9-22. Graphs showing the difference in history of the corpus leteum of ovulation and the corpus luteum of pregnancy in the sow. (After Corner; From Patten: Foundations of Embryology. Courtesy McGraw-Hill Book Co.)

attained by days 14 to 16; then it degenerates rapidly. The bovine corpus luteum changes from a light brown to gold by day 7, then to a golden yellow by day 14. Between days 14 and 20 the corpus luteum progressively changes from yellow to orange to a brick red. The brick red color remains for several cycles as the old corpus gradually regresses. The color of the corpus luteum of the cow or mare is more intense than that of the other species because of a yellow pigment, lutein. The corpora lutea of the ewe and sow are devoid of this lipochrome pigment, hence the lighter color.

Corpus Luteum Function

The production of progesterone by the CL is estimated by determining its levels in the peripheral plasma of the animal. This gives an indication of the level of hormone that the entire body, including the target organs of the genital tract, is subjected to.

Since hormonal levels in the blood are dependent upon a variety of factors, including secretion and metabolic clearance rates, frequency of sampling, and assay system used, the values provided are to serve only as reference and general guidelines. Figure 9-23 represents the pattern of progesterone levels in the peripheral plasma of four cows.

The circulating level of progesterone in other species is given in Table 9-2. Notice the variability from polytocous species to monotocous species of the highest level during diestrus, but the levels of progesterone during the follicular phase are similar for the species examined.

Should pregnancy ensue, then the progesterone level slowly continues to rise after mid-

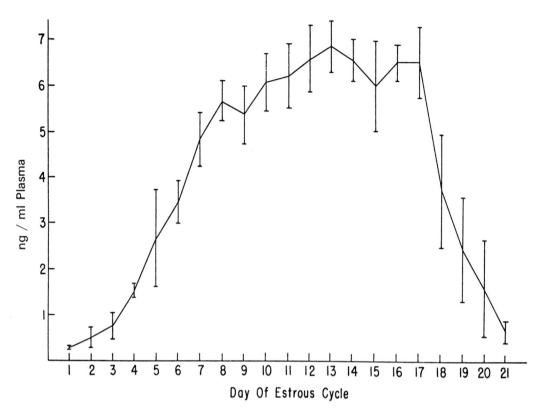

Fig. 9-23. Progesterone concentration in jugular venous plasma from four cows with 21-day estrous cycles. Vertical bars represent the standard error of the mean. (From Stabenfeldt, G. H., Ewing. L. L., and McDonald, L. E.: J. Reprod. Fertil. *19*:433, 1969.)

cycle in all species. The hormonal levels during pregnancy are presented in Chapter 18.

GROSS OVARIAN CHANGES DURING THE ESTROUS CYCLE

Few organs change their gross appearance or even their physiological function from day to day like the cycling ovary. Figure 9-24 will help the reader to visualize these important changes. These studies were made on a polyestrous, polytocous (litter bearing) animal, the sow. Ovarian changes in monotocous species like the cow or mare would be less dramatic because of the single follicle. A

Table 9-2   *Progesterone Levels in Peripheral Plasma During the Follicular and Luteal Phases*

Species*	Follicular Phase ng/ml	Luteal Phase ng/ml
Cow	0.4	6.6
Gilt	0.5	12.0
Ewe	0.25	3.7
Mare	0.4	7.7 to 9.5
Bitch	< 1.0	23.0
Queen	< 1.0	24.6 to 25.8

*Notice higher levels in the polytocous species.
Compiled from different sources.

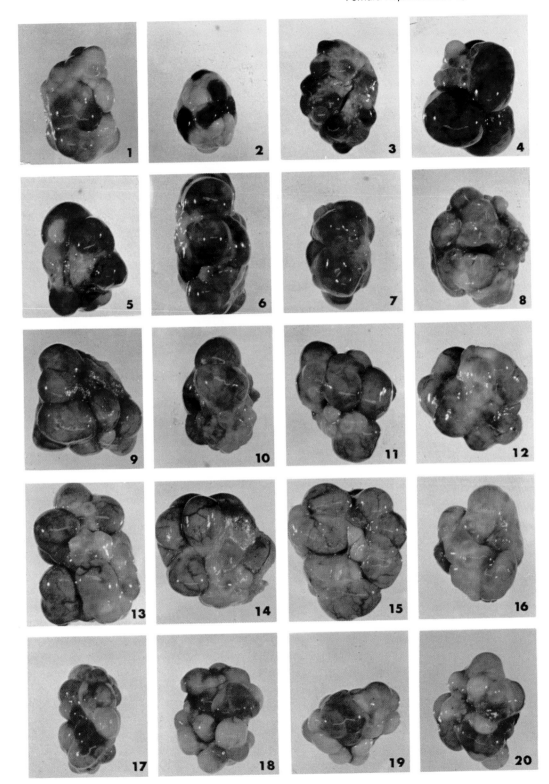

Fig. 9-24. Cyclic changes in the sow's ovary during the 20-day estrous cycle. Photograph 1 is day 0 of the cycle or the first day of estrus. Photographs 1 and 2 are ovaries obtained during estrus, photographs 3 and 4 (days 3 and 4) during metestrus, photographs 5 to 16 during diestrus. Photographs 17 to 20 are during proestrus. See the text for more complete discussion of these photographs. (From Akins, E. L., and Morrissette, M. C.: Am. J. Vet. Res. *29*:1953, 1968.)

typical ovary was selected at slaughter for each day of the 20-day cycle. Unfortunately each day represents a different ovary so there is a lack of ovarian uniformity.

Photograph 1 represents the first day of estrus and several large fluid-filled (mature, graafian) follicles can be seen in the lower left corner. Notice how these protrude above the surface. Fusion of follicles appears to have occurred, but the cavities remain distinct. The centermost follicle shows some blood discoloration. The right side of the ovary contains several blanched corpora albicans from the previous cycle. These are essentially nonfunctional, but the size has not decreased a great deal. These corpora albicans are similar to the follicles in size. There are no ovulation sites yet on this ovary.

Photograph 2 (day 2) shows two corpora hemorrhagica (top and left). These are the site of the first ovulations. These blood-filled and ruptured follicles are somewhat collapsed. Luteal cell growth has begun, but the new corpora lutea will not be well-developed for 2 days. Several blood-tinged follicles fill the center, and these appear ready to ovulate. The old corpora albicantia appear a bit more regressed. This is the last day of estrus.

Day 3 (photograph 3) shows more ovulation sites. A few follicles have not ovulated. Ovulation sites are developing into more organized luteal masses. Corpora albicantia from the previous cycle are less noticeable, very soft, and degenerate.

By day 4 the blood-clot-filled follicles have been reorganized into functional luteal tissue interspersed by a rapidly developing blood supply. The large corpora are liver-like in consistency and color. Progesterone production is rising. A few small follicles are present which may persist until the next estrus or degenerate.

By days 5 and 6 the corpora are more distinct and have a lighter color because the blood clots have been resorbed. Diestrus or the "period of the corpus luteum" has begun. The corpora are still growing and progesterone output is rising.

Days 7 and 8 witness corpora lutea that are more meaty and lighter in color. Diestrus is well underway, and the corpora lutea are functional.

Days 9, 10, 11, and 12 reveal a similar picture whereby the corpora lutea are fully formed, functional, meaty, distinct, encapsulated, and endowed with a good blood supply. Most of the pooled blood from the ovulation site has been resorbed. More small follicles are appearing, but their size is small. Day 12 is critical in the life of the corpora lutea of the sow. If viable embryos are present in the uterus, then the corpora lutea will continue their function. If viable embryos are not present, these corpora lutea will initiate irreversible regression which will be expressed macroscopically later in the cycle.

Days 13 and 14 are similar to the previous 4 days. Macroscopic evidence of luteolysis become apparent by days 15 and 16 and some blanching of the corpora luteal vessels may be seen on day 15. Progesterone production is falling by day 15. By day 16 the corpora lutea have lost most of their vascularity, shrinkage in size has begun, and the ovary is smaller.

By day 17 there is marked follicular enlargement and hyperemia. By days 17 or 18 proestrus has begun, and the estrogenic phase of the cycle will last for 4 to 5 days. The waning corpora are evident and their white color and soft texture signal the end of their function. Although complete regression of these corpora albicantia will take another 15 to 20 days, they are nearly functionless.

Days 19 to 20 represent rising estrogen secretion by the growing follicles. Fluid is being accumulated in the follicles.

One should recall that cyclic changes are occurring in the genital tract concomitant with these dramatic ovarian changes. The most marked changes occur in the uterus, but epithelial and glandular changes also occur throughout the tract.

The ovaries of other litter-bearing animals such as the bitch resemble to some degree the grape-cluster appearance of the sow, but the bitch usually has fewer ovulation sites. The monotocous animals like the cow, ewe, and mare would usually have only one ovary involved in each cycle, but the individual growth and regression of a follicle and corpus luteum resembles that of a single follicle in the sow.

Uterine Changes During the Estrous Cycle

The steroid hormone-dependent organs of the female reproductive system undergo profound changes in growth and differentiation as puberty approaches. Once puberty is reached and estrous cycles occur, the tubular genital tract is sequentially exposed during each cycle to estrogens, the dominant hormones during the follicular phase of the cycle, and then to progesterone, the dominant hormone during the luteal phase of the cycle. The reproductive organs of the female undergo macro- and microscopic changes, which are induced by either estrogens or progesterone. At the end of the follicular phase and the beginning of the luteal phase of the cycle, as well as at the end of the luteal phase and beginning of the subsequent follicular phase, the reproductive organs respond to the transitional dominance from estrogens to progesterone and back to estrogens with changes that reflect the combined effects of both hormones.

Estrogen Influence

Estrogens favor retention of water and electrolytes throughout the genital tract (Table 9-3). The most prominent morphological changes noted in the uterus during the estrous cycle are in the endometrium and its associated glands. During estrus the endometrial cells increase in height and show intense mitotic activity and the glandular elements of the endometrium secrete a fluid mucus which flushes the tract. Under estrogenic influence, the capillary bed in the endometrium grows, increasing the blood supply to the uterus. The increase in blood supply results in further growth and thickening of the endometrium due to cell proliferation and edema.

Progesterone Influence

After ovulation, as the corpus luteum develops and begins secreting progesterone, the superficial endometrial cells further increase in size and the glandular elements of the endometrium multiply and secrete. This period is sometimes called the "secretory phase" because the uterine glands respond to progesterone by glandular development and secretion of a thick material, "uterine milk," into the uterine lumen to nourish the embryo. The subepithelial layer becomes infiltrated with neutrophils and eosinophils as the cycle progresses, and the edema lessens. By midcycle, high columnar cells predominate in the surface epithelium and invasion of the superficial stroma with eosinophilic leukocytes becomes maximal.

Falling Progesterone and Rising Estrogen Influence

If a viable embryo is not present by the end of diestrus, the corpus luteum initiates retrogressive changes and the synthesis of progesterone is severely impaired. The increasing estrogenic influence is reflected in the tubular genitalia by changes in the surface epithelium, which becomes low and cuboidal. Marked vacuolar degeneration of the epithelial cells is characteristic of the declining progesterone effect at this stage of the cycle. Thus the major changes noted during the estrous cycle appear to be the cyclic manifestations of stromal edema, neutrophilic and eosinophilic infiltrations of the subepithelial areas, and changes in the growth of surface and glandular epithelium.

THE ANTERIOR PITUITARY AND THE OVARY

Two separate gonadotropins that specifically stimulate the ovary are present in the anterior pituitary. One promotes follicular growth in the ovary, whereas the second substance has little effect on the ovary unless the follicle-stimulating factor is administered first. Since the early investigations, the terms follicle-stimulating hormone (FSH) and

Table 9-3 Mucosal Changes in the Reproductive Tract of the Cow During the Estrous Cycle

Area of tract	Proestrus	Estrus	Postestrus
Vestibule and posterior vagina	Congestion; edema	Congestion; edema Leukocyte infiltration; extravasation of blood	9 days: cornification 2 days: mucus-secreting cells 8–11 days: leukocyte infiltration, extravasation of blood
Anterior vagina	Large, wide mucous cells; 2–3 layers of epithelial cells; stroma edematous	Tall, narrow, columnar mucous cells; 2–3 layers epithelial cells; stroma edematous; leukocytes abundant	2 days: several layers epithelial cells 8–11 days: vacuolar and degenerate epithelium 9–16 days: cornified cells in smears rise rapidly; leukocytes present in all smears
Cervix	Mucus-secreting cells	Cells loaded with mucus, many emptying; edema and hyperemia	1–2 days: loaded cells disappear; regeneration of mucous membrane; less congestion 3 days on: cells filled with mucus, but low; few cells emptying mucus; stroma compact; little or no congestion
Uterus	Cells tallest; cell length to nucleus length 4:1; marked edema	Congested blood vessels; edema of stroma; cells tall 2:1; glands straight with large lumens	Cells vacuolize just after heat 2 days: cells lowest, 1.5:1 cell to nucleus 2 days: glandular growth starts 1–8 days: increased glandular secretion 8–11 days: glandular hypertrophy 8–12 days: glandular-cells height increases; greatest coiling of glands
Oviducts	Cilia present and active; edema; granules in epithelial cells; cells $33\,\mu$ high; cytoplasmic projections from cells	Cilia present and active; edema; granules in epithelial cells; cells $45\,\mu$ high	Cilia present and active 1–2 days: edema and granules in cells 1–5 days: epithelial height $44\,\mu$ 3–4 days: mucus-like material in oviducts 6–15 days: epithelial height $27\,\mu$

From Salisbury, G. W., and VanDemark, N. L.: Physiology of Reproduction and Artificial Insemination of Cattle. San Francisco, W. H. Freeman and Co., 1961.

luteinizing hormone (LH) have become commonplace in the literature.

A third pituitary gonadotropin, now known to be prolactin, stimulates corpora lutea of the rat to produce progesterone. This luteotropic effect of prolactin is only known for the rat. The ovarian follicles in mammals are dependent upon FSH and LH for follicular growth and maturation. Both FSH and LH are essential for the synthesis of estrogen.

Rising blood levels of estrogen suppress the pituitary release of FSH and facilitate release of LH. Purified LH in itself has no conspicuous effects on the growing ovarian follicle. Thus, it is well established that FSH promotes ovarian growth and follicular maturation and that LH is essential for synthesis of estrogen and ovulation in most species and for the initial development of the corpus luteum in some species.

Estrogens in large amounts inhibit FSH secretion. Large quantities of estrogen completely inhibit the secretion of gonadotropic hormones. Low physiological levels of estrogen cause a positive feedback on gonadotropin output. Injection of low doses of certain estrogenic substances can facilitate ovulation in cattle, sheep, rabbits, and rats. It also has been reported that progesterone in a low dosage can cause the release of LH. Thus it seems apparent that both steroids, when present at a critical level at a certain time in the hypothalamic-hypophyseal axis may be essential to the ovulatory process in mammals.

Apparently FSH and LH are synthesized continuously and stored in the pituitary gland from where they are released throughout the estrous cycle. The proportions and levels of each of these gonadotropins change during the different stages of the cycle. In relation to the amount of hormone released, the levels reached in the peripheral circulation, and the periodicity of the release of these hormones, one can distinguish at least three major forms: basal levels, pulses, and surges. Basal levels refer to a low and relatively constant level of the hormone in the blood. Pulses refer to a sharp and increased concentration of the hormone in the blood above the preceding plasma concentration, lasting for short periods, usually less than one hour. A surge is defined as a large increase in the concentration of a hormone in the blood, significantly above the basal level, lasting for more than one hour. A brief recapitulation of the cyclic hormone changes is in order. Figure 9-25 shows a typical cycle in the cow. On day 16 a luteolysin (probably prostaglandin $F_{2\alpha}$, see following pages) from the nonpregnant progesterone-dominated endometrium reaches the ovary by a local route and induces luteolysis. Progesterone levels plummet, thereby allowing an outpouring of FSH, since the block is released. The FSH levels are pulsatile, but the clearest and most constant peaks are on days 17 and 18. FSH in synergy with LH facilitates follicular growth and estrogen production. The declining levels of progesterone and rapidly rising levels of estrogen induce behavioral estrus. Rising estrogen triggers a release of an "ovulatory surge" of LH on the day of estrus. Estrogen levels then decline, but the new CL starts progesterone pro-

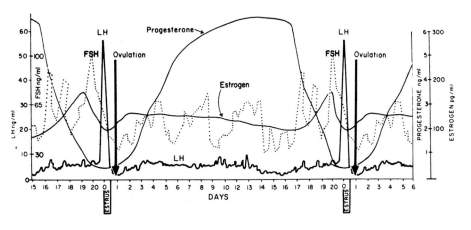

Fig. 9-25. Cyclic hormonal changes in the cow.

duction which rises during the next few days and holds gonadotropin release at low levels. If luteotropic signals are not given by day 16, the CL irreversibly regresses and a new cycle will follow.

Prostaglandins

Nobel Laureate von Euler, in 1934, coined the name *prostaglandin* (PG) for a substance found in human semen. Since 1960, considerable interest has been shown in this group of 20 carbon unsaturated fatty acids which have been found in many mammalian tissues. The precursors of PG are essential dietary fatty acids. The trivial names of the PGs are by letter and subscript number as shown in Figure 9-26. Prostaglandins have a wide variety of actions as follows: PGE_2 and $PGF_{2\alpha}$ (induction of labor, abortion, and destruction of the corpus luteum); PGA_1 (gastric secretion inhibition); PGE_1 and PGE_2 (bronchial dilation); PGA_1 (vasodilation and diuresis); and PGE_1 (inhibition of platelet aggregation). PGF and PGE differ only in a ketone or hydroxyl group at C-9 and a double bond between C-5 and C-6.

Consideration will be given primarily to the role of $PGF_{2\alpha}$ in animal reproduction. PGF is assigned the letter F because it was found to be soluble in phosphate (spelled *fosfat* in Swedish), whereas PGE was found to be soluble in ether.

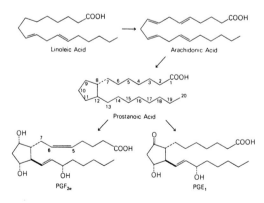

Fig. 9-26. $PGF_{2\alpha}$ has an hydroxyl at carbon 9, whereas PGE has a ketone. Both arise through many steps not shown from the essential dietary 18 carbon linoleic and 20 carbon arachidonic fatty acids.

The prostaglandins in general and $PGF_{2\alpha}$ in particular, are rapidly metabolized in the body, namely in the lungs. However, there are species differences in the degree and rate of metabolism of exogenous prostaglandins. For instance, in the ewe, 99% of the $PGF_{2\alpha}$ that was injected in the pulmonary artery was metabolized during a single passage through the lungs, regardless of the stage of the cycle, whereas in the sow only about 18% of exogenous prostaglandin was metabolized during a single passage through the lungs.[30] Interestingly, as will be discussed later in this chapter, the luteolytic activity of uterine $PGF_{2\alpha}$ is exerted through local utero-ovarian pathways in the sheep, a species in which most of the $PGF_{2\alpha}$ is metabolized during a single passage through the lungs, while the luteolytic activity of uterine $PGF_{2\alpha}$ is mainly systemic in the sow. It is tempting to speculate that in the mare, little if any of the $PGF_{2\alpha}$ is metabolized during a single passage through the lungs, since $PGF_{2\alpha}$ is a very effective luteolysin even given in small doses, and the pathway of uterine luteolytic control is systemic in this species.

Prostaglandins in Luteolysis

It is now generally accepted the $PGF_{2\alpha}$ is the natural *luteolysin* for the majority of the domestic species. Indomethacin, a potent inhibitor of prostaglandin synthesis, extends the functional lifespan of the corpus luteum in several species if given at the time of diestrus when prostaglandins are secreted by the uterus. Oxytocin may also be involved in the release of $PGF_{2\alpha}$ by the uterus. Exogenous oxytocin given to heifers early in diestrus induces luteal regression and shortens the length of the estrus cycle, whereas the administration of antibodies to oxytocin delays luteolysis. Figure 9-27 displays a postulated mechanism by which estradiol induces the formation of oxytocin receptors in the endometrial cells. Oxytocin would then activate these receptors, resulting in the synthesis, pulsatile secretion, and release of $PGF_{2\alpha}$.

Several mechanisms have been proposed to explain the luteolytic activity of $PGF_{2\alpha}$.

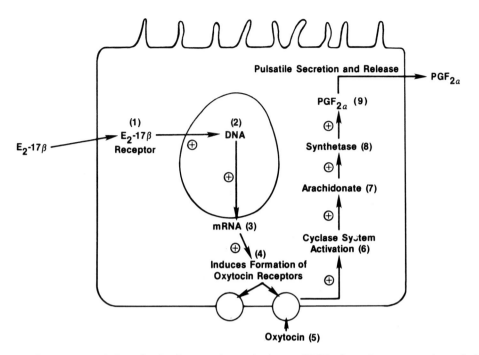

Fig. 9-27. Receptor regulation of pulsatile secretion and release of $PGF_{2\alpha}$ from the uterus at the end of the luteal phase of the cycle. (Drawn and adapted from Fig. 1 in: J. A. McCracken, Res. Reprod. *16*:1, 1984.)

Among these are (1) constriction of the utero-ovarian vessels causing ischemia and starvation of the luteal cells; (2) interference with progesterone synthesis; (3) competition with LH for the receptor site, or (4) destruction of LH receptor sites.

For all the species so far studied, including the domestic species, the ovarian artery is coiled and follows a tortuous course along the major (ewe and cow) or minor (mare, sow, bitch, queen) branches of the utero-ovarian vein draining the uterus. The ovarian artery is intertwined and in close apposition with a complex vascular network of venules from the utero-ovarian vein. This vascular arrangement favors the passage of substances from the venous blood draining the uterus to the arteries supplying the ovary. In fact, luteolytic substances from the uterus, likely $PGF_{2\alpha}$, are now generally believed to reach the ovary in species such as the ewe and cow by transfer, diffusion or some other means, from the venous efferent to the arterial affluent circulation. For these species, the uterine horn controls the corpus luteum on the ipsilateral

ovary through a local luteolytic pathway in the nonpregnant animal and through a local luteotropic pathway when a viable embryo is present in the ipsilateral horn (Fig. 9-28). The local utero-ovarian pathway demonstrated for the cow and ewe has not been established for the goat. By the contrary, intrauterine devices, which induce luteolysis through a local pathway in cows and ewes, appear to act by a systemic route in goats.

The reader is encouraged to review the vascular anatomy of the uterus and ovaries for the domestic species, published in Veterinary Scope. [57]

$PGF_{2\alpha}$ induces abortion when given during early pregnancy and will induce labor when given during late pregnancy in most species. Abortion during the early periods of pregnancy is probably due to luteolysis since progesterone production falls sharply. Induction of labor during late pregnancy may depend on the action of PGs on the myometrium in addition to possible effects on the corpus luteum.

The ability of $PGF_{2\alpha}$ to induce luteolysis in

cattle, sheep, mares, and other species has stimulated study of its use as an agent to control and synchronize estrus in livestock species.

MAINTENANCE OR REGRESSION OF THE CORPUS LUTEUM

In polyestrous domestic animals, corpora lutea develop after ovulation and function for only 14 to 18 days, unless pregnancy occurs to signal the corpora lutea to continue functioning. The question then raised is *how does the corpus luteum know that a 2-week-old, often unimplanted blastocyst is in the uterus?* Or conversely, why does the corpus luteum regress in an infertile cycle?

There appear to be marked species differences in the control of luteal function. Much early work was done on the rat which now appears to be an atypical species. For purposes of simplicity this discussion will be confined to the sow, mare, goat, ewe, and cow. The bitch and queen also seem to be atypical species. Corpora lutea of nonpregnant bitches continue to function for approximately the same length of time as for the pregnant bitch, a condition termed *pseudopregnancy*. In the bitch, $PGF_{2\alpha}$ does not induce complete regression of the corpus luteum when given in single doses, even when given at doses which are toxic to the bitch. The corpora lutea of the queen are also resistant to $PGF_{2\alpha}$. This phenomenon will be discussed under "Reproductive Patterns of Dogs and Cats," Chapters 16 and 17.

The study of the factors that control the formation, functional life, secretory activity, and regression of the corpus luteum in the cycling animal must include both the *luteotropic* and *luteolytic* influences or signals, and also, the temporal, sequential interplay of these influences. Luteotropic influences to the corpus luteum are provided by pituitary gonadotropins, mainly LH, and after a fertile mating has occurred, by the embryo in most species.

Pituitary Effect

The pituitary is needed in most species to produce luteotropin at ovulation to form the corpus luteum. LH is probably the luteotropic substance of most domestic animals, although the mere act of ovulation favors luteal development in most species. For most species in which hypophysectomy has been successfully performed, the corpus luteum does not form when hypophysectomy is done before the ovulatory surge of LH. If hypophysectomy is performed after the ovulatory surge of LH, the corpus luteum forms and, depending upon the species, either remains functional for a few days to regress early in the diestrus (ewe, heifer) or remains functional for the normal length of the diestrus, regressing at the expected time (sow). Administration of LH or LH-like hormones, such as hCG, at appropriate times during diestrus to ewes, heifers, goats, mares, and sows prolongs the functional lifespan of the corpus luteum of the cycle. On the other hand, the administration of antiserum containing high titers of biologically active antibodies to LH during middiestrus shortens the lifespan of the corpus luteum and luteal regression is induced in ewes, goats, heifers, and mares, but not in the sow. The corpora lutea of the cycle in the sow are somehow independent of further pituitary LH luteotropic control once the initial luteotropic stimulus is given by the ovulatory surge of LH. However, antibodies to LH, when given in early pregnancy can induce luteal regression in the sow. Antiserum to LH also interferes with luteal function in the bitch and drugs that block the release of prolactin from the pituitary also suppress corpus luteum activity in this species, suggesting that the corpora lutea of the bitch are under the control of both pituitary hormones. There is no information available for the queen, regarding pituitary control of CL function.

Uterus Effect

Loeb demonstrated in 1923 that the uterus exerted some form of control on ovarian function by studying the effects of hysterectomy on corpus luteum maintenance in the rabbit. By now, a wealth of experimental evidences have accumulated since 1923 that point to the uterus as the center to control the corpora luteal life span during the estrous cycle.

Studies in several domestic species indicate that the nonpregnant uterus produces a substance, probably $PGF_{2\alpha}$, which has a "lytic" influence on the corpus luteum. With the exception of the bitch, which is a special case to be discussed in Chapter 16, and the queen for which no information was available at the time of the writing of this chapter, the complete removal of the uterus during middiestrus in the cycling cow, ewe, goat, mare, and sow prolongs the lifespan of the corpus luteum of that cycle for a length of time approaching that of pregnancy for the species. Another interesting aspect of the utero-ovarian relationship, in relation to the mechanisms of uterine control of corpus luteum function in the domestic species, is the local pathway of uterine control for some of the species versus systemic pathway of control for the others. In mares, total removal, but not partial removal of the uterus, prolongs the lifespan of the corpus luteum of the cycle. This is attributable to the vascular anatomy of the uterus and ovaries for this species, which favors the systemic distribution of the uterine luteolytic factors to the ovary carrying the corpus luteum. The uterus as a whole contributes the amount of uterine luteolysin necessary to cause regression of the corpus luteum. In the cow and ewe there is a local effect of the uterus on the corpus luteum and unilateral hysterectomy, implying the removal of only one of the uterine horns during middiestrus will or will not prolong the lifespan of the CL, depending on which of the uterine horns is removed with respect to ovary carrying the corpus luteum. If the horn removed is adjacent or *ipsilateral* to the ovary carrying the corpus luteum, the corpus luteum will be maintained functional, as it would after total removal of the uterus. If the horn removed on the side *contralateral* to the ovary carrying the corpus luteum, the corpus luteum regresses at the expected time in the cycle, as it would in the intact animal. This differential response to total or to partial hysterectomy is also attributable to the vascular anatomy of the uterus and ovaries, which in these two species favors the local transfer of uterine luteolysin to the ovary via a local, venous-arterial pathway.

In the sow, both the systemic and the local pathways of uterine control appear to participate in the regression of the corpora lutea. Experimental evidence indicates that a mini-

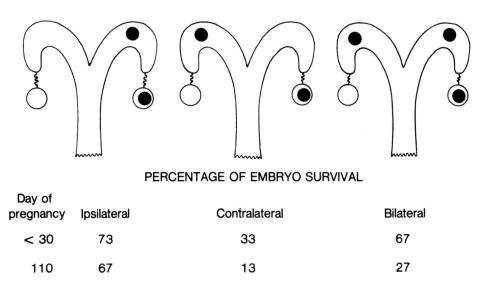

PERCENTAGE OF EMBRYO SURVIVAL

Day of pregnancy	Ipsilateral	Contralateral	Bilateral
< 30	73	33	67
110	67	13	27

Fig. 9-28. Embryo survival in heifers when a single embryo (black dot in the horn) is transferred to the horn ipsilateral or contralateral to the ovary carrying the corpus luteum (black dot in the ovary), or when a single embryo is transferred to each horn. (Adpated from: M. R. Del Campo et al.: Reprod. Nutr. Develop. *23*:303, 1983.)

mum amount of uterine tissue is needed in both horns for bilateral luteal regression. If as little as one-fourth of the ovarian end of each horn is left intact and the vascular connections have not been impaired, the corpora lutea of both ovaries will regress, even though three-fourths of each horn was eliminated. On the other hand, if unilateral, partial hysterectomy is performed and a horn is extirpated or less than one-fourth of that uterine horn is left *in situ*, while the horn in the other side is left intact, the corpora lutea in the *ipsilateral* ovary will be maintained, whereas the corpora lutea in the other ovary, *ipsilateral* to the intact horn, will regress.

In the control of the estrous cycle, the mechanism that "turns off" the corpus luteum appears to be of much greater practical significance than the pituitary mechanism(s) that "turns on" ovulation, as well as initiates growth and function of the corpus luteum.

It may be concluded, therefore, that luteolysin(s), likely $PGF_{2\alpha}$ from the nonpregnant uterus, induces the regression of the corpus luteum at the end of the cycle. Luteal degeneration can be shown through morphological studies of luteal cell degeneration as well as through analysis of their progesterone content and by the declining levels of progesterone in the blood. The uterus manifests its maximal "luteolytic" influence on the corpus luteum when under maximal influence of progesterone from the corpus luteum.

Exogenous $PGF_{2\alpha}$ effectively induces luteal regression and shortens the length of the estrous cycle only when the corpus luteum is fully formed and secreting progesterone. Exogenous $PGF_{2\alpha}$ does not induce luteal regression when given during the first 4 to 5 days of diestrus in cows, ewes, goats, and mares. The sow is a particular case in that $PGF_{2\alpha}$ induces luteal regression only on days 11 or 12 of diestrus, at a time when the corpora lutea of the sow have already initiated retrogressive changes if viable embryos are not present in the uterus. On this basis, the use of $PGF_{2\alpha}$ has no practical application in the cycling sow because the sow will come to

estrus at the expected time, whether $PGF_{2\alpha}$ is administered or not.

Corpora lutea can be made to regress not only by the abrupt effect of $PGF_{2\alpha}$, but also by a lack of pituitary-tropic effect on the corpus luteum, as previously discussed. Regression of luteal tissue in the latter case is gradual.

There also appears to be a third way in which corpora lutea may regress. In hysterectomized ewes, persistent corpora lutea diminish in progesterone concentration by 150 days, which is the length of gestation in the intact ewe. If hysterectomized ewes are made to ovulate and new corpora lutea form, then these will also persist but will diminish in progesterone content in another 150 days. This effect suggests that "aging" may be a factor in corpora luteal regression. Similarly, the corpora lutea of the bitch appear to be independent of uterine control insofar as their regression is concerned. Corpora lutea of pregnant, nonpregnant, mated or nonmated bitches regress at about the same time, suggesting that aging or the lack of extrauterine luteotropic stimuli may be contributing factors to their demise by the end of pregnancy or pseudopregnancy.

Local Uterus-Corpus Luteum Effect

Progesterone production in the ewe plummets on day 15 much like the decrease on day 17 in the cow. This decrease appears to be due to $PGF_{2\alpha}$ from the nonpregnant progesterone-dominated endometrium. By local circulation, the $PGF_{2\alpha}$ is transferred from the uterine vein to the ovarian artery by the countercurrent pathway shown in Figure 9-29. Figure 9-30 shows what happens in the ewe. Similar responses also occur in the cow. In subfigure "a" the normal corpus luteum of nonpregnancy lasts until day 15 with an intact uterus. In subfigure "b" total hysterectomy prolongs the function of the corpus luteum for many months, since the source of $PGF_{2\alpha}$ has been removed. Subfigure "c" shows that transplantation of the ovaries to the neck prolongs the life of the corpus luteum for many weeks because the $PGF_{2\alpha}$ countercurrent system has been interrupted. In sub-

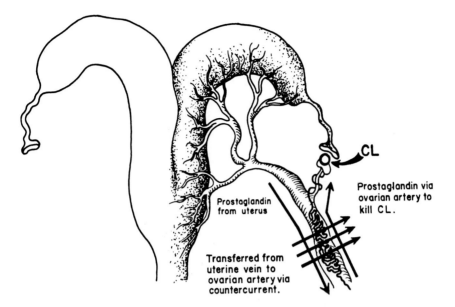

Fig. 9-29. Prostaglandins transfer from uterus to uterine vein, then countercurrent transfer to ovarian artery, and thence to the CL in the ewe and possibly other species.

figure "d" the same principle is shown because removal of the uterine horn adjacent to the ovary causes the corpus luteum to live for many days, since local transfer of $PGF_{2\alpha}$ is interrupted and a less efficient systemic route must be utilized. Finally in subfigure "e" removal of the contralateral uterine horn does not affect corpus luteal life because the ipsilateral uterine horn produces $PGF_{2\alpha}$ which reaches the corpus luteum by the local route like that in subfigure "a." Available evidence lends support to this route in the ewe, sow, and cow.

Understanding of both the local and systemic pathways of uterine control of luteal function has physiologic and pharmacologic implications. For instance, the mare which has a systemic pathway of uterine control of luteal function requires much smaller doses of $PGF_{2\alpha}$, regardless of the route of administration, to effectively induce luteolysis than does the cow. However, if $PGF_{2\alpha}$ is infused into the uterus of the cow, which has a local pathway of uterine control, the required dose of $PGF_{2\alpha}$ is about 10 times lower than that needed when the parenteral route is used. In this case, the effective dose of $PGF_{2\alpha}$ for the cow is about the same as that needed for the mare.

It is not clear whether the interaction of the embryo with the endometrium prevents the secretion and/or release of the uterine luteolysin or the embryo produces a luteotropin that counteracts, at the ovarian level, the luteolytic activity of uterine factors. In sheep, luteotropic signals from the embryo reach the ipsilateral ovary through local venous-arterial pathways, similar to that described for $PGF_{2\alpha}$. Furthermore, the experimental transfer of embryos to the uterine horn ipsilateral to the ovary carrying the corpus luteum results in pregnancy in sheep and heifers, whereas the transfer of embryos to the horn contralateral to the ovary with the corpus luteum often results in embryonicc mortality (Fig. 9-28). Embryos from several species at certain stages of embryonic development are known to produce LH-like factors, and also to secrete estrogens, which are needed for implantation. These may form part of the embryonic luteotropic signal that counteracts the uterine luteolysin or prevents its activity. Intrauterine infusion of embryonic extracts prolongs luteal maintenance in some species. Recent evidence

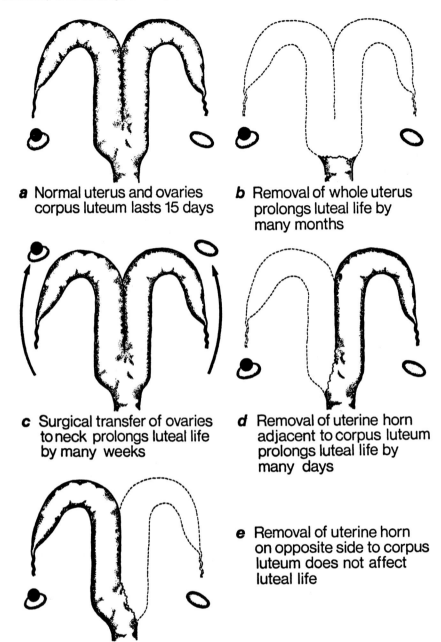

a Normal uterus and ovaries corpus luteum lasts 15 days

b Removal of whole uterus prolongs luteal life by many months

c Surgical transfer of ovaries to neck prolongs luteal life by many weeks

d Removal of uterine horn adjacent to corpus luteum prolongs luteal life by many days

e Removal of uterine horn on opposite side to corpus luteum does not affect luteal life

Fig. 9-30. The local lytic effect of the uterus on the corpus luteum in sheep. For the sake of simplicity, the corpus luteum is always shown in the left ovary. (From Reproduction in Mammals, edited by C. R. Austin and R. V. Short. Cambridge University Press, 1972.)

suggests that the embryo may suppress the pulsatile release of ovarian oxytocin, and as a consequence, interferes with the release of $PGF_{2\alpha}$ from the uterus (see Fig. 9-27).

As discussed previously in this chapter, the presence of a viable embryo in the uterus is needed in single-bearing species at a critical time, before the end of diestrus, to prevent luteal regression. In the sow, and probably in other litter-bearing species, more than 4 embryos are required to establish and maintain pregnancy. Apparently 4 embryos or less are unable to overcome completely the luteolytic effect normally exerted by a nongravid uterus. It is possible that when fewer than 4 embryos are present during the 2nd to 3rd weeks of pregnancy, more than one fourth of the internal uterine surface is not occupied by the trophoblasts and thus production of $PGF_{2\alpha}$ causes luteolysis. It has also been shown in swine that if embryos are confined to one uterine horn, the unilateral pregnancy so established is not maintained unless the nonpregnant horn is removed before the 14th day of pregnancy.

Other Uterine Effects

Uterine infections prevent luteal regression in the ewe and cow. Perhaps uterine infections mimic pregnancy and cause persistent corpora lutea by preventing secretion of the luteolytic factor ($PGF_{2\alpha}$) from the endometrium.

In the mare, chronic uterine infections cause prolonged luteal function, but acute uterine infections trigger corpus luteum degeneration and cycle shortening. Another line of evidence for uterine involvement in luteal life has been shown by studies with intrauterine devices (IUD) in sheep, cattle, and swine. These IUD's were similar to the contraceptive devices used in the human female. Estrous cycles were shortened by the IUD's in cattle and sheep but not affected in swine. It has been shown that these devices cause luteal degeneration through local mechanisms operating directly between the uterine horn and the adjacent ovary. For years, equine practitioners have used intrauterine infusion of 500 to 1,000 ml of sterile, physiological saline solution to initiate estrus in anestrous mares. In 2 to 4 days, estrus usually follows. The mechanism is not known, but may be similar to that postulated for the IUD.

OVARIAN HORMONES

The ovary produces two main steroid hormones, estradiol-17β and progesterone, which bring about changes in the genital tract and some other parts of the body. There are several pathways, precursors, and metabolites in the process of steroid biosynthesis (Fig. 9-31). In this chapter, the discussion will be restricted to the major end-products of ovarian steroid biosynthesis: estradiol-17β,

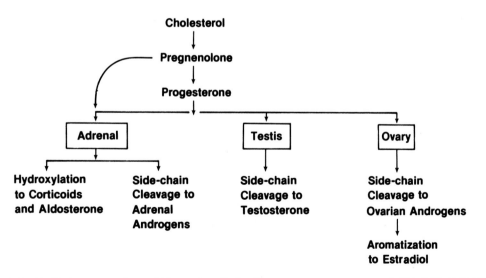

Fig. 9-31. Unified concept of steroid formation. Notice the common precursors and side-chain cleavages to originate end-products. *Adapted from* Ryan, K. J.: Steroid Hormones and Prostaglandins. *In* Principles and Management of Human Reproduction, D. E. Reid et al, (eds.) Philadelphia, W. B. Saunders Co., 1972, pp. 4–27.)

the natural estrogenic hormone, two physiologically important circulating metabolites of estradiol-17β, estriol and estrone, and progesterone, the hormone secreted by the corpus luteum. Figure 9-32 shows the structure of several natural and synthetic steroids.

Peptide Factors Produced by the Ovary

In addition to the steroid hormones, the ovary is involved in the secretion of peptide factors such as oocyte maturation inhibitor (OMI), inhibin, gonadocrinin, and relaxin. OMI appears to be secreted by the granulosa cells of primordial and developing follicles and is responsible for maintenance of the oocyte at the dictyate stage of meiosis. It is not yet clear whether the ovulatory surge of LH inhibits the production of OMI or blocks its transfer from the cells of the cumulus to the oocyte (see Fig. 7-10). Inhibin is a polypeptide factor apparently produced by the granulosa cells, which selectively controls the secretion and release of FSH by the adenohypophysial cells. Thus, inhibin is involved in the regulation of the growth of ovarian follicles. Gonadocrinin is a small peptide, similar to GnRH in activity, but produced locally in the ovarian follicle by the granulosa cells. The physiologic role of gonadocrinin has not been clearly determined and specific receptors for GnRH have not been found in the follicles of cows, ewes, and sows. However, experimental evidences in other species suggest that gonadocrinin would, in a paracrine fashion, locally control steroidogenesis by the thecal cells (see Fig. 8-4) by decreasing LH receptors and by interfering with the cAMP system of the follicular cells. Relaxin is a polypeptide factor considered to be a hormone of pregnancy, responsible for relaxation of the pelvic structures and cervix needed for normal parturition. Relaxin is also present in significant amounts in the blood of nonpregnant gilts and sows. Granulosa cells of the ovarian follicle appear to be the source of relaxin in the nonpregnant animal. The role of relaxin in the nonpregnant animal remains unclear.

Estrogens

Estrogens have been isolated from the ovaries, adrenals, placenta, and even the testes of the male, especially the stallion. Table 9-4 shows the concentration of estrogens in different organs of female mammals.

Estrogens are produced by the theca interna and granulosa cells of the ovarian follicle under the synergistic control of FSH and LH, and possibly under the local influence of intrafollicular factors such as inhibin and gonadocrinin. LH receptors are present on the thecal and interstitial cells of the ovary, but the granulosa cells of the developing follicles appear to

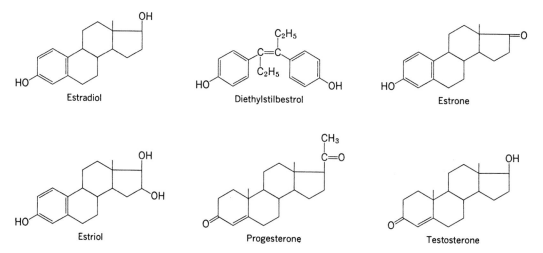

Fig. 9-32. The structure of some steroid hormones.

Table 9-4   Estrogens Found in Endocrine Organs of Female Mammals

Species	Organ	Estrone	Estradiol-17-β	Estradiol-17-α	Estriol	6-α-OH-Estradiol-17-β
Sow	Ovary	+	+	−	−	−
Cow	Ovary, follicular fluid	7.3 µg/100 ml	68.5 µg/100 ml	−	−	−
Mare in estrus	Ovary, follicular fluid	16.9 µg/100 ml	252 µg/100 ml	−	−	−
	Ovary	+	+	−	−	+
Woman	Ovary, luteal tissue of pregnancy	24–89 µg/100 ml	7–64 µg/100 ml	−	24 µg/100 ml	−
Sow	Placenta	+	−	−	−	−
Cow	Placenta	+	+	+	−	−
Ewe	Placenta	−	−	+	−	−
Goat	Placenta	−	−	+	−	−
Woman	Placenta	+	+	−	+	−
Cow	Adrenal	+	−	−	−	−

From Van Tienhoven, A.: *Reproductive Physiology of Vertebrates:* Philadelphia, W. B. Saunders Co., 1968.

be the only follicular cells to have measurable receptors for FSH. As the follicle matures, LH receptors begin to develop in the granulosa cells reaching their highest concentration in the mature follicle, prior to ovulation. Thus, the appearance of receptors to LH in both thecal and granulosa cells marks a major event enabling the follicle to respond to the rising levels of LH during the preovulatory surge. The interaction between the thecal and granulosa cells is required for follicular steroidogenesis. Figure 9-33 shows an operational model for interaction between thecal and granulosa cells during steroidogenesis in the domestic species, with the possible exception of the mare. In this model, LH stimu-

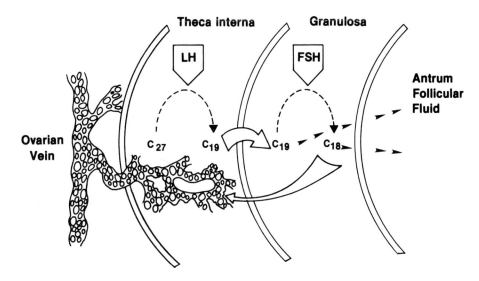

C_{27}=Cholesterol; C_{19}=Androgen; C_{18}=Estrogen

Fig. 9-33. Biosynthesis of estrogen in the preovulatory follicle. (Adapted From: S. G. Hillier: J. Endocrinology *89*:3P, 1981.)

lates the biosynthesis of androgens from cholesterol by the thecal cells. The androgens then diffuse across the basement membrane of the follicular wall and a portion of these androgens reach the antrum. The granulosa cells uptake the androgens diffusing across the basement membrane and aromatize them to estrogens under the influence of FSH. A portion of these estrogens accumulate in the follicular fluid filling the antrum, but the majority diffuse into the capillaries of the thecal layer to be distributed into the systemic circulation. In the mare, the theca interna is thought to be the major site of estrogenic biosynthesis by the follicle, thus the model represented by Figure 9-33 may not be applicable to the mare. Ovarian androgens, which diffuse into the capillary bed of the follicle, can be detected in the systemic circulation. Countercurrent transfer of androgens and other steroids from the venous to the arterial blood occurs at the ovarian pedicle in some species, providing additional androgenic substrate for follicular steroidogenesis and estrogen biosynthesis.

The main physiologic roles of estradiol-17β and estrogens in general are the development and maintenance of the functional structure of the female sex organs by stimulating protein synthesis and mitosis of estrogen-dependent organs. The secondary sex characteristics of the female, including changes in body conformation and growth, hair or plumage distribution, and mammary gland development are under estrogenic control. From this point of view, estrogens in general and estradiol-17β in particular, are feminine hormones. After progesterone priming, estrogens are responsible for the induction of sexual receptivity to mating of the female. In most of the domestic species, estrogen alone or increasing blood levels of estrogen in association with declining levels of progesterone induce behavioral estrus. In the queen, estrogenic hormone alone appears to be sufficient to induce sexual receptivity, whereas the bitch requires declining plasma levels of estrogen and increasing levels of progesterone for the full expression of behavioral estrus.

Perhaps the most dramatic organic changes induced by estrogens are those of the uterus, vagina, and vulva. Estrogens secreted by the developing follicles during the cycle, or the exogenous administration of estrogens, induce pronounced vascularization, increased blood flow and hyperemia, water and salt retention, and edema of the uterus, vagina, and vulva. Swelling of the vulva is an external sign of the edema of the tract associated with estrus. Estrogens cause an increased uterine tone, which can be ascertained through rectal palpation of the uterus in large animal species. The myotropic effect of estrogens is expressed by increased myometrial contractions during proestrus and estrus. At this time, the myometrium is sensitized by estrogens to respond to oxytocin and prostaglandins. Prolonged exposure to pharmacologic doses of estrogens may cause uterine disturbances including hyperplasia of the glandular epithelium of the uterus and excessive mucus secretion. Ewes grazed on subterranean clover in Australia develop infertility due to the high and prolonged intake of ginestein, a plant proestrogen which is converted to estrogens during ruminal digestion.

Estrogens increase antibody levels in the uterus and enhance local protection against infection. Estrogens are responsible for the marked cornification of the vaginal epithelium in some of the species, such as the bitch.

Estrogens induce ductal development of the mammary glands in all of the domestic species. In addition, estrogens also induce mammary alveolar development in the heifer.

Estrogens inhibit the growth of bones and favor ossification of the epiphyses, interrupting the postpubertal growth of the female.

While progesterone dominance is necessary for the maintenance of pregnancy, localized estrogenic action is necessary for embryonic implantation. Blastocysts from several species, including the sheep, cow, and possibly pig, produce estrogens. These estrogens act locally to counteract the anti-inflammatory activity of progesterone at the site of implantation, and create a localized hyperemic area where embryo-uterine attachment can occur.

Administration of estrogens to animals is a common clinical practice for the control and treatment of a variety of conditions affecting the reproductive system. However, estrogens like any other hormonal factor, must be used with caution and the understanding of their actions and associated undesirable side effects is essential. Estrogens are routinely used in veterinary clinical practice for the control of mismating, to induce early abortion in dogs, for the treatment of urinary incontinency of spayed bitches, or for the treatment of hypertrophy of the prostate. However, doses given are often unnecessarily large and the treatment excessively prolonged. As a consequence, a fatal condition may develop because estrogens are myelotoxic for dogs. Dogs and particularly bitches over 5 years old are prone to react with bone marrow depression, impaired erythropoiesis, and aplastic anemia. Species differences must also be considered when prescribing treatment with estrogens. For instance, estrogens are luteolytic when given in pharmacological doses during middiestrus to cows and ewes. Luteal regression occurs and the animal returns to estrus within 3 to 7 days after estrogen treatment. In the sow, however, exogenous estrogens are luteotropic and prolong the lifespan of the corpora lutea. In mares, exogenous estrogens do not affect the lifespan of the corpus luteum, but they prolong the interestrous interval by interfering with follicular development and ovulation.

The role of estrogens is especially important in ruminants because of the protein anabolic effect as seen when a small amount of a synthetic nonsteroid estrogen, diethylstilbestrol, is fed to fattening beef cattle. The U.S. Food and Drug Administration has banned the use of estrogenic growth promoters because of public health implications. Research is continuing in the search for other nonestrogenic anabolic substances such as the mycotoxin zearalanol.

Extraovarian Sources of Estrogens

The adrenal glands produce estrogens, but under normal conditions, in quantities that are insufficient to replace the normal ovarian production of estrogens. Thus, atrophy of the female estrogen-dependent organs follows ovariectomy.

In the pregnant animal, the placenta is an important physiologic source of estrogens, as well as of other endocrine factors, including progesterone, gonadotropins, and GnRH-like factors.

Progesterone

Progesterone is the primary progestational hormone produced by the corpus luteum of the cycling animal and by the corpus luteum and the placenta of some species during pregnancy. Progesterone is needed for the maintenance of pregnancy in all species whether supplied by the corpus luteum, by the placenta or both. Abortion will ensue if progesterone is lacking or secreted in insufficient amounts to maintain pregnancy. Pregnancy can be maintained by exogenous administration of progesterone to bilaterally ovariectomized animals of those species whose placenta does not produce progesterone (see Chapter 18).

In the cycling animal, the main source of progesterone is the luteal cells of the corpus luteum, although progesterone has been isolated from the adrenal cortices of several species.

The corpus luteum of domestic species is formed by cells with distinct morphologic characteristics. The corpus luteum of the cow, ewe, and sow contains two major cell types: large and small lutein cells, which differ in their steroidogenic capabilities, even though both types contain the same enzymatic machinery (3β-hydroxysteroid dehydrogenase) and capacity to secrete progesterone. An emerging model (Fig. 9-34) suggests that under the influence of LH, the small lutein cells have the capability to uptake and store cholesterol. Upon further stimulation by LH, the small lutein cells respond by secreting progesterone in short pulses. The large lutein cells, which are more attenuated than the small lutein cells in their response to LH stimulation, uptake cholesterol from the small lutein cells (Fig. 9-34) and, thus, would be able to secrete more progesterone for pro-

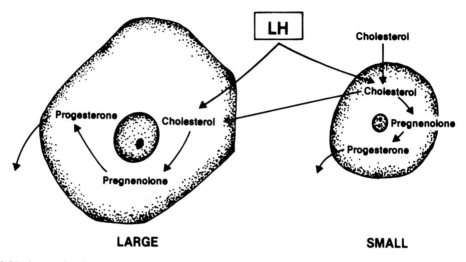

Fig. 9-34. Interaction between LH and small and large luteal cells in the synthesis of progesterone. (Adapted from different sources.)

longed periods. The small lutein cells are often interposed between the large lutein cells and blood capillaries. Cell to cell relationships, including gap junctions, may facilitate the diffusion of cholesterol and other precursors from one cell type to the other. Thus, the role of LH, at this level, would be to mobilize cholesterol stored in the small to the large lutein cells. The origin, either granulosa or thecal, of these cells is controversial. Some evidences suggest that the large lutein cells originate from cells of the granulosa while the small lutein cells originate in the theca layer. The small luteal cells would eventually become large luteal cells, as the corpus luteum develops and ages.

The effects of progesterone are usually seen only after the target tissue has been subjected to a period of estrogen stimulation. This *priming by estrogen* leads to a synergistic response. Progesterone acts on the uterus to cause quietening of the myometrium and induces secretion of uterine milk by the endometrial glands. The uterine glands increase not only in depth but especially in branching and tortuosity.

Large doses of progesterone inhibit gonadotropin output of the pituitary gland. In some cycling animals (cow, ewe, mare, sow) this may regulate the length of diestrus because as soon as the corpus luteum fails to secrete progesterone, a burst of FSH follows, which causes the development of the follicles.

Declining blood levels of progesterone to less than 1.0 ng/ml, in synergistic action with rising levels of estrogens, brings about behavioral estrus in most of the domestic species. In the prepubertal ewe and heifer, the progesterone secreted from a short-lived corpus luteum is needed to establish the cyclic pattern of gonadotropin release. In seasonal breeders, such as the goat and ewe, progesterone is required before a full response to estrogen can be seen. This requirement may explain silent heat in the ewe during the first estrous cycle of each breeding season. In the absence of progesterone from the previous corpus luteum, the first surge of estrogen is unable to elicit heat. Progesterone also appears to facilitate the estrogen-induced behavioral receptivity in the female. The influence of progesterone on lactation is important—it acts on the mammary glandular tissue much as it acts on the uterine glands.

The most dramatic role of progesterone probably occurs during *pregnancy*. As the name of the steroid implies, it *favors gestation*, at least in early pregnancy in all species. The early rise in progesterone following the development of the corpus luteum prepares the uterus for pregnancy at every cycle. Progesterone acts on the endometrium to inhibit myometrial activity and cause preparation for nidation, regardless of whether an embryo is present.

Progesterone production by the corpus luteum and/or placenta may be essential for pregnancy maintenance due to its ability to inhibit cell-mediated responses involved in tissue rejection. Progesterone may be nature's immunosuppressant of the mother's rejection mechanism of the fetus, since the fetus contains paternal antigens that would be incompatible with those of the mother (Fig. 9-35). Immunosuppression by progesterone may be likened to the immunosuppressant activity already described for the glucocorticoids.

Progesterone favors an economy of body metabolism, and during pregnancy the female uses nutrients more efficiently. Appetite is stimulated during pregnancy, presumably due to the influence of progesterone, but there is also a tendency toward less physical activity. The combination of these effects favors weight gain in the pregnant animal. Psychic effects of progesterone favor maternal behavior in the female such as nest building.

The physiological half-life of progesterone is only *22 to 36 minutes* in the cow. Thus, a constant secretion is essential to maintain the circulating levels.

Gonadal Steroid Transport and Mechanism of Action

Transport of estrogens (estradiol particularly) and progestins (progesterone particularly) in the serum is similar. Both are weakly yet extensively bound to albumin. This accounts for most of the circulating sex steroids. Of the remainder, progesterone is strongly bound to transcortin, whereas estrogen is weakly bound to the sex steroid binding globulin (SSBG).

Most of the steroid (90 to 95% of the estrogen) is transported in a bound form which is a protection from liver and kidney metabolism. A small amount circulates in the free form which enters the target cell (Fig. 9-36). Actually, the free steroid enters all cells but is retained only in those which have the appropriate receptors (target cells). As the level of free steroid falls, bound steroid is released to maintain the free steroid level.

Once a sex steroid enters the target cell, it performs its function as depicted in Figures 9-36 and 9-37. Once protein synthesis is induced, then the target cell functions. For example, a glandular cell could secrete, mitosis could be stimulated in an epithelial cell, psychic estrus could be induced if the target cell was a neuron, or hypertrophy could be induced in a myometrial cell.

Gonadal Hormones During Senility

Few domestic animals, except pet animals, are retained until old age. Gonadal hormone production usually declines as the animal ages

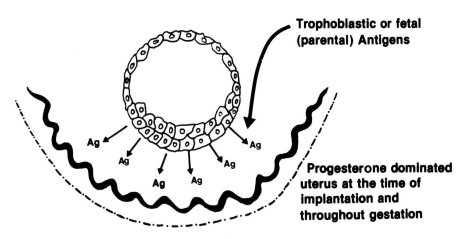

Fig. 9-35. Progesterone and probably other steroid hormones in high local concentrations exert local immunosuppressive activities in the uterus. These activities include: anti-inflammatory reaction, inhibition of lymphocytes and macrophage activation.

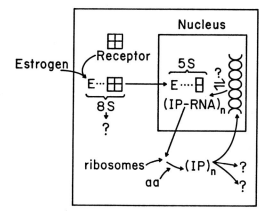

Fig. 9-36. Hypothetical model for estrogen interaction with uterine cell. E, estrogen; ⊞ , cytoplasmic receptor; ⊟ , nuclear receptor; ⋈ , genetic apparatus; IP, induced protein; *aa*, amino acids. (Reproduced from Handbook of Physiology, Section 7: Endocrinology, American Physiological Society, Baltimore, Williams & Wilkins, 1973.)

and the protein anabolic effect is lost. Consequently the addition of androgen or estrogen to "geriatric pills" may be indicated to counteract the "wasting disease" of old age. Commercial efforts to synthesize androgens or estrogens possessing mainly the anabolic effects with minimal androgenic or estrogenic effects have been moderately successful.

ESTRUS DURING PREGNANCY

Folliculogenesis is depressed during pregnancy because of the accompanying high levels of progesterone. This is true in all domestic animals except the mare where an unusual situation prevails leading to follicle growth and even ovulation early in pregnancy. This will be described in detail in the chapter on patterns of reproduction in the horse.

The placenta produces estrogen which might account for the occurrence of sexual receptivity during pregnancy. Estrus during pregnancy has been observed in all species, but has been most studied in the cow. Natural copulation is not apt to have an adverse effect on the pregnancy, but the artificial insemination of the pregnant cow should be avoided.

Estrus in the pregnant ewe is associated with follicular growth, but ovulation usually does not occur. Estrus has been reported during pregnancy in other species but, except in the mare, ovulation usually does not occur.

POSTPARTUM ESTRUS

Occurrence of estrus after parturition and the endocrinology controlling this event are quite different among the domestic species. Perhaps the situation in the human should be mentioned, since this demonstrates an evolutionary trait which is protective of the maternal organism. The corpus luteum is maintained by the stimulus of lactation. The ovary usually does not grow follicles or ovulate as long as the young are suckling. The human female, especially in primitive societies and underdeveloped areas of the world, has long utilized this mechanism for conception control. The young are sometimes nursed for several years for this reason.

In domestic animals, the other extreme is the sow which, for reasons not fully understood, experiences estrus within 3 to 6 days after parturition even though she is nursing a litter. Follicles have not grown, ovulation does

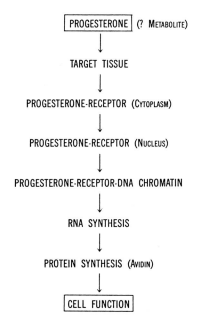

Fig. 9-37. Summary of the biochemical sequence of events occurring during progesterone action in the cells of target tissues. (Reproduced from Handbook of Physiology, Section 7: Endocrinology. American Physiological Society. Baltimore, Williams & Wilkins, 1973.)

not occur, and pregnancy does not follow. Thereafter, as long as the sow nurses the litter, the ovaries remain inactive, and heat does not occur until after the pigs are weaned. After weaning, the suppressive effect of lactation is removed and *estrus with ovulation* occurs within a week. This is a favorable time to breed the sow. Early weaning or loss of the litter soon after delivery is also followed by estrus and ovulation.

Most ewes are seasonal breeders; consequently the ovaries apparently remain inactive until the next breeding season. In the breeds which have been selected to produce two crops of lambs each year there is need for breeding soon after lactation ceases. As soon as weaning occurs, these breeds usually show a cyclic activity in the ovaries accompanied by estrus and ovulation.

The mare ordinarily shows estrus 6 to 12 days after parturition which is termed the "foal heat." Follicles have grown, ovulation occurs, and it is possible for the mare to become pregnant if she is bred. However, conception rate is usually poor because complete uterine involution does not occur for approximately 30 days. *Breeding at this time would not be wise management.*

The first standing estrus in the cow usually occurs 40 to 50 days after parturition, but a careful examination of the ovaries reveals that the first ovulation usually occurs 25 to 30 days postpartum. This means that the first follicular growth and ovulation are accompanied by *silent estrus*. Although the cow is a nonseasonal breeding animal, there are some effects of seasons on the postpartum estrous interval, since the winter months lengthen and the summer months shorten the interval.

The bitch and the cat tend to be seasonal breeders; consequently there is no tendency toward an early postpartum heat even after weaning. The uterus of the bitch involutes slowly, actually taking up to 4 months to return to the prepregnancy state.

PSEUDOMENSTRUATION

Several domestic animals shed blood from the uterus which eventually shows up in the vaginal secretions. It is important not to confuse this with menstruation in primates. For example, the cow sheds some blood from the uterus following ovulation, during the metestrus period. This is due to intensive endometrial stimulation by estrogen during proestrus and estrus leading to fragility of the vascular system and diapedesis. A similar condition occurs in the bitch, but usually the blood is shed earlier in proestrus. Again the cause is thought to be overstimulation of the endometrium by estrogen from the growing follicles.

FERTILITY—INFERTILITY—STERILITY—FECUNDITY—PROLIFICACY

There is considerable misuse of these terms, but the following definitions were agreed upon by a committee concerned with nomenclature of reproductive diseases.[72]

Fertility is a successful reproduction. *Infertility* is temporary loss of fertility. *Sterility* is permanent loss of fertility. *Fecundity* or *prolificacy* (usually considered to be synonymous) is the degree of reproduction appropriate for the species and is usually used in polytocous species to indicate relative litter size. Fertility, infertility, and sterility are applied to both sexes, but fecundity and prolificacy usually are reserved for the female.

REFERENCES

1. Abel, J. H., Jr., Verhage, H. G., McClellan, M. C., et al. (1975): Ultrastructural analysis of the granulosa-luteal cell transition in the ovary of the dog. Cell Tissue Res. *160*:155.
2. Adams, N. R., and Martin, G. B. (1983): Effects of oestradiol on plasma concentrations of luteinizing hormone in ovariectomized ewes with clover disease. Aust. J. Biol. Sci. *36*:295.
3. Akbar, A. M., Reichert, L. E., Jr., and Dunn, T. G. (1974): Serum levels of follicle-stimulating hormone during the bovine estrous cycle. J. Anim. Sci. *39*:360.
4. Alila, H. W., and Hansel, W. (1984): Origin of different cell types in the bovine corpus luteum as characterized by specific monoclonal antibodies. Biol. Reprod. *31*:1015.
5. Almquist, J. O., and Amann, R. P. (1976): Reproductive capacity of dairy bulls. XI. Puberal characteristics and post puberal changes in production of semen and sexual activity of Holstein bulls ejaculated frequently. J. Dairy Sci. *59*:986.
6. Anderson, L. L., Rathmacher, R. P., and Melampy,

R. M. (1966): The uterus and unilateral regression of corpora lutea in the pig. Am. J. Physiol. *210*:611.

7. Aron, C. (1979): Mechanisms of control of the reproductive function by olfactory stimuli in female mammals. Physiol. Rev. *59*:229.

8. Aten, R. F., Willams, A. T., Behrman, H. R., et al. (1986): Ovarian gonadotropin-releasing hormone-like protein(s): demonstration and characterization. Endocrinology *118*:961.

9. Azalon, N., and Marcus, S. (1975): Estrus synchronization and conception rate in dairy cattle treated with progestin-impregnated vaginal sponges. Theriogenology *3*:95.

10. Ball, G. D., and Day, B. N. (1982): Bilateral luteal maintenance in unilaterally pregnant pigs with infusions of embryonic extracts. J. Anim. Sci. *54*:142.

11. Bazer, F. W., Roberts, R. M., and Thatcher, W. W. (1979): Actions of hormones on the uterus and effect on conceptus development. J. Anim. Sci. *49* (Suppl. 2):35.

12. Bell, E. T., Bailey, J. B., and Christie, D. W. (1973): Studies on vaginal cytology during the canine estrous cycle. Res. Vet. Sci. *14*:173.

13. Bellve, A. R., and McDonald, M. F. (1968): Directional flow of fallopian tube secretion in the Romney ewe. J. Reprod. Fertil. *15*:357.

14. Bernard, C., Valet, J. P., Béland, R., et al. (1983): Prediction of bovine ovulation by a rapid radioimmunoassay for plasma LH. J. Reprod. Fertil. *68*:425.

15. Betteridge, K. J., Eaglesome, M. D., Randall, G. C. B., et al. (1980): Collection, description and transfer of embryos from cattle 10–16 days after oestrus. J. Reprod. Fertil. *59*:205.

16. Black, D. L., and Duby, R. T. (1965): Effect of oxytocin, epinephrine and atropine on the oestrous cycle of the cow. J. Reprod. Fertil. *9*:3.

17. Brinkley, H. J. (1981): Endocrine signaling and female reproduction. Biol. Reprod. *24*:22.

18. Brown, J. L., and Reeves, J. J. (1983): Absence of specific luteinizing hormone releasing hormone receptors in ovine, bovine and porcine ovaries. Biol. Reprod. *29*:1179.

19. Buhr, M. M., McKay, R. M., and Grinwich, D. L. (1986): Luteolytic action of prostaglandins in swine and effects of cloprostenol on luteinizing hormone receptors and membrane structure on porcine corpora lutea. Canad. J. Anim. Sci. *66*:415.

20. Carter, C. S., and Davis, J. M. (1977): Biogenic amines, reproductive hormones and female sexual behavior: a review. Behav. Rev. *1*:213.

21. Casida, L. E., Woody, C. O., and Pope, A. L. (1966): Inequality in function of the right and left ovaries and uterine horns of the ewe. J. Anim. Sci. *25*:1169.

22. Chemineau, P. (1983): Effect on oestrus and ovulation of exposing creole goats to the male at three times of the year. J. Reprod. Fertil. *67*:65.

23. Chemineau, P. (1986): Sexual behavior and gonadal activity during the year in the tropical creole meat goat. I. Female oestrous behaviour and ovarian activity. Reprod. Nutr. Dévelop. *26*:441.

24. Conaway, C. H. (1971): Ecological adaptation and mammalian reproduction. Biol. Reprod. *4*:239.

25. Concannon, P. (1980): Effects of hypophysectomy and of LH administration on luteal phase plasma progesterone levels in the beagle bitch. J. Reprod.

Fertil. *58*:407.

26. Cooke, R. G., and Knifton, A. (1980): Removal of corpora lutea in pregnant goats. Effects of intrauterine indomethacin. Res. Vet. Sci. *29*:77.

27. Cooke, R. G., and Homeida, A. M. (1985): Suppression of prostaglandin F-2α releases and delay of luteolysis after active immunization against oxytocin in the goat. J. Reprod. Fertil. *75*:63.

28. Crafts, R. C. (1948): The effects of estrogens on the bone marrow of adult female dogs. Blood *3*:276.

29. Cronin, G. M., Hemsworth, P. H., and Winfield, C. G. (1982): Oestrous behaviour in relation to fertility and fecundity of gilts. Anim. Reprod. Sci. *5*:117.

30. Davis, A. J., Fleet, I. R., Harrison, F. A., et al. (1979): Pulmonary metabolism of prostaglandin $F_{2\alpha}$ in the conscious nonpregnant ewe and sow. J. Physiol. *301*:86P.

31. Del Campo, C. H., and Ginther, O. J. (1972): Vascular anatomy of the uterus and ovaries and the unilateral luteolytic effect of the uterus: guinea pigs, rats, hamsters, and rabbits. Am. J. Vet. Res. *33*:2561.

32. Del Campo, C. H., and Ginther, O. J. (1973): Vascular anatomy of the uterus and ovaries and the unilateral luteolytic effect of the uterus: horses, sheep and swine. Am. J. Vet. Res. *34*:305.

33. Del Campo, C. H., and Ginther, O. J. (1973): Vascular anatomy of the uterus and ovaries and the unilateral luteolytic effect of the uterus: Angioarchitecture in sheep. Am. J. Vet. Res. *34*:1377.

34. Del Campo, C. H., and Ginther, O. J. (1974): Vascular anatomy of the uterus and ovaries and unilateral luteolytic effect of the uterus: histologic structure of uteroovarian vein and ovarian artery in sheep. Am. J. Vet. Res. *35*:397.

35. Del Campo, C. H., and Ginther, O. J. (1974): Arteries and veins of uterus and ovaries in dogs and cats. Am. J. Vet. Res. *35*:409.

36. Del Campo, M. R., Rowe, R. F., Chaichareon, D., et al. (1983): Effect of the relative locations of embryo and corpus luteum on embryo survival in cattle. Reprod. Nutr. Dévelop. *23*:303.

37. Del Campo, M. R., Rowe, R. F., French, L. R., et al. (1977): Unilateral relationship of embryos and the corpus luteum in cattle. Biol. Reprod. *16*:580.

38. Dobson, H., and Kamonpatana, M. (1986): A review of female cattle reproduction with special reference to a comparison between buffaloes, cows and zebu. J. Reprod. Fertil. *77*:1.

39. Douglas, R. H., and Ginther, O. J. (1973): Luteolysis following a single injection of prostaglandin $F_{2\alpha}$ in sheep. J. Anim. Sci. *37*:990.

40. Dufour, J., Whitmore, H. L., Ginther, O, J., et al. (1972): Identification of the ovulating follicle by its size on different days of the estrous cycle in heifers. J. Anim. Sci. *34*:85.

41. Dukelow, W. R. (1978): Laparoscopic research techniques in mammalian embryology. In Methods in Mammalian Reproduction, edited by J. C. Daniel. Academic Press Inc., New York, pp. 437–460.

42. Dyrmundsson, O. R. (1973): Puberty and early reproductive performance in sheep. I. Ewe lambs. Anim. Breed. Abst. *41*:273.

43. Edqvist, L.-E., Settergren, I., and Astrom, G. (1975):

Peripheral plasma levels of progesterone and fertility after prostaglandin $F_{2\alpha}$ induced oestrus in heifers. Cornell Vet. *65*:120.

44. Ellinwood, W. E., Nett, T. M., and Niswender, G. D. (1979): Maintenance of the corpus luteum of early pregnancy in the ewe. I. Luteotropic properties of embryonic homogenates. Biol. Reprod. *21*: 281.

45. Endland, B. G., Webb, R., and Dahmer, M. K. (1981): Follicular steroidogenesis and gonadotropin binding to ovine follicles during the estrous cycle. Endocrinology *109*:881.

46. Eppig, J. J., and Downs, S. M. (1984): Chemical signals that regulate mammalian oocyte maturation. Biol. Reprod. *30*:1.

47. Erickson, B. H., Reynolds, R. A., and Murphree, R. L. (1976): Ovarian characteristics and reproductive performance of the aged cow. Biol. Reprod. *15*:555.

48. Erickson, G. F., Magoffin, D. A., Dyer, C. A., et al. (1985): The ovarian androgen producing cells: a review of structure/function relationships. Endocrine Rev. *6*:371.

49. Espey, L. L. (1978): Ovarian contractility and its relationship to ovulation: a review. Biol. Reprod. *19*:540.

50. Fernandez-Pardal, J., Gimeno, M. F., and Gimeno, A. L. (1986): Catecholamines in sow graafian follicles at proestrus and at diestrus. Biol. Reprod. *34*:439.

51. Fitz, T. A., Mayan, M. H., Sawyer, H. R., et al. (1982): Characterization of two steroidogenic cell types in the ovine corpus luteum. Biol. Reprod. *27*:703.

52. Flechon, J. E., Pavlok, A., and Kopecný, V. (1984): Dynamics of zona pellucida formation by the mouse oocyte. An autoradiographic study. Cell Biol. *51*: 403.

53. Foster, D., and Ryan, K. (1979): Mechanism governing onset of ovarian cyclicity at puberty in the lamb. Ann. Biol. Anim. Biochim. Biophys. *19*:1369.

54. Fulkerson, W. J., Sawyer, G. J., and Crothers, I. (1983): The accuracy of several aids in detecting oestrus in dairy cattle. Appl. Anim. Ethol. *10*:199.

55. Garcia-Villar, R., Toutain, P. L., Schams, D., et al. (1983): Are regular activity episodes of the genital tract controlled by pulsatile releases of oxytocin? Biol. Reprod. *29*:1183.

56. Geisert, R. D., Renegar, R. H., Thatcher, W. W., et al. (1982): Establishment of pregnancy in the pig: I. Interrelationships between preimplantation development of the pig blastocysts and uterine endometrial secretions. Biol. Reprod. *27*:925.

57. Ginther, O. J. (1976): Comparative anatomy of uteroovarian vasculature. Vet. Scope *20*:2.

58. Ginther, O. J., and Del Campo, C. H. (1974): Vascular anatomy of the uterus and ovaries and the unilateral luteolytic effect of the uterus: cattle. Am. J. Vet. Res. *35*:193.

59. Gonzalez-Padilla, E., Niswender, G. D., and Wiltbank, J. N. (1975): Puberty in beef heifers. I. The inter-relationship between pituitary, hypothalamic and ovarian hormones. J. Anim. Sci. *40*:1091.

60. Gonzalez-Padilla, E., Ruiz, R., LeFever, D., et al. (1975): Puberty in beef heifers. III. Induction of fertile estrus. J. Anim. Sci. *40*:1110.

61. Guillemot, M., and Guay, P. (1982): Ultrastructural features of the cell surfaces of uterine and trophoblastic epithelia during embryo attachment in the cow. Anat. Rec. *204*:315.

62. Gwynne, J. T., and Strauss III, J. F. (1982): The role of lipoproteins in steroidogenesis and cholesterol metabolism in steroidogenic glands. Endocrine Rev. *3*:299.

63. Hafez, E. S. E. (1987): Reproduction in Farm Animals, 5th Ed. Philadelphia, Lea & Febiger.

64. Hallford, D. M., Wettemann, R. P., and Thurman, E. J. (1975): Luteal function in gilts after prostaglandin $F_{2\alpha}$. J. Anim. Sci. *41*:1706.

65. Hansel, W., and Wagner, W. C. (1960): Luteal inhibition in the bovine as a result of oxytocin injections, uterine dilation and intrauterine infusions of seminal and preputial fluids. J. Dairy Sci. *43*:796.

66. Haresign, W., Foxcroft, G. R., and Lamming G. E. (1983): Control of ovulation in farm animals. J. Reprod. Fertil. *69*:383.

67. Head, J. R., and Billingham, R. E. (1986): Concerning the immunology of the uterus. Am. J. Reprod. Immunol. Microbiol. *10*:76.

68. Heap, R. B., Perry, J. S., Gadsby, J. E., et al. (1975): Endocrine activities of the blastocyst and early embryonic tissue in the pig. Biochem. Soc. Trans. *3*: 1183.

69. Hillier, S. G. (1981): Regulation of follicular oestrogen biosynthesis: A survey of current concepts. J. Endocrinol. *89*:3P.

70. Hogg, J. T. (1984): Mating in bighorn sheep: Multiple creative male strategies. Science *225*:526.

71. Hsue, A. J. W., and Schaeffer, J. M. (1985): Gonadotropin-releasing hormone as a paracrine hormone and neurotransmitter in extra-pituitary sites. J. Steroid Biochem. *23*:757.

72. Hubbert, W. T., Dennis, S. M., Adams, W. M., et al. (1972): Recommendations for standardizing bovine reproduction terms. Cornell Vet. *62*:216.

73. Hunter, R. H. F. (1980): Differentiation, puberty, and the oestrous cycle. Chapter 1, *In* Physiology and Technology of Reproduction in Female Domestic Animals, Academic Press, Inc., New York, p. 1.

74. Hunter, R. H. F., and Wilmut, I. (1984): Sperm transport in the cow: peri-ovulatory redistribution of viable cells within the oviduct. Reprod. Nutr. Dévelop. *24*:597.

75. Hunter, R. H. F., and Nichol, R. (1986): A preovulatory temperature gradient between the isthmus and ampulla of pig oviduct during the phase of sperm storage. J. Reprod. Fertil. *77*:599.

76. Hurtgen, J. P., and Leman, A. D. (1980): Seasonal influence on the fertility of sows and gilts. J. Am. Vet. Med. Assoc. *177*:631.

77. Imakawa, K., Day, M. L., Zalesky, D. D., et al. (1986): Regulation of pulsatile LH secretion by ovarian steroids in the heifer. J. Anim. Sci. *63*:162.

78. Inskeep, E. K. (1973): Potential uses of prostaglandins in control of reproductive cycles of domestic animals. J. Anim. Sci. *36*:1149.

79. Johnson, A. D., and Foley, C. W., Eds. (1974): The Oviduct and its Functions. New York, Academic Press.

80. Kesner, J. S., Convey, G. M., and Anderson, C. R.

(1981): Evidence that estradiol induces the preovulatory LH surge in cattle by increasing pituitary sensitivity to LHRH and then increasing LHRH release. Endocrinology *108*:1386.

81. King, G. J., and Robertson, H. W. (1974): A two-injection schedule with prostaglandin F$_{2\alpha}$ for the regulation of ovulatory cycle of cattle. Theriogenology *1*:123.

82. Knickerbocker, J. J., Thatcher, W. W., Bazer, F. W., et al. (1986): Proteins secreted by Day-16 to -18 bovine conceptuses extend corpus luteum function in cows. J. Reprod. Fertil. *77*:381.

83. Korach, K. S. (1981): Selected biochemical actions of ovarian hormones. Env. Health Persp. *38*:39.

84. Kotwica, J., Williams, G. L., and Marchello, M. J. (1982): Counter current transfer of testosterone by the ovarian vascular pedicle of the cow: Evidence for a relationship to follicular steroidogenesis. Biol. Reprod. *27*:778.

85. Kruip, T. A. M., Cran, D. G., Van Beneden, T. H., et al. (1983): Structural changes in bovine oocytes during final maturation in vivo. Gamete Res. *8*:29.

86. Lauderdale, J. W. (1975): The use of prostaglandins in cattle. Ann. Biol. Anim. Biochim. Biophys. *15*:419.

87. Lehrer, A. R., Fischler, H., Schindler, H., et al. (1974): Telemetry of uterine motility in the cycling ewe. J. Anim. Sci. *38*:89.

88. Lemon, M., and Mauleon, P. (1982): Interaction between two luteal cell types from the corpus luteum of the sow in progesterone synthesis in vitro. J. Reprod. Fertil. *64*:315.

89. Levasseur, M.-C. (1979): Thoughts on puberty. The gonads. Ann. Biol. Anim. Biochim. Biophys. *19*:321.

90. Levasseur, M.-C. (1983): Utero-ovarian relationships in placental mammals: role of uterus and embryo in the regulation of progesterone secretion by the corpus luteum. A review. Reprod. Nutr. Dévelop. *23*:793.

91. Lipner, H., and Cross, N. L. (1968): Morphology of the membrana granulosa of the ovarian follicle. Endocrinology *82*:638.

92. Lord, E. M., Sensabaugh, G. F., and Stites, D. P. (1977): Immunosuppressive activity of human seminal plasma. I. Inhibitory in vitro lymphocyte activation. J. Immunol. *118*:1704.

93. MacLusky, N. J., and Naftolin, F. (1981): Sexual differentiation of the central nervous system. Science *211*:1294.

94. Mahi-Brown, C. A., and Yanagimachi, R. (1983): Parameters influencing ovum pickup by oviductal fimbria in the golden hamster. Gamete Res. *8*:1.

95. McCracken, J. A. (1971): Prostaglandin F$_{2\alpha}$ and corpus luteum regression. Ann. N. Y. Acad. Sci. *180*:456.

96. McCracken, J. A. (1984): Update on luteolysis-receptor regulation of pulsatile secretion of prostaglandin F$_{2\alpha}$ from the uterus. Res. Reprod. *16*:1.

97. McDonald, L. E., McNutt, S. H., and Nichols, R. E. (1953): On the essentiality of the bovine corpus luteum of pregnancy. Am. J. Vet. Res. *145*:539.

98. McNatty, K. P., Gibb, M., Dobson, C., et al. (1981): Changes in the concentration of gonadotrophic and steroidal hormones in the antral fluid of ovarian

follicles throughout the oestrous cycle of the sheep. Aust. J. Biol. Sci. *34*:80.

99. McNatty, K. P., Heath, D. A., Henderson, K. M., et al. (1984): Some aspects of thecal and granulosa cell function during follicular development in the bovine ovary. J. Reprod. Fertil. *72*:39.

100. Mohammad, W. A., Grossman, M., and Vatthauer, J. L. (1984): Seasonal breeding in United States dairy goats. J. Dairy Sci. *67*:1813.

101. Moor, R. M., and Rowson, L. E. A. (1966): The corpus luteum of the sheep; functional relationship between the embryo and the corpus luteum. J. Endocrinol. *34*:233.

102. Moor, R. M., and Rowson, L. E. A. (1966): Local maintenance of the corpus luteum in sheep with embryos transferred to various isolated portions of the uterus. J. Reprod. Fertil. *12*:539.

103. Moor, R. M., and Seamark, R. F. (1986): Cell signaling, permeability, and microvasculatory changes during antral follicle development in mammals. J. Dairy Sci. *69*:927.

104. Moore, L. G., and Watkins, W. B. (1982): Embryonic suppression of oxytocin-associated neurophysin release in early pregnant sheep. Prostaglandins *24*:79.

105. Mori, Y., and Kano, Y. (1984): Changes in plasma concentrations of LH, progesterone and oestradiol in relation to the occurrence of luteolysis, oestrus and time of ovulation in the shiba goat. J. Reprod. Fertil. *72*:223.

106. Moyle, W. R., Kuczek, T., and Bailey, C. A. (1985): Potential of a quantal response as a mechanism for oscillatory behavior: implications for our concepts of hormonal control mechanisms. Biol. Reprod. *32*:43.

107. Murdoch, W. J. (1985): Follicular determinants of ovulation in the ewe. Dom. Anim. Endocrinol. *2*:105.

108. Nalbandov, A. V. (1964): Reproductive Physiology. San Francisco, W. H. Freeman & Co.

109. Niswender, G. D., Reimers, T. J., Diekman, M. A., et al. (1976): Blood flow: a mediator of ovarian function. Biol. Reprod. *14*:64.

110. Niswender, G. D., Sawyer, H. R., Chen, T. T., et al. (1980): Action of luteinizing hormone at the luteal cell level. Adv. Horm. Res. *4*:153.

111. Niswender, G. D., Schwall, R. H., Fitz, T. A., et al. (1985): Regulation of luteal function in domestic ruminants—New Concepts. Rec. Prog. Horm. Res. *41*:101.

112. Noonan, J. J., Adair, R. L., Halbert, S. A., et al. (1978): Quantitative assessment of oxytocin-stimulated oviduct contractions of the ewe by optoelectronic measurements. J. Anim. Sci. *47*:914.

113. Northey, D. L., and French, L. R. (1980): Effect of embryo removal and intrauterine infusion of embryonic homogenates on the lifespan of the bovine corpus luteum. J. Anim. Sci. *50*:298.

114. Odell, W. D., and Swerdloff, R. S. (1974): The role of the gonads in sexual maturation. *In* The control of the onset of puberty, edited by M. M. Grumbach, G. D. Grave, and F. E. Mayer. New York, John Wiley and Sons, Inc., p. 313.

115. Okkens, A. C., Dieleman, S. J., Bevers, M. M., et al. (1985): Evidence for the non-involvement of the uterus in the lifespan of the corpus luteum in the

cyclic dog. Vet. Quart. *7*:169.

116. Okkens, A. C., Dieleman, S. J., Bevers, M. M., et al. (1986): Influence of hypophysectomy on the lifespan of the corpus luteum in the cyclic dog. J. Reprod. Fertil. *77*:187.

117. Olson, P. N., Bowen, R. A., Behrendt, M. D., et al. (1984): Concentrations of testosterone in canine serum during late anestrus, proestrus, estrus, and early diestrus. Am. J. Vet. Res. *45*:145.

118. Olson, P. N., Bowen, R. A., Behrendt, M. D., et al. (1984): Concentrations of progesterone and luteinizing hormone in the serum of diestrous bitches before and after hysterectomy. Am. J. Vet. Res. *45*: 149.

119. O'Shea, J. D. (1981): Structure-function relationships in the wall of the ovarian follicle. Aust. J. Biol. Sci. *34*:379.

120. Paape, S. R., Shille, V. M., Seto, H., et al. (1975): Luteal activity in the pseudopregnant cat. Biol. Reprod. *13*:470.

121. Pant, H. C., Hopkinson, C. R. N., and Fitzpatrick, R. J. (1977): Concentration of oestradiol, progesterone, luteinizing hormone and follicle-stimulating hormone in the jugular venous plasma of ewes during the oestrous cycle. J. Endocrinol. *73*:247.

122. Perkins, S. N., Cronin, M. J., and Veldhuis, J. D. (1986): Properties of β-adrenergic receptors on porcine corpora lutea and granulosa cells. Endocrinology *118*:998.

123. Pope, W. F., Maurer, R. R., and Stormshak, F. (1982): Intrauterine migration of the porcine embryo: influence of estradiol-17β and histamine. Biol. Reprod. *27*:575.

124. Rajakoski, E. (1960): The ovarian follicular system in sexually mature heifers. Acta Endocrinol. *34*: (Suppl. 52)1.

125. Reimers, T. J., Smith, R. D., and Newman, S. K. (1985): Management factors affecting reproductive performance of dairy cows in the Northeastern United States. J. Dairy Sci. *68*:963.

126. Ricketts, A. P., and Flint, A. P. F. (1980): Onset of synthesis of progesterone by ovine placenta. J. Endocrinol. *86*:337.

127. Roche, J. F. (1976): Calving rate of cows following insemination after a 12-day treatment with Silastic coils impregnated with progesterone. J. Anim. Sci. *43*:164.

128. Rodgers, R. J., O'Shea, J. D., and Findlay, J. K. (1985): Do small and large luteal cells of the sheep interact in the production of progesterone. J. Reprod. Fertil. *75*:85.

129. Ross, G. T. and Lipsett, M. B. (1978): Homologies of structure and function in mammalian testes and ovaries. Internat. J. Androl. Suppl. *2*:39.

130. Rothchild, I. (1981): The regulation of the mammalian corpus luteum. Rec. Progr. Horm. Res. *37*: 183.

131. Rowson, L. E. A., Tervit, R., and Brand, A. (1972): The use of prostaglandins for synchronization of oestrus in cattle. J. Reprod. Fertil. *29*:145.

132. Ryan, K. J. (1972): Steroid hormones and prostaglandins. *In* Principles and Management of Human Reproduction, edited by Reid, D. E., Ryan, K. J., and Benirschke. Philadelphia, W. B. Saunders Co., p. 4.

133. Sawyer, H. R., Moeller, C. L., and Kozlowski, G. P. (1986): Immunocytochemical localization of neurophysin and oxytocin in ovine corpora lutea. Biol. Reprod. *34*:543.

134. Schams, D., and Prokopp, S. (1979): Oxytocin determination by RIA in cows around parturition. Anim. Reprod. Sci. *2*:267.

135. Schams, D., Schallenberger, E., Gombe, S., et al. (1981): Endocrine patterns associated with puberty in male and female cattle. J. Reprod. Fertil., Suppl. *30*:103.

136. Schams, D., Schallenberger, E., Hoffmann, B., et al. (1977): The oestrous cycle of the cow: hormonal parameters and time relationships concerning oestrus, ovulation, and electrical resistance of the vaginal mucus. Acta Endocrinol. *86*:180.

137. Schams, D., Schallenberger, E., Menzer, C., et al. (1978): Profiles of LH, FSH and progesterone in postpartum dairy cows and their relationship to the commencement of cyclic functions. Theriogenology *10*:453.

138. Schramm, W., Einer-Jensen, N., and Schramm, G. (1986): Direct venous-arterial transfer of ^{125}I-radiolabelled relaxin and tyrosine in the ovarian pedicle in sheep. J. Reprod. Fertil. *77*:513.

139. Schramm, W., Einer-Jensen, N., Schramm, G., et al. (1986): Local exchange of oxytocin from the ovarian vein to ovarian arteries in sheep. Biol. Reprod. *34*:671.

140. Schultz, R. M. (1985): Roles of cell-to-cell communication in development. Biol. Reprod. *32*:27.

141. Schwall, R. H., Sawyer, H. R., and Niswender, G. D. (1986): Differential regulation by LH and prostaglandins of steroidogenesis in small and large luteal cells of the ewe. J. Reprod. Fertil. *76*:821.

142. Schwall, R. H., Gamboni, F., Mayan, M. H., et al. (1986): Changes in the distribution of sizes of ovine luteal cells during the estrous cycle. Biol. Reprod. *34*:911.

143. Sequin, B. E., Morrow, D. A., and Oxender, W. D. (1974): Intrauterine therapy in the cow. J. Am. Vet. Med. Assoc. *164*:611.

144. Shamesh, M., and Hansel, W. (1983): Hormone production by the early bovine embryo. J. Steroid Biochem. *19*:979.

145. Sharpe, R. M. (1982): Cellular aspects of the inhibitory actions of LH-RH on the ovary and testis. J. Reprod. Fertil. *64*:517.

146. Sheldrick, E. L., Mitchell, M. D., and Flint, A. P. F. (1980): Delayed luteal regression in ewes immunized against oxytocin. J. Reprod. Fertil. *59*:37.

147. Siiteri, R. K., and Stites, D. P. (1982): Immunologic and endocrine interrelationships in pregnancy. Biol. Reprod. *26*:1.

148. Siiteri, P. K., Febres, F., Clemens, L. E. et al. (1977): Progesterone and maintenance of pregnancy: Is progesterone nature's immunosuppressant? Ann. N. Y. Acad. Sci. *286*:384.

149. Smith, I. D., Bassett, J. M., and Williams, T. (1970): Progesterone concentrations in the peripheral plasma of the mare during the oestrus cycle. J. Endocrinol. *47*:523.

150. Smith, M. S., and McDonald, L. E. (1974): Serum levels of LH and progesterone during the estrous cycle, pseudopregnancy and pregnancy in the dog.

Endocrinology *94*:404.

151. Spicer, L. J., and Echternkamp, S. E. (1986): Ovarian follicular growth, function and turnover in cattle: a review. J. Anim. Sci. *62*:428.

152. Squires, E. L., Douglas, R. H., Steffenhagen, W. P., et al. (1974): Ovarian changes during the estrous cycle and pregnancy in mares. J. Anim. Sci. *38*:330.

153. Squires, E. L., Hillman, R. B., Pickett, B. W., et al. (1980): Induction of abortion in mares with equimate: effect on secretion of progesterone, PMSG and reproductive performance. J. Anim. Sci. *50*:490.

154. Stabenfeldt, G. H. (1974): Physiologic, pathologic and therapeutic roles of progestins in domestic animals. J. Am. Vet. Med. Assoc. *164*:311.

155. Stabenfeldt, G. H., Edqvist, L.-E., Kindahl, H., et al. (1978): Practical implications of recent physiological findings for reproductive efficiency in cows, mares, sows, and ewes. J. Am. Vet. Med. Assoc. *172*:667.

156. Stabenfeldt, G. H., Hughes, J. P., and Evans, J. W. (1972): Ovarian activity during the estrous cycle of the mare. Endocrinology *90*:1379.

157. Stabenfeldt, G. H., Hughes, J. P., and Evans, J. W. (1974): Spontaneous prolongation of luteal activity in the mare. Equine Vet. J. *6*:158.

158. Staigmiller, R. B., England, B. G., Webb, R., et al. (1982): Estrogen secretion and gonadotropin binding by individual bovine follicles during estrus. J. Anim. Sci. *55*:1473.

159. Stormshak, F., Kelley, H. E., and Hawk, H. W. (1969): Suppression of ovine luteal function by 17β-estradiol. J. Anim. Sci. *29*:476.

160. Szego, C. M. (1984): Mechanisms of hormone action: parallels in receptor-mediated signal propagation for steroid and peptide effectors. Life Sci. *35*:2383.

161. Tesoriero, J. V. (1984): Comparative cytochemistry of the developing ovarian follicles of the dog, rabbit, and mouse: Origin of the zona pellucida. Gamete Res. *10*:301.

162. Thatcher, W. W., Bartol, F. F., Knickerbocker, J. J., et al. (1984): Maternal recognition of pregnancy in cattle. J. Dairy Sci. *67*:2797.

163. Thibault, C., Courot, M., Martinet, L., et al. (1966): Regulation of breeding season and estrous cycles by light and external stimuli in some mammals. J. Anim. Sci. *25*:(Suppl.)119.

164. Thompson, F. N., Abrams, E., and Miller, D. M. (1983): Reproductive traits in nubian dairy goats. Anim. Reprod. Sci. *6*:59.

165. Tyslowitz, R., and Dingemanse, E. (1941): Effect of large doses of estrogen on blood picture of dogs. Endocrinology *29*:817.

166. Van de Wiel, D. F. M., Bar-Ami, S., Tsafriri, A., et al. (1983): Oocyte maturation inhibitor, inhibin and steroid concentrations in porcine follicular fluid at various stages of the estrous cycle. J. Reprod. Fertil. *68*:247.

167. Verhage, H. G., Beamer, N. B., and Brenner, R. M. (1976): Plasma levels of estradiol and progesterone in the cat during polyestrus, pregnancy, and pseudopregnancy. Biol. Reprod. *14*:579.

168. Walles, B., Edvinsson, L., Owman, C., et al. (1976): Cholinergic nerves and receptors mediating contraction of the Graafian follicle. Biol. Reprod. *15*:565.

169. Warren, J. E., Jr., Hawk, H. W., and Williams, W. F. (1974): Interaction of stage of the breeding season and intrauterine devices on estrous cycle length in the ewe. J. Anim. Sci. *38*:363.

170. Wathes, D. C. (1984): Possible actions of gonadal oxytocin and vasopression. J. Reprod. Fertil. *71*:315.

171. Wathes, D. C., Swan, R. W., and Pickering, B. T. (1984): Variations in oxytocin, vasopressin and neurophysin concentrations in the bovine ovary during the oestrous cycle and pregnancy. J. Reprod. Fertil. *71*:551.

172. Wei, L. L., and Horwitz, K. B. (1985): The structure of progesterone receptors. Steroids *46*:677.

173. Wenzel, J. G. W., and Odend'hal, S. (1985): The mammalian rete ovarii: a literature review. Cornell Vet. *75*:411.

174. Wiltbank, J. N., Kasson, C. W., and Ingalls, J. E., (1969): Puberty in crossbred and straightbred beef heifers on two levels of feed. J. Anim. Sci. *29*:602.

175. Wolfenson, D., Thatcher, W. W., Drost, M., et al. (1985): Characteristics of prostaglandin F measurements in the ovarian circulation during the oestrous cycle and early pregnancy in the cow. J. Reprod. Fertil. *75*:491.

176. Wolff, L. K., and DeMonty, D. E., Jr. (1974): Physiologic response to intense summer heat and its effect on the estrous cycle of nonlactating and lactating Holstein-Friesian cows in Arizona. Am. J. Vet. Res. *35*:187.

177. Wolgemuth, D. J., Celenza, J., Bundman, D. S., et al. (1984): Formation of the rabbit zona pellucida and its relationship to ovarian follicular development. Develop. Biol. *106*:1.

178. Woods, G. L., and Ginther, O. J. (1983): Intrauterine embryo reduction in the mare. Theriogenology *20*:699.

179. Zamboni, L., Bézard, J., and Mauléon, P. (1979): The role of the mesonephros in the development of the sheep fetal ovary. Ann. Biol. Anim. Biochim. Biophys. *19*:1153.

Artificial Insemination

S. M. HOPKINS and L. E. EVANS

10

Artificial insemination (AI) in the broadest sense is defined as the transfer of male gametes to reach the oocyte by means other than natural mating. This includes the insemination of the female with fresh, extended or frozen semen and the in vitro fertilization of oocytes. The other important component of AI involves the examination of the male for normal structural development and analysis of the ejaculate for semen quality. Together the two components provide for the collection and transfer of acceptable numbers of normal spermatozoa to the oocyte.

The driving force behind AI in any form is to disseminate superior genes within the population at a reasonable cost. The important genetic traits, depending on the species, include meat production, milking gains, athletic performance, and correct conformation.

The cattle industry relies almost exclusively on the use of frozen semen, whereas other domestic species are usually bred with fresh or extended, non-frozen semen. There are political, economic, and genetic obstacles to the widespread use of AI in species other than cattle. The political block to the development of frozen AI protocols in horses is the refusal of several of the equine breed associations to allow registry of AI produced offspring. Consequently little data can be obtained about use of frozen semen in horses under field conditions.

Another major obstacle is the lack of economic drive for the development of AI. The potential offspring must command a price which makes research and the use of AI important to the industry. An example would be the canine breeds which permit AI with fresh and frozen semen. The economic return to those involved with collection, processing, and distribution of semen generally has been insufficient to support development of that industry. Additionally, the current conception rates are relatively low, further aggravating a poor economic return.

One of the natural limitations of AI in all species involves the identification of genetic merit. The dairy industry computes a Predicted Difference (PD) index, which is a measure of the bull's ability to genetically transmit production increases or decreases to his progeny. The PD is averaged with the Cow Index (CI) and together these two parameters can be used to predict the potential genetic gain of their offspring. These indices are based on production records rather than pedigree or body type and indicate true genetic merit. Unless the industries dealing with the other species develop comparable means of identifying individuals of superior genetics, there is no reasonable assurance that their offspring will perform above average. This also includes identifying potentially lethal or defective genes before they are spread throughout the population.

There is the potential for advances to be made within the AI industries in all species. There must, however, be sufficient funding, guidelines, and controls to make the venture economically feasible and genetically sound.

DISEASE CONTROL THROUGH AI

Artificial insemination has the potential to reduce disease transmission between breeding animals. This includes not only the venereal and reproductive diseases which are transmittable through mating, but other pathogens spread via contact. These include a wide variety of parasitic, protozoal, viral, and microbial organisms.

The cattle industry has established guidelines to minimize the transfer of venereal pathogens through AI. These guidelines take two approaches: the identification of pathogen free males and the treatment of extended semen with antibiotics.

The National Association of Animal Breeders (NAAB)* has established rules for isolation and testing of bulls in order to provide

*NAAB: P.O. Box 1033, Columbia, Missouri 65205-1033

a reasonable assurance that the semen is free from specific bacterial and protozoal organisms. The tests involve serology for brucellosis, leptospirosis and paratuberculosis; immune reaction for tuberculosis and darkfield examination and culture for vibriosis and trichomoniasis. Preparing semen for export, however, may require that the bull undergo additional tests which are established by the regulatory agencies of the particular country. Unfortunately, there is not a standard series of tests applicable to all countries. In addition, some states in the U.S. have their own requirements. For example, Wisconsin has regulations similar to those of the NAAB. The majority of the other states do not have any male health stipulations for semen produced for domestic use.

These tests, although extensive, may not be fully adequate for protection due to disease incubation, sampling techniques, or test interpretation. While the regulations stipulate retesting at 6- to 12-month intervals, depending on the particular disease, it is quite possible, for example, that a bull which tests negative for leukosis may subsequently seroconvert and shed the virus before the next annual retest. Similarly, although tested bulls are maintained in an isolation facility, diseases such as leptospirosis can be shed by rodents or other mammals which may have contact with the bulls. Consequently, the health tests only offer reasonable assurance for disease avoidance.

As a safeguard against diseases borne by bull semen, antibiotics are added to both the neat and extended ejaculate. The antibiotics have been selected for efficacy against organisms causing trichomoniasis, vibriosis, and ureaplasmosis and may have activity against other bacteria. Dilution of the semen during the process of extension provides additional protection against disease transmission. Dilution may lower the number of infective organisms to a level below that which is required for host infection.

In the cattle industry, the use of disease testing in bulls, antibiotics in the semen, and proper hygiene during collection and processing have made the likelihood of disease transmission from bull semen remote.

In the equine species, extended, non-frozen semen is treated with antibiotics in order to decrease transmission of pathogenic and non-pathogenic organisms. With natural mating, bacterial contamination of a mare's uterus is common, and immunologically competent mares are able to clear contaminants before the embryo enters the uterus, about 6 days post ovulation. Mares with decreased uterine resistance benefit from antibiotics in extended semen since they cannot effectively remove the bacterial contaminants found in an ejaculate and may develop endometritis.

There are no definite requirements in the other domestic species, although many organizations routinely use antibiotics in a similar fashion as the cattle industry. There is, however, a lack of information in these species regarding the effects of antibiotics on fertility.

SEMEN COLLECTION

The collection of semen from domestic animals employs the use of an artificial vagina (AV), electroejaculator (EE), or digital massage (DM).

Artificial Vagina

Each species requires its own type of AV, however, the basic construction, preparation, and usage have many similar traits. The temperature of the interior of the AV is maintained by placing hot water between an interior liner and outer casing. The inner liners are made of rubber and have a smooth to coarse texture depending on the species to be collected and the individual male's preference. The outer casing can be either rigid or soft. The water at the appropriate temperature is placed into the AV through a valve, then air is blown in to create the proper pressure.

The AV is lubricated with sterile jelly at the service end in order to permit atraumatic intromission. The collection end of the AV has a director cone to which the semen collection vial is attached. For some species the collection vial is encased in an insulating water jacket.

Electroejaculation

There are different types of commercial electroejaculators available with rectal probes specially designed for the individual species. They are, however, similar in their basic construction and function. The control unit has an electrical power supply which may be generated by a 12 volt rechargeable battery, clipped to a car or truck battery or plugged into a standard 120V AC line. DC power to the probe is supplied by a single or multiple power step control and regulated by a variable stimulator knob. Depending on the species, the power is applied for either short (2 to 3 seconds) or long (7 to 15 seconds) periods of time followed by a rest period and re-stimulation. This stimulating sequence is followed successively at higher power settings until ejaculation occurs.

Digital Manipulation

Digital manipulation for ejaculation in the boar or dog involves imitation of the female cervical or vaginal response, respectively. The penis is protruded by stimulating the male with an estrous, or with a nonestrous, but restrained female. The penis is grasped and appropriate pressure applied. If performed properly, the typical ejaculatory pattern that would occur during natural mating will also take place under digital manipulation.

COLLECTION TECHNIQUES

Bovine

From a practical standpoint and based on consistency of response, collection of semen from bulls is performed by EE or the use of an AV. Digital massage of the accessory reproductive structures produces variable responses and is rarely employed.

EE is used most widely for performing breeding soundness examinations under field conditions. The AV, however, is preferred for semen collection where the ejaculate will be processed and frozen. The ejaculate from an AV is more uniform, concentrated, and generally less subject to contamination.

The characteristics of bull semen collected by EE differ from those of semen collected with the AV. EE usually produces samples of greater volume, higher pH and lower concentrations of sperm and fructose per ml. The characteristics of three fractions of semen collected by EE or AV are shown in Table 10-1. EE stimulates the release of additional accessory gland fluids along with the sperm-rich fraction, while AV collections have less accessory gland fluids. The fertility of neat semen collected by EE compares favorably with that of semen collected by AV. However, the survival of frozen spermatozoa from semen collected by AV is generally superior to that collected by EE. Occasionally, intractable bulls or males unable to mount are collected by EE for the production of frozen semen.

Collection via electroejaculation requires a minimum of practice and is fairly simple to perform. Most commercially available ejaculators are suitable for bovine collection (Fig. 10-1). There are differences in rectal probe sizes and electrode orientation. A probe with three ventrally located electrodes is considered superior to a four electrode model because of decreased stimulation of the sur-

rounding muscle masses (Fig. 10-2). Consequently, with ventral electrodes the bull reacts with less muscular rigidity and firmer foot placement.

Collection procedures may vary somewhat between bulls due to their temperament and physical condition. Usually the bull is restrained in a chute capable of handling these powerful animals. A rope is then placed under the chest behind the front legs and secured to the chute. This prevents the bull from dropping suddenly during the collection procedures, which could result in the animal choking or injury to the semen collector's arm. Finally a bar is placed behind the bull to limit back to front motion as well as kicking. The animal should then be identified by tattoo, metal eartag, or brand if possible. The probe is lubricated, inserted into the evacuated rectum with the electrodes placed ventrally and an assistant holds the yoke to prevent the bull from expelling the probe.

The person stimulating the bull may also collect the ejaculate into a suitable sterile and warm container. Stimulation is provided in 'steps' alternating with a rest interval. Stimulation is usually of 2 to 3 seconds' duration

Table 10-1   Characteristics of Three Fractions of Bull Semen Collected by Artificial Vagina (AV) or by Electroejaculation (EE)

	Presperm		Sperm-rich		Postsperm	
	AV	EE	AV	EE	AV	EE
Sperm count (millions/ml)	4 ± 2	8 ± 4	1062 ± 124	572 ± 80*	19 ± 8	132 ± 65
No. samples	18	9	16	9	5	9
Fructose (mg/dl)	3 ± 2	76 ± 38[†]	602 ± 50	444 ± 77	139 ± 64	503 ± 85*
No. samples	18	9	16	9	5	9
Nitrogen (μg/ml)	11 ± 3	27 ± 6*	59 ± 13	48 ± 10	38 ± 13	49 ± 11
No. samples	18	9	15	9	4	9
Free amino acids (mg/dl)	17.4 ± 6.9	27.2 ± 8.5	86.0 ± 11.1	67.6 ± 13.3	47.6 ± 7.0	50.4 ± 13.1
No. samples	14	9	12	9	4	9
pH	7.45 ± 0.10	7.97 ± 0.45	6.73 ± 0.09	7.30 ± 0.11*	7.80 ± 0.05	7.63 ± 0.16
No. samples	18	9	16	9	5	9

From Faulkner, L. C., et al.: J. Dairy Sci. 47:824, 1964
*Significant from AV collection at 1 % level
[†]Significant from AV collection at 5 % level
± Refers to standard deviation

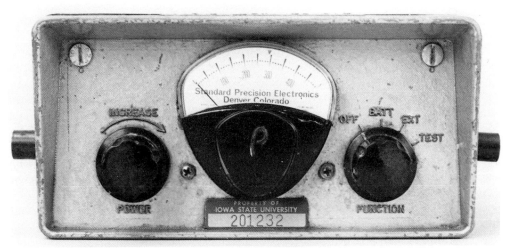

Fig. 10-1. Battery-operated, electroejaculator control unit.

and the rest period is generally 1/2 to 1 second. Increasing voltage is applied with each successive step until ejaculation occurs and an adequate sample is obtained, or maximum power is reached. If maximum stimulation is applied without ejaculation, the animal may not be suitable to collect by EE, but should be tried again after a 10- to 15-minute rest.

During the stimulation process, the bull's penis should become erect and extend past the preputial orifice in order to obtain the ejaculate with minimal contamination. If the bull fails to protrude his penis, extension may be assisted by pushing on the sigmoid flexure to straighten the penis. There are organic diseases such as traumatic adhesions, corpus cavernosal shunts, and anatomic defects which may prevent extension of the penis.

The ejaculate should be maintained at 37°C during the collection and evaluation process. Specific criteria for semen analysis will be discussed later in this chapter.

Collection by an AV requires a tractable, trained animal and more extensive facilities for handling both the bull and mount steer.

The AV should be selected for proper length. It is desirable for the bull to ejaculate

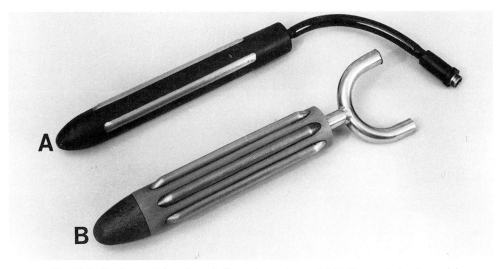

Fig. 10-2. Bovine rectal probes. A. Four-electrode model. B. Three-electrode model

while the tip of the penis is within the director cone rather than on the liner. The higher temperature of the liner may be lethal to sperm. Conversely, if the casing is too short the bull's penis may dislodge the collection vial resulting in loss of the ejaculate. A standard bovine casing is 41 × 7.5 cm in length and width, which is suitable for mature animals (Fig. 10-3). Younger bulls should be collected with an AV made from a casing and liners which have been shortened (1/2 to 2/3 the length for mature bulls, Fig. 10-4). Also there seems to be a lower incidence of avulsion tears of the glans penis from the prepuce with a shortened soft molded rather than a larger hard rubber casing. The AV is partially filled with water, the temperature of which should be 42 to 46°C at the time of collection. Time between collections and ambient temperature will determine how hot the water should be at the time of filling since cooling of the AV will take place. The first 10 to 15 cm of the AV is lubricated with a non-spermicidal lubricant, then air is added through a valve in the outer casing to supply the correct amount of pressure. An insulated cover is placed over the director cone and water jacket in order to protect against thermal shock following collection.

The bull must be prepared before the actual collection takes place in order to maximize ejaculate output. This includes psychic stimulation by walking past other bulls or restraining the male in close prox-

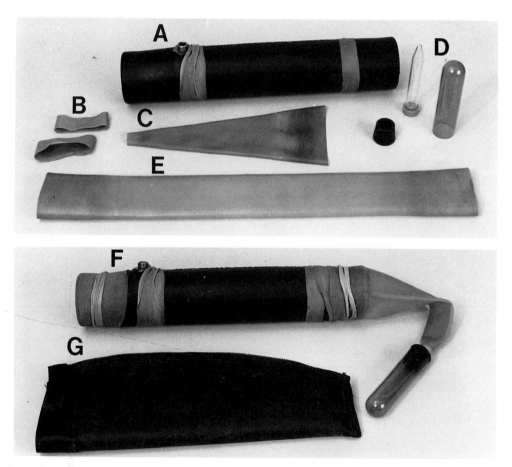

Fig. 10-3. Unassembled bovine AV. Moulded rubber casing (A). Rubber bands (B) used to attach coarse liner (E) and director cone (C) to the casing. The sterile test tube and insulating water jacket (D). The assembled AV (F), and the insulating cover (G).

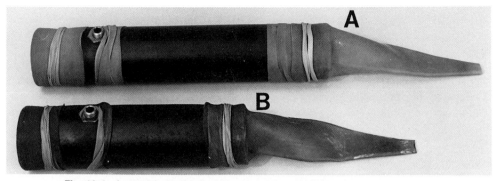

Fig. 10-4. Assembled, standard-length bovine AV (A) and shortened AV (B).

imity to another bull. This will increase the volume and concentration of the ejaculate. In addition, the bull is allowed to mount 1 to 3 times before actual collection in order to decrease the volume of accessory sex gland secretion in semen. When the bull is firmly on the mount animal, the penis is deviated and as the bull thrusts, excess seminal fluid is ejected. This procedure also increases the sperm concentration in the collected ejaculate. If the ejaculate is too dilute, it would be unsuitable for extension because there would be too few spermatozoa to achieve satisfactory conception rates.

For collection, the bull mounts the steer, the penis is again deviated then directed into the AV. If the pressure, temperature, and consistency of the liner are correct, the bull will lunge, complete intromission, and ejaculate in only a few seconds.

If additional ejaculates are desired, the bull is rested for a minimum of 10 to 15 minutes and the process repeated with a new AV. The AV is changed at each collection to prevent contamination of the ejaculate by previous debris or dead cells.

Equine

For practical purposes, semen is collected from the stallion with an AV, both for semen evaluation and for extended or frozen semen production. Stallions can be collected with an electroejaculator if they are anesthetized, but this procedure is reserved for diagnostic cases involving reproductive dysfunctions. Condoms have been used in the past and are still available, but are rarely used in clinical situations.

There are three common types of equine AVs available and the model used is based on the collector's personal preference.

The AV consists of a rigid plastic casing with liners or two layers of soft rubber with a small leather harness for carrying support (Fig. 10-5). The rigid AVs use rubber liners and a disposable collecting cone, whereas the cone is an integral component of the soft AV. The rigid models are prepared as the bovine AV in that the rubber liner and cones are secured to the exterior casing with rubber bands, then the AV is filled with water, lubricated, and air is added to achieve the proper pressure. The recommended temperature at the time of collection for all models is between 45° to 50°C. Water, lubricant and air are similarly placed in the soft AV, and the leather carrying harness is attached.

Plastic bottles are used to collect the ejaculate with or without an integral filter which removes the gel fraction of the stallion's ejaculate. An insulating cover is placed over the cone and bottle to control thermal changes in the ejaculate.

A mount animal (mare), or a mounting phantom to which the stallion is trained, is used for collection. The phantom is a padded horizontal tube on which the stallion is trained to mount. The training process requires a variable period of time, but is useful when

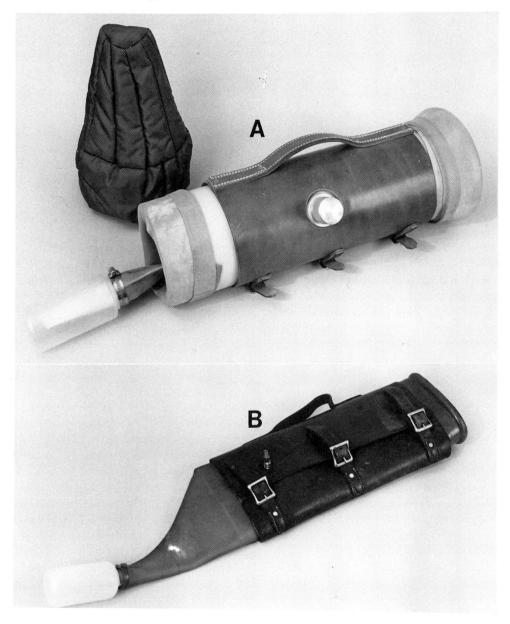

Fig. 10-5. Assembled rigid equine AV (A) and molded rubber equine AV (B).

frequent collections of a stallion are required. The mount mare should be in estrus in order to provide a controllable animal.

The mount animal is prepared by thoroughly washing the perineal area with an iodine based scrub, followed by liberal water rinses. This helps prevent contamination of the glans penis if the stallion contacts the hindquarters of the mare. The mare's tail is either clipped or wrapped to prevent abrasion of the stallion's penis and entanglement in the coarse hairs of the tail during collection.

After preparation, the mare is restrained in a stock while the stallion is allowed to 'tease' her. Teasing allows additional evaluation of the mount mare's response to a particular stallion and generally produces a favorable response in the male resulting in a greater volume of ejaculate and increased sperm output. During teasing, the stallion undergoes erection and extension of the penis. After the stallion has been stimulated, he is backed away from the mare and the penis is washed. The procedure involves grasping the penis behind the glans and gently washing the distal half of the penis with wet cotton pledgets containing iodine cleanser. The smegma from the preputial diverticulum is also removed and the penis rinsed liberally with clean water to remove the iodine, which is spermicidal and may be irritating to the penile mucosa of the stallion. Washing of the stallion also requires a period of training and should always be approached with caution.

The actual collection involves moving the mare to an open area and restraining her with a nose or ear twitch. In addition a foreleg may be held up to hinder kicking. After the stallion mounts, the foreleg is dropped so that the mare can support herself and the male.

Once the mare is restrained, the stallion is allowed to approach the mare from the rear and slightly toward the left side. The collector follows the stallion handler as the stallion approaches the left rear side of the mare. After the stallion mounts, the collector deviates the penis towards the left by using a hand on the shaft of the penis rather than the sensitive glans penis.

As the stallion moves further onto the mare, the penis is guided into the AV and the stallion will begin thrusting motions in order to complete intromission. At ejaculation 'flagging' occurs which is an up and down motion of the stallion's tail. This motion ceases after ejaculation and the stallion begins to dismount. The mare is turned partially toward the stallion as he dismounts in order to prevent injury if the mare should kick.

Generally the entire AV is taken to the laboratory and the collection bottle removed at that time.

Ovine

Semen is collected from rams by EE or with an AV, depending on their previous training. Rams can be taught to service an AV while mounting a ewe, but more commonly EE is employed, because of the infrequency of ram use in AI.

To electroejaculate a ram, two different approaches may be considered. One approach allows the ram to remain standing behind a gate or to be restrained by assistants. A three-electrode ram probe is inserted into the rectum of the animal collected in a similar fashion as used in the bull. A major weakness of this technique involves the frequent failure of the ram to extend his penis while under stimulation, which results in ejaculation within the preputial sheath. This produces a sample of low volume which is heavily contaminated with bacteria, cells and debris.

The lateral recumbency approach allows exteriorization of the penis but requires more physical restraint. Basically, the ram is cast so that he is sitting on his haunches with his shoulders held between the standing operator's knees. The increased abdominal pressure helps the operator to gently exteriorize the penis by retracting the prepuce. Once the tip of the penis is exposed, it is grasped with a piece of gauze and the ram is then placed in lateral recumbency. Next, the probe is inserted into the rectum and the pattern of stimulation follows that of a bull. The operator holding the penis collects the semen into a suitable warm sterile container. Rams generally ejaculate at lower voltages compared to a bull, but occasionally require higher settings.

To collect semen with an AV, a ewe is placed into a stanchion, which consists of a head catch and side restraining bars. The mount animal need not be in estrus for collection of a trained ram. The ram will respond to an immobile ewe, whether due to restraint or estrus. The ram is allowed to approach from the rear with minimal restraint and mount the female. The AV is similar in design to that used on bulls except that it is of smaller diameter and shorter (5.5 × 20 cm). Some models have an attachment for a rubber bulb for the addition of air in order to obtain the correct pressure. Generally the AV temperature should be between 42° to 44°C. The collection procedure used in the ram is similar to that used in the bull.

Caprine

Collection of semen from a buck by EE is primarily used for semen evaluation, although satisfactory samples could be processed for freezing.

First, the buck is restrained and the rectum emptied of contents by gentle lavage using warm water. The procedure may be performed standing or in lateral recumbency; however, both techniques require adequate restraint due to movement and extreme vocalization.

The probe is placed in the rectum with the three electrodes directed ventrally and the buck is stimulated for 2 to 4 seconds, followed by a rest phase of 2 to 3 seconds. Increasing levels of current are administered; with successive stimulations the penis is extended and ejaculation takes place. As in other species the extension process is variable and ejaculation may take place within the prepuce, yielding a poor sample.

The AV used for bucks is similar to those for the ovine species. The construction includes the molded rubber housing with an inner liner, director cone, collection tube, insulating water jacket and outer covering. The unit is filled so that the internal temperature of the AV is 40° to 45°C at the time of collection. Air is used to provide the proper pressure.

In most cases, an untrained buck requires the use of an estrual doe. Trained bucks, however, will readily mount a restrained, nonestrual doe. The collector stands to one side as the buck is led up to the doe. After sniffing and testing the female, the buck mounts and extends the penis. The collector, by grasping the prepuce deviates the penis laterally into the AV. At the time of ejaculation, the buck produces a pronounced pelvic thrust followed by dismount. The AV should be maintained on the penis during the dismount due to the continued expulsion of semen.

Porcine

Swine semen may be collected for evaluation, insemination or freezing by either EE, DM or AV. Due to the normally large volume of the ejaculate, collections by any technique gives satisfactory results. Generally DM is the preferred technique and the use of a swine AV is not commonly employed. DM gives equivalent results compared to the AV and is also easier to perform.

The DM or gloved hand technique involves collection on a mount sow or a phantom (Fig. 10-6). Training the boar to collect on the phantom requires replacement of an estrous animal after several collections or the observation of another boar mounting the phantom. Frequently the presence of another boar's scent will stimulate untrained boars to mount the phantom.

After the boar mounts, the spiral portion of the glans penis is firmly grasped with a gloved hand. This mimics the pressure and stimulation of the sow's cervix. The semen is directed into a thermos as ejaculation of the sperm rich fraction begins.

The principles behind the use of an AV in the boar are similar to those used with other species. The casing is 22.5 × 3.75 cm in length and width and uses a latex rubber liner. The casing is filled with water and air so at the time of collection, the interior of the AV is between 45° to 50°C. The boar is 'locked' into the AV by grasping the spiral tip through the long rubber collection cone. Ejaculation may last up to 15 minutes. Boars ejaculate large volumes, so the collection bottle should hold 450 to 500 ml.

After ejaculation is complete, the pressure used to hold the glans is released and the boar will dismount.

The collection of boar semen by EE requires the use of general anesthesia, since physical restraint would be inadequate to control the boar and exteriorize the penis. The most frequently used anesthetic is Thiamylal which is an ultrashort acting barbiturate. Thiamylal is safe when administered in the proper dose (1 g per 300 pounds, IV) to a normal animal. Deaths, however, have been reported in boars with lung damage from chronic respiratory disease or in genetic carriers of porcine stress syndrome.

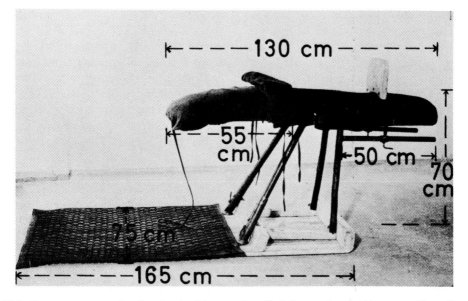

Fig. 10-6. Dummy sow, made of galvanized iron and stuffed, has a changeable cover. The adjustable wooden block, top right, prevents the boar from getting too far forward during collection of semen. (From Aamdal, J.: *In* The Artificial Insemination of Farm Animals, 3rd ed., edited E. J. Perry. New Brunswick, New Jersey, Rutgers University Press, 1960.)

To administer the anesthetic, the animal is restrained with a nose rope or snare and Thiamylal is administered via an ear vein or through the anterior vena cava. The anesthetic is given as a bolus and the animal becomes recumbent in about 10 seconds.

Fecal material is removed from the rectum with a gloved hand prior to probe insertion. The boar probe has longitudinal circular rather than linear electrodes as for the other species (Fig. 10-7). After placement, the person operating the ejaculator applies a light level of stimulation. This provides some penile erection and facilitates exteriorization. To complete exteriorization, a long atraumatic forcep is inserted into the prepuce, the glans penis is engaged and gently exteriorized. After the penis has been extended it is grasped with a hand-held gauze and the tip is directed into a collection container. The

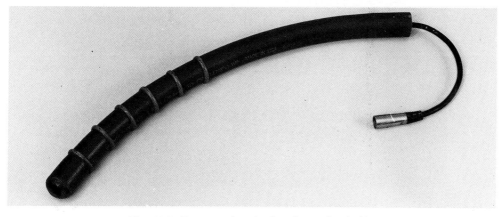

Fig. 10-7. Boar rectal probe for electroejaculation.

container is usually a thermos containing a sterilized plastic bag to hold the ejaculate and the mouth of the thermos is covered by gauze in order to filter out the gel portion of the boar semen. The stimulation technique differs from that used in other species in that power is administered for 5 to 7 seconds followed by a rest phase of 5 to 10 seconds. The long rest period is necessary because the progressively higher stimulations interfere with the intercostal muscles and respiration.

The boar will normally ejaculate sperm-poor fluids during the lighter stimulations which is discarded. The sperm-rich fraction intermixed with gel follows next and the total volume to be collected will depend on whether the sample is for analysis, insemination or freezing.

Canine

Semen collection for the canine species most commonly involves DM and less frequently an AV. With either technique, collection of semen is facilitated by the presence of an estrous bitch. The female is restrained to prevent movement in an area which provides secure footing. The male is brought up to the female on a short leash and allowed nasal-genital contact.

Initially the penis is massaged through the prepuce in order to stimulate erection. After partial erection has commenced, the sheath is gently retracted behind the bulbus glandis and the penis cleaned with a cotton pledget saturated with warm water. Digital pressure is then applied behind the bulbus glandis to complete erection. The male frequently begins to ejaculate while the penis is being handled. Some dogs may require additional stimulation for ejaculation. Gentle message of the tip of the glans penis may elicit further erection leading to ejaculation.

There are three fractions to the ejaculate (Fig. 10-8). The first fraction is clear and nearly sperm free, the second fraction is sperm-rich and the final portion is watery and sperm

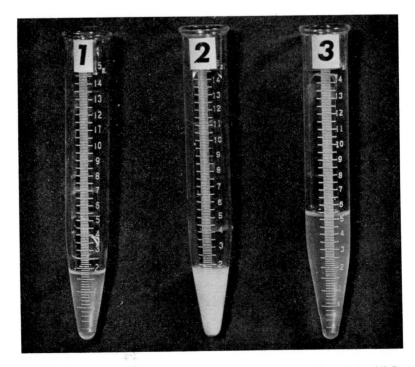

Fig. 10-8. The three fractions of the dog's ejaculate shown are from left to right: (1) first fraction, (2) second fraction, (3) third fraction. (From Boucher, J. H., et al.: Cornell Vet. *48*:73, 1958.)

poor. The sperm-rich fraction can be collected with a warm funnel into a sterile test tube. A styrofoam cup makes a useful insulated collection receptacle or the appropriate sized, sterile syringe case may be used. In some instances, the penis may be inserted into the syringe case as erection begins and this provides additional pressure and stimulation to the dog. However, the use of this procedure should be discouraged and care must be taken that the sharp edges of the case are dulled or covered to avoid trauma to the penis.

The ejaculate should be maintained at 35°C during collection and evaluation.

Following ejaculation, the male should be checked periodically to be sure that detumescence and retraction of the penis has taken place.

To employ an AV, which may be as simple as a director cone attached to a collection tube (Fig. 10-9), the male is stimulated as previously decribed. After partial erection and exterior-ization of the penis, the director cone is placed over the penis and the collector's hand applies pressure around the cone behind the bulbus glandis. The ejaculatory pattern is identical, except that the first and second fractions are commonly collected together.

Feline

Semen can be collected from felines by EE or the AV. There has not been a great demand for collected feline semen so the techniques, although adequate, are not routinely employed.

To collect semen by EE, the tom is anesthetized, then placed in lateral recumbency. The electronic control unit and probes are usually custom made since there is not a commercial source of this equipment. After insertion of the probe the collection tube is placed on the exposed penis and electrical stimulation is applied in a rapid series of pulses. A rest phase is permitted between the pulse series, then stimulation is reapplied at a

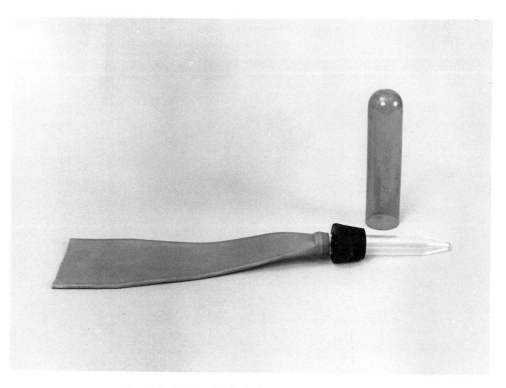

Fig. 10-9. Canine AV, including protective waterjacket.

higher power setting. The specifics for EE in the tom have been recently investigated (see Chapter 17).

Collection with an AV (Fig. 10-10) requires a trained tom and an estrous queen. The feline AV can be made from a rubber bulb and glass tube. A water jacket is used over the AV for 45°C temperature control. As the male mounts the queen, the AV is directed over the penis and ejaculation takes place.

Avian

DM is the preferred method for collecting semen from poultry. Collection begins by massaging the back of the bird, beginning behind the wings and stroking gently toward the tail with the thumb and forefinger making a slight upward movement at the base of the tail. This motion stimulates erection of the copulatory organ. Repetitive stroking may be required on untrained birds. An alternative method is to massage the bird's abdomen. In either case, a thumb and forefinger part the feathers around the vent and gentle pressure is exerted on the ejaculatory ducts. Collection of semen from the turkey is essentially the same as for the rooster.

EQUIPMENT MAINTENANCE

Depending on the species there may be many disposable products used with AV collections, eliminating the need for post-use cleaning. These include plastic test tubes, director cones and in the case of the stallion, secondary inner liners. Rubber items must be cleaned and sanitized after each use. First the liner is rinsed and scrubbed to remove gross contamination, then washed with iodine or a mild detergent. After washing, the liners and cones are rinsed with tap and then with distilled water. Then the goods are rinsed with alcohol or boiled for sterilization and allowed to air dry in a dust-free environment. Glassware is washed in a similar fashion and then dry-heat sterilized (160°C for 2 hours). Reuseable plastic items are cleaned and sterilized with alcohol or dry-heat depending on their type of construction. Steam sterilization is not routinely used due to the possibility of depositing salts on the containers which may be spermicidal. Ethylene oxide gas sterilization can be used, but is frequently unavailable, expensive, and requires airing time (up to 30 days) to remove all traces of this very toxic oxide.

EE equipment is cleaned of fecal matter after the final collection. Mucus buildup on the electrodes can be removed by lightly cleaning with an abrasive cleanser.

ANALYSIS OF SEMEN

The semen is brought to the laboratory and the collection container is placed in a waterbath, incubator, or dri-block heater at 35° to

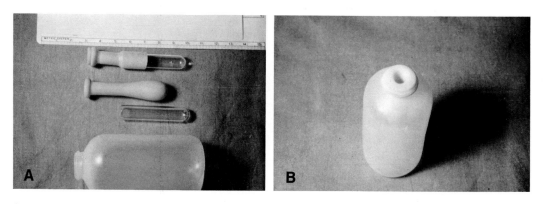

Fig. 10-10. Semen collection from the cat. A, Components of artificial vagina. B, Assembled artificial vagina. (From Sojka, N. J., Jennings, L. L., and Hamner, C. E.: Artificial insemination in the cat (*Felis catus* L.). Lab. Anim. Care *20*(2):199, 1970.)

37°C for temperature stability. In general the ejaculate will be examined for spermatozoal motility and normal-abnormal spermatozoal morphology. Semen should be stored and handled in a 35° to 37°C environment until analysis is completed and processing begins. Some species tolerate semen cooling better than others; for example, semen from the dog and pig can be held at room temperature for several hours without addition of extenders, if allowed to cool slowly. Sensitivity of spermatozoa to temperature change is governed by the protective action of the secretory fluid in the ejaculate and the integrity of the sperm cell membrane at a given temperature. Integrity of the membrane is strongly influenced by its basic lipid-protein composition and the ratio of cholesterol to phospholipids forming the membrane bi-layer.

To date the most comprehensive analysis protocols and standards have been developed for bovine semen. The analysis of semen from other species is similar to that used for bovine semen; however, the parameters have not been as closely correlated with fertility. Semen evaluations alone cannot identify or rank individuals, which have a satisfactory ejaculate, as being average or superior in their fertilizing ability. Such rankings can only be determined through breeding trials.

The motility of the spermatozoa is estimated by microscopic examination at 40 to 100× magnification. Normal bovine semen will display rapidly swirling patterns with 70% or more of the cells in vigorous forward motion. If large amounts of seminal fluid are released and discarded prior to collection of semen from a bull by an AV, then the concentration of cells/ml will be greatly increased. The gross microscopic motility pattern (swirls) will be enhanced due to the higher concentration. On the other hand, if EE is employed and excessive seminal fluid is collected with the sperm-rich fraction, the sample will be diluted and the sperm will not form strong wave patterns. To estimate individual sperm cell motility, an aliquot of the ejaculate is mixed with warm physiologic extender in order to further dilute the semen

sample. A drop of the sample is placed on the slide, coverslipped, and evaluated for percent progressive motility on an individual basis, rather than on a gross motility level. This technique, although more accurate, is not always employed due to the time consuming nature of the procedure. Samples that fall below the suggested standards for use in AI are eliminated. Photomicroscopy or videomicroscopy may be used to further assess individual cell motility.

Spermatozoa morphology is assessed with microscopic examination of a small drop of semen which has been mixed with a stain, smeared on a slide, and air dried. Eosin-nigrosin is the most common stain used for sperm cell examination; however, other acceptable stains include india ink or Wright's.

Sperm abnormalities are classified as primary or secondary according to their importance relative to fertility. It was thought that primary abnormalities arose within the testes and secondary ones in the efferent duct system; however, primary and secondary abnormalities can arise from both areas, so it is common to use major or minor defects relative to their effects on fertility. Depending on the total number of major and minor abnormalities, the morphology score is rated as satisfactory or unsatisfactory.

Scrotal circumference (SC) is assessed in the bull as part of the selection process. The SC is a measure of the bull's capacity to produce spermatozoa, since sperm production per gram of testes is fairly constant. Bulls with extremely small testes produce so few cells that they are subfertile or sterile. Also a bull with small testes as a yearling will experience some increase in SC as he grows, but will continue to produce an ejaculate of low concentration. If an animal does not have a satisfactory SC by 16 to 18 months of age, he probably should not be used for breeding. There is a tendency for bulls with a large SC to undergo puberty earlier and develop a greater servicing capacity. These are desirable heritable characteristics, and all things being equal, bulls with a large SC should be preferentially selected over animals with a smaller SC.

Semen analysis in swine is closely related to the procedures used for bulls. The main differences is that the scrotal size is determined by measuring the length and width of individual testes. A yearling boar should have a testicular size of at least 11 cm in length by 7 cm in width for each testis. A motility estimate of 70% or greater is considered satisfactory. A total of 20% or more of major abnormalities or greater than 40% minor abnormalities would render the boar as suspect fertility.

Semen analysis in the stallion is based on motility, morphology and concentration. Measurement of testicular size is not consistently employed and has not been correlated with fertility.

Unless the stallion semen was collected into an AV with a filter, the gel fraction should be removed from the ejaculate by syringe aspiration or gravity filtration. This is necessary to prevent trapping of the spermatozoa in the gel and hindering motility estimates.

Concentration can be estimated by employing a hemocytometer to count cells/unit area of diluted semen and then with appropriate formulas determine concentration of sperm cells/ml of the ejaculate. An alternative technique is to assess the color of the ejaculate and correlate this to an approximation of cells/ml. The average ejaculate contains approximately 150×10^6 cells/ml.

Generally stallion ejaculates are not as dense as bovine samples, so motility estimates are performed on a warm slide with a coverslip over the sample. The percentage of motile sperm are then estimated, with greater than 70% motile considered satisfactory. The ejaculate should also have more than 70% morphologically normal cells.

Analysis in the ram is based on motility and morphology, in addition to satisfactory scrotal circumferences. General guidelines require that a ram evaluated during the mating season have greater than 70% motility and less than 25% major morphologic abnormalities. Semen evaluation out of the breeding season will generally show an increase in abnormal cells and a decrease in motility and SC.

Semen parameters in the buck are similar to other species except that a motility estimate of greater than 75% and less than 25% of the cells with major defects represent a satisfactory ejaculate. Currently other parameters are not employed in the examination of caprines.

Semen analysis in the dog is based on motility where 70 to 80% of the cells should show a rapid forward motion and a morphologic estimate of no more than 25% major abnormalities.

There are no specific recommendations for semen analysis in the feline species other than those determined in a series of tests in which the average motility was 78%. The range of abnormal defects was 1 to 10%.

SEMEN EXTENSION AND CRYOPRESERVATION

Diluting semen in a buffered extender containing antibiotics helps to maintain sperm viability for a short term before use or freezing. Generally only canine and feline females are inseminated with fresh, non-extended semen.

Extenders differ in composition depending upon the species, use, temperature at which the diluted semen is to be stored, and the duration of storage desired. All extenders are based on a particular buffer, which has provided the best results for a given species. Buffers modulate the change in extender pH due to the metabolic products of the stored sperm. In addition, carbohydrates are added to provide an energy source for sperm glycolysis. Egg yolk or milk-based fractions are added to provide phospholipids, which promote membrane stabilization at cooler temperatures and limit premature acrosomal membrane activation. Antibiotics are used to control growth of bacteria which may have been picked up during the collecting process.

Some extenders will maintain sperm viability at room temperatures, while others are refrigerated at 4° to 5°C to help control bacterial growth and slow the metabolic rate of the spermatozoa.

Bovine

Semen freezing is most advanced in the bovine species and has served as a basic model for processing semen of other species. There are variations in extenders, the use of freezing point depression compounds, and freezing rates, but the principles of cryopreservation in all species are similar to those used in freezing bovine semen. The information concerning the optimum parameters for semen cryopreservation are not standardized within or between species and different sources conflict over the best procedures. The procedure described herein is employed on a commercial basis in our laboratory.

First the fresh bovine ejaculate is evaluated for volume, motility, and morphology. To be satisfactory for further processing, the sample must have a minimum of 80% gross motility and 70% or greater of normal morphology. Samples of lower quality are discarded.

An aliquot of semen is diluted 100 fold with normal saline solution and the concentration of cells/ml is determined with a calibrated spectrophotometer (optical density). Satisfactory samples receive antibiotics in accordance to the recommendations of the NAAB for pathogen control. The antimicrobial activity of the antibiotics is hindered by the presence of milk or egg yolk phospholipids. Consequently the antibiotics are added to the neat semen and allowed to incubate for 10 to 15 minutes in order to maintain maximal efficacy.

After equilibration with the antibiotics, the semen is added to an extender which is at the same temperature (37°C). This extension is only half the final desired dilution. The extended semen is then placed in an isothermal water jacket, which is in turn placed in a 5°C cold cabinet and allowed to cool over a minimum period of 1.5 hours. At the end of the 1.5 hours, the samples are removed from the water jackets and cooled an additional minimum of 30 minutes.

After the extended semen has been held at 5°C for a minimum of 1 hour, the sample is diluted to the final desired concentration with glycerolated extender. Glycerol is a freezing point depressing compound which helps prevent ice and solute damage to the cells during the freeze-thaw process. Glycerol at the final recommended levels is slightly toxic to sperm if added in one step, so the glycerolated extender is mixed gradually with the semen over 1 hour. After the final addition, the semen is packaged into 0.5-ml plastic french straws, sealed, and frozen in static nitrogen vapor at a starting temperature of $-160°C$.

After freezing, the straws are immersed into liquid nitrogen until the time of thawing. Thawing is achieved by placing the straw into a 37°C waterbath for 30 to 60 seconds. All post-thaw evaluations are performed at 37°C. Semen from this laboratory must meet the minimum criteria as outlined in Table 10-2 before it is acceptable for distribution to producers.

There are limits to the predictability of potential fertility by laboratory assessment and true fertility can only be determined by breeding results. There is a tendency, however, for semen with progressively higher motility and intact acrosomes to have a higher level of fertility.

Equine

Frozen stallion semen is used commercially only on a limited basis. Freezing uniformity and post-thaw results, especially motility and conception rates, have been erratic.

On a research basis, only stallion ejacu-

Table 10-2   Post Thaw Analysis: Minimum Standards

	0 hr	2 hr
Motility (%)	30	20
Progressive Linear Motility[1]	2	1
Percent Intact Acrosomes	—	> 50

[1]PLM is an estimate of the rate of forward motion. The range is from 0 to 4 with 0 assigned to no motion and 4 indicating extremely rapid linear movement.

lates which have better than 50% progressive motility and more than 50×10^6 spermatozoa/ml are used. In one method, the semen is extended in a sodium-citrate-ethylenediamine tetraacetic acid (EDTA) glucose medium cooled to 20°C and centrifuged for washing and concentrating the sperm sample. The semen pellet is then resuspended in lactose-egg yolk EDTA extender with a glycerol concentration of 4%. The final extended semen has a concentration of 200 to 800×10^6 motile, normal cells/ml, and is packaged into 0.55 ml Continental plastic straws. Recently, it has been claimed that dilution of stallion ejaculates to 25×10^6 motile spermatozoa/ml improves longevity and spermatozoal motility.

Freezing is accomplished in a forced nitrogen vapor unit by cooling from 20°C to −15°C at 10°C/min, followed by cooling at 25°C/min from −15°C to −120°C. The straws are then immersed in liquid nitrogen for storage.

Thawing is accomplished by placing the straw in 75°C water for 7 seconds then transferring it into 35°C water for at least 30 seconds.

Results of one insemination trial revealed that the frozen-thawed semen produced a conception rate that varied from 75 to 100% of the rate of fresh semen. These results were based on a limited trial and do not represent average conception rates expected in a commercial situation.

Ovine

There are several variations in the protocol for freezing of ram semen including sperm concentration, % glycerol, equilibration times and rate of freezing.

One of the popular techniques involves a two step dilution rate. The total amount of glycerolated and non-glycerolated extender is calculated so the final sperm concentration will be 900×10^6 cells/ml in 4% glycerol. The ejaculate is then diluted with 3/5 of the calculated volume using non-glycerolated lactose extender at 30°C. Following cooling to 4°C, the remaining 2/5 of the volume of

I.N.R.A. extender* with glycerol is added in one step. The semen is allowed to equilibrate with the glycerol for 20 to 150 minutes, placed into straws, and frozen in liquid nitrogen vapor at an initial temperature of −75°C to −125°C. Storage is in liquid nitrogen. Thawing is accomplished in 37°C water for 30 seconds. The minimum insemination dose is 180×10^6 motile cells/straw. The conception rate reported in one trial with this technique was 73.5%.

Caprine

Cryopreservation of buck semen employs milk or egg yolk extenders, glycerol, and packaging in 0.5-ml french straws with 100 million cells/ml. Initial cooling is to 4°C in non-glycerolated extender. The glycerolated portion is slowly added and allowed to equilibrate over 2 hours before freezing in nitrogen vapor. Thawing is accomplished in a 35°C water bath for 10 to 20 seconds prior to insemination.

Porcine

Swine semen freezing is a multistep process due to the sensitivity of the sperm membranes to temperature fluctuations and the depressing effect of glycerol on fertility. Specifics are beyond the scope of this chapter; however, highlights of one method will be described.

The collected ejaculate is added to a predilutor and cooled to 18°C over 4 hours. The semen is then centrifuged at 18°C for 10 minutes and the pellet resuspended in a cooling diluter containing egg yolk. The semen is then cooled from 18° to 5°C. Prior to freezing, the semen is diluted to a final concentration of 1.2 $\times 10^9$ spermatozoa/ml in a deep-freeze diluter containing 4% glycerol. The semen is then frozen in 5-ml tubes.

The freezing program involves four different cooling rates to −100°C followed by immersion into liquid nitrogen. Thawing recommenda-

*I.N.R.A. extender: A.N.V.A.R., A.13 rue Madeleine Michelis, 92200 Neuilly-sur-Seine, France

tions vary widely depending on the processor.

As a general rule, frozen boar semen results in lower pregnancy rates and litter sizes compared to breeding with fresh extended semen.

Canine

Canine semen can be frozen and its use is recognized by the American Kennel Club (AKC). The highest and most consistent pregnancy rates follow uterine insemination. Uterine insemination most often requires a surgical approach.

In one procedure, the ejaculate to be frozen is equilibrated at body temperature for 15 minutes. Room temperature extender (Pipes-citrate-egg yolk) containing glycerol is added dropwise to obtain a dilution ratio of 1:1. The extended semen is then cooled in a 5°C refrigerator for 30 minutes. An additional aliquot of extender cooled to 5°C is added dropwise to obtain a dilution of 1:2 (semen-extender). The semen is then placed in 0.5 ml french straws and frozen in nitrogen vapor 8″ above the liquid phase. Storage is in liquid nitrogen.

To thaw, the straws are placed in 37°C water for 50 seconds and insemination should be done within 10 minutes of thawing.

Feline

The use of frozen feline semen has not been adequately documented.

INSEMINATION PROCEDURES

The objective of artificial insemination is to deposit a prescribed number of normal, motile sperm cells in the female tract so they reach the oocyte at a time which will permit normal sperm capacitation followed by fertilization (Table 10-3).

The domestic species, except the bitch and queen, being bred with fresh semen, require uterine deposition for normal conception rates.

For practical considerations, cattle are exclusively inseminated with frozen-thawed semen. Horses, pigs, sheep, dogs and occasionally goats are inseminated with fresh-extended semen and only in limited cases, with frozen semen. Dogs and cats are generally bred with fresh-non-extended semen.

Bovine

Semen produced for cattle is generally extended in a milk or egg-yolk buffer and packaged in glass ampules or 0.25 or 0.5 ml plastic french straws (Fig. 10-11). The bovine AI industry has primarily phased out ampules due to more efficient storage capabilities and improved insemination instruments for plastic straws.

Regardless of the packaging, the semen is stored in small liquid nitrogen tanks (Fig. 10-12). These tanks have a static loss of nitrogen and must be periodically refilled to main-

Table 10-3   Mean Seminal Characteristics and Reproductive Data for Domestic Mammals

Species	Bovine	Equine	Ovine	Caprine	Porcine	Canine	Feline
Volume (ml)	5	60	1	8	200	10	06
Concentration (million/ml)	1,200	150	3,000	2,400	270	300	1,730
*Total sperm/ ejaculate	6,000	9,000	3,000	1,920	54,000	3,000	86.5
Motility (%)	70	70	75	80	60	85	78
Normal Morphology (%)	80	70	90	90	70	80	90
Time of Insemination, day of estrus	Middle to end	Third day[1]	Toward end	Toward end	First or second day[2]	Second and fourth day	During estrus[3]

[1]Insemination repeated at 48-hour intervals until ovulation.
[2]Gilts on first day, sows on second day. Repeat insemination if animal still standing to be mounted 12 hours later.
[3]Induced ovulation
*Spermatozoa in millions

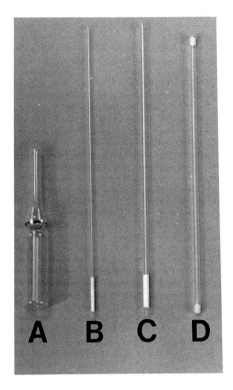

Fig. 10-11. (A) One ml glass ampule. (B) 0.25 ml french straw (C) 0.5 ml french straw (D) Continental straw

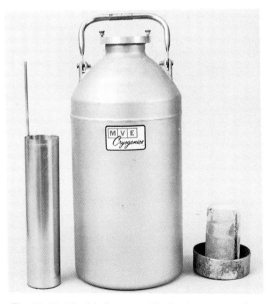

Fig. 10-12. Liquid nitrogen shipping/storage tank.

tain proper cryogenic temperatures. The length of time semen can remain viable if properly stored is unknown, but semen collected over 40 years ago has provided acceptable fertility. There is, however, a gradual decrease in viability for semen maintained at cryogenic temperatures.

When handling stored semen, whether transferring from tank to tank or removing a unit from a goblet that contains other units, the exposure time to elevated temperatures (room temperature to −80°C) must be limited to seconds. If the semen is allowed to warm to above −80°C, recrystallization which damages the spermatozoa can occur.

The thawing procedure for ampules is not the same as for straws because of differences in the surface to volume ratio of the container. Straws are generally thawed rapidly in a 37°C waterbath for 30 to 60 seconds, while ampules are thawed more slowly in an ice water bath for 10 minutes. The physical chemistry involved in freezing and thawing of semen is outside the scope of this chapter, but involves rate of freezing, size of intracellular ice crystals, changes in intracellular osmolarity during freezing and thawing, and the degree of dehydration of the cell. Generally if freezing is slow, then thawing must be slow and visa versa.

Once a unit is thawed, it is removed from the warm water or ice bath and dried. The unit was identified while still in the liquid nitrogen tank and is now double checked to prevent insemination with the wrong bull's semen.

Straws are loaded into an insemination gun after the sealed tip has been removed (Fig. 10-13). A rigid plastic sheath is placed over the gun used for insemination. While loading the gun, transporting it to the breeding site, and manipulating the gun into the vagina, the semen should not be exposed to severe temperature change or rapid temperature fluctuations. A temperature range of 15°C to 37°C for post-thaw semen is compatible with satisfactory pregnancy rates.

When ampules are used, the neck of the ampule is broken off and the semen is aspi-

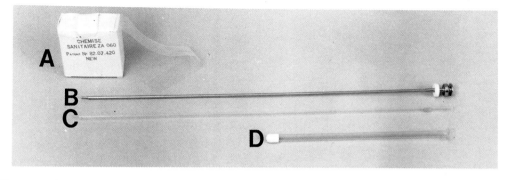

Fig. 10-13. Insemination gun for french straws. The straw is inserted into the stainless steel gun (B), and a plastic sheath (C) is placed over the gun to hold in the straw. (A) and (D) are two types of additional protective sheaths used to prevent vaginal contamination of the plastic sheath (C).

rated into an insemination pipette (Fig. 10-14). The column of semen should remain unbroken when drawn into the pipette. If the column is broken by air bubbles, then some of the semen tends to remain in the pipette following insemination.

The insemination procedure involves passing the AI gun or pipette through the cow's vagina while fixing the female's tract with rectal manipulation (Fig. 10-15). Once the pipette reaches the external cervical os, the cervix is manipulated by the hand in the rectum to guide the pipette through the 3 to 5 cervical rings. The site of deposition is at the level of the internal cervical os. Depositing the semen only part way through the cervix or deeper into the uterine horns, decreases conception rates.

The success of AI within a breeding pro-gram depends upon several factors including the accuracy of estrus detection, semen quality, cow fertility, and the expertise of the AI technician.

Estrus detection is one of the major factors controlling conception rates with AI. For example if 95% of the animals are accurately detected in heat and bred properly and the fertility level of the herd is 50% (first service conception rate), then 47.5% of the animals will become pregnant. If, however, only 70% of the animals are properly detected then only 35% become pregnant. On the other hand if estrus detection is excellent (95%), but the insemination procedure is poorly handled, then the number of pregnancies/insemination will still be poor.

In dairy cattle the goals are an estrus detection rate of 85% for cows and 95% for

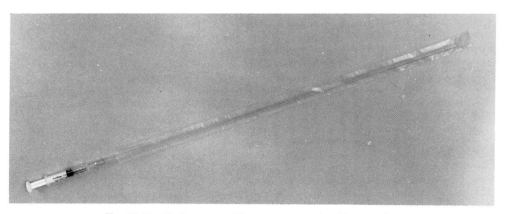

Fig. 10-14. AI pipette used for semen contained in ampules.

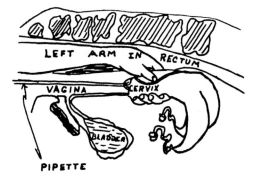

Fig. 10-15. The rectovaginal approach for cervical insemination of the cow.

heifers within a 24-day period of observation.

A cow in estrus will stand to be mounted by other cows, prepared teasers, or a bull. Accompanying the mounting behavior are variable degrees of restlessness, vocalization, mucus discharge, and edema of the vulva. These ancillary signs become apparent as the animal approaches estrus, become more fre-quent and intense during estrus, and decline following estrus. The only accurate way to assess estrus is to note when the cow stands to be mounted. Generally the optimum breeding period is 10 to 16 hours after the cow begins to stand for mounting (Fig. 10-16). Aids in es-trus detection include observation of non-stanchioned cows 2 to 3 times daily and the use of heat detector animals such as teaser bulls or androgenized cows. Milk or serum progesterone assays and electronic devices that measure the conducting potential of the vaginal mucus can also be used to identify cows or heifers that may be in estrus.

Estrus synchronization procedures which shorten the interval that females must be ob-served, or which allow for timed matings, have also been used in AI of cattle.

Heifers are generally bred at an approxi-mate body weight and age that is particular for the breed. Postpartum dairy cows are usually rebred the first time between 45 and 60 days after calving and beef cows at 50 to 80 days after calving.

WHEN TO BREED — *"Timing Guide" for the average cow*

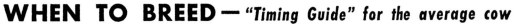

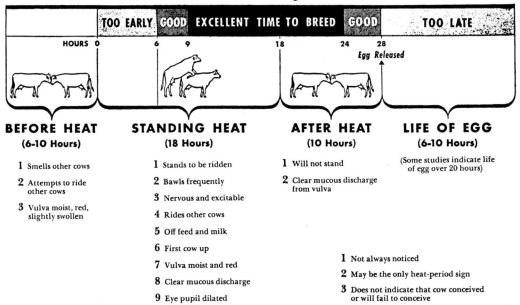

Fig. 10-16. Many cattle owners have testified to the value of becoming thoroughly familiar with this type of timing guide. (From The Artificial Insemination of Farm Animals, 3rd ed., edited by E. J. Perry. New Brunswick, New Jersey, Rutgers University Press, 1960.)

Equine

The optimum insemination dose for the mare is 100 to 500 $\times$ 10^6 progressively motile normal sperm. Generally the semen is extended in a milk-based diluent at a semen to extender ratio of 1:1 to 1:3.

Estrus detection in mares requires the use of a stallion in order to elicit the estrual response. The estrous cycle is about 20 to 21 days long during the breeding season. The luteal phase (progesterone dominated) lasts about 15 days and the follicular phase (estrogen dominated) has an average duration of 5.5 days. As the mare approaches late diestrus–early estrus, her reaction to the stallion progressively changes from rejection to submission. Estrual signs include raising of her tail, squatting, urinating and vulvar 'winking' when being teased by the stallion. Additionally rectal palpation will reveal advanced follicular growth (greater than 35 mm in diameter), an edematous uterus, and relaxed cervix. The mare ovulates 24 to 48 hours before the end of estrus. Consequently, most management systems begin breeding on the 2nd or 3rd day of estrus. The average lifespan of stallion semen in the female reproductive tract is 48 hours, so mares are inseminated every 2 days until ovulation is detected by rectal palpation or estrus ceases.

The mare is prepared for insemination by securing her in a set of stocks. The tail is wrapped and tied out of the way or held by an assistant. Wrapping helps prevent tail hairs from being pulled into the vagina during insemination and keeps them off the perineum during washing. Next the perineal area is washed with iodine detergent and rinsed with water. Generally 3 to 5 wash-rinse cycles are necessary for proper hygiene.

During the cleaning process, an assistant has aspirated the appropriate amount of extended semen into a syringe. The inseminator puts on a sterile plastic shoulder-length glove, applies some sterile lubricant to the glove, and gently passes the insemination pipette (Fig. 10-17) through the vagina and guides the tip of the pipette through the cervix. The semen is then gently expelled into the uterus over a period of 15 to 30 seconds.

Ovine

Most ewes are bred by natural service. There is, however, a slowly developing trend to use fresh extended or frozen ram semen on a limited basis. The semen is generally frozen in french straws on a 'custom' basis where the ram is brought to a center for collection and returned after a requisite number of units are produced.

A major limitation to successful AI in sheep is the difficulty of traversing the cervix with insemination instruments. Vaginal or

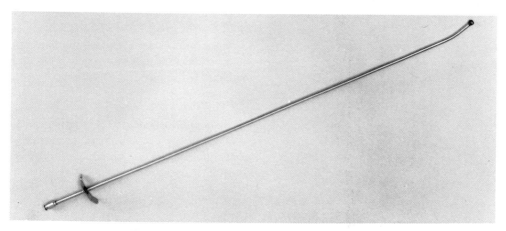

Fig. 10-17. Chambers catheter used for equine AI.

shallow cervical deposition results in a pregnancy rate of less than 30%, whereas intrauterine deposition can achieve levels similar to natural breeding.

The insemination process requires a vaginal speculum and light source for cervical visualization. This can be done in a restrained standing ewe or one placed on a tilt table which elevates the hindquarters. The AI gun is specifically designed for use in sheep and consists of a stainless steel tube with plunger. The unit of semen is placed in the stainless steel tube over which a plastic sheath with a bendable tip is added. The tip is slightly bent for use in virgin ewe lambs and more severely bent in older animals. The bent tip helps in threading of the cervix in a higher proportion of the females.

Estrus detection is critical in sheep AI. A teaser male (vasectomized) is used to identify the estrous females. The teaser has a marking harness (Fig. 10-18) or grease paint on the chest, which leaves a colored dye on the ewe's wool. Insemination should be done 12 to 24 hours after the onset of estrus.

Ewes can be synchronized so that the majority are in estrus within a 24- to 48-hour interval. Techniques include the use of a progestogen or prostaglandin in order to regulate the lifespan of the corpus luteum. Breeding can be performed at a preset time following synchronization. Conception rates have often been lower in the 1st synchronized estrus.

Caprine

Goats are (occasionally) inseminated with frozen semen. Restraint is necessary, the degree of which depends on the animal's temperament. This will vary from the use of a collar to the stanchioning of the female in a head catch.

The perineal area is cleaned with water and a lubricated speculum is passed into the vagina. Mucus that is cloudy or turbid indicates the doe is in late estrus which is the optimum time for insemination.

The type of instrument used for insemination depends on the packaging of the semen. A shortened plastic pipette is used for ampules, while the sheep AI gun is suitable for straws.

The cervical os is located with the aid of a light and the tip of the AI gun is entered into the os. Gentle pressure is used to pass the gun past the cervical rings. Often complete penetration of the cervix is not possible so the semen is deposited intracervically. When complete penetration is possible, part of the semen is placed in the uterus and part within the cervix. This is to prevent the inadvertent deposition of the entire unit of semen within only one horn.

Conception rates are generally lower than natural service but a 60% conception rate is possible with optimum conditions.

Porcine

Swine are inseminated with either fresh extended or frozen semen. With accurate estrus detection and optimal breeding time, the conception rate of fresh extended semen equals that obtained with natural breeding. Frozen semen usually results in a lower conception rate and litter size.

Normally the sow or gilt is inseminated

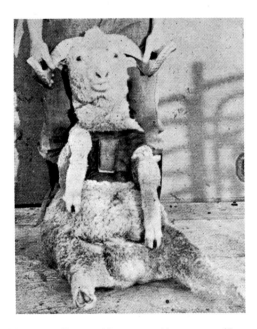

Fig. 10-18. Removable ewe marking crayon. (From Radford, H. M., et al.: Aust. Vet. J. *36*:57, 1960.)

with 2 to 4 × 10^9 motile spermatozoa extended to a volume of 80 to 100 ml or 6 to 12 × 10^9 cells if frozen-thawed semen is employed.

The proestrous female displays increased sexual activity and will stand for mounting at the onset of estrus. Standing estrus lasts 24 to 36 hours with gilts and 30 to 60 hours with sows. Gilts should be mated 12 to 18 hours after the onset of estrus and again 12 hours later if still standing. Sows are bred 24 hours from the onset of estrus again 12 to 18 hours later. To facilitate estrus detection, a boar is walked by or allowed into the pen with the females to identify those which will stand to be mounted or stand to back pressure applied by the handler.

Actual insemination involves the use of a spirette, or a disposable pipette with a small bent tip (Fig. 10-19). The vulva is cleaned with a paper towel and the lubricated spirette is inserted along the dorsal vaginal wall to the external cervical os. When resistance is detected with the spirette it is gently rotated counter clockwise so that the spiral end advances and locks into the cervix (Fig. 10-20). A pipette will advance past one or two cervical rings with manipulation, but will not lock into the cervix. The semen is injected slowly into the uterus with a syringe or collapsible plastic bottle.

Canine

AI in the canine generally is based on the use of fresh, unextended semen. Generally, the entire sperm rich fraction is deposited into the anterior vagina of the estrous female.

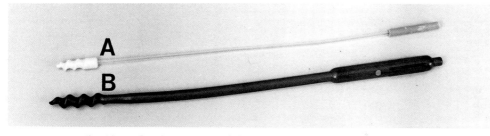

Fig. 10-19. Porcine spirettes. (A) disposable and (B) non-disposable.

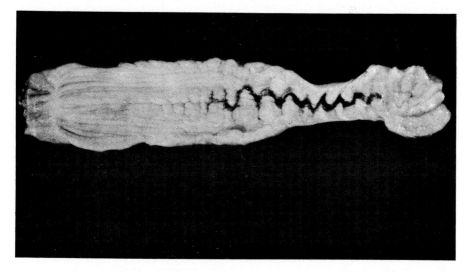

Fig. 10-20. Longitudinal section through the vagina and uterine cervix of a sow. The curved course of the cervical canal is stained. (Aamdal, J.: *In* The Artificial Insemination of Farm Animals. 3rd ed., edited by E. J. Perry. New Brunswick, New Jersey, Rutgers University Press, 1960.)

A plastic pipette is passed dorso-cranially into the vagina of the bitch to the external cervical os. Intracervical or intrauterine insemination via the vagina is nearly impossible. The semen is slowly injected, followed by elevation of the bitch's hindquarters for 5 minutes. Elevation helps prevent the premature loss of semen from the vaginal tract. Vaginal stimulation with a gloved finger may aid in the transport of semen into the uterus via genital contractions and altering vaginal pressures.

The use of transvaginal insemination with frozen semen has produced extremely erratic results in conception rate and litter size. The most consistent results are obtained through surgical interuterine insemination of frozen semen containing 100×10^6 spermatozoa.

Feline

The queen is inseminated vaginally with a minimum of 5×10^6 spermatozoa. The insemination pipette is passed through the vagina to the area of the cervix, and the insemination dose is expelled. The time of breeding coincides with the maximum hypertrophy of the vaginal epithelial cells. Consequently, a vaginal wash is performed to check that the queen is in estrus prior to insemination.

After insemination, the queen must be given LH or human chorionic gonadotrophin to induce ovulation.

Avian

The recommended insemination dose of neat semen is 0.1 ml for chickens and 0.025 ml for turkeys with a minimum of 300×10^6 spermatozoa. The vagina of the hen is everted, the inseminating syringe is inserted to a depth of about 3 cm and the semen is deposited (Fig. 10-21). Pressure on the abdomen is released and the vagina is allowed to retract. The inseminator gently blows on the vent to induce rhythmic contractions of the vaginal wall. Late afternoon is the recommended time for insemination in order to avoid the presence of a hard-shelled egg in the uterus.

Insemination is repeated at weekly intervals in chickens and every 2 to 3 weeks in turkeys. The inseminated sperm enter the utero-vaginal host gland where it is stored and released over time, providing the capability for 1 to 3 weeks of normal fertilization. Semen may last longer than the period recommended between breedings; however, the fertility level begins to decline. Inseminating equipment is depicted in Figure 10-22.

AGING OF GAMETES

The physiology described in other chapters on neural, endocrine and behavioral patterns for a particular species provide for the successful union of male and female gametes. The female must be in the proper stage of her estrous cycle and sufficient semen must be deposited at the correct time.

Semen in the domestic species must have adequate time to undergo capacitation within the female reproductive tract in order to be capable of fertilization. In addition the ovum has only a limited lifespan within the oviduct during which it can be fertilized (Table 10-4).

Any influence which disrupts the normal patterns can prevent conception. This is a factor of importance when using AI since insemination may occur during suboptimal times. The effects of suboptimal timing most commonly are expressed in a lack of conception and a return to estrus by the female. Fertilization may occur, but the embryo may not develop due to the damage of the gametes through aging (Table 10-5).

Timing of inseminations for a female depend on accurate estrous detection or repetitive breedings until ovulation takes place. The disadvantage of repetitive breedings lies in the increased costs of semen and labor in order to obtain conception. Use of synchronization programs, however, for timed breedings invariably have lower conception rates, when compared to natural breeding or insemination after the detection of estrus. In cattle, the animal is in estrus for 12 to 18 hours with the optimum insemination time being 10 to 16 hours after the onset of estrus. The majority of cows begin estrus during the evening hours, making the exact onset difficult to ascertain. Processed bull semen, especially if frozen, has

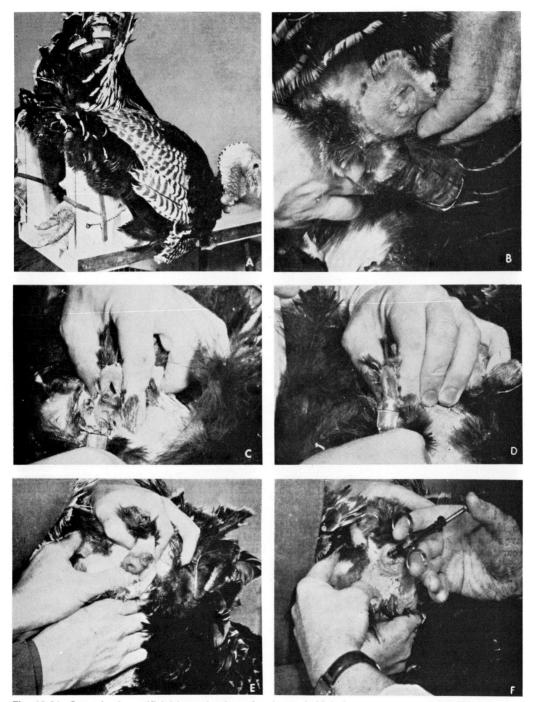

Fig. 10-21. Steps in the artificial insemination of turkeys. *A*, Male is secured on a special stand. As an alternative, the male may be held on a table or other suitable support. *B*, Position of hands for stimulating the ejaculatory reflex in males. *C*, Male is ready to ejaculate: the vent becomes partly everted, revealing the turgid phallic and lymph folds. Massaging should stop. *D*, The semen is being collected into a vial. *E*, Left oviduct of a laying hen is everted with little pressure from below the cloacal region. *F*, After the syringe is inserted into the oviduct, the vagina and the cloaca should be allowed to become withdrawn to their normal position. (From Johnson: Artificial Insemination of Turkeys. Publ. No. 897, 1953. Courtesy Canada Department of Agriculture.)

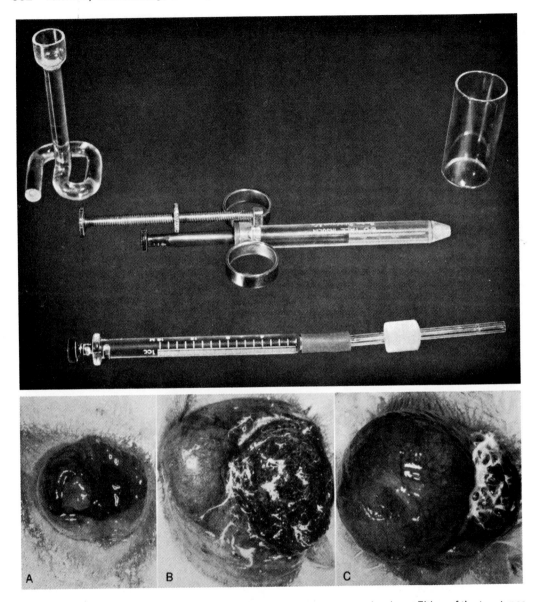

Fig. 10-22. *Top*, Equipment used in artificial insemination of chickens and turkeys. Either of the two types of beakers should prove to be satisfactory for relatively small flocks. The two types of syringes have specific uses. The nut on the threaded rod and metal grips of upper syringe facilitate delivery of accurate dosage in mass-mated flocks. The detached glass tube on the lower syringe is useful in pedigree breeding: each tube contains semen from an individual male. (From Johnson: Artificial Insemination of Turkeys, 1953. Publ. No. 897. Courtesy Canada Department of Agriculture.)

Bottom, Oviductal occluding plate in turkeys. The establishment of a satisfactory level of fertility in the turkey breeding flock may be delayed or even prevented by presence of oviductal occluding plate in a high proportion of females at the time of the initial mating or AI. This membranous plate, located between the vaginal and the shell-gland portions of the oviduct, forms a physical barrier to the spermatozoa. In the female turkey nearing sexual maturity the plate, at first small and inconspicuous (*A*, light-colored tissue on the left), balloons (*B*), and then finally becomes perforated (*C*) just before the laying of the first egg. (From Harper: Poult. Sci., *42*:482, 1963.)

Table 10-4 Effects of Aging of the Ovum in Cattle

Hours from Ovulation to Insemination	Fertility Observed at 2–4 Days		Fertility Observed at 21–335 Days	
	No. of Cows	% with Fertile Ova	No. of Cows	% with Normal Embryo
2–4	4	75	4	75
6–8	4	75	10	30
9–12	5	60	13	31
14–16	4	25	8	0
18–20	5	40	6	17
22–28	1	0	11	0

From G. R. Barrett: Time of Insemination of Conception Rates in Dairy Cows. Ph.D. Thesis, Univ. of Wisconsin, 1948.

Table 10-5 Influence of Postovulatory Aging of Eggs in the Uterine Tubes on Fertilization and on Embryonic Survival at 25 Days Postinsemination

Estimated Age of Eggs at Fertilization Hours	Fertilized Eggs		Viable Embryos	
	%	± (SE)*	% Survival	± (SE)*
0 (control)	90.8	(4.5)	87.9	(2.9)
4	92.1	(2.7)	72.9	(14.9)
8	94.6	(2.3)	60.5	(13.2)
12	70.3	(7.8)	53.3	(15.7)
16	48.3	(8.4)	27.9	(14.5)
20	50.9	(7.5)	32.3	(15.2)

Adapted from Hunter, R. H. F.: Br. Vet. J. *133*:461, 1977.
*Standard error of the mean.

a shorter lifespan for fertility. Consequently, one bull's semen may work successfully if used 10 hours after the onset of heat, whereas another bull may fertilize the ovum only if used closer to 16 hours after the beginning of estrus.

In the mare, multiple breedings with fresh-extended semen are the rule, owing to the inability to accurately predict the time of ovulation. Consequently, female gamete aging does not appear to be a factor in most cases. Stallion semen is susceptible to extension and particularly storage, and probably does not survive as long in the uterus as fresh spermatozoa. The general result of semen storage for more than 24 hours is lower conception rates.

Similar situations affecting gamete surviv-al exist in the other domestic species.

Improving techniques for estrous detection and predicting ovulation time would enhance the use of the AI in all the domestic species. Improved procedures for semen cryopreservation and insemination are necessary before breeders of the other species will have results comparable to the cattle breeders using AI.

REFERENCES

Disease Control

1. Andersen, J. B. and Warming, M. (1980): Danish legislative measures for the prevention and control of disease transmission through AI in cattle. *In* 9th Int. Cong. Anim. Reprod. and Art. Insem. 16th–20th June 1980, Madrid, Spain. Volume III. p. 228.

2. Back, D. G., Pickett, B. W., Voss, J. L., et al. (1975): Effect of antibacterial agent on the motility of stallion spermatozoa at various storage times, temperatures and dilution ratios. J. Anim. Sci. *41*:137.

3. Bowen, R. A., Howard, T. H., Entwistle, K. W., et al. (1983): Seminal shedding of bluetongue virus in experimentally infected mature bulls. Am. J. Vet. Res. *44*(12):2268.

4. Brickon, R. D., Luedke, A. J., and Walton, T. E. (1980): Bluetongue virus in bovine semen: viral isolation. Am. J. Vet. Res. *41*(3):439.

5. Cameron, R. D. A. (1976): Characteristics of semen changes during Brucella ovis infection in rams. Vet. Rec. *99*:231.

6. Carmichael, L. E. (1976): Canine brucellosis. An annotated review with selected cautionary comments. Theriogenology *6*:105.

7. Doak, G. (1986): CSS Implementation of New Antibiotic Combination. 1986 NAAB Technical Conference, Milwaukee, WI.

8. Dubey, J. P., and Sharma, S. P. (1980): Prolonged excretion of Toxoplasma gondii in semen of goats. Am. J. Vet. Res. *41*(5):794.

9. Hall, C. E., and McEntee, K. (1981): Reduced post-thawing survival of sperm in bulls with mycoplasmal vesiculitis (Mycoplasma bovigenitalium). Cornell Vet. *71*(1):111.

10. Harbi, M. S. M. A., Elhassan, S. M. and Ahmed, M. A. (1983): Isolation and identification of Mycoplasma bovigenitalium from imported semen of bulls. Vet. Rec. *113*(5):114.

11. Hashimoto, K., Kishima, M., Nakano, Y., et al. (1981): Isolation of Ureaplasmas sp. from bovine frozen semen, preputial washings and cervicovaginal mucus. National Institute of Animal Health Quarterly, Japan *21*(4):189.

12. Holzmann, A., Laber, G. and Gumhold, G. (1984): Tiamulin, a new antibiotic for eliminating mycoplasms from bovine serum: Investigations on spermatozal toxicity. Theriogenology *22*:237.

13. Hopkins, S. (1986): Vaccination to Maximize Bovine Fertility. *In*: Current Therapy in Theriogenology. 2nd Ed., Edited by D. Morrow, Philadelphia, W. B. Saunders Co., p. 408.

14. Howard, T. H., Vasquez, L. A. and Amann, R. P. (1982): Antibiotic control of Campylobacter fetus by three extenders of bovine semen. J. Dairy Sci. *65*(8):1596.

15. Humphrey, J. D., Little, P. B., Barnum, D. A., et al. (1982): Occurrence of Haemophilus somnus in bovine semen and in the prepuce of bulls and steers. Can. J. Comp. Med. *46*(2):215.

16. Jurmanova, K., Weznik, Z., Cerna, J., et al. (1983): Demonstration and role of mycoplasms and ureaplasmas in bull semen and the control of mycoplasma infections in bulls. Archiv fur Experimentelle Veterinarmedizin *37*(3):421.

17. Kahrs, R. F., Gibbs, E. P. J., and Larsen, R. E. (1980): Diagnostic techniques for identifying viruses in bovine semen. *In*: Proceedings of the Second International Symposium of Veterinary Laboratory Diagnosticians, June 24–26, 1980, Volume II. Lucerne, Switzerland. p. 274.

18. Kahrs, R. F. and Little, R. C. (1980): Detection of viruses in bovine semen. (Influence of preparative centrifugation on isolation of IBR virus). Proceedings of the Annual Meeting of the American Association of Veterinary Laboratory Technicians *23*: 251.

19. Kaja, R. W. and Olson, C. (1982): Non-infectivity of semen from bulls infected with bovine leukosis virus. Theriogenology *18*(1):107.

20. Kobisch, M. and Goffaux, M. (1980): Isolation of Mycoplasma from boar semen. *In*: Proceedings of the International Pig Veterinary Society Congress. Copenhagen, Denmark, p. 217.

21. Krogh, H. V., Pedersen, K. B. and Blom, E. (1983): Haemophilus somnus in semen from Danish bulls. Vet. Rec. *112*(19):460.

22. LaFaunce, N. A., and McEntee, K. (1982): Experimental Mycoplasma bovis seminal vesiculitis in the bull. Corn. Vet. *72*(2):150.

23. Larsen, A. B., Stalheim, O. H. V., Hughes, D. E., et al. (1981): Mycobacterium paratuberculosis in the semen and genital organs of a semen-donor bull. J. Am. Vet. Med. Assoc. *179*(2):169.

24. Larsen, R. E. and Leman, A. D. (1980): Effect of pseudorabies on semen quality in the boar. *In*: 9th International Congress on Animal Reproduction and Artificial Insemination 16th–20th June 1980, Madrid, Spain. Volume III. p. 224.

25. Larsen, R. E., Shope, R. E. Jr., Leman, A. D., et al. (1980): Semen changes in boars after experimental infection with pseudorabies virus. Am. J. Vet. Res. *41*(5):733.

26. Pursel, V. G., McVicar, J. W., George, A. E., et al. (1980): Guideline for international exchange of swine semen and embryos. *In*: 9th International Congress on Animal Reproduction and Artificial Insemination, 16th–20th June, 1980, Madrid, Spain. Volume II p. 301.

27. Rae, A. G. (1982): Isolation of mycoplasma from bovine semen. Vet. Rec. *111*(20)462.

28. Ramachandra, R. N., Rao, M. S., Raghavan, R. R., et al. (1981): Bacterial load and bacteriological study of frozen bull semen. Ind. J. Comp. Micro. Immun. Infect. Dis. *2*:35.

29. Rideout, M. I., Burns, S. J., and Simpson, R. B. (1982): Influence of bacterial products on the motility of stallion spermatozoa. J. Reprod. Fertil. No. 32, Supplement, 35.

30. Romanowksi, W., Marre, H., and Pfeilsticker, J. (1980): Hygiene at A. I. centers in special consideration of leukosis. *In*: 9th International Congress on Animal Reproduction and Artificial Insemination, 16th–20th June, 1980, Madrid, Spain. Volume III. p. 258.

31. Rutherford, R. N. and Curnock, R. M. (1984): The use of sheep artificial insemination as an aid to the control of scrapie (Abstract). Animal Production *38*(3):547.

32. Schultz, R. D., Adams, L. S., Letchworth, G., et al. (1982): A method to test large number of bovine semen samples for viral contamination and results of a study using this method. Theriogenology *17*(2): 115.

33. Sellers, R. F. (1983): Transmission of viruses by artificial breeding techniques: a review. J. Royal Soc. Med. *76*(9):772.

34. Shin, S. (1986): New Antibiotic Combination for

Controlling Ureaplasma, Mycoplasmas, *Haemophilus somnus, Campylobacter fetus* and Leptospirosis in frozen Bovine Semen. Proc. 11th NAAB Technical Conference.

35. Sone, M., Ohmura, K. and Bamba, K. (1982): Effects of various antibiotics on the control of bacteria in boar semen. Vet. Rec. *111*(1):11.

36. Stalheim, O. H. V. (1980): Standardized procedures for the microbiologic examination of semen. *In*: Proceedings of the Second International Symposium of Veterinary Laboratory Diagnosticians, June 24–26, 1980, Volume II. Lucerne, Switzerland p. 306.

37. Storz, J., Carroll, E. J., Stephenson, E. H., et al. (1976): Urogenital infection and seminal excretion after inoculation of bulls and rams with chlamydiae. Am. J. Vet. Res. *37*:517.

38. Truscott, R. B. (1983): Factors associated with the determination of antibiotic activity in bovine semen. Can. J. Comp. Med. *47*(4):480.

39. Wierzbowski, S., Nowakowski, W., Furowicz, A., et al. (1980): Biochemical and toxic properties of potentially pathogenic microorganisms isolated from bull semen. *In*: 9th International Congress on Animal Reproduction and Artificial Insemination, 16th–20th June 1980, Madrid, Spain. Volume III. Madrid, Spain.

40. Wierzbowski, S., Nowakowski, W. Furowicz, A., et al. (1980): The biological value of bull semen having staphylococcal and blue pus bacillus. *In*: 9th International Congress on Animal Reproduction and Artificial Insemination, 16th–20th June 1980, Madrid, Spain. Volume III. p. 222.

Collection of Semen

41. Almquist, J. D., Branas, R. J., and Barber, K. A. (1976): Post-puberal changes in semen production of charolais bulls ejaculated at high frequency and the relation between testicular measurements and sperm output. J. Anim. Sci. *42*:670.

42. Ball, L. (1976): Electroejaculation. *In*: Applied Electronics for Veterinary Medicine and Animal Physiology, edited by W. R. Klemm. Springfield, Charles C Thomas, p. 394.

43. Ball, L., Ott, R. S., Mortimer, R. G., et al. (1983): Manual for breeding soundness examination of bulls. J. Soc. Theriogenology *12*:1983.

44. Bongso, T. A., Jainudeen, M. R. and Zahrah, S. (1982): Relationship of scrotal circumference to age, body weight and spermatogenesis in goats. Theriogenology *18*:513.

45. Braun, W.F., Thompson, J. M. and Ross, C. V. (1980): Ram scrotal circumference measurements. Theriogenology *13*:221.

46. Cameron, R. D. A. (1977): Semen collection and evaluation in the ram: The preparation of spermatozoa for morphological examination. Australian Vet. J. *53*:384.

47. Cooper, D. M. (1963): Modern trends in animal health and husbandry. Artificial insemination of poultry. Br. Vet. J. *119*:194.

48. DeSilva, P. L. G. (1963): Artificial insemination in the fowl. 2. Technique of insemination. Ceylon Vet. J. *11*:13.

49. Dowsett, K. F., and Pattie, W. A. (1980): Collection of semen from stallions at stud. Aust. Vet. J. *56*(8):373.

50. Elmore, R. G., Bierschwal, C. J. and Youngquist, R. S. (1976): Scrotal circumference measurements in 764 beef bulls. Theriogenology *6*:485.

51. Foote, R. H. (1974): Artificial insemination. *In*: Reproduction in Farm Animals, 3rd ed., edited by E. S. E. Hafez. Philadelphia, Lea & Febiger, p. 409.

52. Hillman, R. B., Olar, T. T., Squires, R. L., et al. (1980): Temperature of the artificial vagina and its effect on seminal quality and behavioral characteristics of stallions. J. Am. Vet. Med. Assoc. *177*(8): 720.

53. Kumi-Diaka, J., Nagaratnam, V., and Rwuaan, J. S. (1980): Seasonal and age-related changes in semen quality and testicular morphology of bulls in a tropical environment. Vet. Rec. *198*(1):13.

54. Morrow, D. (1980): Breeding soundness evaluation in bulls. *In*: Current Therapy in Theriogenology, edited by D. Morrow. Philadelphia, W. B. Saunders Co., p. 330.

55. Ott, R. S. (1986): Breeding soundness examination of bulls. *In*: Current Therapy in Theriogenology, Vol. 2, edited by D. Morrow. Philadelphia, W. B. Saunders Co., p. 125.

56. Ott, R. S., and Menon, M. A. (1980): Breeding soundness examination of rams and bucks. A review. Theriogenology *13*:155.

57. Pickett, B. W., and Back, D. G. (1973): Procedures for preparation, collection, evaluation and insemination of stallion semen. Colorado State Univ. Exp. Sta. and Anim. Reprod. Lab. Gen. Ser. 935.

58. Pickett, B. W. and Back, D. G. (1973): Procedures for preparation, collection, evaluation, and insemination of stallion semen. Information Series No. 2-1, Animal Reproduction Lab., Colorado State University, Ft. Collins, pp. 3, 14, 22.

59. Pickett, B.W., Gebauer, M. R., Seidel, G. E., Jr., et al. (1974): Reproductive physiology of the stallion: spermatozoal losses in the collection equipment and gel. J. Am. Vet. Med. Assoc. *165*:708.

60. Pineda, M. H. (1977): A simple method for collection of semen from dogs. Canine Pract. *4*:14.

61. Platz, C. C., Follis, T., Demorest, N., et al. (1976): Semen collection, freezing and insemination in the domestic cat. Proc. 8th Int. Cong. Anim. Reprod. Art. Insem., *4*:1053.

62. Platz, C. C., Wildt, D. E., and Seager, S. W. J. (1978): Pregnancy in the domestic cat after artificial insemination with previously frozen spermatozoa. J. Reprod. Fertil. *52*:279.

63. Seager, S. W. J., and Fletcher, W. S. (1973): Progress on the use of frozen semen in the dog. Vet. Rec. *92*:6.

64. Tischner, M., Kosiniak, K., and Bielanski, W. (1974): Analysis of the pattern of ejaculation in stallions. J. Reprod. Fertil. *41*:329.

65. Woodard, A. E., Ogasawara, F. X., Abplanalp, H., et al. (1976): Effect of semen dose, frequency of insemination, age, and productivity of the male on duration and levels of fertility and hatchability in the turkey. Poult. Sci. *55*:1367.

Analysis of Semen

66. Bielanski, W. (1975): The evaluation of stallion semen in aspects of fertility control and its use for artificial insemination. J. Reprod. Fertil. Suppl. *23*:19.
67. Brotherton, J. (1975): The counting and sizing of spermatozoa from ten animal species using a coulter counter. Andrologia *7*:169.
68. Brown, K. I., and Graham, E. F. (1971): Effect of semen quality on fertility in turkeys. Poult. Sci. *50*:295.
69. Buckland, R. B. (1971): Comparison of chicken semen diluents and evaluation of various methods of estimating fertility. Can. J. Anim. Sci. *51*:252.
70. Cochran, R. C., Judy, J. K., Parker, C. F., et al. (1985): Prefreezing and post thaw semen characteristics of five ram breeds collected by electroejaculation. Theriogenology *23*:431.
71. Dott, H. M. (1975): Morphology of stallion spermatozoa. J. Reprod. Fertil. Suppl. *23*:41.
72. Dott, H. M. and Foster, G. C. (1975): Preservation of differential staining of spermatozoa by formol citrate. J. Reprod. Fertil. *45*:57.
73. Dowsett, K. F., Osborne, H. G. and Pattie, W. A. (1984): Morphological characteristics of stallion spermatozoa. Theriogenology *22*:463.
74. Dowsett, K. F. and Pattie, W. A. (1982): Stallion semen characteristics and fertility. J. Reprod. Fertil. Suppl. *32*:1.
75. Gibson, C. D. (1983): Clinical evaluation of the boar for breeding soundness: physical examination and semen morphology. Comp. Cont. Educ. Pract. Vet. *5*(5): S244.
76. Hammitt, D. (1985): The relationship between heterospermic fertility *in vivo* and *in vitro* tests of spermatozoan quality and function. Ph.D. Thesis, Iowa State University, Ames.
77. Harasymowycz, J., Ball, L., and Seidel, G. E., Jr. (1976): Evaluation of bovine spermatozoal morphologic features after staining or fixation. Am. J. Vet. Res. *37*:1053.
78. Hulet, C. V. (1977): Prediction of fertility in rams: Factors affecting fertility, and collection, testing and evaluation of semen. Vet. Med./Small Anim. Clin. *72*:1363.
79. Johnson, L., Berndtson, W. E., and Pickett, B. W. (1976): An improved method for evaluating acrosomes of bovine spermatozoa. J. Anim. Sci. *42*:951.
80. Linford, E., Glover, F. A., Bishop, C., et al. (1976): The relationship between semen evaluation methods and fertility in the bull. J. Reprod. Fertil. *47*:283.
81. Makler, A. (1980): The improved 10 mm chamber for rapid sperm count and motility evaluation. Fertil. Steril. *33*:337.
82. Makler, A., Fisher, M., and Lissak, A. (1984): A new method for rapid determination of sperm concentration in bull and ram semen. Theriogenology *21*:543.
83. Pickett, B. W., Sullivan, J. J., and Seidel, G. E., Jr. (1975): Reproductive physiology of the stallion. V. Effect of frequency of ejaculation on seminal characteristics and spermatozoal output. J. Anim. Sci. *40*:917.

84. Pickett, B. W., Voss, J. L. and Squires, E. L. (1983): Factors affecting quality and quantity of stallion spermatozoa. Comp. Cont. Educ. for the Pract. Vet. *5*(5):S259.
85. Swierstra, E. E. (1973): Influence of breed, age, and ejaculation frequency on boar semen composition. Can. J. Anim. Sci. *53*:43.
86. Taha, M. B., Noakes, D. E. and Allen, W. E. (1983): The effect of the frequency of ejaculation on seminal characteristics and libido in the Beagle dog. J. Sm. An. Pract. *24*(5):309.
87. Taha, M. B., Noakes, D. E. and Allen, W. E. (1981): The effect of season of the year on characteristics and composition of dog semen. J. Sm. Anim. Pract. *22*(4):177.
88. Voss, J. L., Pickett, B. W., and Squires, E. L. (1981): Stallion spermatozoal morphology and motility and their relationship to fertility. J. Am. Vet. Med. Assoc. *178*:287.
89. White, I. G. (1974): Mammalian semen. *In*: Reproduction in Farm Animals, 3rd ed., edited by E. S. E. Hafez. Philadelphia, Lea & Febiger, p. 101.

Semen Extension and Cryopreservation

90. Almquist, J. O. and Rosenberger, J. L. (1979): Effect of thawing time in warm water on fertility of bovine spermatozoa in plastic straws. J. Dairy Sci. *62*:772.
91. Berndtson, W. E. and Pickett, B. W. (1980): Evaluation of frozen semen. *In*: Current therapy in Theriogenology, edited by D. A. Morrow. Philadelphia, W. B. Saunders Co., p. 347.
92. Brown, J. L., Senger, P. L. and Hillers, J. K. (1982): Influence of thawing time and post-thaw temperature on acrosomal maintenance and motility of bovine spermatozoa frozen in .5-ml french straws. J. Anim. Sci. *54*:938.
93. Cochran, J. D., Amann, R. P., Froman, D. P., et al. (1984): Effects of centrifugation, glycerol level, cooling to 5°C freezing rate and thawing rate on the post-thaw motility of equine sperm. Theriogenology *22*:25.
94. Colas, G. (1975): Effect of initial freezing temperature, addition of glycerol and dilution on the survival and fertilizing ability of deep frozen ram semen. J. Reprod. Fertil. *42*:277.
95. Cristanelli, M. J., Squires, E. L., Amann, R. P. et al. (1984): Fertility of stallion semen processed, frozen and thawed by a new procedure. Theriogenology *22*:39.
96. Darin-Bannett, A. and White, I. G. (1977): Influence of cholesterol content of mammalian spermatozoa on susceptibility to cold shock. Cryobiology *14*:466.
97. DeAbreu, R. M., Berndtson, W. E., Smith, R. L., et al. (1979): Effect of post-thaw warming on viability of bovine spermatozoa thawed at different rates in french straws. J. Dairy Sci. *62*:1449.
98. Drobnis, E. Z., Nelson, E. A., and Burrill, M. J. (1980): Effect of several processing variables on motility and GOT levels for frozen goat semen. Proc. Western Section, Am. Soc. Anim. Sci. J. Anim. Sci. Suppl 1, *51*:439.
99. Entwistle, K.W. and Martin, I. C. A. (1972): Effects

of the number of spermatozoa and of volume of diluted semen on fertility in the ewe. Australian J. Agr. Res. *23*:467.

100. Graham, E. F., Crabo, B. G. and Brown, K. I. (1971): Effect of some zwitter ion buffers on the freezing and storage of spermatozoa 1. Bull. J. Dairy Sci. *55*:372.

101. Holt, W. V., and North, R. D. (1985): Determination of lipid composition and thermal phase transition temperature in an enriched plasma membrane fraction from ram spermatozoa. J. Reprod. Fertil. *73*:285.

102. Larsson, K. (1978): Deep-freezing of boar semen. Cryobiology *15*:352.

103. Lee, A. G. (1977): Lipid phase transitions. Biochimica et Biophysica Acta *472*:237.

104. Loomis, P. R., Amann, R. P., Squires, E. L., et al. (1983): Ferility of stallion spermatozoa frozen in EDTA-lactose egg yolk extender and packaged in 0.5 ml straw. J. Anim. Sci. *56*:687.

105. Lundgren, B. (1980): Influence of long term storage on fertility of deep frozen bull semen. Nordisk Vet. *32*(10):427.

106. Moore, H. D. M., and Hibbitt, K. G. (1977): Fertility of boar spermatozoa after freezing in the absence of seminal vesicular proteins. J. Reprod. Fertil. *50*:349.

107. Morris, G. R., Burtan, L. J. and Pitt, C. J. (1984): Sperm losses during deep-freeze processing of bull semen. Theriogenology *21*:1001.

108. Pace, M. M. and Sullivan, J. J. (1978): A biological comparison of the 0.5-ml ampule and 0.5-ml French straw for packaging bovine spermatozoa. Proc. 7th NAAB Tech. Conf. Artif. Insemin. Reprod. p. 22.

109. Pickett, B. W. and Voss, J. L. (1975): The effect of semen extenders and sperm number on mare fertility. J. Reprod. Fertil. Suppl. *23*:95.

110. Pistenma, D. A., Snapir, N. and Mel, H. C. (1971): Biophysical characterization of fowl spermatozoa. I. Preservation of motility and fertilizing capacity under conditions of low temperature and low sperm concentrations. J. Reprod. Fertil. *24*:153.

111. Province, C. A., Amann, R. P., Pickett, B. W., et al. (1984): Extenders for the preservation of canine and equine spermatozoa at 5°C. Theriogenology *22*: 409.

112. Quinn, P. J. (1981): The fluidity of cell membranes and its regulation. Prog. Biophy. Molec. Biol. *38*:1.

113. Robbins, R. K., Saacke, R. G. and Chandler, P. T. (1976): Influence of freeze rate, thaw rate and glycerol level on acrosomal retention and survival of bovine spermatozoa frozen in french straws. J. Anim. Sci. *42*:145.

114. Rodriguez, O. L., Berndtson, W. E., Ennen, B.D., et al. (1975): Effects of the rates of freezing, thawing and level of glycerol on the survival of bovine spermatozoa in straws. J. Anim. Sci. *41*:129.

115. Saacke, R. G. (1982): What happens when a sperm is frozen and thawed? Proc. 9th Technical Conference on Artif. Insem. and Reprod. p. 6.

116. Salamon, S., and Visser, D. (1974): Fertility of ram spermatozoa frozen-stored for 5 years. J. Reprod. Fertil. *37*:433.

117. Senger, P. L., Becker, W.C. and Hillers, J. K. (1976): Effect of thawing rate and post-thaw temperature on

motility and acrosomal maintenance in bovine semen frozen in plastic straws. J. Anim. Sci. *42*:932.

118. Senger, P. L., Mitchell, J. R., and Almquist, J. O. (1982): Freezing semen—comparing the .25 and .5 ml french straws. Proc. 9th Technical Conference on Artif. Insem. Reprod. p. 32.

119. Senger, P. L., Mitchell, J. R. and Almquist, J. O. (1983): Influence of cooling rates and extenders upon post-thaw viability of bovine spermatozoa packaged in .25 and .5 ml french straws. J. Anim. Sci. *56*:1261.

120. Shinitizky, M. (1984): Physiology of Membrane Fluidity. Vol. 1. Boca Raton, Florida, CRC Press.

121. Smith, F. (1984): Update in freezing canine semen. Proc. Soc. Therio. Sept. 26–28, Denver, CO.

122. Sullivan, J. J. (1978): Characteristics and cryopreservation of stallion spermatozoa. Cryobiology *15*: 355.

123. White, I. G. and Darin-Bennett, A. (1976): The lipids of sperm in relation to cold shock. VIII International Congress on Animal Reproduction and Artificial Insemination, Cracow, p. 951.

124. Wilmut, I., and Polge, C. (1977): The low temperature preservation of boar spermatozoa. 1. The motility and morphology of boar spermatozoa frozen and thawed in the presence of permeating protective agents. Cryobiology *14*:471.

125. Wilmut, I., and Polge, C. (1977): The low temperature preservation of boar spermatozoa. 2. The motility and morphology of boar spermatozoa frozen and thawed in diluent which contained only sugar and egg yolk. Cryobiology *14*:479.

126. Wilmut, I., and Polge, C. (1977): The low temperature preservation of boar spermatozoa. 3. The fertilizing capacity of frozen and thawed boar semen. Cryobiology *14*:483.

Insemination Procedures

127. Asbury, A. C. (1984): Uterine defense mechanisms in the mare: The use of intrauterine plasma in the management of endometritis. Theriogenology *21*: 387.

128. Ball, G. D., Leibfried, M. L., Lenz, R. W., et al. (1983): Factors affecting successful *in vitro* fertilization of bovine follicular oocytes. Biol. Reprod. *28*:717.

129. Berndtson, W. E. and Pickett, B. W. (1980): Factors affecting fertility: artificial insemination program for beef cattle. Bov. Pract. *1*(3):35.

130. Berndtson, W. E., Pickett, B. W. and Rugg, C. D. (1976): Procedures for field handling of bovine semen in plastic straws. Proc. 6th NAAB Tech. Conf. Artif. Insem. Reprod. p. 51.

131. Brackett, B. G., Keefer, C. L., Troop, C. G., et al. (1984): Bovine twins resulting from *in vitro* fertilization. Theriogenology *21*:224.

132. Bristol, F. (1981): Studies on estrous synchronization in mares. Proc. Soc. Theriogenology p. 258.

133. Chenoweth, P. J., Spitzer, J. C. and Ramge, J. C. (1980): Beef cattle breeding programs employing synchronization of estrus and artificial insemination. Southwestern Vet. *33*(1):31.

134. Cooper, W. L. (1980): Artificial breeding of horses. Vet. Clin. North Am., Large An. Pract. *2*(2):267.

135. Critser, E. S., Leibfried, M. L. and First, N. L.

(1984): The effect of semen extension, cAMP and caffeine on *in vitro* fertilization of bovine oocytes. Theriogenology *21*:625.

136. DeSilva, P. L. G. (1962): Artificial insemination of poultry. 1. Collection of semen from the cock. Ceylon Vet. J. *10*:124.

137. Douglas-Hamilton, D. H., Osol, R., Osol, G., et al. (1984): A field study of the fertility of transported equine semen. Theriogenology *22*:291.

138. Edwards, D. F., and Azzinbud, E. (1980): Bibliography on the timing of artificial insemination in cattle, sheep and pigs by measurement of vaginal conductivity (1962–1980). Bibliography Reprod. *36*(5):425, 549.

139. Evans, J. W. (1982): Breeding management and foal development. Equine Research, Tyler, Texas.

140. Gomez, W. R. (1977): Artificial insemination. *In*: Reproduction in Domestic Animals, 3rd ed., edited by H. H. Cole and P. T. Cupps, New York, Academic Press, Inc. p. 257.

141. Hughes, J. P., and Loy, R. P. (1970): A. I. in the equine. Cornell Vet. *60*:463.

142. Hunter, R. H. F. (1977): Physiological factors influencing ovulation, fertilization, early embryonic development and establishment of pregnancy in pigs. Br. Vet. J. *133*:461.

143. Kenney, R. M., Bergman R. V., Cooper, W. L., et al. (1975): Minimal contamination techniques for breeding mares: Technique and preliminary findings. Proc. Am. Assoc. Equine Pract. 327.

144. Morcom, C. B. and Dukelow, W. R. (1980): A research technique for the oviductal insemination of pigs using laparoscopy. Lab. An. Sci. *30*(6):1030.

145. Ott. R. S. (1981): Use of a teaser bull in a beef cattle artificial insemination program. J. Am. Vet. Med. Assoc. *179*(7):694.

146. Park, Y. W., and Hunter, A. G. (1977): Effect of repeated inseminations with egg yolk semen extender on fertility in cattle. J. Dairy Sci. *60*:1645.

147. Pickett, B. W., and Back, D. G. (1973): Procedures for Preparation, Collection, Evaluation, and Insemination of Stallion Semen. Information Series No. 2-1, Animal Reproduction Lab, Colorado State University, Ft. Collins, p. 19.

148. Rossdale, P. D., and Ricketts, S. W. (1980): The Stallion. *In*: Equine Stud Farm Medicine, 2nd Ed. London, Bailliere Tindall, p. 158.

149. Schams, D., Schallenberger, E., Hoffman, B., et al. (1977): The oestrous cycle of the cow: Hormonal parameters and time relationships concerning oestrus, ovulation and electrical resistance of the vaginal mucus. Acta Endocrinol. *86*:180.

150. Schindler, H., and Amir, D. (1973): The conception rate of ewes in relation to sperm dose and time of insemination. J. Reprod. Fertil. *34*:191.

151. Seager, S. W. J., and Platz, C. C. (1977): Artificial insemination and frozen semen in the dog. Vet. Clin. North Am. *7*:757.

152. Seager, S. W. J., Platz, C. C., and Fletcher, W. S. (1975): Conception rates and related data using frozen dog semen. J. Repro. Fertil. *45*:18.

153. Smith, R. D. (1986): Estrous Detection. *In*: Current Therapy in Theriogenology, 2nd Ed. Edited by D. Morrow. Philadelphia, W. B. Saunders Co., p. 153.

154. Stover, D. G., and Sokolowksi, J. H. (1978): Estrous behavior of the domestic cat. Feline Practice *8*:54.

155. Sturman, H., Bakhar, A. and Smuel, Z. B. (1980): The rate of incidence and damage caused by insemination of cows not in estrus in large dairy herds in Israel. In 9th International Congress on Animal Reproduction and Artificial Insemination, 16th–20th June 1980, Madrid, Spain, Volume III. p. 236.

156. Takeda, K., Sone, M. and Bamba, K. (1981): Two-step insemination apparatus for pigs. Vet. Rec. *108*(7):146.

157. Watson, E. D. and MacDonald, B. J. (1984): Failure of conception in dairy cattle: progesterone and oestradiol-17B concentration and the presence of ovarian follicles in relation to the timing of artificial insemination. Br. Vet. J. *149*(4):398.

158. Wenkoff, M. (1986): Estrous Synchronization in Cattle, In: Current Therapy in Theriogenology, 2nd Ed. Edited by D. Morrow. Philadelphia, W. B. Saunders Co.

159. Williams, J. K. and Evans L. E. (1983): Estrous synchronization and artificial insemination in sows: a field study. I. S. U. Vet. *45*(1):29.

160. Woodard, A. E., and Abplanalp, H. (1975): The effects of three systems of housing turkey breeder males on semen quality and quantity. Poult. Sci. *54*:872.

Gamete Aging

161. Austin, C. R. (1975): Sperm fertility, viability and persistence in the female tract. J. Reprod. Fertil., Suppl. *22*:75.

162. Longo, F. J. and So, F. (1982): Transformations of sperm nuclei incorporated into aged and unaged hamster eggs. J. Androl. *3*:420.

163. Vander Vliet, W. L. and Hafez, E. S. E. (1974): Survival and aging of spermatozoa: A review. Am. J. Obstet. Gynecol. *118*:1006.

Patterns of Reproduction

L. E. MCDONALD

11

THERE are great variations in the patterns of reproduction of animals. Table 11-1 summarizes some pertinent facts concerning reproductive patterns of the common domestic animals, laboratory animals and exotic animals. It is felt that a detailed description of the reproductive patterns of cattle, horses, sheep, swine, dogs, and cats is necessary. Chapters 12 through 17 will deal with the reproductive patterns of these 6 species. This chapter treats the interspecies information (Table 11-2).

Reproductive patterns of animals in their natural environments differ greatly from those of highly domesticated animals which have become accustomed to a protected environment. The reproductive pattern of the animal under natural conditions, far removed from a domestic environment, tends toward *a pattern by which the young are delivered at the time of the year when temperature and feed are optimal.* Thus parturition in the temperate zone is usually early in the growing season so the young can mature as much as possible before adverse changes occur in climate or feed supply. At the other extreme are those animals which have been privileged to enjoy domestication and selection for many generations in a protected environment where shortages of feed or severe climatic changes do not occur. An example of the latter is the domestic cow.

BREEDING SEASONS

All females show seasonal cyclic changes in ovarian activity, but it is the degree of ovarian activity or inactivity which is influenced by the environment. Restricted breeding seasons are the more natural state for all animals except those whose natural habitat is the tropics. Loss of breeding season tendencies is really a response of the animal to its association with man. Since this loss of response to the seasons can sometimes adversely affect fertility, we must remain cognizant of those factors which elicit the seasonal response. Some of these factors are length of daylight, temperature, nutrition, presence of the other sex (pheromones), and several other environmental factors.

The cat, mink, ferret, and skunk are seasonal breeders, coming into estrus only at a certain time of the year. This time of estrus, to which is added the gestation period, allows delivery of the young at an optimal time of the year. These animals also have another unusual safeguard in their reproductive patterns, since under wild conditions the male and female may not come into contact at frequent intervals for purposes of copulation.

389

Table 11-1   Summary of Female Reproductive Patterns

	Puberty (months)	Estrous Cycle Length (days)	Estrus Duration (days)	Ovulation Time in Relation to Estrus	Gestation Length (days)	Litter Size Average	Breeding Season (Northern Hemisphere)	(Southern Hemisphere)	
Antelope, roan					300	1	nonseasonal		
Ass, donkey	12	21–28	2–7	last ⅓	365	1	Mar.–Aug.	Oct.–Apr.	Foal heat 2–8 days postdelivery.
Badger, Am.	12–24				variable	1–5	Aug.–Sept.		Breed Aug.–Sept., implant Feb., deliver April.
Bear, N. Am. black	36				ca. 210	1–4			Breed June, implant Nov., deliver Jan.–Feb.
Beaver, Am.	24				ca. 90	1–6	Jan.–Feb.		Nonseasonal in captivity.
Bison, Am. buffalo	24	21	2		270	1	Jul.–Sept.		Seasonal polyestrus.
Bobcat					50	1–6	Feb.–Apr.		Polyestrus. Foal heat 1 day postdelivery.
Camel, two-humped					406	1		nonseasonal	
Cat, domestic	7–12	10–20	1–7 / 4 w male / 9–10 wo male	24–48 hr. postcoitus	63	4–5	Spring-fall		Seasonal, induced ovulation. Sterile coitus gives pseudopregnancy.
Chimpanzee	8–11				227	1		nonseasonal	Menstruation 4 days at beginning of 34-day cycle. Ovulate day 16.
Chinchilla		24	2		111	1–4		nonseasonal	12 hr. postparturient estrus.
Chipmunk, western	12				31	4–8	April		Eastern chipmunk is polyestrus, March–Aug.
Cattle, domestic	6–18	21	½	12–16 hr. after	280	1		nonseasonal	Right ovary sheds 60% ova.
Coyote, northern	24				63	6	Feb.–Apr.		Variable gestation due to delayed implantation. Same as for Va. deer.
Deer, mule	12–24	ca. 28	4		204	1–2	Oct.–Nov.		
Dog	6–12		7–9	first ⅓	58–63	ca. 1–8	Spring-fall		Pseudopregnancy for 2 mo. if not pregnant Monestrus.
Elephant, African	96–144	42	3–4		660	1		nonseasonal	Jan.–Feb. main breeding season. Indian elephant similar.
Elk, moose	16–24	30			245	1–2	Sept.–Oct.		
Ferret				30 hr. postcoitus first ½	42	5–13	Mar.–Aug.		Pseudopregnancy follows sterile coitus.
Fox, red or silver	12–14		2–4		52	4–5	Dec.–Mar.		No estrus during lactation. Pseudopregnancy follows sterile coitus. Monestrus.
Giraffe	36	14			435	1	Jul.–Sept.		Some report nonseasonal.
Gnu, wildebeest	36				250		Mar.		
Goat, domestic	4–8	21	1–3		150	1–3	Sept.–Nov.		Seasonal polyestrus.
Gorilla	60	45			258				
Ground hog, woodchuck	24				32	4	Feb.–Mar.		
Guinea pig	2	16½	½	last ¼	67	0–4		nonseasonal	Laboratory G P is polyestrus, nonseasonal.
Hamster	2	4	1	last ½	21	6–12	nonseasonal in lab		Pseudopregnancy follows sterile coitus.
Hippopotamus	48	30	4–7		237	1–2		nonseasonal	

Species								
Horse	20		7	last 1/3	330	1	Mar.–Aug.	Seasonal polyestrus.
Hyena					210	2–4		Nonseasonal in zoo.
Jaguar	22				100	1–2	Aug.–Sept.	Nonseasonal in zoo.
Kangaroo, gray					38	1	Sept.–Jan.	
Leopard					90	2–4	nonseasonal	Polyestrus.
Lion	40	21	7		108	2–4	nonseasonal	Nonseasonal in zoo.
Llama					330	1–2	Spring-fall	
Marmot			1/2		33	7	Apr.	
Mink	10			40–50 hr. postcoitus	45–70	4–5	Mar.	Delayed implantation. Induced ovulation. Seasonal Polyestrus.
Mole, Am.	12			postcoitus	28	4	Feb.–Mar.	Induced ovulation. Vagina closed until estrus.
Monkey, S. Am. spider					139	1–2	nonseasonal	Menstruation 4 days beginning of 25-day cycle.
Mouse, lab.	32	4–6		first 1/3		5–6		Pseudopregnancy follows sterile coitus. Nonseasonal in South. Some report 29-day estrus cycle.
Muskrat		3–5			29	6–7	Apr.–Jul.	
Opossum, common Va.	6	28	1–2	first 1/2	12	5–13	Jan.–Nov.	Two litters/yr. in South. Young born immature.
Panda					90	1–2	Dec.–Jan.	
Pig, domestic	5–10	21	2–3	last 1/2	114	4–14	nonseasonal	Frequently postpartum nonovulatory estrus.
Porcupine, N. Am.	14				112	1	Nov.	
Porpoise	12				315	1	Jul.–Aug.	
Prairie dog					30	5–6	Jan.–Apr.	
Rabbit, domestic lab.	5–8		somewhat continuous	10 hr. postcoitus	31	2–10	nonseasonal	Pseudopregnancy (16 day) following sterile coitus. Induced ovulation.
Rabbit, cottontail	10				30	2–7	Jan.–Aug.	Several litters/year.
Raccoon	10	4–6	3	postcoitus	63	3–4	Jan.–Mar.	Induced ovulation.
Rat, lab. albino	1–2		1	last 1/3	21	7–9	nonseasonal	Inactive corpus l. unless coitus. Pseudopregnancy follows sterile coitus.
Reindeer, caribou	18				225	1	Sept.–Oct.	Monestrus.
Rhinoceros, black Afr.					540	1	nonseasonal	
Sheep, bighorn	28				180	1–3	Nov.–Dec.	Breeds mostly Nov.–Dec.
Sheep, domestic Eng.	6–12	16 1/2	1 1/2	last 1/2	150	1–3	Aug.–Nov.	Mediterranean breeds nonseasonal polyestrus.
Skunk	10				62	4–7	Mar.	
Squirrel, Am. red	10–20				40	3–6	Feb.–Jul.	Canada 1 litter, U.S. 2 litters/yr.
Tiger	50				113	2–5	nonseasonal	
Walrus					330	1	June	
Whale, sperm					500	1	Feb.–June Aug.–Dec.	
Wolf	24				61	2–7	Jan.–Mar.	
Wolverine	24					2–4	Apr.–Oct.	Implantation delayed several months.
Zebra					345	1	Jul.–Sept.	

Adapted from Asdell, S. A.: Patterns of Mammalian Reproduction, 2nd. ed. Ithaca, N. Y., Comstock-Cornell Press, 1964.

Table 11-2   Estrous Cycle Normal Values

Species	Length of Cycle (days)	Duration of Heat or Estrus	Ovulation Type	Ovulation Time
Cow	21	14–18 hr.	Spontaneous	12–16 hr. after *end* of estrus
Mare	19–23	4–7 days	Spontaneous	Last 2 days of estrus
Sow	21	2–3 days	Spontaneous	Last day of estrus
Ewe	16	1–2 days	Spontaneous	Last day of estrus
Bitch	2–3 estrous periods per year	7–9 days	Spontaneous	First 1–3 days of estrus
Cat	2–3 estrous periods per year	4 days with male if copulation 9–10 days without male	Induced	One day after mating No ovulation if no copulation

Therefore, these species have developed the mechanism of *induced ovulation* and have retained it despite domestication attempts (Table 11-3). Wastage of ova is thereby prevented, since ovulation awaits copulation. During the nonbreeding season the ovaries are quiescent, and the animal is in *anestrus.*

Other species, such as the mare and ewe (English breeds), have a breeding season which likewise favors delivery of the young at the optimal time of the year. These species show several estrous cycles (polyestrus) during the breeding season if pregnancy does not interrupt, but the breeding season is limited to such length that the animal usually delivers the young in the spring of the year. The bitch usually has one to three breeding seasons, but the season that is most frequently the productive one is late winter, thereby causing the young to be born in the spring of the year. The bitch has only one estrous cycle with each breeding season; consequently she is *seasonally monestrus.*

Many years of protective environments under highly domesticated conditions have permitted the cow and sow to disregard the effects of seasons on their breeding patterns. Likewise, the Mediterranean breeds of sheep are nonseasonal breeders, but this pattern is probably associated with the mild climate in which the breeds have developed. These animals are not seasonal breeders, although peaks of reproductive capacity still exist which coincide with what would have been the breeding season under adverse or primitive conditions.

Table 11-3   Classification of Animals According to Breeding Season and Ovulation Characteristics

I. Spontaneous ovulation
  A. Seasonal breeding animals
    1. Polyestrous—more than one estrous cycle each season
      Mare—spring and usually extended
      Ewe—fall (English)
      Goat—fall
      Ass—spring
    2. Monestrous—single heat/season
      Dog
  B. Nonseasonal or continuous breeding animals
    Cow
    Sow
    Guinea Pig
    Man
    Monkey
    Rat
    Ewe (Mediterranean)
II. Induced ovulation (reflex), (copulation or cervical stimulation necessary)
  A. Seasonal breeding animals
    Mink
    Cat
    Ferret
    Skunk
    12-lined ground squirrel
    Wild rabbit
  B. Nonseasonal breeding
    Lab rabbit

The influences of season, feed supply, or other environmental factors on the reproductive patterns of animals are *most vivid in the female.* Similar but less pronounced changes occur in the male. During the nonbreeding season, especially in wild seasonal breeding animals, there is a quiescence of the male gonads sometimes leading to cessation of spermatogenesis and gonadal hormone production. In those wild animals with a specific breeding season, the reproductive activity in the male during the breeding season is accompanied by striking behavioral changes frequently referred to as "rutting." Nature has been kind to the male in these species, since there would be great expenditure of energy in the futile quest of estrous females during the nonbreeding season if the male sex apparatus remained functional along with the attendant behavioral changes. In all species thus far studied, the pattern of reproductive function in the male is in keeping with the pattern of development in the female of that species. Usually the male has a more extended breeding season than the female of the species.

Obviously the regulation of these patterns of reproduction in the different species is under hormone influence (Fig. 11-1). The hypothalamic releasing hormones (GnRH) and pituitary gonadotropins appear to be somewhat central in the hormonal control of the cyclic changes. But strong outside influences *modulate this hypothalamic-pituitary influence.* The most measurable one is the effect of light. The length of the daylight period is the best way for nature to inform the hypothalamic-pituitary control mechanism of the season of the year. Other important modulators are feed supply and environmental temperature.

Effects of Light

Professor Marshall's experiments at Cambridge on sheep were some of the earliest to point out that some seasonal breeders are "short day" breeders (sheep), and other species are "long day" breeders (mare). In the northern hemisphere, ewes breed in the fall (September-November) and 5 months later deliver lambs in the spring. If these ewes are transported to the southern hemisphere, most will reverse their breeding season and breed in March or April. Artificial manipulation of the photoperiod in a closed environment can

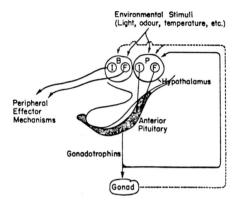

Fig. 11-1. Diagram to depict both facilitative (F) and inhibitory (I) hypothalamic mechanism, influencing sexual behavior (B) as well as pituitary function (P). These mechanisms serve independently as target areas for the gonadal, and possibly for the gonadotropins, in the production of sexual behavior and in the feedback system regulating the anterior pituitary mechanisms. The particular regions involved vary greatly among species. (From Johnson et al.: *In* The Behaviour of Domestic Animals, 1962 London, courtesy Bailliere, Tindall & Cox.)

cause the ewe to breed when the length of the daylight hours is decreasing.

Birds and the mare respond to lengthening daylight hours. Birds have such a short incubation period that egg laying and growth of the young can occur within the same spring. Mares have a rather extended breeding season. Probably the evolutionary effects of environmental manipulation by man are being partially manifested in the mare. Nonetheless, after December 21 in the northern hemisphere, the mare's ovaries begin to awaken. Follicular development increases, and the breeding season arrives by February or later, depending on the latitude. Since the mare has a gestation period of nearly a year, conception one spring means delivery the next spring. Seasonal breeding species raised near the equator tend to disregard the seasonal effect.

The overall effect of the photoperiod is not as clear cut as the above discussion implies. Experimental manipulation of the ewe's breeding seasons has not been entirely successful, possibly because there are other factors such as temperature, genetic makeup, and nutrition.

Although the domestic cow is nonseasonal, she has only partially freed herself from the effects of seasonal change. The cow experiences more "silent heat" cycles during the winter, and the winter season is the least fertile of the estrous cycles (see Table 11-4). Likewise, anestrus is reported to be more common in winter.

The normal route of the light stimulus is from the retina by the optic nerve to the CNS and thence to the hypothalamus. At this point a humoral substance (releasing hormone) affects gonadotropin release. Because animals with severed optic nerves can respond to light changes, it is thought that alternate routes, such as directly through the cranium, may exist for light transfer.

Effects of Temperature

The effects of temperature are less clearcut than the effects of light. Lowering the environmental temperature for sheep has given mixed results, although in general, protection of the ewe from high summer temperature favors an earlier onset of the breeding season.

Most nonseasonal breeding species, such as the cow, may experience "silent estrus" during prolonged periods of summer heat. There is some logical speculation that this is due to a disengagement of the pituitary-thyroid axis. The effects of thyroidectomy on the heifer are ovulation but silent heat. Perhaps the effect of high temperatures on the ewe is similar to the effect of thyroid hypofunction observed in cows. Ambient temperatures that are high for long periods may raise testicular temperatures and adversely affect spermatogenesis, androgen production, and libido.

Extremely cold temperatures may interrupt breeding in continuous breeding species. Extremely cold temperature may delay or shorten the breeding season in seasonal breeding species. Extremes of temperature act as modulators of the natural pattern for the species.

Effects of Feed Supply

An enhanced diet will cause any animal to show vigor. This response is seen especially in herbivores or omnivores when the spring grazing season arrives. An examination of the ovaries will reveal increased follicular activity regardless of the pattern of reproduction. Monotocous species like the cow and mare experience some ovarian response, but the polytocous species like the sow will respond to increased nutrient intake and digestibility by shedding more ova. The procedure of increasing the feed quantity and quality several weeks before breeding is called "flushing." Litter size in sows often can be increased several piglets (Fig. 11-2).

In sheep, "flushing" several weeks before and during the breeding season will increase the rate of twinning and even encourage triplet births. Such husbandry practices are recommended in all species—even the cow and mare show increased fertility.

Undernutrition of farm animals will delay but not eliminate puberty, delay the breeding season onset, decrease folliculogenesis, and

Table 11-4 Effect of Season on the Fertility of Cows of Various Ages Bred by Artificial Insemination in New York

Age of Cows (months)	Season			
	Winter	Spring	Summer	Fall
Under 39	Low	2nd high	2nd low	High
39–63	2nd low	High	Low	2nd high
63–90	Low	High	2nd low	2nd high
Over 90	High	2nd high	2nd low	Low
All cows	Low	High	2nd low	2nd high

From Salisbury, G. W., and VanDemark, N. L.: Physiology of Reproduction and Artificial Insemination of Cattle. San Francisco, W. H. Freeman and Co., 1964. Prepared from data of Mercier and Salisbury: J. Dairy Sci. *30*:817, 1947.

lower fertility. Protein and vitamin A are particularly critical, but TDN level is also important. Special species responses will be discussed in the chapter on each species.

Effects of Psychologic Factors

Sexual behavior is closely tied to the psychological state of the animal. The male may refuse to copulate in an unnatural environment. Conversely, removal of a bull to a "new environment" often increases his reproductive potential. Pennsylvania workers have exhausted the ejaculation response in the bull to a single cow or dummy. Bringing a new cow into the same breeding chute arouses a new and additional response in the "exhausted" bull leading to several additional ejaculations. An estrous bitch may refuse one male but immediately thereafter accept another male.

The addition of a ram to a flock of ewes in late summer will hasten the onset of the breeding season several days. Putting a boar in a pen adjacent to sows will hasten the next estrus in many sows. Cows respond similarly to a bull's presence. These responses are due mainly to the male's pheromones.

Illius et al. have studied the ram in different social environments and found testosterone profiles not to vary in rams reared in isolation, in an all male group, or in a mixed sex group.[8] Older rams kept near ewes had larger testes, increased testosterone output, and greater sexual and aggressive activity. Other workers have found copulation to increase testosterone output in bulls, rabbits, and man, but not in rams.

French workers have recorded the "sounds" of a boar communicating with an estrous sow. The playback of this record will cause sows in estrus to leave the herd and come to the "call." This has been used in artificial insemination procedures as a means of locating the estrous sows for insemination.

Artificial environments affect some species adversely, even though temperature, light, and feed supply are ideal. For example, reproductive failure is an increasing problem in swine reared in confinement.

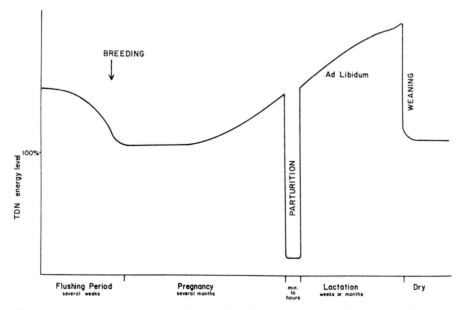

Fig. 11-2. Level of energy recommended for the dam. Breeding season: high level to stimulate ovarian function (flushing). First half of pregnancy: maintenance level to prevent embryonic deaths. Last half of pregnancy: higher level to coincide with growth of fetus. Parturition: low level before, during, and after. Lactation: high level to prevent dam's weight loss. Weaning: low to discourage lactation.

PHEROMONES

Pheromones are chemical substances produced on the exterior surfaces of animals. These "chemical messengers" do not meet Starling's definition of a hormone but must be recognized as members of the broader concept of a "hormone or external chemical messenger." These odoriferous substances serve as communication media between animals. Olfactory stimuli are manifold, but these are one group. Certain pheromones of animals, such as the odor of a boar or a male goat, can be recognized by man. Apparently most species and both sexes elicit odors recognizable by the opposite sex or even other species.

Some of the pheromones are used to communicate information concerned with reproduction and these are termed *sex pheromones*. The usual source of sex pheromones is modified skin glands. The boar has such glands in the perineum, whereas the external genitalia of the cow and bitch are common sources. The urine apparently contains pheromones.

Male dogs are attracted from great distances by an estrous female. Likewise, the boar and bull apparently seek out the estrous female from a large herd by olfaction, at least in part. Perhaps some of the response of ewes and sows to apposition with the male, previously described, may be elicited via pheromones.

Most of the responses described have been recognized for many years in domestic animals. Only recently have scientists focused attention on this important area. For example, removal of the olfactory bulb from sows (anosmic) causes their estrous cycles to cease or become irregular. The ovaries contain vesicular follicles, but apparently not enough LH is released to cause ovulation.

The experiment of Bruce reawakened the scientific world to the importance of pheromones.[2] The "Bruce effect" occurs when pregnant mice are put in the vacant but soiled cages of strange males. The pregnancy fails because the corpora lutea degenerate. This degeneration can be overridden by administering luteotropin (prolactin in rats). The phero-

mone concerned is in the urine of the strange male. After a proper "get acquainted" period the female will mate with the no longer "strange" male and have a normal pregnancy.

Before copulation the boar secretes a sex pheromone in his saliva foam that is attractive to the sow and induces the "immobilization reflex." This offensive urine-like odor is detectable by humans and is referred to as "boar taint," since it adversely affects the flavor of boar meat. It has been identified by Claus as a steroid, 5 α-androst-16-en-3-one, which is synthesized like androgens in the testes. The occurrence of the boar taint steroid is unfortunate because boars convert feed to protein more efficiently than females or castrates. The anabolic hormone, testosterone, and the boar taint steroid are produced in parallel amounts by the LH-stimulated testes. Attempts to selectively block boar taint steroid production or to neutralize it have failed.

Although humans can detect a boar sex pheromone, humans are unable to detect the sex pheromones of the cow or bitch in estrus. Kiddy et al. studied the ability of dogs which had previous experience in olfactory detection of explosives to seek out cows in estrus.[9] After training with cow's vaginal fluids, these dogs were 87% correct in detecting estrous cows. This interspecies detection of pheromones may provide valuable help in identifying estrus in farm animals when artificial insemination is to be used.

Most perfumes used by human females mimic the odor of the musk deer. Needless to say, the perfume industry is following the research on sex pheromones.

SUMMARY

The veterinary medical student is plagued with much variability in species norms. On the positive side, though, are the interesting and challenging aspects of comparative reproduction. As the patterns of the several species are considered and compared (Table 11-5), a broad appreciation can be developed for the utility of such differences, the impact of evolutionary forces, and the response of the species to a changing environment. Finally,

Table 11-5   Average Delivery Dates Following Particular Breeding Dates

Date of Breeding	Mares 330 days	Cows 280 days	Ewes 150 days	Sows 114 days	Queens Bitches 63 days
Jan. 1	Nov. 26	Oct. 7	May 30	Apr. 24	Mar. 4
" 11	Dec. 6	" 17	June 9	May 4	" 14
" 21	" 16	" 27	" 19	" 14	" 24
" 31	" 26	Nov. 6	" 29	" 24	Apr. 3
Feb. 10	Jan. 5	" 16	July 9	June 3	" 13
" 20	" 15	" 26	" 19	" 13	" 23
Mar. 2	" 25	Dec. 6	" 29	" 23	May 3
" 12	Feb. 4	" 16	Aug. 8	July 3	" 13
" 22	" 14	" 26	" 18	" 13	" 23
Apr. 1	" 24	Jan. 5	" 28	" 23	June 2
" 11	Mar. 6	" 15	Sept. 7	Aug. 2	" 12
" 21	" 16	" 25	" 17	" 12	" 22
May 1	" 26	Feb. 4	" 27	" 22	July 2
" 11	Apr. 5	" 14	Oct. 7	Sept. 1	" 12
" 21	" 15	" 24	" 17	" 11	" 22
" 31	" 25	Mar. 6	" 27	" 21	Aug. 1
June 10	May 5	" 16	Nov. 6	Oct. 1	" 11
" 20	" 15	" 26	" 16	" 11	" 21
" 30	" 25	Apr. 5	" 26	" 21	" 31
July 10	June 4	" 15	Dec. 6	" 31	Sept. 10
" 20	" 14	" 25	" 16	Nov. 10	" 20
" 30	" 24	May 5	" 26	" 20	" 30
Aug. 9	July 4	" 15	Jan. 5	" 30	Oct. 10
" 19	" 14	" 25	" 15	Dec. 10	" 20
" 29	" 24	June 4	" 25	" 20	" 30
Sept. 8	Aug. 3	" 14	Feb. 4	" 30	Nov. 9
" 18	" 13	" 24	" 14	Jan. 9	" 19
" 28	" 23	July 4	" 24	" 19	" 29
Oct. 8	Sept. 2	" 14	Mar. 6	" 29	Dec. 9
" 18	" 12	" 24	" 16	Feb. 8	" 19
" 28	" 22	Aug. 3	" 26	" 18	" 29
Nov. 7	Oct. 2	" 13	Apr. 5	" 28	Jan. 8
" 17	" 12	" 23	" 15	Mar. 10	" 18
" 27	" 22	Sept. 2	" 25	" 20	" 28
Dec. 7	Nov. 1	" 12	May 5	" 30	Feb. 7
" 17	" 11	" 22	" 15	Apr. 9	" 17
" 27	" 21	Oct. 2	" 25	" 19	" 27

one can speculate on the manipulative role that man will play with his newly found resources for environment control and hormone synthesis. Animal behavior, or ethology, is a rapidly developing field. The sexual behavior of individual species will be described in Chapters 12 through 17.

REFERENCES

1. Akhlebininskii, K. S., and Ishutov, A. A. (1974): Tests for the study of pheromones in cows. Zhivot-novodstvo *3*:78.
2. Bruce, H. M. (1966): Smeel as an exteroceptive factor. Environmental influences on reproductive processes. J. Anim. Sci. *25*(Suppl):83.
3. Claus, R. (1976): Investigations on boar taint physiology. Int. Pig Vet. Congress, Ames, Iowa.
4. Dutt, R. H. (1960): Temperature and light as factors in reproduction among farm animals. J. Dairy Sci. *43*(Suppl.):123.
5. Farner, D. S., and Follett, B. K. (1966): Light and other environmental factors affecting avain reproduction. J. Anim. Sci. *25*(Suppl):90.
6. Hale, E. B. (1966): Visual stimuli and reproductive behavior in bulls. J. Anim. Sci. *25*(Suppl.):36.
7. Illius, A. W., Haynes, N. B., and Lamming, G. E. (1976): Effects of ewe proximity on peripheral plasma testosterone levels and behavior in the ram. J. Reprod. Fertil. *48*:25.

8. Illius, A. W., Haynes, N. B., Purvis, K., et al. (1976): Plasma concentrations of testosterone in the developing ram in different social environments. J. Reprod. Fertil. *48*:17.

9. Kiddy, C. A., Mitchell, D. S., Bolt, D. J., et al. (1978): Detection of estrus-related odors in cows by trained dogs. Biol. Reprod. *19*:389.

10. Marshall, F. H. A. (1937): On the change over in the oestrous cycle in animals after transference across the equator, with further observations on the incidence of the breeding seasons and the factors controlling sexual periodicity. Proc. Roy. Soc., B *122*:413.

11. Mills, J. N. (1966): Human circadian rhythms. Physiol. Rev. *46*:128.

12. Paleologov, A. M. (1977): Detecting estrus in cows by a method based on bovine sex pheromones. Vet. Rec. *100*:319.

13. Pepelko, W. E., and Clegg, M. T. (1965): Influence of season of the year upon patterns of sexual behavior in male sheep. J. Anim. Sci. *24*:633.

14. Sambraus, H. H., and Waring, G. H. (1975): Effect of urine from estrous cows on libido in bulls. Z. Saeugetierkd. *40*:49.

15. Schinckel, P. G. (1954): The effect of the ram on the incidence and occurrence of estrous in ewes. Aust. Vet. J. *30*:189.

16. Shorey, H. H. (1976): Animal Communication by Pheromones. New York, Academic Press, Inc.

17. Thibault, C., Courot, M., Martinet, L. et al. (1966): Regulation of breeding season and estrous cycles by light and external stimuli in some mammals. J. Anim. Sci. *25*(Suppl):119.

Reproductive Patterns of Cattle*

S. M. HOPKINS

12

The domestic female bovine (Bos taurus) has a nonseasonally polyestrous reproductive cycle. Estrus normally occurs at approximately 21-day intervals for cows and 20 days for heifers (range 17 to 25 days, Fig. 12-1).

*Much information concerned with reproduction in cattle has been covered in Chapter 9 (Female Reproduction), Chapter 8 (Male Reproduction), Chapter 10 (Artificial Insemination), and Chapter 2 (Pituitary Gland). The reader is encouraged to refer to these chapters in order to permit conciseness.

The estrous cycle is conventionally divided into 4 phases: estrus (Day = 0), metestrus (Day = 1 to 3), diestrus (Day = 4 to 18), and proestrus (Day = 19 to onset of estrus), based on the presence of ovarian cyclic structures (follicles, corpora lutea), uterine and vaginal changes, and overt behavioral changes.

During estrus the female exhibits psychic manifestations indicating sexual receptivity. The ovaries contain one and occasionally two graafian follicles which have matured to preovulatory size. The corpus luteum (CL) of the preceding diestrous period has become non-secretory and decreased in volume. During estrus, the uterus shows a marked turgidity and is edematous. Concurrently, the vaginal mucosa is congested and the mucosal cells of the vagina and cervix have high levels of secretory activity.

Ovulation occurs after estrus, when the psychic and behavioral manifestations of estrus have abated and the animal is no longer sexually receptive.

In addition to the recently ovulated follicle, there may also be anovulatory follicles which were functionally immature and failed to ovulate following the preceding estrus. Also, the ovaries may contain the nonfunctional CL from a preceding cycle which is now termed a corpus albicans (CA). The walls of the follicle which ovulated collapse, forming an ovulatory depression. Over the

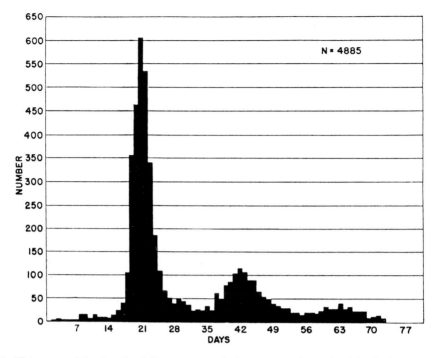

Fig. 12-1. Histogram of the length of the estrous cycle in cows, as determined by the interval between services in artificial insemination. (From Moeller and VanDemark: J. Anim. Sci. *10*:988, 1951.)

next 50 to 62 hours the granulosa and thecal cells proliferate and/or increase in size and enter their active secretory phase.

During diestrus the CL continues to increase in mass and reaches the mature size by day 7 of diestrus. During the diestrous phase, follicular development and regression can be detected through rectal palpation of the ovaries. It is only after the CL of the cycle regresses during proestrus, 2 to 3 days before the onset of the next estrus, that the follicle destined to ovulate in the next estrus begins its final maturation.

In relationship to their spermatogenic activity, bulls are non-cyclic. Depending on the geographic area, however, there may be periods of decreased spermatozoal motility, morphology, and concentration, accompanied by changes in the biochemical characteristics of the ejaculate. These changes are often related to heat stress and observed during periods of high humidity and temperature. The degree of spermatogenic de-

pression varies among individuals, breeds, and the level and duration of the stress.

PUBERTY AND SEXUAL MATURITY

Puberty in the female is the onset of reproductive cyclicity and in the male is defined as the age at which a bull calf produces an ejaculate containing spermatozoa. Puberty is the consequence of a series of cumulative hormonal events in both males and females. In the bovine species, the onset of puberty is more closely associated to body weight rather than age. Both the bull calf and heifer must reach their breed average weight before puberty ensues. The male tends to undergo pubertal changes prior to heifers of the same breed.

Female

The ovaries of prepubertal heifers are active and contain growing follicles before the heifer displays estrual activity. These follicles usually regress and become atretic. Waves of follicular development and regression continue until puberty. The resultant production of ovarian estrogens is unable to stimulate the release of gonadotropin releasing hormone (GnRH) due to the high threshold level in the prepubertal heifer. As the heifer grows, however, the threshold for estrogenic stimulation of GnRH release decreases and, as a consequence, LH is released from the pituitary in a pulsatile pattern.

The onset of puberty is regulated by the maturity of the hypothalamic adenohypophysial axis rather than by inability of the pituitary to produce gonadotropins, or by an ovarian insensitivity to their effects (see Chapter 9). As puberty approaches, the frequency of LH peaks increases, followed by a transient rise in the progesterone levels. In many cases, the mature-like preovulatory surge of LH is associated with behavioral estrus during this pubertal period.

The initiation of puberty is also influenced by the nutritional level received by the calves during the prepubertal period. At low energy levels, the onset of puberty is significantly delayed. The onset of puberty may range from 5 to 20 months, with an average of 9 to 11 months. Sorenson et al.[93] found that for Holstein heifers maintained at a high level of energy intake, the first estrus occurred at 7 to 10 months of age, 6 to 9 months earlier than for heifers of the same breed which were poorly fed. Poorly fed animals have a delayed puberty and do not display estrus until they reach a body weight similar to the body weight at first estrus observed in well-fed animals of that breed (Table 12-1).

THE ESTROUS CYCLE

The four phases of the bovine estrous cycle are reflected in gross morphologic changes of the reproductive tract and in behavioral changes. These phases are also related to specific endocrinologic events occurring before, during, and after the ovulatory surge of gonadotropins and during the luteal phase of the cycle. The major endocrinological events of the bovine estrous cycle are depicted in Figure 12-2.

Pregonadotropin Surge Period

The pregonadotropin surge period begins with the decline in progesterone secretion by the CL. This period is traditionally described as proestrus. The exact mechanisms of luteal regression in the bovine are not fully understood, but appear to be influenced by estrogens, oxytocin, and prostaglandins. For the purposes of this chapter we will consider that these three hormones act in concert to decrease progesterone secretion and cause retrogressive changes in the luteal cells.

The frequency of pulsatile LH release increases after the decline in the negative feedback caused by decreasing blood levels of progesterone. This results in a rise of LH levels in the peripheral circulation. There is a subsequent rise in the estradiol levels which become maximal at the time of estrus. This estrogen production probably stems from increased steroidogenic activity in the pool of developing follicles. Recent evidence suggests that this early production of estradiol is independent of the increasing LH levels.

Table 12-1   Age and Weight at First Estrus in Holstein Heifers Fed at Three Energy Levels

	Age, in Weeks and Months, at 1st Estrus				Weight, in Pounds at 1st Estrus*	
TDN Intake	Range	Av.	Range	Av.	Range	Av.
Low (60%)	59–80	72	13.6–18.5	16.6	430–575	540
Normal (100%)	37–55	49	8.5–12.7	11.3	440–650	580
High (140%)	29–43	37	6.7–9.9	8.5	460–640	580

From Sorensen *et al.*: Cornell Univ. Agr. Expt. Sta. Bull. 936, 1959.
*Estimated from growth curves presented.

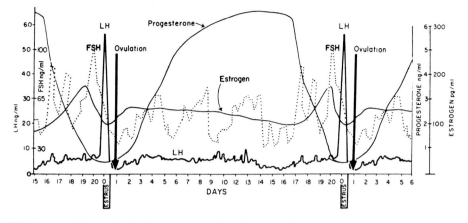

Fig. 12-2. Hormonal levels during the estrous cycle of the cow. (FSH values from Schams, D., et al.: 1977, 1978.)

The retrogressive changes in the CL and progressively decreasing secretory activity removes the negative feedback action of progesterone, enabling the ovaries to increase levels of estradiol in order to stimulate the surge of gonadotropins. Apparently, estradiol increases the capability of the pituitary gland to respond to GnRH, while also increasing the amount of LH and FSH released under GnRH stimulation. When estradiol levels exceed a threshold value, the hypothalamus responds with a surge of GnRH that produces a protracted release of LH and FSH by the pituitary. This entire pregonadotropin surge period occurs during the proestrus phase of the cycle.

The ovarian follicles can be readily palpated along with the regressing CL during the proestrual period. The decline in progesterone and rise in estrogen levels are responsible for the increases in turgidity and edema associated with the tubular portions of the reproductive tract.

Gonadotropin Surge Period

The peak gonadotropin surge begins as maximal estradiol levels stimulate the secretion and pulsatile release of GnRH which in turn induces a prolonged surge of LH and FSH. These high levels of estradiol also bring about behavioral estrus, including the 'standing to be mounted behavior' characteristic of estrus and necessary for mating. The palp-

able changes of the ovaries, associated with the gonadotropin surge, are not readily distinguishable from those of the late pregonadotropin surge, making successful breeding by artificial insemination, on the sole basis of palpation findings, highly erratic. The mature graafian follicle is detectable through rectal palpation, as well as the regressed CL or corpus albicans. The uterus is also turgid and palpation stimulates additional myometrial activity. Vaginal discharge of mucus is copious and the mucus is thin. The LH and FSH surges also induce the final stages of oocyte maturation, just prior to ovulation, to metaphase II. The levels of estradiol fall after the LH and FSH surge and the psychic manifestations of estrus abate. The ovarian and uterine structural changes characteristic of metestrus occur during the late gonadotropin surge period where LH levels are declining towards a baseline level. Ovulation occurs 24 to 30 hours after the initial maximal gonadotropin surge. At the time of ovulation, the levels of estradiol, progesterone and LH are low. Progesterone production increases to levels above 1 ng/ml by day 3 of the estrous cycle. This denotes the end of metestrus or of the gonadotropin surge period.

Sexual Behavior

The behavioral changes in the estrous cow are short in duration (12 to 22 hours) but high in intensity. During the restricted 12- to 22-hour period of estrus, the female bellows, attempts to mount other cows or bulls, but will stand to be mounted by bulls or cows. The latter is the usual criterion of estrus in the cow, and reported variations in the length of estrus may simply reflect differences in the criteria used to detect estrus. The heifer is in heat fewer hours than the mature cow. Appetite declines in estrous cows and milk production may drop. This period of frenzied activity varies among cows, but usually is more dramatic and intense in the bovine than in other farm species.

The bull detects the estrous cow by pheromones released from the vaginal secretions, by auditory communication from the bellowing cow, or by visual communication when he observes increased activity of the estrous cow, including the mounting of other cows. Upon approaching the estrous cow, the bull nuzzles the external genitalia and rear quarters for several minutes and then reacts by standing rigidly with the head extended and the upper lip raised, displaying the "flehmen" reaction. Often the bull will approach the cow at a right angle and rest his head over the middle of the cow's back, whereupon the estrous cow reacts by standing quietly. After several minutes of such activity, the bull approaches the rear quarters of the cow, mounts, presses his forelimbs into her flanks, presses the chin firmly on the cow's back, and makes a single pelvic thrust. The cow usually arches the back and elevates the tail to facilitate intromission and ejaculation in the anterior vagina. The bull dismounts shortly after ejaculation and often leaves the cow at this point. The actual act of copulation lasts only a few seconds during which the bull's rear feet may have momentarily left the ground during the pelvic thrust. Depending on the bull, a refractory period usually follows during which the male shows little interest in the estrous cow. Some bulls have an enormous capacity for frequent copulations, particularly if there is additional stimulation from other estrous cows. A single breeding or insemination near the end of estrus is satisfactory for a good conception rate, although several breedings often occur during natural mating.

Estrual activity is less intense in beef cows. Breed differences also occur in bull libido. Dairy bulls are more active than beef bulls and the Brahman bull is often sexually sluggish.

Estrus Detection

Overt signs of estrus in the female are divided into pre-estrual, estrual, and post-estrual manifestations. These signs include mucus discharge, vulvar edema, vocalization, increased activity, decreased milk production, and the mounting of other cows. The cow in estrus will stand to be mounted by bulls, steers, or other cows or heifers. Artificial insemination based only on external changes yields significantly lower pregnancy rates as compared to breeding the cow on the basis of standing to be mounted.

For the purpose of artificial insemination, it is recommended that the females that are open be observed at least twice daily. This will allow for detection of 90% of the animals in estrus. However, this percentage may vary considerably, depending on the knowledge and ability of the observer. Also, 60 to 70% of this estrual activity takes place between 6 pm and 6 am when cows are allowed to roam freely. Consequently, aids to detect estrual activities have been developed to assist visual observation. These aids include pressure sensitive devices or ink, sexually aggressive 'teaser' animals, electronic probes, pedometers, and video tapes. The pressure devices or ink are placed on the tailhead of the female. When she stands to be mounted, the indicator smears or changes color indicating standing behavior has occurred. Similarly, teaser males or testosterone-primed females, which display libido similar to that of an intact male, can be used to seek out receptive females by their acceptance to be mounted. A 'chin ball marker' will leave an ink mark upon the withers of ridden cows, indicating that standing and acceptance to mounting have occurred.

Electronic probes can be used to measure the electrical conductivity of the cervical mucus. There is a decrease in the resistance of the cervical mucus around the time of estrus when compared to the resistance during the pregonadotropin surge. This technique has merit only if the normal electrical patterns of individual animals are established during 1 or 2 previous cycles. There is simply too much variation between animals to assign a minimum level of vaginal mucus resistance relative to the optimum breeding time.

The increase in levels of activity in cows approaching estrus can be determined by a pedometer. A diestrual animal has a typical daily pattern of eating, moving, and resting. Any increase in the amount of mobility often indicates which animals should be preferentially observed for standing behavior.

Video monitors and recorders can also be used on animals which are allowed to roam within a confined area. The videotapes can be reviewed to identify those animals which stood to be mounted within a given period. This system works effectively but is expensive and requires visible identification tags on the cows, which are clearly recognizable on the video monitor.

The average cycle length is 20 to 21 days, so on any given day 1/20 or 5% of randomly cycling animals should be in estrus. The estrus detection efficiency for a herd can be calculated by dividing the number of cows found in estrus over a 24-day period by the total number of eligible cows. Estrus detection is important since the optimal time for breeding cattle by artificial insemination is during the last half of standing estrus.

Duration of Estrus

Trimberger and Frincher[100] found that estrus averaged 17.8 hours in dairy cows and 15.3 hours in dairy heifers, with an equal distribution throughout the day and night. He reported that animals that first showed estrus in the afternoon stayed in heat for 2 to 4 hours longer than those animals that first showed estrus in the morning. It is known that copulation, administration of LH or LH-like gonadotropic hormones, GnRH, oxytocin, or progesterone will shorten estrus. Ovulation is delayed by the administration of atropine at the beginning of estrus. Atropine blocks the impulses to the hypothalamus which in turn interferes with the release of LH.

Genital tract stimulation affects the length of estrus and ovulation time. Breeding estrous heifers to a vasectomized bull shortens estrus to about 8 hours as compared to 10 hours for nonbred heifers. Proper stimulation with the pipette during artificial insemination has a similar effect. Copulation causes oxytocin release and lactating cows may have a let-down of milk. Dripping of milk is particularly noticeable in the dairy cow. Oxytocin release may also influence the time to ovulation.

Fertilization Time

The cow has such a short period of sexual receptivity that breeding or artificial insemination times are restricted relative to the time of ovulation (Fig. 12-3). Trimberger[99] determined that insemination was most successful when performed near midestrus or by the end of estrus (Table 12-2). Fertility begins to decline soon after the end of heat (heat is a term frequently used for estrus). Table 12-3 shows that the peak of fertility is reached when insemination occurs from 13 to 18 hours before ovulation. Insemination near the time of ovulation results in poor fertilization. The oocyte must be fertilized within 6 hours after ovula-

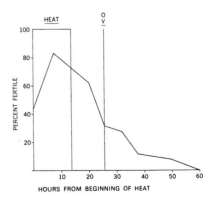

Fig. 12-3. The effect of the time of insemination upon the chance of conception in the cow. The duration of heat and the time of ovulation (OV) are shown. (Asdell: Patterns of Mammalian Reproduction. Comstock Publishing Company, Inc.)

Table 12-2 *The Effect on Fertility of Inseminating Cows at Different Times*

Time of Insemination	% Fertile
Beginning of heat	44.0
Midheat	82.5
End of heat	75.0
6 hours after end	62.5
12 hours after end	32.0
18 hours after end	28.0
24 hours after end	12.0
36 hours after end	8.0
48 hours after end	0

From data of Trimberger and Davis: Univ. Neb. Res. Bull. 129, 1943.

tion if a high rate of fertility is to occur. Aging of spermatozoa for 15 to 20 hours is not as critical as the aging of oocytes, which after 6 to 8 hours post-ovulation become unfertilizable or unable to produce viable embryos that will develop to term.

The fertilized oocyte or embryo usually enters the uterus 72 to 96 hours from the onset of estrus.

Luteal Phase

By the end of the gonadotropin surge period, the secretion of progesterone by the developing CL increases. Progesterone secretion dominates the luteal phase. During the early luteal phase, the CL increases in size and weight to reach a mature size at day 7. Progesterone levels continue to rise and are maximal at day

Table 12-3 *The Effect of Ovulation Time on Fertility (Cows)*

Time of Insemination	% Fertile
Over 24 hours before ovulation	53.3
19 to 24 hours before ovulation	73.3
13 to 18 hours before ovulation	85.7
7 to 12 hours before ovulation	78.5
6 hours or less before ovulation	57.1
2 hours or less after ovulation	30.0
6 hours after ovulation	40.0
12 hours after ovulation	25.0

Asdell, S. A.: Patterns of Mammalian Reproduction. New York, Cornell University Press, 1964.

10. The luteal phase is traditionally called the diestrous period.

If the animal was bred and a normal developing embryo enters the uterus, then a postulated pregnancy recognition factor is released prior to day 16 of diestrus. This factor prevents the regression of the CL, which is necessary to support pregnancy through the continued secretion of progesterone. In the unbred animal or in the bred animal with a non-viable embryo, the CL regresses, terminating the luteal phase and initiating the next pregonadotropin surge period.

Estrous Cycle Length

The length of the estrous cycle is variable but averages 21 days in the cow with a standard deviation of 4 days. The length of the cycle is slightly shorter for heifers; it lasts 20 days with a standard deviation of 3 days. These data are similar to both dairy and beef animals.

There are reports which indicate that up to 30% of all estrous cycles are less than 17 or greater than 25 days in length. As a result considerable variations can be expected, even under normal conditions.

Uterine Therapy and Cycle Length

The length of the estrous cycle can be shortened or lengthened by uterine infusions of irritating iodine solutions or antibiotics, such as tetracycline, when given on different days of the estrous cycle. Uterine infusion given during days 3 to 9 of the cycle (estrus = day 0) may significantly shorten the time for the female to return to estrus, whereas treatment on days 14 to 17 prolongs the luteal period (Fig. 12-4). Uterine irritants cause endometrial damage and probably favor prostaglandin release about 3 days after infusion. The CL is generally refractory to prostaglandin-induced lysis from the time of ovulation to day 5 or 6 of the cycle. Irritating infusions at day 3 frequently result in luteolysis on day 6, whereas infusions earlier than day 3 generally fail to induce luteolysis. Intrauterine infusion on day 15 apparently does not induce release

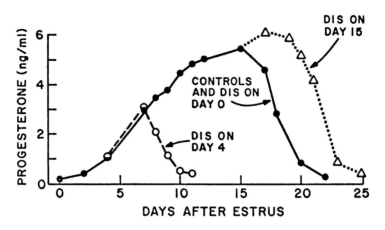

Fig. 12-4. Serum progesterone concentrations in cows (groups 1, 2, and 3) given intrauterine injection of dilute iodine solution (DIS) on days 0, 4, and 15 of the estrous cycle. (From Seguin et al.: Am. J. Vet. Res. *35*:57, 1974.)

of luteolysin and results in a lengthening of the luteal phase. This information demonstrates that the uterus contributes to the decline in progesterone by producing luteolytic factors. The declining progesterone levels (Fig. 12-4) are usually followed by the release of LH due to the removal of the negative feedback of progesterone (Fig. 12-5).

OVARY

Oogenesis with the oocyte arrested at the dictyate stage of meiosis is completed by the time of birth. The newborn heifer has approximately 150,000 oocytes within each ovary. This number declines during the prepubertal period. The mature cow may have only 60,000 oocytes in the ovaries, and an aged cow may have as few as 1,000. Only a small number of these oocytes are lost through ovulation. Most oocytes become atretic or degenerate during the reproductive life of the cow.

Prepubertal heifers may have rather large follicles on the ovary; some follicles may be as large as 12 mm in diameter. After puberty,

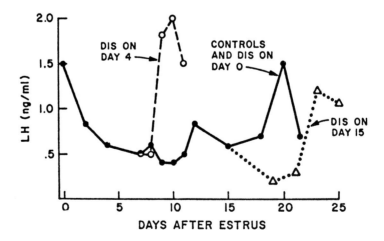

Fig. 12-5. Serum luteinizing hormone values in cows (groups 1, 2, and 3) given intrauterine injection of dilute iodine solution (DIS) on days 0, 4, and 15 of the estrous cycle. (From Seguin et al.: Am. J. Vet. Res. *35*:57, 1974.)

follicles reach diameters greater than 16 mm and only one oocyte will be normally shed at each estrous period.

At the time of ovulation there is slight hemorrhage at the point of rupture, and the ruptured walls of the follicle protrude. Most of the liquor and the cumulus cells leave the follicle, but the granulosa and thecal cells remain intact within the crater.

Immediately after ovulation, the corpus hemorrhagicum begins to organize and develop. Cells from the theca interna and from the granulosa layers, begin rapid division and growth. Within 3 to 5 days the granulosa cells have enlarged to 20 μm in diameter. Organizational changes continue during the first week of the life of the CL. Considerable amounts of progesterone are produced and released from the CL beginning on day 3 or 4 of the cycle. During the second week of the CL life, the physical changes are minimal, and the output of progesterone is maximal. Degenerative changes begin to develop by day 17 unless a "pregnancy recognition factor" is provided by the embryo. The functional activities of the CL cease before physical degeneration is evident. The nonfunctional CL of the previous cycle sometimes is nearly as large as the newly formed corpus hemorrhagicum and often the ovary will contain corpora albicans from previous cycles, in varying stages of physical degeneration and resorption.

The mature CL is round or ovoid, usually about 20 to 25 mm in diameter, and weighs about 5 g. As much as one half of the luteal mass may protrude above the surface of the ovary. During pregnancy there is little increase in weight or size of the CL over that of a nonpregnant cycle. The CL is encapsulated but highly vascularized. Manual enucleation of the CL from the ovary, though easily performed by manipulation through the rectal wall, may result in considerable hemorrhage conducive to ovarian adhesions to the oviduct. A pregonadotropin surge usually follows enucleation of the CL and estrus occurs 3 to 6 days later. Removal of the CL or the ovaries from a pregnant cow will cause abortion during the first 220 days of pregnancy. However, removal of the CL after days 220 to 230 of pregnancy usually does not interfere with pregnancy, but may hasten delivery and favors retention of the placenta. The fetal-maternal unit or placentome apparently secretes enough progesterone to maintain pregnancy after day 230 in nonadrenalectomized animals.

The mature CL of the cow contains a yellow lipochromic pigment which gives it a light brown to yellow appearance. Because of this coloration, the CL is frequently referred to as the "yellow body." As the CL ages and begins degeneration, the color darkens until it finally becomes deep orange to brown. After complete degeneration the CL is termed a corpus albicans (CA) due to its white color.

OVIDUCT

The oviduct of the cow is approximately 25 cm in length. The fimbria and funnel shape of the ovarian end enhance the ability of the oviduct to capture follicular fluid and oocytes. The secretion and muscular activities of the oviduct are influenced by the gonadal hormones. The oocyte moves into the ampulla within 2 hours after ovulation, but spends approximately 40 to 80 hours moving along the length of the oviduct. Fertilization occurs within the upper or middle regions of the ampulla.

Folds of mucus membranes of the oviduct tend to act as a sphincter-like constriction at the junction of the oviduct and uterus, the utero-tubal junction. Gonadal hormones influence the muscular activity of the isthmus and probably control transport of the embryo to the uterus. Elevated progesterone levels due to multiple ovulations or after exogenous progesterone administration appear to hasten embryo entry into the uterus. Elevated estrogen levels apparently do not affect transport rate.

UTERUS

Gonadal hormones induce cyclic changes in the epithelium of the uterus. Under the influence of estrogen there is congestion and edema of the uterine mucosa with a predominance of mucin-filled columnar epithelial cells. On the day after estrus, edema of the mucosa lessens, but a breakdown occurs in some of the congested uterine blood vessels. This allows an extravasation of blood or diapedesis of erythrocytes, which may cause a blood-tinged vaginal mucus. This post-estrual hemorrhage is commonly observed in heifers but seldom in the cow. The appearance of blood-tinged mucus on the tail 2 to 3 days after estrus in the heifer is due to the post-estrual hemorrhage. The post-estrual hemorrhage of the bovine is not related to the menstruation of primates and should not be referred to as such. Some cattle breeders believe that the appearance of this blood-tinged mucus indicates fertilization failure. There is no scientific basis for such a belief.

Marked glandular development of the uterus follows estrus. Under the influence of estrogens, during proestrus and estrus, there is a period of straight lumen glandular growth often referred to as the proliferative phase. Within 3 to 5 days after estrus, progesterone rises and stimulates the endometrial glands to grow, branch, coil, and secrete. This period is often referred to as the secretory phase. The uterus normally has 80 to 125 caruncles which are devoid of glands.

Following ovulation, the secretory activity of CL acts on the estrogen-primed uterus to prepare it for pregnancy. The growth processes of uterine muscles, glands, vasculature, and epithelium are enormously stimulated. This process is repeated every 3 weeks unless interrupted by pregnancy.

If pregnancy occurs, the uterine gland secretions nourish the preimplantation embryo for the first 30 days of its uterine life. At about 35 days of gestation, the chorioallantoic membranes gradually begin to establish a weak attachment to the uterus. Until attachment, the floating embryo survives on the uterine luminal fluids or "uterine milk." The uterine fluid contains proteins, salts, hormones, mucus from the uterine glands, desquamated epithelial cells, and some blood cells. It is a nutritious medium for the young, developing embryo. Unfortunately, it is also a good medium for many microorganisms and is a perfect incubator for pathogenic organisms.

CERVIX

The cervix is the transition from the vagina to the uterus. It is closed during diestrus or pregnancy but is a potential opening during estrus. Closure is only relative, since it is occluded by a thick mucous secretion stimulated by progesterone. Under the influence of estrogen, at estrus, there is a relaxation of the cervical folds. Liquefaction of the cervical mucus at estrus permits uterine drainage, the insertion of an insemination pipet, or the movement of the ejaculate after copulation. It should be remembered that the cervix establishes the transition from the frequently contaminated vagina to the semi-sterile environment of the uterus. In addition, the cervix serves to retain abnormal spermatozoa from the ejaculate following natural breeding.

VAGINA AND VULVA

The secretory and epithelial changes of the vagina are cyclic, responding to varying levels of estrogen and progesterone in a fashion similar to that of other parts of the tract. Attempts to identify the stages of the estrous cycle by a vaginal smear or biopsy have met with little success in the cow.

The vulva responds to varying levels of estrogen and progesterone. During proestrus and estrus, under estrogen domination, the vulva is slightly swollen and congested. This edema recedes after estrus and the vulva becomes small during early pregnancy when progesterone is dominant. As parturition approaches, the vulva again becomes edematous and relaxed. This response is associated with rising levels of placental estrogen and relaxin from the CL.

CLINICAL OVARIAN DYSFUNCTION

It is not within the scope of this book to cover clinical aspects of reproduction, but at this point an understanding of the reproductive cycle may be enhanced by a brief description of some common ovarian abnormalities in the cow. Ovarian dysfunction may be classified into three general groups: anestrus; subestrus; and pathologic ovarian changes.

Anestrus

Anestrus or the lack of cyclicity is normal in the prepubertal, pregnant, or postpartum animal. Only when anestrus extends past the normal time of puberty, or exceeds the normal postpartum interval, is it considered to be abnormal. These animals are classified as anestrous because of the lack of reproductive cyclicity, which is necessary in order to breed the female. Of animals which have been cycling and were bred, pregnancy is the most frequent cause of anestrus.

The two major causes of anestrus in heifers are abnormal reproductive tracts and nutritional deficiencies. The nutritional component has been discussed previously in this chapter under puberty. The best therapy for pubertal anestrus is to provide adequate nutrition to the heifers. If, however, the heifer is near the breed-weight average for puberty, she can often be induced to undergo her pubertal estrus with exogenous hormones. Synthetic progestagens are given as implants in order to mimic the progesterone increase which usually occurs prior to the pubertal estrus. The implant is then removed 9 days later, resulting in a gonadotropin surge similar to normal pubertal heifers.

The percentage of animals which have abnormal reproductive tracts is generally small. These animals are identifiable by rectal palpation of the uterus and oviducts and should be eliminated from the breeding herd.

A major cause of anestrus in cows is associated with prolonged postpartum intervals. These animals have calved and their uteri have involuted; however, they do not initiate follicular activity or growth, and fail to ovulate. As a result they are not rebred in a timely fashion and constitute a major, direct economic loss to the producer.

Lactation usually exacerbates the problems caused by a poor diet; however, lactation can directly influence the length of the anestrous period. Research has shown that a mastectomized postpartum cow will return to cyclicity within a few weeks. A lactating animal will normally have a longer anestrous period unless milking, or suckling ceases. It appears that, either through machine milking or the suckling of the calf, there is a negative influence on the release of gonadotropic hormones. The negative effect appears to be related to the amount of milk produced and has been shown to relate directly to a lower pulsatile release of LH.

Another pathologic condition common in dairy cows is cystic follicular degeneration or cystic ovarian disease. Although the exact mechanism is not well defined, the follicles which develop in a cycle fail to ovulate, yet continue to grow, sometimes reaching 5 to 6 cm in diameter. The normal preovulatory follicle is less than 2.5 cm in diameter. Cystic follicular degeneration can be successfully treated with exogenous hormones. LH or GnRH cause luteinization and return to cyclicity. There appears, however, to be a heritable component to this disease and the incidence of this problem can increase within the herd.

Subestrus

Subestrus is a nonspecific term which indicates the inability to identify cows that are cycling, but do not express detectable estrus. The economic importance is obvious when artificial insemination is contemplated since the subestrous cow is not bred and the number of days she remains open (time from calving to the next conception) increases. In most cases, the major cause is due to the herd manager, who does not spend an adequate amount of time observing the animals. As a consequence a brief estrus is missed. Observation failure is further hampered by the fact that the natural mounting behavior lasts only a few seconds and freely roaming cattle demonstrate most estrual activity at night.

Subestrous cows may have a significantly shorter estrus period than the average cow. Some cows have an estrus period of less than 16 hours and up to 1/4 of these animals may be in heat for 8 hours or less. These animals often display normal homosexual mounting behavior but are not detected due to the shorter estrual period.

Of special consideration is the effect of high ambient temperature and humidity on cyclicity. Thermal stress causes a pronounced decrease in the duration of estrus and in the intensity of behavioral changes. These animals cycle but are much more difficult to detect and artificially inseminate. An additional component is that thermal stress has a negative effect on the male, and on the normal development of the embryo. During the hot summer months thermal stress can have an extremely pronounced detrimental effect on cattle reproduction.

FREEMARTINISM

The freemartin is a sterile heifer which has been born twin to a male. Sterility occurs in greater than 90% of these heifers. The male is fertile, although there is evidence of lowered fertility. The physical cause of infertility is incomplete development of the female genital tract. The tubular genital tract of the freemartin heifer is poorly developed even to the extent that segments of the tract are missing (Fig. 12-6). The external genitalia resemble those of the normal female, although the vagina is usually shorter. The gonads, when present, resemble testes more closely than ovaries, but they frequently are nonfunctional; consequently, a freemartin heifer is in anestrus. The clitoris is sometime overly developed and the mammary glands fail to develop. All freemartins have small seminal vesicles located laterally to the incompletely developed cervix. These are diagnostic aids for this condition if the animal is large enough to be palpated.

Diagnosis of Freemartinism

Since greater than 90% of the heifers born twin to a bull are permanently sterile, the possibilities of a potentially fertile heifer arising from twinning is less than 1 in 10. In valuable breeding animals, it is important to know if the female is potentially fertile since freemartinism is congenital rather than heritable. Caution in breeding such females is

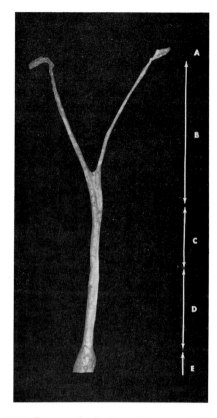

Fig. 12-6. Freemartin. Rudimentary gonad (A); oviduct and horn (B); cervix and body (C); vagina (D); anterior segment of vestibulum (E). (From Zemjanis, R.: Animal Reproduction. Baltimore, Williams & Wilkins, 1962.)

needed, however, because twinning is an undesirable heritable trait in cattle.

The appearance of the external genitalia of the newborn freemartin heifer is relatively normal, yet the internal genitalia are abnormal. A diagnosis can be made in several ways. The easiest method is to insert a 10-ml test tube into the vagina of the newborn heifer. If the tube passes only 2 or 3 inches into the vagina, the heifer is probably a freemartin. In a normal newborn heifer the test tube can be inserted into the vagina for its full length. Observation should also be made of the clitoris, since it is often enlarged in the freemartin.

Another diagnostic method is to send blood samples from each of the twins to a typing laboratory to determine if the two are chimeras. Such blood typing procedures are sometimes used to help establish parentage, especially in artificial insemination programs. If the heifer is mature enough to permit rectal examination of the genital tract, this should indicate whether the internal components of the tract are properly developed. A vaginal speculum can also be inserted to examine the posterior part of the tubular genital tract to determine cervical development.

THE MALE

In the bull puberty is earliest in the lighter dairy breeds and occurs relatively late in the heavy beef breeds. A range of 7 to 12 months would cover the onset of puberty in most well-nourished bulls. Puberty is delayed by undernutrition in the male as in the female. Underfeeding delays the onset of puberty, but it is difficult to completely prevent puberty by starvation. Bulls on a total digestable nutrient (TDN) intake of only 60 to 70% reached puberty at 14 to 15 months of age.

Limited use of the bull may begin soon after puberty; maximal semen production and reproductive capacity, however, are reached by 4 years of age and begin to decline after 7 years of age. Few bulls remain in the breeding

herd beyond 8 to 10 years of age, although some bulls may remain fertile until 20 years of age. The latter is rare.

Erection and copulation in the bull are associated with enormous increases in the blood pressure within the penis, as discussed in Chapter 8. The correlations between testicular size and spermatozoal production (quantity and quality) are described in Chapter 10.

Prepubertal males show an increase in the amplitude of LH peaks up to about 3 months of age, when the amplitude of these LH peaks begins to decline. The frequency of LH pulses increases until 4 months of age. From 7 through 13 months of age, the plasma levels of LH increase in a linear fashion. Initially, the Leydig cells require a high level of LH for testosterone secretion. This threshold begins to decline at about 6 months of age. Leydig cells are steroidogenically active after about 3 months of age for androstenedione production and by 7 months testosterone production ensues. Apparently, there is an interaction between these testicular steroids and the hypothalamic-hypophysial axis which results in increased sensitivity to LH through maturation. The roles of follicle stimulating hor-

Table 12-4 *Age and Physical Measurements of Holstein Bulls on Low-, Medium-, and High-Energy Intakes at the Time the First Ejaculate Contained Motile Spermatozoa*

			First Ejaculation			
	Feeding Level (% required TDN)	No. Bulls	Age (weeks)	Weight (lb)	Withers Height (in.)	Heart Girth (in.)
Cornell	60	3	56	503	43.3	55.5
	75	6	47	526	45.3	57.1
	100	12	43	578	45.6	57.2
	140	6	36	599	45.7	58.2
	160	6	39	688	46.1	60.2
Pennsylvania	70	8	61	523	44.9	56.7
	100	8	45	643	44.9	60.2
	115	6	41	675	46.1	61.0
	130	8	44	784	46.8	64.2
Illinois	60	6	52	352	40.9	48.5
	100	6	45	588	45.7	58.2

From Salisbury, G. W., and VanDemark, N. L.: Physiology of Reproduction and Artificial Insemination of Cattle. San Francisco, W. H. Freeman and Co., 1964.

mone and prolactin relative to the onset of puberty in the male have not yet been defined.

The process of spermatogenesis in the prepubertal bull has been described by Abdel-Raouf[1] to consist of four stages which occur between 2 and 11 months of age. Following puberty, changes in spermatogenesis are primarily qualitative. Following the onset of puberty, seminal evaluation reveals an increase in spermatozoal motility, concentration, and the percentage of normal spermatozoa in ejaculates obtained over time during the postpubertal period. Concurrently, there is also a decline in the number of proximal cytoplasmic droplets.

Testicular development and scrotal circumference are closely associated with the onset of puberty. In bulls, puberty is associated with a scrotal circumference of 25.9 to 26.3 cm. This relationship seems to be consistent across various breeds. The normally developing testes reach 90% of their adult size by 24 months of age.

Nutrition influences the onset of puberty of the male in a similar fashion as described for the female (Table 12-4). Balanced high-energy diets fed until puberty appear to be beneficial in terms of later spermatozoal numbers and seminal quality. High energy diets given to bulls after puberty can be detrimental and cause decreases in both spermatozoal reserves and ejaculate quality.

REFERENCES

1. Abdel-Roouf M. (1960): The postnatal development of the reproductive organs in bulls with special reference to puberty. Acta Endocrinol. (Suppl.) *49*:9.
2. Akbor, A. M., Reichert, L. E., Dunn, T. G., et al. (1974): Serum levels of follicle stimulating hormone during the bovine estrous cycle. J. Anim. Sci. *39*: 360.
3. Anderson, L. L. (1982): Relaxin localization in porcine and bovine ovaries by assay and morphologic techniques. Adv. Exp. Med. Biol. *143*:1.
4. Archbald, L. F., Schultz, R. H., Fahning, M. L., et al. (1973): Sequential morphologic study of the ovaries of heifers injected with exogenous gonadotropins. Am. J. Vet. Res. *34*:21.
5. Asdell, S. A. (1964): Patterns of Mammalian Reproduction. New York, Cornell University Press.
6. Batta, S. K. (1975): Effect of prostaglandin on steroid biosynthesis. Steroid Biochem. *6*:1075.
7. Beck, T. W., and Convey, E. M. (1977): Estradiol control of serum luteinizing hormone concentrations in the bovine. J. Anim. Sci. *45*:1096.
8. Beckett, S. D., Walker, D. F., Hudson, R. S., et al. (1974): Corpus cavernosum penis pressure and penile muscle activity in the bull during coitus. Am. J. Vet. Res. *35*:761.
9. Blockey, M. A. de B. (1972): Puberty, oestrus and ovulation in cattle, sheep, and pigs. Victorian Vet. Proc. *30*:58.
10. Bond, J., McDowell, R.E., Curry, W. A., et al. (1960): Reproductive performance of milking shorthorn heifers as affected by constant high environmental temperature. J. Anim. Sci. *19*:1317 (Abst.)
11. Brewster, J. E., and Cole, C. L. (1941): The time of ovulation in cattle. J. Dairy Sci. *24*:111.
12. Carenzi, C., Casati, M., and Crimella, C. (1973): Chimerism and freemartinism in a cattle sextuplet. Folia Vet. Lat. *3*:438.
13. Carruters, T. D., and Hafs, H. D. (1980): Suckling and four times daily milking: influence on ovulation, estrus and serum luteinizing hormone, glucocorticoids and prolactin in post-partum Holsteins. J. Anim. Sci. *50*:919.
14. Casida, L. E., and Chapman, A. B. (1951): Factors affecting the incidence of cystic ovaries in a herd of Holstein cows. J. Dairy Sci. *34*:1200.
15. Chenault, J. R., Thatcher, W. W., Kalra, P. S., et al. (1975): Transitory changes in plasma progestins estradiol, and luteinizing hormone approaching ovulation in the bovine. J. Dairy Sci. *58*:709.
16. Committee on Bovine Reproductive Nomenclature (1972): Recommendations for standardizing bovine reproductive terms. Cornell Vet. *62*:216.
17. Convey, E. M., Beck, T. W., Neitzel, R. R., et al. (1977): Negative feedback control of bovine serum luteinizing hormone (LH) concentration from completion of the preovulatory LH surge until resumption of luteal function. J. Anim. Sci. *45*:792.
18. Convey, E. M., Kesner, J. S., Padmanabhan, V., et al. (1981): Luteinizing hormone releasing hormone-induced release of luteinizing hormone from pituitary explants of cows killed before or after oestradiol treatment. J. Endocrinol. *88*:17.
19. Dixon, S. N., and Gibbons, R. A. (1979): Proteins in the uterine secretions of the cow. J. Reprod. Fertil. *56*:119.
20. Dobson, H. (1978): Plasma gonadotropins and oestradiol during oestrus in the cow. J. Reprod. Fertil. *52*:51.
21. Dobson, H., Hopkinson, C. R. N., and Ward, W. R. (1973): Progesterone, 17-beta-oestradiol and LH in relation to ovulation in cows. Vet. Rec. *93*:76.
22. Eley, R. M., Thatcher, W. W., and Bazer, F. W. (1979): Luteolytic effect of estrone sulfate on cyclic beef heifers. J. Reprod. Fertil. *55*:191.
23. Erickson, B. H. (1966): Development and senescence of the postnatal bovine ovary. J. Anim. Sci. *25*:800.
24. Erickson, B. H., Reynolds, R. A., and Murphree, R. L. (1976): Ovarian characteristics and reproductive performance of the aged cow. Biol. Reprod. *15*:555.
25. Estergreen, V. L., Frost, O. L., Gomes, W. R., et al. (1967): Effect of ovariectomy on pregnancy maintenance and parturition in dairy cows. J. Dairy Sci. *50*:1293.

26. Farris, E. J. (1954): Activity of dairy cows during estrus. J. Am. Vet. Med. Assoc. *125*:117.

27. Fields, M. J., Fields, P. A., Castro-Hernandex, A., et al. (1980): Evidence for relaxin from corpora lutea of late pregnant cows. Endocrinology *107*:869.

28. Garverick, H. A., Erb, R. E., Niswender, G. D., et al. (1971): Reproductive steroids in the bovine. III. Changes during the estrous cycle. J. Anim. Sci. *32*: 946.

29. Gerneke, W. H. (1965): Chromosomal evidence of the freemartin condition in sheep. J. S. Afr. Vet. Med. Assoc. *36*:99.

30. Ginther, O. J., and Meckley, P. E. (1972): Effect of intrauterine infusion on length of diestrus in cows and mares. Vet. Med. Small Anim. Clin. *67*:751.

31. Goodsaid-Zalduondo, F., Rintoul, D.A., Carlson, J. C., et al. (1982): Luteolysis-induced changes in phase composition and fluidity of bovine luteal cell membranes. Proc. Natl. Acad. Sci. *79*:4322.

32. Gripper, J. N., and Littlewood, H. F. (1969): Uterine irrigation as a means of producing oestrus in the cow. Vet. Rec. *85*:641.

33. Hansel, W., and Convey, E. M. (1983): Physiology of the estrous cycle. J. Anim. Sci. *57*:Suppl. 2, 404.

34. Hansel, W., and Snook, R. B. (1970): Pituitary ovarian relationship in the cow. J. Dairy Sci. *53*:945.

35. Hansel, W., and Trimberger, G. W. (1951): Atropine blockage of ovulation in the cow and its possible significance. J. Anim. Sci. *10*:719.

36. Hansel, W., Shemesh, W. M., Hixon, J., et al. (1975): Extraction, isolation and identification of a luteolytic substance from bovine endometrium. Biol. Reprod. *13*:30.

37. Harms, R. G., and Malven, P. V. (1969): Modification of bovine luteal function by exogenous oxytocin and progesterone. J. Anim. Sci. *29*:25.

38. Hixon, J. E., and Hansel, W. (1979): Effects of prostaglandin $F_{2\alpha}$ estradiol and luteinizing hormone in dispersed cells preparations of bovine corpora lutea. *In*: C. P. Channing and J. M. Marsh (Eds.). Ovarian Follicular and Corpus Luteum Function. Plenum Publishing Corp., New York, pp. 613–620.

39. Hoffmann, B., Gunzler, O., and Hamburger, R. (1976): Milk progesterone as a parameter for fertility control in cattle; Methodological approaches and present status of application in Germany. Br. Vet. J. *132*:469.

40. Horton, E. W., and Poyser, N. L. (1976): Uterine luteolytic hormone: A physiological role for prostaglandin $F_{2\alpha}$. Physiol. Rev. *56*:595.

41. Illari, G., and Calisti, V. (1949): The mucous plug of pregnancy and the estrous secretion in cows (Trans. title) Zootec. Vet. *3*:549. Abst. *In*: Anim. Breeding Abstr. *17*:33.

42. Jost, A. (1970): Hormonal factors in the sex differentiation of the mammalian fetus. Phil. Trans. R. Soc. Lond. B. *259*:119.

43. Kesner, J. S., and E. M. Convey (1982): Interaction of estradiol and luteinizing hormone releasing hormone on follicle-stimulating hormone release in cattle. J. Anim. Sci. *54*:817.

44. Kesner, J. S., Convey, E. M., and Anderson, C. R. (1981): Evidence that estradiol induces the preovulatory LH surge in cattle by increasing the pituitary sensitivity to LHRH and then increasing LHRH

45. Killian, G. J., and Amann, R. P. (1972): Reproductive capacity of dairy bulls, changes in reproductive organ weights and semen characteristics of Holstein bulls during the 1st 30 weeks after puberty. J. Dairy Sci. *55*:1631.

46. Kindahl, H., Granstrom, E., and Edqvist, L-E. (1977): Progesterone and 15-keto-13,14-dihydroprostaglandin $F_{2\alpha}$ levels in peripheral circulation after intrauterine iodine infusions in cows. Acta Vet. Scand. *18*:274.

47. Laing, J. A. (1970): Anoestrus and suboestrus in cattle. I. Functional abnormalities causing infertility in cattle. Vet. Rec. *87*:34.

48. Lamond, D. R., Dickey, J. R., Hendrick, D. M., et al. (1971): Effect of a progestin on the bovine ovary. J. Anim. Sci. *33*:77.

49. Leclerc, A., Guay, P., Malo, R., et al. (1972): Relationship between reproduction and the presence of microorganisms in the external opening of the cervix in the cow. Can. Vet. J. *13*:234.

50. Lineweaver, J. A., and Hafez, E. S. E. (1970): Ovarian responses in gonadotropin-treated calves. Am. J. Vet. Res. *31*:2157.

51. Liptrap, R. M., and McNally, P. J. (1976): Steroid concentration in cows with corticotropin-induced cystic ovarian follicles and the effect of prostaglandin F_2 and indomethacin given by intrauterine injection. Am. J. Vet. Res. *37*:369.

52. Lombard, L., Morgan, B. B., and McNutt, S. H. (1950): The morphology of the oviduct of virgin heifers in relation to the estrous cycle. J. Morphol. *86*:1.

53. Lutwak-Mann, C. (1954): Note on the chemical composition of bovine follicular fluid. J. Agric. Sci. *44*:477.

54. Lynn, J. E., McNutt, S. H., and Casida, L. E. (1966): Effects of intrauterine bacterial inoculation and suckling on the bovine corpus luteum and uterus. Am. J. Vet. Res. *27*:1521.

55. McDonald, L. E., Nichols, R. E., and McNutt, S. H. (1952): Studies on corpus luteum ablation and progesterone replacement therapy during pregnancy in the cow. Am. J. Vet. Res. *13*:446.

56. McLaren, A. (1976): Mammalian Chimaeras. Cambridge, Cambridge University Press.

57. Macmillan, K. L. (1973): The effect of benzyl alcohol on the oestrous cycle of cattle. Aust. Vet. J. *49*:267.

58. McNutt, G. W. (1924): The corpus luteum of the ox ovary in relation to the estrous cycle. J. Am. Vet. Med. Assoc. *65*:556.

59. Matton, P., Adelakoun, V., Couture, Y., et al. (1981): Growth and replacement of the bovine ovarian follicles during the estrous cycles. J. Anim. Sci. *52*:813.

60. Marion, G. B., Smith, V. R., Wiley, T.E., et al. (1950): The effect of sterile copulation on time of ovulation in dairy heifers. J. Dairy Sci. *33*:885.

61. Mellin, T. N., and Erb, R. E. (1965): Estrogens in the bovine. J. Dairy Sci. *48*:687.

62. Moller, K. (1970): A review of uterine involution and ovarian activity during the postparturient period in the cow. N. Z. Vet. J. *18*:83.

63. Moor, R. M. (1977): Sites of steroid production in ovine Graafian follicles in culture. J. Endocrinol.

release. Endocrinology *108*:1386.

73:143.

64. Morrow, D. A., Roberts, S. J., and McEntee, K. (1969): Postpartum ovarian activity and involution of the uterus and cervix in dairy cattle. I. Ovarian activity. II. Involution of uterus and cervix. III. Days nongravid and services per conception. Cornell Vet. *59*:173.

65. Morrow, D. A., Swanson, L. V., and Hafs, H. D. (1970): Estrous and ovarian activity in pubertal heifers. J. Anim. Sci. *31*:232.

66. Morrow, D. A., Swanson, L. V., and Hafs, H. D. (1976): Estrous behavior and ovarian activity in prepubertal heifers. Theriogenology *6*:427.

67. Nadaraja, R., and Hansel, W. (1976): Hormonal changes associated with experimentally produced cystic ovaries in the cow. J. Reprod. Fertil. *47*:203.

68. Nakahara, T., Domeki, I., and Yamauchi, M. (1971): Synchronization of estrous cycle in cows by intrauterine injection with iodine solution. Natl. Inst. Anim. Health Qt. *11*:219.

69. Nalbandov, A., and Casida, L. E. (1939): The best time for insemination of dairy cows. Wisconsin Agr. Expt. Sta. Bull. *446*:15.

70. Nalbandov, A., and Casida, L. E. (1942): Ovulation and its relation to estrus in cows. J. Anim. Sci. *1*:189.

71. Northey, D. L., and French, L. R. (1980): Effect of embryo removal and intrauterine infusion of embryonic homogenates on the lifespan of the bovine corpus luteum. J. Anim. Sci. *50*:298.

72. Olds, D., and VanDemark, N. L. (1957): Composition of luminal fluids in bovine female genitalia. Fertil. Steril. *8*:345.

73. Oxenreider, S. L., and Wagner, W.C. (1971): Effect of lactation and energy intake on postpartum ovarian activity in the cow. J. Anim. Sci. *33*:1026.

74. Padmanabhan, V., Leung, K., and Convey, E. M. (1982): Ovarian steroids modulate the self-priming effect of luteinizing hormone-releasing hormone on bovine pituitary cells in vitro. Endocrinology *110*: 717.

75. Plasse, D., Warnick, A. C., and Koger, M. (1970): Reproductive behavior of Bos indicus females in a subtropical environment. IV. Length of oestrous cycle, duration of estrus, time of ovulation, fertilization and embryo survival in grade Brahman heifers. J. Anim. Sci. *30*:63.

76. Radford, H. M., Nancarrow, C. D., and Mattner, P. E. (1978): Ovarian function in suckling and nonsuckling beef cows post partum. J. Reprod. Fertil. *54*:49.

77. Rahe, C. H., Owens, R. E., Fleeger, J. L., et al. (1980): Pattern of plasma luteinizing hormone in the cyclic cow: dependence upon the period of the cycle. Endocrinology *107*:498.

78. Rajakoski, E. (1960): The ovarian follicular system in sexually mature heifers. Acta Endocrinol. *34*: (Supp. 52) 1.

79. Rao, A. V., and Kesava, M. A. (1971): Variation of body temperature in cows during certain stages of estrus cycles. Indian Vet. J. *48*:1237.

80. Reid, J. T. (1959): Effect of energy intake upon reproduction in farm animals. J. Dairy Sci. *43*: (Suppl.) 103.

81. Roche, J. F., and Prendville, D. J. (1979): Control of estrus in dairy cows with a synthetic analogue of prostaglandin F$_2$ alpha. Theriogenology *11*:153.

82. Rosati, P., and Pelagalli, G. V. (1970): Blood supply of the ovary with reference to the developing Graafian follicle and corpus luteum research in Bos taurus. Acta Soc. Ital. Sci. Vet. *23*:260.

83. Saiduddin, S., Rowe, R. F., Thompson, K. W., et al. (1971): Effect of ovariectomy on pituitary gonadotrophins in the cow. J. Dairy Sci. *54*:432.

84. Salisbury, G. W., and VanDemark, N. L. (1961): Physiology of Reproduction and Artificial Insemination of Cattle. San Francisco, W. H. Freeman and Co.

85. Schams, D., Schallenberger, E., Hoffmann, B., et al. (1977): The oestrous cycle of the cow: hormonal parameters and time relationships concerning oestrous, ovulation, and electrical resistance of the vaginal mucus. Acta Endocrinol. *86*:180.

86. Schams, D., Schallenberger, E., Menzer, C., et al. (1978): Profiles of LH, FSH and progesterone in postpartum dairy cows and their relationship to the commencement of cyclic functions. Theriogenology *10*:453.

87. Seguin, B. E., Morrow, D. A., and Louis, T. M. (1974): Luteolysis, luteostasis, and the effect of prostaglandin F$_{2a}$ in cows after endometrial irritation. Am. J. Vet. Res. *35*:57.

88. Seguin, B. E., Morrow, D. A., and Oxender, W. D. (1974): Intrauterine therapy in the cow. J. Am. Vet. Med. Assoc. *164*:609.

89. Shemesh, M., and Hansel, W. (1975): Levels of prostaglandin F (PGF) in bovine endometrium, uterine venous, ovarian arterial and jugular plasma during the estrous cycle. Proc. Soc. Exp. Biol. Med. *148*:123.

90. Shemesh, M., and Hansel, W. (1975): Arachidonic acid and bovine corpus luteum function. Proc. Soc. Exp. Biol. Med. *148*:243.

91. Short, R. V. (1962): Steroid concentrations in normal follicular fluid and ovarian cyst fluid from cows. J. Reprod. Fertil. *4*:27.

92. Short, R. E., Bellows, R. A., and Wiltbank, N. H. (1970): Unilateral ovariectomy and CL removal in the bovine. J. Anim. Sci. *31*:230.

93. Sorenson, A. M., Hough, W. H., Armstrong, D. T., et al. (1959): Causes and prevention of reproductive failures in dairy cattle. I. The influence of underfeeding and overfeeding on growth and development of Holstein heifers. Cornell Univ. Agric. Exp. Sta. Bull. 936.

94. Stabenfeldt, G. H. (1970): Recent advances in bovine reproductive physiology. Bovine Pract. *5*:2.

95. Stabenfeldt, G. H., Edqvist, L.-E., Kindahl, H., et al. (1978): Practical implications of recent physiologic findings for reproductive efficiency in cows, mares, sows, and ewes. J. Am. Vet. Med. Assoc. *172*:667.

96. Stafford, M. J. (1972): The fertility of bulls born co-twin to heifers. Vet. Rec. *63*:146.

97. Takeuchi, S., Ota, M., Sugawara, S., et al. (1971): Influence of uterine irrigation soon after parturition on the fertility in dairy cattle. Tohoku J Agric. Res. *22*:169.

98. Tan, G. J. S., Tweedale, R., and Biggs, J. S. G. (1982): Effects of oxytocin on the bovine corpus luteum of early pregnancy. J. Reprod. Fertil. *66*:75.

99. Trimberger, G. W. (1948): Breeding efficiency in dairy cattle from artificial insemination at various intervals before and after ovulation. Nebraska Agric. Expt. Sta. Res. Bull. No. 153.

100. Trimberger, G. W., and Frincher, M. G. (1956): Regularity of estrus, ovarian function and conception rates in dairy cattle. Cornell Univ. Agric. Expt. Sta. Bull. No. 911.

101. Veis, A. (1980): Cervical dilatation: A proteolytic mechanism for loosening the collagen fiber network. *In*: F. Naftolin and P. G. Stubblefield (Ed.) Dilation of the Uterine Cervix. Raven Press, New York, pp. 195–202.

102. Villa-Godoy, A., Ireland, J. J., Wortman, J. A., et al. (1981): Luteal function in heifers following destruction of ovarian follicles at three stages of diestrus. J. Anim. Sci. *52*(Suppl. 1):372.

103. Wagnon, K. A., Rollins, W. C., Cupps, P. T., et al. (1972): Effects of stress factors on the oestrous cycles of beef heifers. J. Anim. Sci. *34*:1003.

104. Walker, D. (1969): Uterine irrigation as a means of producing oestrus in the cow. Vet. Rec. *85*:724.

105. Whitmore, H. L., Tyler, W. J., and Casida, L. E. (1974): Incidence of cystic ovaries in Holstein-Friesian cows. J. Am. Vet. Med. Assoc. *168*:693.

106. Williamson, N. B., Morris, R. S., Blood, D. C., et al. (1972): A study of oestrus detection methods in a large commercial dairy herd. I. The relative efficiency of methods of oestrus detection. II. Oestrus signs and behavior patterns. Vet. Rec. *91*: 50.

107. Wiltbank, J. N. (1966): Modification of ovarian activity in the bovine following injection of oestrogen and gonadotrophin. J. Reprod. Fertil., Suppl. *1*:1.

108. Wishart, D. F., and Snowball, J. B. (1973): Endoscopy in cattle: observation of the ovary in situ. Vet. Rec. *92*:139.

109. Wordinger, R. J., Ramsey, J. B., Dickey, J. F., et al. (1973): On the presence of a ciliated columnar epithelial cell type within the bovine cervical mucosa. J. Anim. Sci. *36*:936.

Reproductive Patterns of Horses*

L. E. McDonald

13

THE domestic mare is seasonally poly-estrus, with the breeding season beginning in late winter or early spring and continuing until pregnancy or fall ensues. The breeding season is shorter near the poles and extended in tropical or semitropical areas where estrus may actually occur throughout the year. The mare appears to be in a transi-

tion from a seasonal breeder to a nonseasonal breeder. The estrous cycle is variable in length but averages about 22 days. Estrus, or heat varies from 2 to 11 days, but averages about 7 days. This is one of the longest periods of estrus of any animal and is possibly associated with the high FSH content of the horse's anterior pituitary gland which is apparently the highest of any domestic animal. Split estrus is common; the mare may not be receptive for 1 to 2 days during the long period of estrus.

SEXUAL MATURITY (PUBERTY)

Little definitive work has been recorded on the onset of puberty in horses. It is reasonable to suspect, though, that the age of puberty is influenced by the nutritional level of the foal (Ellis and Lawrence[11]) similar to that which has been recorded in cattle.

Puberty in the Female

In general, the stallion reaches puberty at 24 months of age and the mare at 18 months of age, subject to variability. Since the onset of puberty in the filly is associated with the usual breeding season, she tends to show her first estrus during the late winter or early spring which follows the time she reaches 18 months of age. This could cause some animals to be 23 to 26 months of age before the first estrus would be possible.

* Much information concerned with reproduction in horses has been covered in Chapter 9 (Female Reproduction), Chapter 8 (Male Reproduction), Chapter 10 (Artificial Insemination), and Chapter 2 (Pituitary Gland). The reader is encouraged to refer to these chapters in order to permit conciseness.

Puberty in the Male

The stallion does not have as marked and definite a breeding season as the filly or mare; hence the onset of puberty is not so closely tied to the spring of the year. The testes descend into the scrotum at about 2 or 3 weeks of age, although in some cases they are descended at birth. The testes begin marked growth at about 1 year of age. Some spermatozoa may be found at this age. During the second year of life the maturation process is continued and mature spermatozoa with the capability of fertilization appear by approximately 2 years of age.

A castrated stallion is called a *gelding*.

BREEDING SEASON

The breeding season of the mare is thought to respond to the influence of light; with the increasing length of daylight after December 21 in the northern hemisphere, the pituitary-gonad axis responds and follicular growth begins. This effect of light is the same in the southern hemisphere, but of course the period during the calendar year is reversed. The breeding season of the mare is not as sharply defined as in the ewe. In fact, all values quoted for length of estrus, estrous cycle, or breeding season are subject to wide variations in the mare—more than any other species. This may reflect the evolutionary state of the mare whereby she is changing from a seasonal to a nonseasonal breeder, and from a monestrus to a polyestrus species.

Ginther[18] compiled data on mares in several countries and found ovulation percentage to be lowest during the shortest daylight months and highest during the longest daylight months. Estrus and ovulation percentages peak during the long daylight months, but estrus occurrence exceeds ovulation occurrence during the short daylight months.

With ideal husbandry, many mares do not show winter anestrus. Artificial light also encourages continuous cycling or early onset of the breeding season. Oxender et al. reported that a 16-hour photoperiod started in early December for anestrous mares caused normal estrous cycles to begin within 2 months.[39]

A definite and restricted breeding season occurs in the wild horse in zones close to the poles. Mares kept in a tropical or semitropical environment fairly well protected from high temperatures are less inclined to show a definite breeding season and tend toward year-round breeding. In such animals the peak of fertility coincides with the usual breeding season. Most of the world horse population is located in intermediate climatic conditions. Therefore, most domestic mares show a defined breeding season, but under unusual environmental conditions estrus may occur at other times of the year.

Nishikawa reports that the injection of gonadotropins from either pregnant mare serum (PMSG) or human pregnancy urine (HCG) will not arouse the anestrous ovary of the mare as it would in the anestrous ewe.[35]

Following delivery, the breeding season usually begins with estrus 6 to 12 days after delivery. This is referred to as a "foal heat" or "9-day heat." Regular estrous cycles continue thereafter at approximately 22-day intervals during the breeding season. See Chapter 9 for a discussion of breeding at the foal heat or first postpartum estrus.

THE ESTROUS CYCLE

The estrous cycle of the mare averages 1 or 2 days longer than that of the cow. Ponies have a cycle about 2 days longer than the mare. Because the mare has a much longer period of estrus (7 days) than the cow, the period of diestrus, which is the period of the corpus luteum, is slightly shorter in the mare. The corpus luteum of the mare is active for about 13 or 14 days of the 22 day cycle. This length of activity of the corpus luteum in the mare is fairly constant from cycle to cycle. So if the period of estrus or heat is markedly altered, then the length of the estrous cycle varies. The period of estrus or sexual receptivity is 1 to 2 days longer during the early part of the breeding season, but about 1 day shorter in the lactating mare. Ovulation is spontaneous, usually occurring during the last half of estrus regardless of the length of estrus. Ovulation usually signals the end of estrus within 1 to 2 days and, in fact, may be the controller of estrus length.

The first day of estrus is considered the beginning of the estrous cycle in the mare (Figs. 13-1, 13-2). The usual criterion for es-

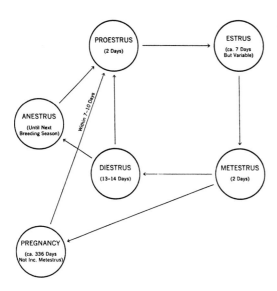

Fig. 13-1. The ovarian cycle of the mare with alternates.

trus is whether the mare will stand for breeding by the stallion. Since courtship behavior in horses is violent, protective measures are ordinarily taken and the actual time of first "standing" is hard to determine. This may account for the variability in the reported length of estrus in the mare.

The drop in progesterone level beginning several days before the onset of estrus permits a rise in FSH which leads to follicular growth, estrogen rise, estrus, and LH rise to cause ovulation (Fig. 13-3).

The total length of the estrous cycle of the mare is usually 1 or 2 days longer than that of the cow. The phases of the estrous cycle of the mare will not be discussed in detail, but differences from the cow will be stressed. The growth of the follicle during proestrus is similar to that in the cow, but the length of sexual receptivity is different. Since the mare is sexually receptive for several days, it is difficult to compare some of the phases. It can be hypothesized that the long and variable length of estrus in the mare may be due to high levels of FSH followed by a longer period of LH release.

The serum LH curve (Fig. 13-3) is elevated for a week in the mare compared to only 1 day in the cow. Ovulation in the mare apparently occurs at the peak of LH release, which in turn forecasts the end of estrus in 1 to 2 days in most mares. Therefore, termination of estrus is somewhat dependent on when ovulation occurs. The use of HCG or GnRH to ensure ovulation soon after breeding apparently improves conception and terminates estrus in 1 to 2 days.

Regardless of the length of estrus, the corpus luteum is functional for a constant length of time. Therefore, most of the variability in the length of the estrous cycle is due to the variability in the length of estrus. The length

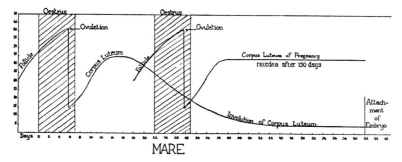

Fig. 13-2. The ovarian cycle in the mare. (From Dukes, H. H.: The Physiology of Domestic Animals. Ithaca, N. Y., Comstock Pub. Assoc., 1955.)

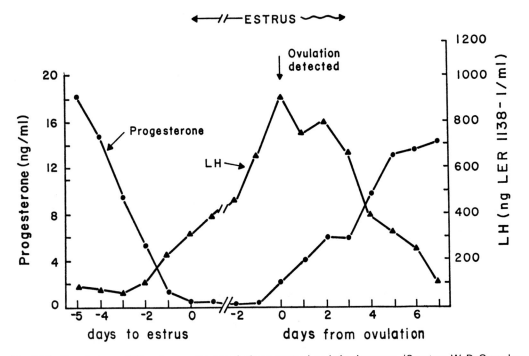

Fig. 13-3. Blood plasma LH and progesterone during a control cycle in six mares. (Courtesy W. D. Oxender and P. A. Noden.)

of estrus is usually longer in old mares or in undernourished mares or early in the breeding season.

Stabenfeldt et al. studied 11 California mares and found considerable variations in follicular and luteal phase lengths, ovulation time, and estrous cycle length. Also they found an incidence of 25% multiple ovulations, which is higher than most other reports which ranged from 4 to 27%. Since fewer than 1% of all pregnant mares deliver live

twin foals, multiple ovulation rates of this magnitude could be a cause of reproductive failure in the mare.

The mare is a "left" ovulator; 55 to 65% of all ovulations occur from the left ovary.

Fertilization Time

Breeding during the first few days of estrus invariably results in low fertility, although the ideal time is unsettled (Table 13-1). It has been found that insemination prior to ovula-

Table 13-1   Time of Insemination and Conception Rate

	Day of Insemination (Ovulation = O)							
	Days before Ovulation					On Day of Ovulation	Days after Ovulation	
	−5	−4	−3	−2	−1	0	1	3
No. of mares inseminated	30	20	89	124	164	256	13	1
Conception rate (%)	10	40	52	65	60	60	54	0

From Hafez, E. S. E.: Reproduction In Farm Animals. Phila., Lea & Febiger, 1962. (Adapted from Sato and Hoshi. J. Jpn. Soc. Vet. Sci., *47*, 545, 1934.

tion is 86% successful, at the time of ovulation 74% successful, and 2 to 10 hours after ovulation only 30% successful. Insemination longer after ovulation is even less successful. In general, *it is most desirable to breed a short time before ovulation*, but since ovulation time and estrous length are so difficult to predict, an average time must be selected, which usually is 4 to 5 days after the onset of estrus. Alternate day breeding is desirable if the stallion is available. In some studs where the breeding operations are carefully monitored, LH, HCG, or GnRH is often used to induce ovulation in order to correlate ovulation more closely with insemination or breeding.

Twin pregnancies and the successful delivery of twins are uncommon. The mare is similar to the cow in that the uterus is not designed to accommodate two fetuses, and it is poor husbandry or medicine to encourage twinning.

Estrus and Sexual Behavior

The mating behavior of the mare is unusual. During estrus she is excitable, whinnies or squeals, seeks other mares or stallions, assumes a urinary stance, urinates frequently, and in general demonstrates considerable interest in courtship. The tailhead is often raised, and the clitoris is exposed by frequent "winking" of the vulva. At the same time she is aggressive and prone to paw, bite, or kick the stallion when approached. Concurrently the stallion shows an aggressive attitude, including a tendency to bite the mare whenever possible. This violent type of courtship makes it exceedingly difficult to determine exactly when the mare is willing to stand for mounting and copulation.

Under domestication the horseman enters into the picture in an attempt to protect the stallion from severe injury. This aggressive violent courtship in practice is limited by teasing the mare with the stallion while they are separated by a board fence. In this way the horseman determines if the mare will stand for mounting and copulation. When this is determined, the mare is usually put into a breeding chute which involves locating her feet slightly lower than ground level and putting hobbles on her rear legs to prevent kicking. Often a nose twitch is applied to prevent her from biting the horseman or the stallion. After suitable teasing of the stallion in order to encourage full erection, the stallion is permitted to approach the mare from the rear, to mount, and to copulate. Intromission is followed by up to one minute of pelvic thrusts and then ejaculation of 70 ml of semen against the cervix and into the uterus.

Obviously there is some limitation on the determination of the exact day of estrus under such restraint. Probably this accounts, in part, for the wide variation reported in the length of estrus in the mare. Copulation does not hasten ovulation in the mare.

Quiet ovulation or silent heat occasionally is reported in the mare. In addition, a *split estrus* is sometimes reported whereby the mare is receptive for several days and then manifests an interval of unreceptivity before returning to sexual receptivity. Because standing estrus is hard to determine, the induction of ovulation after breeding seems to improve conception. For this reason, HCG or GnRH is often administered at the time of breeding. Michel and Rossdale[30] found hCG caused greater ovulation and pregnancy rates than GnRH.

Since the follicle of the mare develops to several centimeters in diameter, it is often desirable to examine the ovaries by rectal palpation to determine when the follicle has grown to full size. In this way some reasonable prediction may be made of impending ovulation.

Corpus Luteum: Function and Control

Following ovulation, the mare remains in behavorial estrus for about 2 days during which development of the corpus luteum occurs in the hemorrhage-filled follicle as described in Chapter 9. Measurable levels of plasma progesterone occur within 24 hours after ovulation and continue to rise for approximately a week, when a plateau is reached which continues for a total corpus luteal lifespan of 14 days in nonpregnancy. $PGF_{2\alpha}$ or its metabolite, 15-keto-13,14-dihydro-$PGF_{2\alpha}$, has been found concurrent with progesterone drop. This suggests that prostaglandins are involved in killing the corpus luteum in the cycling mare. The role of uterine $PGF_{2\alpha}$ is reinforced by the fact that the hysterectomized mare has continued corpus luteal function for several months. Intra-uterine saline infusion will kill the corpus luteum in the cycling mare through its premature release of $PGF_{2\alpha}$ from the uterus.[31,32] For unknown reasons, the corpus luteum is not subject to lysis by PG for 4 or 5 days following ovulation.

Acute endometritis during the luteal phase of the cycle will also induce premature lysis of the corpus luteum and shorten the cycle, but the mechanism is unknown unless it is the release of luteolysin. In contrast to this, chronic endometritis will often prolong the life of the corpus luteum for several months. The cause of this effect is also unknown, although one can hypothesize that the chronic infection interferes with formation and release of luteolysin.

Control of Estrus

Control of estrus in the mare is a desirable procedure which is useful in the management of the breeding program. Such control permits a more programmed use of valuable stallions, artificial insemination, the control of conception date and thereby parturition date, and transportation of mares for breeding at a predetermined time. Control of estrus became possible when $PGF_{2\alpha}$ was found to be an effective luteolytic substance after day 4 or 5 of corpus luteal life in the cycling mare. Even before PG was commercially available, veterinarians recognized that release of endogenous luteolysin would induce estrus after saline uterine irrigation. Although the indirect approach still has limited merit, the direct usage of PG is widespread. With the exception of the first 4 or 5 days after ovulation, but for the following 10 days, the corpus luteum of most mares will respond to $PGF_{2\alpha}$ or analogues (Prostin $F_{2\alpha}$, Upjohn; Equimate, ICI). The mare will usually show estrus about 4 days following treatment with the usual estrous length, ovulation time, and conception rate. Lack of luteolysis and estrus after PG administration in some mares may be due to (1) larger PG dose requirements or (2) the presence of young corpora lutea from a midcycle ovulation which is not susceptible to PG lysis.

Prolonged Diestrus

During the breeding season it is common for a mare in good genital health to experience periods of persistent or prolonged function of the corpus luteum for 1 or 2 months in the absence of pregnancy. The reason for the persistent function of the corpus luteum is unknown, but for some reason, luteolysis does not occur at the proper time even though the mare is not pregnant. One wonders if it is an inadequate synthesis or release of luteolysin (PG). Such a prolongation of corpus luteal function should not be considered true anestrus because the ovary is functioning. The problem is created by the prolonged and needless function of the corpus luteum. Folliculogenesis often continues with occasional ovulation but without estrus. Such periods during the breeding season severely cripple the breeding program. PG administration is a good way to kill the persistent corpus luteum and cause estrus and ovulation to return.

Another oddity in the reproductive physiology of the mare is her inclination to ovulate during midcycle without showing standing estrus. The reason for this is unknown. During the next 4 to 5 days after the new ovulation, this corpus luteum would not be responsive to luteolysis by PG. Such ovarian activity would be confusing during rectal palpation of the ovaries.

GESTATION LENGTH

Gestation in the mare varies from 329 to 345 days, with a standard deviation of 9.5 days. The lighter breeds have longer gestation periods. Pregnancies terminating in winter are also found to be about 20 days shorter which is significant. Male fetuses are carried approximately 2 days longer than female fetuses, and twins about 10 days less than singles. A mare carrying a mule foal has a gestation period about 10 days longer than if bred to a stallion. The ass has a gestation period about 20 days longer than horses. Hence it is seen that the mare carrying a mule foal has a gestation period about midway between the periods of the horse and the ass. An ass bred to a stallion (the foal is called a hinny) likewise has a gestation period midway between the two parents. This suggests that the fetus has some influence on the length of the gestation period.

Implantation of the embryo is delayed in the mare. Not until the conceptus is about 3 inches in diameter and 35 to 60 days after fertilization do cells from the allantochorionic girdle burrow into the endometrium and form the endometrial cups. The PMSG-producing cells are actually fetal in origin. Implantation proceeds gradually after days 35 to 45 and may not be profound until day 60.

Events during gestation in the mare are illustrated in Figure 13-4.

OVARY

The ovary of the mare has several features which distinguish it from that of the cow or other domestic animals. Perhaps the most interesting is the ovulation fossa or groove from which the eggs are liberated. The ovary develops differently in the mare, since the cortical tissue which contains the germinal epitheluim and is the source of follicles is located only adjacent to the ovulation fossa. Consequently, the follicles grow in the fossa area, and the eggs are ovulated there.

During proestrus the Graafian follicles enlarge in the mare. Mature follicles range in size from 1 to 3 cm in diameter, but the follicle which eventually ruptures grows to 5 to 6 cm. Rectal palpation of these large follicles is quite easy because of their size. Ovulation is spontaneous in the mare, and hemorrhage into the cavity is much greater than in the cow. In fact, the developing corpus luteum looks like a blood clot. This is gradually organized and invaded by luteal tissue and becomes buff-colored. In contrast to the cow, little of the corpus luteum protrudes above the surface of the ovary in the mare. In general, the organization, development, and function of the corpus luteum for the cycling mare is similar to those in the cow for the first 12 days.

During early pregnancy the endometrial cups of the uterus, which are composed of fetal placental cells that have detached themselves and invaded the endometrium, begin secretion of a milky material which is high in FSH-like hormone (PMSG). The mare's blood level of PMSG rises from day 40, peaks

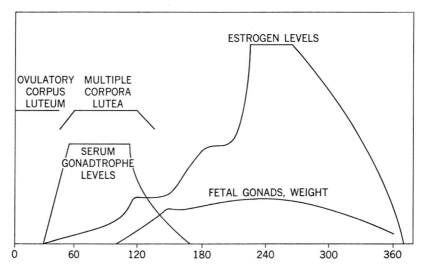

Fig. 13-4. Diagram of events during gestation in the mare. (From Asdell, S. A.: Patterns of Mammalian Reproduction. New York, Cornell University Press, 1964.)

at day 60 of pregnancy, declines after day 80, and reaches low levels by day 140. PMSG has become the commercial source of FSH-like hormone. This high circulating level of FSH-like hormone acts on the ovaries of the mare that produced it. New follicles grow, and several ovulate even though the mare is carrying a normal fetus. Ova may be recovered from the uterine tubes. PMSG apparently contains some LH-like hormone which favors ovulation. Refer to Chapter 2 for a review of non-pituitary gonadotropins.

The new ovulation sites luteinize and develop multiple corpora lutea. Follicles that do not ovulate also luteinize. These *accessory corpora lutea* become functional and function until about days 180 to 200 of pregnancy, after which these secondary and primary corpora lutea regress.[44] During the remainder of pregnancy there is no functional luteal tissue in the ovary.

Progesterone rises to a peak at days 90 to 100 and then declines until days 180 to 200 when a second rise of *progestins* (progesterone and its 5α and 5β metabolites) occurs and lasts until parturition. The sources of the first progesterone rise are the primary and accessory corpora lutea, and the source of the second rise of *progestins* is the placenta.[14] This explains why ovariectomy in the mare after day 150 of pregnancy does not interrupt pregnancy, since the placenta takes over the responsibility of progestin production.

After about day 100 to 120 considerable stimulation of the fetal gonads occurs. Although follicles do not develop on the ovary of the fetus, the testes or ovaries enlarge tremendously. This enlargement was once thought to be due to the PMSG which transgressed the placenta into the fetal circulation, but it now appears that changes in the fetal gonad occur after PMSG levels have declined. The cause is currently unknown.

The development of the fetal gonads, both male and female, continues until about the sixth month when they are composed almost entirely of connective tissue and are actually larger than the maternal ovaries. The fetal gonads then decrease in size and by term are only 1/10 of the maximum size that was attained during pregnancy.

Small breeds appear to have higher levels of PMSG, although there is considerable variation. A mare bred to a jack (mule fetus) produces low levels of PMSG, since the endometrial cups disappear prematurely. A mare carrying twins has an unusually high level of PMSG if both uterine horns develop endometrial cups.

PMSG is mainly FSH-like in activity, although it possesses some luteinizing hormone-like properties. It causes luteinization of induced multiple ovulation sites in cattle and sheep. The hormone is commercially prepared in a purified form. It appears to be a glycoprotein. It does not pass the renal filter; hence it is confined to the blood. This is in contrast to another nonpituitary gonadotropin, hCG, which concentrates in the urine of pregnant women.

UTERINE TUBE

The uterine tube of the mare is 20 to 30 cm long, 4 to 8 mm thick at the ampulla, and 2 to 3 mm thick near the uterus. The response of the uterine tube of the mare to gonadal hormones and oxytocin is similar to that of other animals. Fertilization usually occurs in the ampulla of the uterine tube, and the zygote spends approximately 6 days traversing it. The unfertilized ova remain in the uterine tube up to several months, slowly degenerating after some parthenogenic cleavage. In fact, a fertilized egg will "jump over" unfertilized ova from previous estrous cycles in order to reach the uterus. This is unique to the mare, insofar as is presently known.[51] There is a dearth of information on the uterine tube of the mare or the manner in which the fimbriated end of the uterine tube seeks the ovary or captures the ovum at the time of ovulation.

UTERUS

The uterus of the mare is bipartite with a prominent uterine body. The uterine horns are less prominent than those in the cow, and the fetus develops in the body as well as in the horns. For this reason the anatomy of the organ is inappropriate for twinning because of the competition for space and lack of separate compartmentalization.

The cyclic response of the endometrium to the gonadal hormones is similar to that in the cow and sow and is described by Kenney.[23] There is no loss of blood from the endometrium during the postestrous period, though, as occurs in the cow. The myometrium of the mare is less responsive to gonadal hormones than that of the cow. Consequently, the estrous uterus of the mare is not "erect" or in tone like that of the cow.

CERVIX

The cervical canal is not well defined in the mare and is not as highly developed as a canal-like organ as it is in the cow. Instead there are a series of large folds reinforced with a powerful sphincter muscle. From the vagina, the cervix looks like a rose. The cervix is relaxed, red, and congested under the influence of estrogen, but contracted, pale, and blanched under the influence of progesterone. Otherwise the cervix responds to cyclic changes in the estrous cycle or pregnancy much as does the cervix of the cow.

VAGINA AND VULVA

The vagina and vulva respond to the influence of estrogen at the time of estrus by epithelial hypertrophy, congestion, reddish coloration, and the secretion of serous fluids. The cyclic response of the epithelium is not as noticeable as that in the rat, bitch, or even the cow. Consequently, a vaginal smear is not a satisfactory means of determining the exact stage of the estrous cycle. Instead, judgment can be based on the gross appearance of the vulva and vagina and especially the cervix.

THE MALE

The stallion is not a seasonal breeder to the extent the mare is. Consequently, semen can be collected throughout the year, and the stallion will show the behavioral responses associated with breeding at any time he is with a mare in estrus. Nonetheless, his behavioral responses are more intense and pronounced during the spring and summer (when androgen levels are highest) which coincide with the breeding season.

The male ejaculates from 50 to 200 ml of fluid, and the number of spermatozoa per ejaculate ranges from 4 to 13 billions. The average ejaculate is about 70 ml and has 8 billion spermatozoa. Since the stallion ejaculates such a large quantity of fluid, it is fairly easy to separate the ejaculate into three fractions based on the order in which they are ejaculated. The first component is a grayish fluid devoid of spermatozoa. The second fraction consists of 30 to 75 ml and is the portion containing most of the spermatozoa. The last fraction is a viscous fluid high in a gelatinous material and low in spermatozoa. The first fraction is the smallest, the second fraction the largest, and the third intermediate in quantity.

The stallion's urine is an unusually rich source of estrogens which probably originate in the testes, although there are traces of estrogen in the urine of geldings. Pregnant mare's urine also contains large quantities of several estrogens and was once a source of estrogens for the pharmaceutical industry. Two estrogens, equilin and equilenin, are found only in the horse family and are formed by a route not involving cholesterol as an intermediate. The successful laboratory synthesis of steroids has antiquated what was once an active enterprise—the collection of pregnant mare's urine for processing.

The cryptorchid testis produces less total androgens, about equal testosterone, but more estrogens than the scrotal testis (Ganjam et al.[15]). The unilateral or bilateral cryptorchid stallion retains libido.

PREGNANCY DIAGNOSIS

Diagnosis of pregnancy in the mare by rectal palpation of the ovaries and uterus is quite accurate 40 to 50 days after conception.

A mouse biological test which depends on PMSG to stimulate the ovaries of 21-day-old immature mice is quite accurate after 35 days of pregnancy. This test requires a supply of mice of a known age.[27]

A qualitative hemagglutination-inhibition test for PMSG in serum is commercially available as a rapid test (MIP test, Diamond Labs.). This test must await the serum rise in PMSG; hence the test is not usable until 35 to 40 days postconception. Cost and accuracy of these methods favor the manual approach at the present time.

Ultrasound appears to be a valuable aid to early pregnancy diagnosis, but a false-negative diagnosis of 16% has been reported (Chevalier and Palmer[8]).

HYBRIDS

There are several equine hybrids such as: horse (stallion) × donkey (jenny) = hinny; donkey (jack) × horse (mare) = mule; zebra × donkey (jenny) = zebronkey; and zebra × horse (mare) = zebrorse. These hybrids of both sexes are infertile because horses, donkeys, and zebras have different chromosome numbers and the hybrids have a number intermediate between their parents. The germ cells of the hybrids proceed through mitosis, but there is a block to meiosis, since *pairing* of homologous chromosomes is impossible due to *uneven chromosome numbers* having come from parents with different chromosome numbers.

Testosterone (Leydig cells) is produced in the male hybrid and libido exists, but the *block to spermatogenesis* causes infertility (Fig. 13-5). Estrogen is not produced by the hybrid ovary,

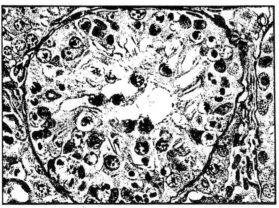

Karyotype of male zebronkey
n=53

Chromosomes from zebra father (n=44)

Y   X

Chromosomes from donkey mother (n=62)

Zebronkey testis

Fig. 13-5. *Top,* Karyotype of male zebronkey, showing chromosomes contributed by each of the parents, illustrating the lack of pairs of homologous chromosomes. *Bottom,* Failure of spermatogenesis in testis of male zebronkey. Large cells near the center of the seminiferous tubule are primary spermatocytes, arrested at the pachytene stage of meiosis as they try in vain to pair homologous chromosomes in preparation for the first reduction division. (From Short, R. V., and Austin, C. R.: Reproduction in Mammals, Book 4, New York, Cambridge University Press; 1972.)

though, since meiosis must occur for the follicle to develop enough to elaborate estrogen. Consequently, very few female mules produce enough sex steroids to exhibit estrus.

REFERENCES

1. Allen, W. E. (1971): The occurrence of ovulation during pregnancy in the mare. Vet. Rec. *88:*508.
2. Allen, W. R., and Rossdale, P. D. (1973): A preliminary study upon the use of prostaglandins for inducing oestrus in non-cycling Thoroughbred mares. Equine Vet. J. *5:*137.
3. Arthur, G. H. (1970): The induction of oestrus in mares by uterine infusion of saline. Vet. Rec. *86:*584.
4. Arthur, G. H. (1975): Influence of intrauterine saline infusion upon the estrous cycle of the mare. J Reprod. Fertil. *23(suppl)*:231.
5. Back, D. G., Pickett, B. W., Voss, J. L., et al. (1974): Observations on the sexual behavior of nonlactating mares. J. Am. Vet. Med. Assoc. *168(8):*717.
6. Bergin, W. C., Gier, H. T., Marion, G. B., et al. (1970): A developmental concept of equine cryptorchism. Biol. Reprod. *3:*82.
7. Campo, C. H. del, and Ginther, O. J. (1973): Vascular anatomy of the uterus and ovaries and the unilateral luteolytic effect of the uterus: horses, sheep, and swine. Am. J. Vet. Res. *34:*305.
8. Chevalier, F. and Palmer, E. (1982): Ultrasound echography in the mare. J. Reprod. Fertil. Suppl. *32:*423.
9. Cole, H. H., and Goss, H. (1943): The Source of Equine Gonadotrophin. Essays in Biology, Berkeley, University of California Press.
10. Douglas, R. H., and Ginther, O. J. (1975): Effects of prostaglandin F$_{2\alpha}$ on the oestrus cycle and pregnancy in mares. J. Reprod. Fertil. *23(suppl.):*257.
11. Ellis, R. N. W. and T. L. J. Lawrence (1978): Energy undernutrition in the weanling filly foal. Br. Vet. J. *134:*205.
12. Evans, M. J., and Irvine, C. H. G. (1975): The serum concentrations of FSH, LH and progesterone in the mare. J. Reprod. Fertil. Suppl. *23:*193.
13. Ganjam, V. K., and Kenney, R. M. (1975): Androgens and oestrogens in normal cryptochid stallions. J. Reprod. Fertil. *23(suppl.):*67.
14. Ganjam, V. K., Kenney, R. M., and Flickinger, G. (1975): Plasma progestagens in cyclic, pregnant and postpartum mares. J. Reprod. Fertil. *23(suppl.):*441.
15. Ganjam, V. K., Kenney, R. M., and Gledhill, B. L. (1974): Increased concentration of androgens in cryptorchid stallion testes. J. Steroid Biochem. *5:*709.
16. Garcia, M. C., and Ginther, O. J. (1978): Regulation of plasma LH by estradiol and progesterone in ovariectomized mares. Biol. Reprod. *19:*447.
17. Ginther, O. J., Carcia, M. C., Squires, E. L., et al. (1972): Anatomy of vasculature of uterus and ovaries in the mare. Am. J. Vet. Res. *33:*1187.
18. Ginther, O. J. (1979): *Reproductive Biology of the Mare.* Published by O. J. Ginther, Cross Plains, Wi. 53528.
19. Ginther, O. J., and First, N. L. (1971): Maintenance of the corpus luteum in hysterectomized mares. Am. J. Vet. Res. *32:*1687.
20. Hughes, J. P., Stabenfeldt, G. H., and Evans, J. W. (1972): Estrous cycle and ovulation in the mare. J. Am. Vet. Med. Assoc. *161:*1367.
21. Hurtgen, J. P., and Whitmore, H. L. (1978): Effects of endometrial biopsy, uterine culture, and cervical dilatation on the equine estrous cycle. J. Am. Vet. Med. Assoc. *173:*97.
22. Kenney, R. M. (1978): Cyclic and pathologic changes of the mare endometrium as detected by biopsy, with a note on early embryonic death. J. Am. Vet. Med. Assoc. *172:*241.
23. Kenney, R. M., Ganjam, V. K., Cooper, W. L., et al. (1975): The use of prostaglandin F$_{2\alpha}$-THAM salt in mares in clinical anoestrus. J. Reprod. Fertil. *23 (suppl):*247.
24. Kirkpatrick, J. F., Wiesner, L., Kenney, R. et al. (1977): Seasonal variation in plasma androgens and testosterone in the North American wild horse. J. Endocrinol. *72:*237.
25. Kooistra, L. H., and Ginther, O. J. (1976): Termination of pseudopregnancy by administration of prostaglandin F$_{2\alpha}$ and termination of early pregnancy by administration of prostaglandin F$_{2\alpha}$ or colchicine or by removal of embryo in mares. Am. J. Vet. Res. *37:*35.
26. Loy, R. G., and Hughes, J. P. (1965): The effect of human chorionic gonadotrophin on ovulation, length of estrus, and fertility in the mare. Cornell Vet. *56:*41.
27. McCaughey, W. J., Hanna, J., and O'Brien, J. J. (1973): A comparison of three laboratory tests for pregnancy diagnosis in the mare. Equine Vet. J. *5:*94.
28. McGee, W. R. (date not given): Veterinary Notes for the Standardbred Breeder. Columbus 5, Ohio, U.S. Trotting Assoc.
29. Mahaffey, L. W. (1950): Studies on fertility in the thoroughbred mare. 1. Introduction. 2. Early postpartum oestrus ("foal heat") Aust. Vet. J. *26:*267.
30. Michel, T. H. and Rossdale, P. D. (1986): Efficacy of hCG and GnRH for hastening ovulation in Thoroughbred mares. Equine Vet. J. *18(6):*438.
31. Neely, D., Hughes, J. P., and Stabenfeldt, G. H. (1974): The influence of intrauterine saline infusion on luteal function and cyclic ovarian activity in the mare. Equine Vet. J. *6:*150.
32. Neely, D. P., Stabenfeldt, G. H., Kindahl, H., et al. (1979): Effect of intrauterine saline infusion during the late luteal phase on the estrous cycle and luteal function of the mare. Am. J. Vet. Res. *40:*665.
33. Nett, T. M., Holtan, D. W., and Estergreen, V. L. (1973): Plasma estrogens in pregnant and postpartum mares. J. Anim. Sci. *37:*962.
34. Nett, T. M., Pickett, B. W., Seidel, G. E., Jr., et al. (1976): Levels of luteinizing hormone and progesterone during the estrous cycle and early pregnancy in mares. Biol. Reprod. *14:*412.
35. Nishikawa, Y. (1959): Studies on Reproduction in Horses. Tokyo, Japan Racing Association.
36. Noden, P. A., Oxender, W. D., and Hafs, H. D. (1974): Estrus, ovulation, progesterone and LH after PGF$_{2\alpha}$ in mares. Proc. Soc. Exp. Biol. Med. *145:*145.
37. Noden, P. A., Oxender, W. D., and Hafs, H. D. (1974): Estrus, ovulation, progesterone and luteinizing hormone after prostaglandin F$_{2\alpha}$ in mares. Proc. Soc. Exp. Biol. Med. *145:*145.
38. Noden, P. A., Oxender, W. D., and Hafs, H. D.

(1978): Plasma luteinizing hormone, progestogens, and estrogens in mares during gestation, parturition, and first postpartum estrus (foal estrus). Am. J. Vet. Res. *39:*1964.

39. Oxender, W. D., Noden, P. A., and Hafs, H. D. (1977): Estrus, ovulation, and serum progesterone, estadiol, and LH concentrations in mares after an increased photoperiod during winter. Am. J. Vet. Res. *38*(2):203.

40. Oxender, W. D., Noden, P. A., and Lewis, T. M. (1974): A review of prostaglandin $F_{2\alpha}$ for ovulation control in cows and mares. J. Vet. Res. *35:*997.

41. Rossdale, P. D., and Short, R. V. (1967): The time of foaling of Thoroughbred mares. J. Reprod. Fertil. *13:*341.

42. Sharma, O. P. (1976): Diurnal variations of plasma testosterone in stallions. Biol. Reprod. *15:*158.

43. Sharp, D. C., Garcia, M. C., and Ginther, O. J. (1979): Luteinizing hormone during sexual maturation in pony mares. Am. J. Vet. Res. *40:*584.

44. Squires, E. L., Douglas, R. H. Steffenhagen, W. P., et al. (1974): Ovarian changes during the estrous cycle and pregnancy in mares. J. Anim. Sci. *38*(2): 330.

45. Stabenfeldt, G. H., Edqvist, L.-E., Kindahl, H., et al. (1978): Practical implications of recent physiologic findings for reproductive efficiency in cows, mares, sows, and ewes. J. Am. Vet. Med. Assoc. *172:* 667.

46. Stabenfeldt, G. H., Hughes, J. P., and Evans, J. W. (1972): Ovarian activity during the estrous cycle of the mare. Endocrinology *90:*1379.

47. Stabenfeldt, G. H., Hughes, J. P., and Evans, J. W. (1974): Spontaneous prolongation of luteal activity in the mare. Equine Vet. J. *6:*158.

48. Steffenhagen, W. P., Pineda, M. H., and Ginther, O. J. (1972): Retention of unfertilized ova in uterine tubes of mares. Am. J. Vet. Res. *33:*2391.

49. Sullivan, J. J., Parker, W. G., and Larson, L. L. (1973): Duration of estrus and ovulation time in nonlactating mares given human chorionic gonadotropin during three successive estrous periods. J. Am. Vet. Med. Assoc. *162:*895.

50. Tolksdorff, E., Jochle, W., Lamond, D. R., et al. (1976): Induction of ovulation during the postpartum period in the Thoroughbred mare with a prostaglandin analogue, Synchrocept™. Theriogenology *6:* 403.

51. van Niekerk, C. H., and Gerneke, W. H. (1966): Persistence and parthenogenetic cleavage of tubal ova in the mare. Onderstepoort J. Vet. Res. *33:*195.

52. Witherspoon, D. M. (1971): The oestrous cycle of the mare. Equine Vet. J. *3:*114.

53. Witherspoon, D. M., and Talbot, R. B. (1970): Ovulation site in the mare. J. Am. Vet. Med. Assoc. *157:* 1452.

Reproductive Patterns of Sheep and Goat*

M. H. PINEDA

14

*Much information concerned with reproduction in sheep and goats has been covered in Chapter 9 (Female Reproduction), Chapter 8 (Male Reproduction), Chapter 10 (Artificial Insemination), and Chapter 2 (Pituitary Gland). The reader is encouraged to refer to these chapters in order to permit conciseness.

SHEEP

The domestic ewe is seasonally polyestrous with interestrous intervals averaging 16 to 17 days during the breeding season. Most estrous cycles in the northern hemisphere occur during the fall and early winter, from September to January. In the absence of fertile matings, ewes cycle 6 to 9 times during the breeding season. In temperate climates, the breeding season is longer and sheep tend to approach a nonseasonal pattern of breeding.

Most of the estrous cycle of the sheep is occupied by the luteal phase. The luteal phase, which includes metestrus and diestrus, lasts for 12 to 14 days. Proestrus is short, lasts for 2 to 3 days, and is not a readily distinguishable phase of the cycle. Estrus lasts an average of 26 hours, with a range of 20 to 36 hours. Ovulation is spontaneous and occurs by the end of estrus. Double and triple ovulations are common in sheep, particularly in those breeds selected for twinning.

After puberty, the ram produces spermatozoa and is capable of fertile matings throughout the year. Rams tend to show seasonality in their libido, as well as in their spermatogenesis and quality of ejaculates. Rams are more sexually active and produce better ejaculates in the fall. Their libido declines noticeably during late winter, spring and summer.

BREEDING SEASON

The breeding season varies considerably within and between breeds. Most domestic breeds such as the Hampshire, Southdown, Shropshire, Romney, and Rambouillet developed in colder climates and are distinctly seasonally polyestric. Breeding during the fall with delivery in the spring of the year, when climatic conditions are more favorable, increases the survival of the newborn lambs. Mediterranean breeds, such as the Merino, Karakul, Persian Blackhead, and to some extent the Dorset developed in moderate climates. These breeds tend to be nonseasonal in their breeding patterns, but may revert to shorter seasonal patterns of breeding when exposed to adverse climates or restricted in either the availability or quality of feed. The most important *regulator* of the onset of the breeding season is the shortening of the daylight period. This begins after June 21 in the northern hemisphere or December 21 in the southern hemisphere. Estrus and ovulation will trail these dates by 60 to 120 days. Ewes will reverse their seasons readily if transferred from one hemisphere to the other.

Ambient temperatures also affect the breeding season; extremely high temperatures of the summer often delay the onset of the first estrus while the presence of the ram hastens the onset of the breeding season. Refer to the discussion on breeding season regulation in Chapter 11.

Theoretically it is possible for nonseasonal breeding ewes to have two lamb crops a year. Under ideal climatic and husbandry conditions this pattern is sometimes approached, but since ewes seldom come into estrus while nursing lambs, it is difficult from the practical point of view to have two gestation periods of approximately 5 months each and two nonpregnant periods of only 1 month within a year. A more practical compromise usually is three lamb crops in 2 years. However, this leads to lack of uniformity of the lambs, since there is considerable variation in the lambing time under such management conditions.

PUBERTY AND SEXUAL MATURITY IN THE FEMALE

Ewe lambs reach puberty by 6 to 7 months of age, but the age of puberty is greatly influenced by breed, nutritional, and environmental factors. Ewe lambs from fast-growing breeds, such as Suffolk, Finnsheep, and Hampshire, tend to have an earlier onset of puberty than ewe lambs from slower growing breeds (Merino). The time of the year at which lambs are born is particularly influential on the age of puberty for lambs of both fast- and slow-growing breeds. Ewe lambs born early in the lambing season tend to reach puberty at 5 months of age and also reach sexual maturity at a younger age than lambs born late in the lambing season. Lambs born late in the lambing season will reach puberty and display estrous cycles during the breeding season of the following year, when they are 12 to 16 months of age.

At the time of puberty, the ewe lamb undergoes one or two ovulations without expressing overt signs of behavioral estrus (silent estrus, see Chapter 9). Similarly, ewes which had cycled the previous year undergo silent estruses at the beginning of the breeding season.

A low plane of nutrition delays the onset of puberty in both female and male lambs, whereas lambs fed properly during their growing period, attain development of their reproductive organs, puberty, and sexual maturity at an earlier age. Breeding ewe lambs during the fall breeding season of their first year is not recommended, unless they have reached a body weight that is at least 50% of their expected adult weight. It is better to breed them the next breeding season, as yearlings. Those bred during the first fall will probably produce more lambs during their lifetime, but the economic feasibility of such a practice is questionable, since conception in ewe lambs is rather poor, with a 50% lamb crop being average.

PUBERTY AND SEXUAL MATURITY IN THE MALE

As for the ewe-lamb, the age of puberty in the ram is affected by breed and by nutritional and environmental influences. Puberty and attainment of sexual maturity is earlier for rams of fast-growing breeds. Male lambs born early in the lambing season may reach puberty by 4 months of age during the first fall, while the onset of puberty may be delayed 9 to 12 months for rams born late in the lambing season, particularly for those lambs exposed to poor feeding and adverse climatic conditions. Fertility is fairly low in these young males, and it is recommended that they be used sparingly. By the next fall, though, the ram will be sexually mature and can be used to near capacity.

A castrated ram is called a *wether*.

THE ESTROUS CYCLE

The stages of the estrous and reproductive cycles of the ewe are depicted in Figure 14-1,

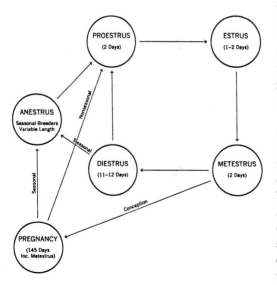

Fig. 14-1. The ovarian cycle of the ewe.

and the changes in levels of reproductive hormones during the estrous cycle are shown in Figure 14-2.

Proestrus

Proestrus lasts for 2 to 3 days in the ewe and is characterized by rapid follicular growth and estrogen secretion, under the stimulation of pituitary gonadotropins. Progressively increasing levels of estradiol in the blood during proestrus are associated with changes in the reproductive organs, including increased blood supply to the tubular genital tract. The ewe does not display overt signs during proestrus. However, as estrus approaches, the vulva swells, the vestibule becomes hyperemic, and the glands of the cervix and vagina secrete a serous secretion which appears as a vaginal discharge.

Estrus and Sexual Behavior

Estrus, based solely on behavioral changes, is difficult to detect in the ewe. Overt signs of estrus are less pronounced in the ewe than in mares, sows, cows, or even in goats. Estrous ewes may "seek out the ram" but, generally, they tend to be passive. Other than vulvar swelling and an occasionally visible mucous discharge from the vulva, the standing of the ewe for mating is the most easily noticed sign of estrus. Successful reproductive management of ewes requires the use of teaser rams. Vasectomized or aproned rams are commonly used to detect estrous ewes. Marking ink can be placed on the ram's brisket to identify estrous ewes by the ink mark left on the rump of the ewe during mounting.

Estrus lasts an average of 26 hours, but may range from 20 to 36 hours during the breeding season. The duration of estrus is influenced by the photoperiod, age of the ewe, and by the presence of rams in the flock. The duration of estrus is shorter and may last as little as 3 to 6 hours at the beginning or end of the breeding season. Estrus is also shorter in ewe-lambs displaying their first overt estrus, whereas the duration of estrus in yearling ewes approaches that of adult ewes. Rams exert an estrous synchronizing effect in

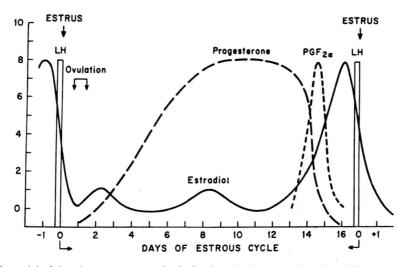

Fig. 14-2. A model of the sheep estrous cycle, indicating the key role played by $PGF_{2\alpha}$ in producing the demise of the corpus luteum. (Reproduced from Caldwell, B. V., Tillson, S. A., et al.: Prostaglandins *1*:217, 1972, with permission.)

ewes. The onset of estrus and breeding season are hastened in ewes exposed to rams before the beginning of the breeding season. Ewes maintained with rams tend to display shorter estruses than ewes not exposed to rams or exposed periodically to rams.

Ovulation

Ovulation is spontaneous and occurs toward the end of estrus. Continued visual and olfactory exposure of ewes to or mating with rams hastens ovulation by facilitating the ovulatory surge of gonadotropins. The wool of rams, but apparently not the urine, contains pheromones that appear to stimulate ovulation.

Double and triple ovulations are common in ewes. These ovulations occur within 2 hours after the first ovulation. The right ovary of the ewe is more active than the left ovary. Approximately 62% of single ovulations and 56% of double or triple ovulations occur from the right ovary.

The first ovulation of the breeding season in adult ewes or the first ovulation at the onset of puberty is silent, not associated with overt signs of behavioral estrus, due to the lack of progesterone, which is needed for the full expression of behavioral estrus in ewes. In the ewe-lamb, the progesterone needed to establish postpubertal estrous cyclicity is provided by short-lived corpora lutea (See Chapter 9). In the adult ewe, due to the prolonged seasonal anestrus and lack of ovulations, corpora lutea are not present. The progesterone needed for the expression of behavioral estrus is provided by corpora lutea formed during the first silent ovulation.

Metestrus

The period of metestrus is only of academic significance in the ewe, since ovulation occurs by the end of estrus. Metestrus defined as the period of formative stage of the corpus luteum is, for all practical purposes, included within diestrus.

The corpus luteum forms rather rapidly in sheep, and blood levels of progesterone are detectable within 2 days after ovulation (Fig. 14-2).

Diestrus

The luteal phase lasts for 12 to 14 days and is the dominant phase of the estrous cycle of the ewe. Viable embryos must be present in the uterus to provide luteotropic signals no later than day 13 of diestrus (day of estrus = day 0). If viable embryos are not present, the corpus luteum regresses rapidly under the influence of prostaglandin $PGF_{2\alpha}$, the uterine luteolysin in sheep, and the ewe undergoes another estrous cycle (Fig. 14-2). This process is repeated during subsequent estrous cycles, until the end of the breeding season, if the ewe does not become pregnant.

The $PGF_{2\alpha}$ released from the nonpregnant uterus reaches the ovary and causes luteolysis through the local utero-ovarian, veno-arterial pathway discussed in Chapter 9. In the sheep, about 99% of exogenous prostaglandins are metabolized during a single passage through the lungs, regardless of the stage of the cycle.[13]

The length of the cycle averages 17 days, with a modal range of 14 to 19 days for most domestic breeds of sheep. The length of the cycle tends to increase toward the end of the breeding season.

Endocrinology of the Cycle

Figure 14-2 depicts the hormonal patterns of LH, estradiol, progesterone, and $PGF_{2\alpha}$ during the estrous cycle of the ewe.

The corpus luteum is the main source of progesterone in the cycling ewe. Blood levels of progesterone are low, less than 1.0 ng/ml during estrus and remain low until day 3 of diestrus. Progesterone levels increase rapidly from day 3 of diestrus, reaching maximal levels by day 8, and remain elevated until days 11 to 12 (Fig. 14-2). If embryos are not present in the uterus, progesterone levels decline rapidly due to the luteal regression induced by $PGF_{2\alpha}$. Ovarian oxytocin stimulates endometrial secretion and release of prostaglandins. Progesterone levels in the peripheral blood decrease to less than 1.0 ng/ml of blood by the last 2 days of diestrus.

Progesterone exerts a blocking effect on the release of pituitary gonadotropins and since estrogens in sheep are secreted by large antral follicles, blood levels of estrogens remain low for most of the luteal phase of the cycle. There appears to be two waves of follicular growth during diestrus in sheep. These are reflected in two peaks in the blood levels of estrogens on days 2 and 8 of diestrus. As the levels of progesterone are declining by the end of dies-

trus, the levels of estrogens in the peripheral blood rise rapidly due to the rapid proestrual follicular growth and secretion. Estrogen levels peak about day 16 of the cycle, just prior to the next behavioral estrus.

The development and secretory activity of the corpus luteum of the sheep depends on the gonadotropic stimulation provided by LH and possibly, prolactin. LH is released from the pituitary gland in episodic pulses at intervals of approximately 3.2 hours for most of diestrus. Due to the low magnitude of the pulses, LH remains at basal levels for most of diestrus, until the preovulatory surge of LH, which occurs approximately within 10 hours from the onset of estrus. During proestrus and estrus, prior to ovulation, the frequency of these episodic pulses of LH increases to intervals of about 1.0 hour. These LH pulses are followed by significant rises in blood levels of estradiol, which is associated with the changes in the reproductive organs and behavior that characterize estrus.

Photoperiod seems to be the major factor controlling the anestrous period during the nonbreeding season that follows the breeding season of sheep. This photoperiodic influence seems to be exerted through hypothalamic modulation of the pulsatile release of gonadotropins from the pituitary. During anestrus the frequency and magnitude of the LH pulses are low.

ANATOMIC CHANGES OF THE REPRODUCTIVE ORGANS

During the nonbreeding season, the ovaries of the ewe undergo follicular development to the antral stages, but ovulation fails to occur and the ewe does not express behavioral estrus. As the breeding season approaches, gonadotropic hormones stimulate the ovarian follicles to mature, secrete estrogens and ovulate. Estrogens secreted by the maturing follicles in turn stimulate the macro- and microscopic changes in the oviducts, uterus, and vagina described in Chapter 9. Follicular growth proceeds rapidly during proestrus and is completed during the preovulatory period of estrus. In the ewe, mature, preovulatory follicles reach a diameter of approximately 1.0 cm.

The ovary of adult ewes may contain as many as 86,000 primordial follicles and 100 to 400 growing follicles, of which 10 to 40 follicles are visible on the surface of the ovary.[15] Single ovulating breeds tend to develop a single follicle at each ovulation, while the other growing follicles undergo atresia. In multiple ovulating breeds, such as the Booroola, several follicles develop and ovulate. It appears that the selection and emergence of a follicle or follicles for ovulation occurs about day 14 of the cycle. The mechanisms for the selection of those follicles which will ovulate, while the other growing follicles undergo atresia, are not known.

The oviducts of the ewe are approximately 15 to 20 cm long and have well-developed mucosal thickenings at their junction with the uterine horns. These mucosal thickenings act like valves and control the passage of spermatozoa from the uterus into the oviduct. The fimbriated end of the sheep's oviduct is well developed and surrounds the ovary at the time of ovulation.

The uterus of the sheep is bipartite and the uterine mucosa, as in the cow, forms a septum that separates the uterine horns. The endometrium of the ewe is highly glandular and contains caruncles, which are nonglandular projections arranged in 4 rows extending from the uterine body to the horns. Externally, the horns are bound by an intercornual ligament.

FERTILIZATION

As for the other domestic species, ram spermatozoa need to be capacitated in the female tract to acquire the capability to fertilize the ewe's oocytes. Fertilization takes place in the ampullary region of the oviduct. After natural or artificial insemination, ram spermatozoa are displaced rather rapidly through the cervix and uterus. The cervix of the ewe controls spermatozoal displacement and possibly also exerts a selective effect on the population of spermatozoa deposited in the anterior vagina. Only a fraction of the spermatozoa deposited in the vagina enter the uterus. The cervical canal is both tortuous and contains non-aligned mucosal folds. Disalignment of these cervical folds prevents intracervical and intrauterine inseminations in the ewe.

The utero-tubal junction further selects spermatozoa entering the oviduct from the uterus. Once in the oviduct, most ram spermatozoa are restricted to the caudal isthmus until ovulation. Two phases of spermatozoal transport within the oviduct have been described for the ewe: (1) a rapid phase that results in the entry of relatively few spermatozoa into the oviducts, within 15 minutes after mating, and (2) a more prolonged phase of transport, which results in the slow accumulation of a functional population of spermatozoa within the ampullary region of the oviduct.

The fertilizable life of the oocyte is considered to be about 10 to 12 hours in the ewe, but may extend up to 24 hours after ovulation. The chances for oocyte aging and associated embryonic losses are reduced in sheep, since ovulation occurs in most ewes by the end of estrus and matings are likely to occur early in estrus. In addition, ram spermatozoa maintain their fertilizing capability in the ewe's oviduct for periods extending up to 48 hours.

Ewe oocytes are released into the oviducts surrounded by cumulus cells. These cumulus cells break down rapidly after ovulation and by the time of fertilization the oocyte is practically free of cumulus cells. Cleavage of the fertilized oocyte to the two-cell stage occurs within 16 hours after fertilization or approximately 24 hours after ovulation. Sheep oocytes have been fertilized *in vitro*, and live offspring have been obtained after transfer of these *in vitro* fertilized oocytes. However, the rate of success has been low and this technology needs to be improved to become profitable. Technological advancements have made it possible to apply micromanipulation, including embryo splitting, gene injection, nuclear transplantation and cell fusion, and cryopreservation to the sheep embryo (see Chapter 19).

PREGNANCY

Sheep embryos enter the uterus at the blastocyst stage by day 3 after ovulation. They remain spherical up to day 4, but undergo rapid elongation prior to attachment to the endometrium. Endometrial attachment of these elongated blastocysts begins from about the 14th day and is completed by 22 days after mating. Transuterine migration of embryos occurs frequently in ewes with two or more ovulations from the same ovary and may occur occasionally in ewes with a single ovulation. Transuterine migration results in better spacing of the embryos and optimal utilization of the uterus for successful pregnancy.

It has long been assumed that placentation in the ewe occurs only between the cotyledons of the chorioallantois and the uterine caruncles. Now it is evident that apposition and attachment occurs over the entire uterine surface,[47] although attachment at the intercaruncular spaces may be tenuous. The placenta of the sheep is diffuse for the first month. As gestation progresses, the attachment is reinforced by the placentomes which interlock the chorionic villi into the crypts of the caruncles. In the sheep, the placental syncytium is formed from fetal cells and is syndesmochorial in structure, lacking a uterine epithelial component.[98] The number of placentomes formed by the fetal cotyledon and the maternal cotyledon or caruncle averages about 90, but may vary from 60 to 100. The placenta of the sheep produces a placental lactogen with prolactin-like activity.

Pregnancy lasts an average of 148 days, but may range from 140 to 159 days, when calculated from the time of mating or artificial insemination to parturition or lambing. The length of pregnancy in sheep is influenced by breed and plane of nutrition, as well as by environmental conditions. Fast-growing breeds, such as the Hampshire, tend to have shorter gestations, averaging 145 days. Slow-growing breeds, such as the Merino, have longer gestations, averaging 151 days. A low plane of nutrition or twin pregnancies also shortens the length of gestation.

Cervical and vaginal stimulations by the lambs at the time of parturition elicit the onset of maternal behavior and selective bonding between mother and lamb. Acceptance of alien lambs can be induced by stimulating the vagina and cervix of nonpregnant ewes previously treated with estrogens and progesterone.[46]

Most ewes do not display estrous behavior during pregnancy. However, ewes that become pregnant early in the breeding season may, on occasion, display some degree of sexual activity.

Lactational anestrus is the norm in sheep. Some ewes display postpartum estrus, within 30 hours after parturition, when lambing occurs early in the breeding season. Pregnancy seldom results from matings which occur during the postpartum estrus. In general, ewes do not return to estrus until after the lambs are weaned. In most cases, estrus is delayed until the next breeding season.

The regression of the corpus luteum of pregnancy proceeds at a lower rate than the regression of the corpus luteum of the cycle. The progesterone secreted by the corpus luteum is needed for the first 50 days of pregnancy in the sheep. If bilateral ovariectomy is performed after day 50 of pregnancy, placental secretion of progestagens is sufficient to prevent abortion.

Pregnancy Diagnosis

The nonreturn to estrus after a recorded mating is a relatively accurate sign of pregnancy in well-managed flocks, but is not accurate in free-mating conditions, since ewes may not cycle for a variety of reasons and remain in a nonpregnant anestrus for the duration of the breeding season.

The use of ultrasound is becoming particularly useful for pregnancy diagnosis in ewes. It allows for accurate diagnosis of pregnancy from the eighth week. Through the use of echonographic ultrasound equipment, accurate diagnosis of pregnancy can be made as early as day 35 after mating.

Determination of blood levels of progesterone is also a useful means for the early diagnosis of pregnancy in high priced ewes that have not returned to estrus by day 18 after mating. High blood levels of progesterone indicate that luteal regression has not occurred and in the majority of cases, this is due to the luteotropic signals provided by embryos in the uterus. Detection of chorionic-somatotropin in the blood after day 40 of gestation is also indicative of pregnancy.

Operators with thin arms can rectally palpate large ewes and diagnose pregnancy. Rectal-abdominal palpation, using rods introduced in the rectum to displace the fetus against the abdominal wall, also is used for pregnancy diagnosis in ewes. However, both procedures are associated with a high incidence of perforated recta, peritonitis, and abortion when performed by untrained individuals.

CONTROL OF REPRODUCTIVE EFFICIENCY

A fertile ewe is customarily defined as an ewe capable of producing at least one lamb per pregnancy. A crop of one lamb per ewe per year is considered the minimal fecundity or prolificacy for the ewe and is referred to as a 100% lamb crop. Sheep breeders seek a prolificacy averaging at least 1.5 lambs per ewe, which represent a lamb crop of 150%.

Many factors, including environment, plane of nutrition, age, breed and selection for high lambing influence prolificacy. The quantity, as well as the quality of feed influences the incidence of estrus, ovulation rates, embryonic survival to term, and the lamb crop. Once the general daily requirements in dietary ingredients are met, a detrimental influence of the plane of nutrition becomes dependent on the lack or excess of a particular component in the diet. Unfortunately, the dietary needs to meet specific requirements for each stage of the reproductive processes of sheep, including pregnancy, are not yet understood.

Breed differences in the fecundity of sheep are shown in Table 14-1. Selection within breeds for higher prolificacy can also be a factor contributing to higher lamb crops (Table 14-2). The ovulation rate, defined as the number of oocytes released at each ovula-

tion is a heritable trait affecting fecundity and the lambing crop. Repeatability of ovulation rate both within a season and between years is high for those ewes which tend to have a high lambing crop. Booroola ewes have ovulation rates of 4 to 5 oocytes. The high ovulation rate and fecundity of the Booroola ewe is due to a gene, which influences the rate

Table 14-1   Fecundity in Sheep

Breed	Lamb Crop, %
Cheviot	89
Scottish Blackface	93
Heath	103
Karakul	110
Corriedale, in Canada	114
Corriedale, in U.S.	118
Southdown	119
Rambouillet, in U.S.	122
Rambouillet, in Canada	124
American Shropshire	124
Oxford Down	127
Columbia	127
Dorset	127
Romney Marsh	128
Navaho	129
Targhee	129
Hampshire Down	132
Dorset Horn	137
Lincoln	140
Suffolk	144
Shropshire	162
Leicester	163
Wensleydale	172
Border Leicester	181
East Friesian Milch Sheep	205
Romanov	238
Finnsheep	300 to 600

From Asdell, S. A.: Patterns of Mammalian Reproduction. Ithaca, N. Y., Comstock Publishing Co. 1964.

Table 14-2   Effect of the Number Born on the Subsequent Fecundity of Romanov Sheep

Ewes Born as	Average Lambs Produced
Singles	2.17
Twins	2.36
Triplets	2.63
Quadruplets	3.01

From Belogradskii, A. P.: Sov. Zooteh. 7:88, 1940.

of ovulation probably by enhancing the sensitivity of follicular cells to pituitary gonadotropin. The trait for high ovulation rate is dominant in the F1 generation of crosses between the Booroola and other breeds.

The influence of other factors, such as age of the dam, is shown in Table 14-3. The lamb crop was greater in ewes that were not bred until 1.5 years of age (effect of age of dam). This superiority existed for the next 3 years, but the overall production of the ewe first bred while a lamb was still greater. Notice that the lamb crop continued to increase through the fifth season in both groups. Prolificacy peaks when the ewe is 4 to 6 years of age.

Because of the restricted breeding season of most breeds of sheep and the economical significance of increasing the lamb crop for the sheep breeder, several schemes have been developed to prolong the breeding season in order to produce lambs at any time of the year, or to increase the crop of lambs by selecting breeds with high ovulation rates.

Induction of Estrus Before the Breeding Season

Stimulation of the ovaries of sheep out of the breeding season using gonadotropins, such as PMSG, has produced satisfactory results particularly when the gonadotropin is given shortly before the normal breeding period and after pretreatment of the ewes with progestagens. Attempts to produce 2 lamb crops per year by exogenous gonadotropic stimulation

Table 14-3 Fecundity of Hampshire Ewes

	Bred and Conceived as Lambs	Bred and Conceived as 1½-Year-Olds
	Lamb Crop %	Lamb Crop %
First season	106	—
Second season	157	195
Third season	176	202
Fourth season	177	175
Fifth season	200	208

From Spencer, D. A., Schott, R. G., Phillips, R. W., and Aune, B.: J. Anim. Sci. *1*:27, 1942.

during the deep anestrus of the nonbreeding season, although possible under ideal conditions of feeding and management, has in general produced unsatisfactory results when applied in large scale. Most failures are attributed to fertilization failure or increased embryonic mortality.

Pretreatment of the ewe with natural or synthetic progestagens is needed to initiate the cyclic release of endogenous gonadotropins (see Chapter 9). Progestagens are usually given for periods of 12 to 16 days, either as subcutaneous implants or in the form of vaginal pessaries. Gonadotropin treatment is given after the withdrawal of the implants or pessaries.

Artificial lighting to alter the natural ratio of light to dark can be used to advance the breeding season for ewes maintained in barns. This approach is generally more expensive and difficult to use on a large scale. Treatments combining artificial lighting with gonadotropic stimulation have also been used.

The social interaction of lambs and ewes with rams is an important component for the reproductive management of sheep. Exposure of ewes and prepubertal ewe-lambs to rams early in the breeding season, hastens the onset of puberty and seasonal estrus. Reproductive management of a flock should incorporate management schemes as well as building design to meet the animal needs for protection, feeding, and social interaction.

Other experimental approaches, such as the use of GnRH to induce surges of LH and cause ovulation in anestrous ewes, active immunization of ewes against androgens to increase ovulatory rates, and hastening the onset of puberty of ewe-lambs by treatment with progestagens and gonadotropins, although successful, are not yet proven to be economically feasible under field conditions.

Estrus Synchronization

Two basic approaches are used to synchronize estrus in ewes: (1) treatment of ewes with progestagens for periods of 12 to 16 days or longer to inhibit the release of gonadotropins and prevent the initiation of the cycle or (2) treatment with $PGF_{2\alpha}$ in single or double treatments with or without progestagens (see Chapter 19, Table 19-13).

THE MALE

The growth of horns is apparently under the influence of gonadal hormones. In some breeds such as the Dorset, both sexes have horns, though the ewes have smaller horns. In Merinos and Rambouillets, only rams have horns. In English breeds neither sex has horns.

Rams reach puberty, as judged by the presence of spermatozoa in their ejaculates, by 5 to 8 months of age. During the prepubertal period there is pulsatile release of pituitary gonadotropins, beginning as early as 1 week of age. Later, as the lamb approaches puberty, a temporal relationship develops between the pulsatile release of gonadotropins, mainly LH, and episodic increases of testosterone production by the testes. These lead to the onset of puberty and the establishment of the adult pattern of gonadotropin secretion (see Chapter 8).

The duration of the cycle of the seminiferous epithelium, spermatogenesis, daily sperm production and output of rams are discussed in Chapters 7 and 8. Rams are capable of spermatogenesis and produce fertile ejaculates throughout the year. The ram's endocrine system responds to photoperiodic changes and the quality of the ejaculates is lower during the nonbreeding season. As the photoperiod decreases, rams respond with an increased frequency of LH pulses and testosterone secretion.

Scrotal volume, circumference, and mean testicular diameter correlate well with spermatozoal production. These parameters are often used as an indication of the breeding capacity of a male, to establish ewe to ram ratios for the flock.

Collection of Semen

Semen is usually collected from the ram with an artificial vagina (AV) or by electroejaculation. The AV method resembles natural mating, but requires training of rams to ejaculate in the AV. In addition, estrous ewes are needed during the period of training to stimulate the ejaculatory responses. The method of electroejaculation is particularly useful to collect semen from untrained rams for breeding soundness examinations. Several electroejaculation protocols have been developed. In general, electroejaculation produces larger volumes of ejaculate than when semen is collected with an AV and tends to produce less total numbers of spermatozoa. Refinements in the protocols of electrical stimulation, number and voltage of stimuli to be given, as well as improvements in the design of rectal probes, make electroejaculation a suitable procedure for the collection of semen from rams.

Spermatogenesis is affected by the temperature of the testes. When wool covers the scrotum of animals, there may be a temporary infertility during the hot summer months. Even in the absence of a wool covering, environmental temperatures above 90°F will usually interfere with spermatogenesis and lower the quality of the ejaculate.

Coitus is rapid with a single thrust or two by the ram causing ejaculation and deposition of semen in the cranial end of the vagina. Rams will copulate frequently with estrous ewes. As many as 26 ejaculations have been recorded for a ram in a single day. In pasture, free-breeding conditions, particularly at the beginning of the breeding season, rams tend to copulate frequently with the first few ewes in estrus, which is conducive to wastage of spermatozoa.

Clearance of Spermatozoa from the Ejaculates of Vasectomized Rams

Rams of lesser genetic quality are commonly vasectomized and used as teasers to detect estrous ewes. Bilaterally vasectomized rams can be used as teasers 7 to 10 days after vasectomy due to the rapid clearance of most spermatozoa from the ejaculates. However, spermatozoal remnants, including a few intact, nonmotile spermatozoa may be found in ejaculates obtained months after vasectomy.

As a precautionary measure, to decrease the chances of undesired pregnancies, it is recommended to flush the vasa deferentia at the time of vasectomy. This approach produces early azoospermic ejaculates in dogs and cats.

With time, vasectomized rams show decreased libido probably because of damage to the Leydig cells caused by the increased intratesticular and intraepididymal pressures, which develop after vasal ligation. Treatment of vasectomized rams with testosterone before and during the breeding season stimulates their teasing activities.

Retrograde Flow of Spermatozoa into the Bladder

There is considerable retrograde flow of spermatozoa into the bladder of rams during electroejaculation[76] (see Chapter 8). The retrograde flow of spermatozoa into the bladder averaged 28% and 21% during the nonbreeding and breeding seasons, respectively,[76] and should be taken into account when evaluating the breeding soundness of rams.

Ram Evaluation and Breeding Management

The examination of rams for breeding soundness prior to their introduction into the flock at the beginning of the breeding season is fundamental to ensure a high lambing crop and financial success for the producer. Rams of high fertility will settle more ewes within a shorter time and produce more lambs over time than rams of low fertility.

A pubertal ram of 6 months of age or older, used sparingly, can serve up to 10 ewes. Yearling rams may serve up to 30 ewes, and adult rams, which may ejaculate up to 3 times daily without depleting their spermatozoal reserves, are usually stocked in a ratio of 2 to 3 rams per 100 ewes. These general recommendations are for pasture breeding and can be modified to achieve maximal breeding efficiency for a given flock. Rams tend to congregate around estrous ewes. The dominant ram copulates frequently and prevents the mating of the other rams. In hand-breeding programs only estrous ewes are presented to the rams. Thus, the stocking ratio of rams to ewes can be reduced to one ram for 60 to 80 ewes.

GOAT

Domestic goats are also seasonally polyestrous and their breeding activity is influenced by photoperiod. Although there are many similarities in the reproductive patterns of sheep and goats, there are distinct genetic and anatomical differences, as well as differences in the physiology of their reproductive processes.

The diploid number of chromosomes is 60 for the goat as compared to 54 for the sheep. Goats and sheep are thought to have evolved from a common ancestor, which probably had 60 chromosomes. The Barbary sheep, thought to represent an intermediate link between sheep and goats, has 58 chromosomes.

The female goat is usually called a doe or a nanny, the male is called a buck or billy goat, and the offspring, a kid.

Mating between rams and does or between billy goats and ewes may result in fertilization; however, these intergeneric embryos do not develop to term. Similarly, the intergeneric transfer of embryos between sheep and goats is not successful due to maternal rejection, which occurs as the placenta begins to develop. Chimaeric sheep-goat embryos resulting from the combination of blastomeres obtained from sheep and goat embryos at different stages of embryonic development or from chronologically similar blastomeres will develop to term and produce live offspring (see Chapter 19).

BREEDING SEASON

The breeding season extends from late summer to early winter for most goat breeds in the continental U.S. Swiss breeds, such as Toggenburg and Saanen, concentrate their breeding activity between late August and early February. Nubian goats tend to concentrate their breeding activity to the early fall. Mediterranean breeds, such as the Creole and Shiba meat goats do not have a definite breeding season. These breeds cycle year round in tropical areas or in geographic areas with temperate climates. The median month of conception in the continental U.S. is October and the median month of kidding is March for Nubian, Toggenburg, Saanen, Alpine, and Lamancha breeds. There are minor variations among breeds according to the geographic location, probably due to influences caused by the photoperiod of the region. For instance, in the southern and south-western states, the median months of conception and kidding for the breeds mentioned above are September and February, respectively.

The length of the estrous cycle averages 21 days, with a range of 19 to 24 days. Estrus in goats lasts an average of 28 hours, with a range of 1 to 3 days. Most breeds of goats apparently do not undergo silent ovulations at the beginning of the breeding season, as is the case for the sheep. However, goats display short cycles with interestrous intervals of about 8 days at the beginning, and occasionally during the breeding season.

Double and triple ovulations are common to goats and the kidding rate is usually greater than 200%.

The male goat is capable of producing fertile ejaculates year around, but as for the ram, the seminal quality as well as the libido of billy goats is affected by the photoperiod. Billy goats exert estrous initiating and synchronizing effects in does at the interface of anestrus and the breeding season. Does tend to cycle earlier and more regularly when exposed to a buck.

PUBERTY AND SEXUAL MATURITY IN THE FEMALE

Does reach puberty around 6 months of age, but as for the ewe-lamb, the onset of puberty is variable and affected by the plane of nutrition, body weight, and month of birth. Puberty in does as in ewe-lambs is a gradual and interactive process involving maturation of the hypothalamic-pituitary-gonadal axis (see Chapter 9). Neither the blocking affect of estradiol on the maturing hypothalamus nor the need for progesterone to establish the cyclic

pattern, which is characteristic for the ewe-lamb, has been conclusively determined for the goat. However, both pubertal and adult goats at the beginning of the breeding season display a short cycle of about 8 days, due to a short luteal phase lasting only 5 to 6 days. The second estrous cycle is usually a cycle of normal length, particularly when the does are exposed to and teased by a buck. This suggests that the hypothalamic-pituitary-gonadal axis of goats, as for sheep, may require progesterone for the initiation of regular cyclic activity, subsequent to the first post-pubertal estrus or at the onset of the breeding season.

PUBERTY AND SEXUAL MATURITY IN THE MALE

Bucks usually reach puberty between 5 and 6 months of age, but in some breeds puberty may occur as early as 4 months of age. The onset of puberty is affected by breed, plane of nutrition, and season of the year.

THE ESTROUS CYCLE

The interestrous interval averages 21 days in goats. The incidence of short cycles, less than 9 days, is relatively high at the beginning of the breeding season, during lactation (particularly in dairy goats), and occasionally during the breeding season in nonlactating goats. Short cycles are due to a shorter luteal phase, lasting only for 5 to 6 days. These short cycles are apparently induced by the teasing activity of the billy goat. A high percentage of goats ovulate within 8 days after exposure to the male and cycle again, on the average, 19 days after this first estrus. Short cycles of less than 17 days may also occur during the breeding season, particularly when does are continuously exposed to bucks. Apparently, the presence and teasing activity of the male goat induces luteolysis in the cycling doe, shortening the luteal phase of the cycle. Blood levels of progesterone fall below detectable levels 5 to 6 days after mating. When matings with fertile bucks are allowed during these male-induced short cycles, the kidding rates remain within normal ranges. The mechanisms involved in this male-induced luteolysis remain to be determined.

Estrus

Estrus lasts an average of 28 hours, with a range of 1 to 3 days. Bucks show interest and will follow does 3 to 5 days before standing estrus occurs, suggesting proestrual activity. Behavioral signs of estrus are more pronounced in goats than in ewes. Riding and mounting of other goats is not common, unless the goats are exposed to a billy goat or billy goat odor, particularly to the scent, probably pheromones, from glands located in the back of the head between the horns. Estrus detection is usually done by observation of does which stand and mate with a fertile buck or by using teasing males painted in their briskets with chin-ball marking ink. In addition, the swelling and reddening of the vulva, in conjunction with rapid flagging of the tail and vocalization, are signs that help to detect estrous goats.

Ovulation

Ovulation occurs 30 to 36 hours after the onset of estrus and is spontaneous although it may be facilitated by the presence and mounting of the buck. The average ovulation rate is 2 to 3 oocytes but may range from 1 to 5 oocytes, depending upon the breed and management conditions. As for the ewe, the right ovary of the goat is more active than the left ovary.

The Corpus Luteum

The day of diestrus by which embryos must be present in the uterus to prevent regression of the corpus luteum has not been precisely determined for the goat. The corpora lutea of goats regress by the end of diestrus if viable embryos are not present and the doe undergoes a subsequent cycle. As for the ewe, the lifespan of corpora lutea of goats is prolonged, for periods approaching those of pregnancy, by bilateral hysterectomy during midcycle.

There are no reported studies related to the utero-ovarian architecture or to the effects of unilateral hysterectomy in the goat. A local uterine luteolytic effect of the nonpregnant horn on the ipsilateral ovary may not exist in the goat. The available experimental evidence suggests that the transfer of uterine luteolytic activity is either systemic or through routes other than the venous drainage from the ipsilateral horn. Intrauterine devices exert a general rather than a local, unilateral shortening effect on the cycle of goats (see Chapter 9).

The corpus luteum is the major, if not the only, source of progesterone for pregnancy in the goat. Bilateral ovariectomy, luteal enucleation, or induced-luteolysis invariably results in abortion at any stage of gestation. In contrast to the ewe, the placenta of the goat does not produce progesterone.

The uterine prostaglandin $PGF_{2\alpha}$ appears to be the natural luteolysin for the goat, as in the ewe, and ovarian oxytocin plays a role in the uterine secretion of $PGF_{2\alpha}$. Administration of indomethacin, a prostaglandin synthetase inhibitor, or immunization against oxytocin suppresses the synthesis of $PGF_{2\alpha}$ and prolongs the lifespan of the corpora lutea of goats.

As demonstrated by studies on hypophysectomized goats, the corpus luteum depends on pituitary gonadotropic stimulation for development and maintenance of secretory activity during both the luteal phase of the cycle and pregnancy. LH appears to be the major luteotropic gonadotropin for the goat and, in contrast to the ewe, prolactin does not appear to play any significant role.

Endocrinology of the Cycle

There is little information regarding the patterns of secretion of reproductive hormones during the estrous cycle of the goat.

Blood levels of progesterone are low, below 1.0 ng/ml during anestrus and early estrus, but increase rapidly after ovulation to reach peak values of 6 to 10 ng/ml by midcycle and decline rather abruptly by the end of diestrus. Blood levels of progesterone remain elevated if the doe becomes pregnant and may reach values of 10 to 12 ng/ml by day 21 of pregnancy. Levels of progesterone in milk from dairy goats parallel those of the blood, but at higher concentrations. Levels of 2 to 4 ng/ml of milk are common during anestrus or estrus, when the levels of progesterone in the blood are below 1.0 ng/ml.

The ovulatory surge of LH is relatively prolonged, lasting for 9 hours, and blood levels of LH may reach peak values of 70 ng/ml. LH remains at basal levels for most of the cycle.

Blood levels of prolactin undergo circannual rhythms in the goat, reaching their highest levels during the breeding season to decline to basal levels during the nonbreeding season.

To date, there are no reported values for levels of estrogens during the estrous cycle of the goat.

ANATOMIC CHANGES OF THE REPRODUCTIVE ORGANS

The anatomic changes of the reproductive organs of the goat resemble those of the ewe. Since double or triple ovulations are common in breeds with high ovulatory rates, the ovary of the doe tends to resemble a cluster of grapes due to either the large follicles or the corpora lutea protruding from the surface of the ovary.

The uterus of the goat has 160 to 180 caruncles, arranged in definite rows. The cervix has concentric mucosal folds which, in contrast to the ewe, are aligned. Alignment of these folds allows for deep intracervical or intrauterine insemination.

PREGNANCY AND PREGNANCY DIAGNOSIS

Gestation lasts an average of 150 days, but may range from 146 to 155 days, depending upon breed, environmental conditions, and number of kids born. Singleton pregnancies, rare in most breeds of goats, tend to have longer gestations than pregnancy of twins or triplets.

Intrauterine migration of embryos is common in goats and in cases of twin, triple, or quadruple pregnancies serves the purpose of a better distribution of the fetuses and utilization of the uterine environment.

Placentation in goats, as in the sheep, is cotyledonary—syndesmochorial. The placentome is formed by apposition of the fetal and maternal cotyledons.

As indicated previously, progesterone secretion by the corpora lutea is needed throughout gestation, since the placenta of the goat does not produce progesterone in amounts sufficient to maintain pregnancy. The placenta of the goat, however, is a rich source of a placental lactogen with prolactin-like activity. This placental lactogen, detectable in the blood from about day 60 of pregnancy, increases progressively throughout the second half of pregnancy to reach concentrations measurable in micrograms per milliliter of blood by the end of pregnancy.

Levels of pituitary prolactin also increase to maximal levels during the second half of gestation and remain high throughout the remainder of gestation, coinciding with the development of the mammary gland.

The nonreturn to estrus by 21 days after mating during the breeding season, is a relatively reliable sign of pregnancy in goats. Other recommended diagnostic procedures include: use of ultrasound to detect heartbeat, accurate after day 40 of pregnancy; abdominal ballottement of the fetuses against the abdominal wall is effective by about day 120 of pregnancy.

CONTROL OF REPRODUCTIVE EFFICIENCY

Several schemes have been developed to extend the breeding season in order to increase the kidding crop or to produce kids, particularly from dairy goats, at any time of the year.

Induction of Estrus Before the Breeding Season

The exposure of yearling does to a male usually advances the breeding season by 3 weeks. Mature does may begin to cycle within 3 to 9 days after exposure to teasing bucks during the onset of the breeding season and mating with fertile males results in pregnancy. Manipulation of the photoperiod by exposing yearling does to artificial lighting during the spring anestrus, followed by exposure to teaser bucks, results in advancing the breeding season by as many as 80 days.

Synchronization of Estrus

During the breeding season, cycling does can be successfully synchronized using $PGF_{2\alpha}$ or synthetic analogs either alone or after treatment of does for 12 to 16 days with progestagen implants or vaginal pessaries.

In the goat, the corpus luteum of the cycle is sensitive to the luteolytic activity of exogenous prostaglandins as early as day 4 of diestrus. Double prostaglandin treatments given 10 days apart effectively synchronize estrus in groups of does for artificial insemination or timed matings.

Prostaglandin $PGF_{2\alpha}$ or synthetic analogs are effective abortifacient agents at any stage of gestation. Abortion usually occurs within 50 hours after prostaglandin treatment. However, abortion or induction of parturition with prostaglandins may be associated with undesirable side effects in goats. A high incidence of deaths by septicemia has been reported after abortion with prostaglandins.

THE MALE

There is little information regarding spermatogenesis and no information regarding daily spermatozoal production for the buck. Young bucks reportedly have a spermatogenic cycle lasting 22 days. Table 14-4 depicts the body weight, scrotal circumference, and some seminal parameters for the Red Sokoto African goat.

Kids are born with the testes located in the scrotum. Prepubertal development of the reproductive organs is rapid and spermatozoa are present in the epididymides as early as 3.5 months of age. The penis is freed from the preputial sheath by 4 to 6 months of age and fertile matings are possible at this age in most breeds. A diverticulum in the dorsal urethra, at the area of opening of the bulbourethral glands, prevents urethral catheterization in the buck.

Table 14-4 Body Weight, Scrotal Circumference, and Seminal Parameters* for the Red Sokoto African Goat

Endpoint	Mean	Range
Body wt, kg	17.80	—
Scrotal circumference, cm	21.80	20.90–22.50
Volume of ejaculate, ml	0.72	0.50–0.90
Spermatozoal concentration per ml × 10^9	0.61	—
Estimated total number of spermatozoa in ejaculate × 10^9 (vol. × conc.)	0.44	—
Total testicular spermatozoal reserves × 10^9	44.32	—
Epididymal spermatozoal reserves × 10^9	59.45	—

*Semen collected with an artificial vagina.
Adapted from: Daudu, C. S., Theriogenology, *21*: 317, 1983.

Collection of Semen

Semen can be collected from the buck with an AV or by electroejaculation. As for the ram, semen collected with an AV has a lower volume and higher spermatozoal concentration than semen collected by electroejaculation.

Buck Evaluation and Breeding Management

Sexual behavior is established early in young bucks. Prepubertal kids display the Flehmen reaction and mounting behavior from about 1 month of age. These responses may be enhanced when the two sexes are reared together. As maturation progresses toward puberty, bucks develop the typical pungent odor of the billy goat. This characteristic odor, usually repugnant to man, is derived from the secretions from the sebaceous glands located between the horns and from the urine. As they grow older, bucks develop the habit of urinating on their own chin hair and forelegs. This billy goat odor exerts a powerful attractive and estrus-stimulating effect in does.

The buck is capable of fertile matings throughout the year, but both quality of semen and libido seem to be influenced by the photoperiod, particularly in geographic areas with pronounced seasonal fluctuations in day light length and temperature. Serum levels of LH and testosterone increase with decreasing day length and reach maximal mean levels of 2.0 ng/ml of LH and 15 ng/ml of testosterone during the middle of the breeding season. In the nonbreeding season, billy goats may show depressed libido and seminal quality and a general lack of interest in does which have been artificially induced to cycle.

In general, the recommendations given for the breeding management of rams are applicable to the buck.

REFERENCES

Sheep

1. Amann, R. P., Nett, T. M., and Niswender, G. D. (1978): Effects of LH, FSH, prolactin and PGF$_{2\alpha}$ on testicular blood flow and testosterone secretion in the ram. J. Anim. Sci. *47*:1307.
2. Baird, D. T. (1978): Pulsatile secretion of LH and ovarian estradiol during the follicular phase of the sheep estrous cycle. Biol. Reprod. *18*:359.
3. Bindon, B. M., Blanc, M. R., Pelletier, J., et al. (1979): Periovulatory gonadotrophin and ovarian steroid patterns in sheep of breeds with differing fecundity. J. Reprod. Fertil. *55*:15.
4. Brinkley, H. J. (1981): Endocrine signaling and female reproduction. Biol. Reprod. *24*:22.
5. Burfening, P. J., Van Horn, J. L., and Blackwell, R. L. (1971): Genetic and phenotypic parameters including occurrence of estrus in Rambouillet ewe lambs. J. Anim. Sci. *33*:919.
6. Buttle, H. L., and Hancock, J. L. (1966): The chromosomes of goats, sheep and their hybrids. Res. Vet. Sci, *7*:230.
7. Carnegie, J. A., McCully, M. E., and Robertson, H. A. (1985): The early development of the sheep trophoblast and the involvement of cell death. Am. J. Anat. *174*:471.
8. Casida, L. E., and Warwick, E. J. (1945): The necessity of the corpus luteum for maintenance of pregnancy in the ewe. J. Anim. Sci. *4*:34.
9. Cottrell, W. O. (1985): Ram management for northeastern flocks. Cornell Vet. *75*:505.
10. Cran, D. G., Moor, R. M., and Hay, M. F. (1980): Fine structure of the sheep oocyte during antral follicle development. J. Reprod. Fertil. *59*:125.
11. Cumming, I. A., Baxter, R., and Lawson, R. A. S. (1974): Steroid hormone requirements for the maintenance of early pregnancy in sheep: A study using ovariectomized adrenalectomized ewes. J. Reprod. Fertil. *40*:443.
12. Cummins, L. J., O'Shea, T. O., Al-Obaidi, S. A. R., et al. (1986): Increase in ovulation rate after immunization of merino ewes with a fraction of bovine follicular fluid containing inhibin activity. J. Reprod.

Fertil. *77*:365.
13. Davis, A. J., Fleet, I. R., Harrison, F. A., et al. (1979): Pulmonary metabolism of prostaglandin F$_{2\alpha}$ in the conscious non-pregnant ewe and sow. J. Physiol. *290*:36P.
14. Driancourt, M. A., Cahill, L. P., and Bindon, B. M. (1985): Ovarian follicular populations and preovulatory enlargement in booroola and control merino ewes. J. Reprod. Fertil. *73*:93.
15. Driancourt, M. A., Gibson, W. R., and Cahill, L. P. (1985): Follicular dynamics throughout the oestrous cycle in sheep. A review. Reprod. Nutr. Develop. *25*:1.
16. Dunlop, A. A., Moule, G. R., and Southcott, W. H. (1963): Spermatozoa in the ejaculates of vasectomized rams. Aust. Vet. J. *39*:46.
17. Dziuk, P. J., and Bellows, R. A. (1983): Management of reproduction of beef cattle, sheep and pigs. J. Anim. Sci. *57*, Suppl. 2:355.
18. Ellinwood, W. E., Nett, T. M., and Niswender, G. D. (1979): Maintenance of the corpus luteum of early pregnancy in the ewe. I. Luteotropic properties of embryonic homogenates. Biol. Reprod. *21*:281.
19. Ellinwood, W. E., Nett, T. M., and Niswender, G. D. (1979): Maintenance of the corpus luteum of early pregnancy in the ewe. II. Prostaglandin secretion by the endometrium in vitro and in vivo. Biol. Reprod. *21*:845.
20. Estes, R. D. (1972): The role of the vomeronasal organ in mammalian reproduction. Mammalia *36*: 315.
21. Fletcher, I. C. (1971): Effects of nutrition, liveweight, and season on the incidence of twin ovulation in South Australian strong-wool Merino ewes. Aust. J. Agric. Res. *22*:321.
22. Foote, W. C., Sefidbakht, N., and Madsen, M. A. (1970): Puberal estrus and ovulation and subsequent estrous cycle patterns in the ewe. J. Anim. Sci. *30*:86.
23. Foster, D., and Ryan, K. (1979): Mechanisms governing onset of ovarian cyclicity at puberty in the lamb. Ann. Biol. Anim. Biochim. Biophys. *19*:1369.
24. Foster, D. L., Lemons, J. A., Jaffe, R. B., et al. (1975): Sequential patterns of circulating luteinizing hormone in female sheep from early postnatal life through the first estrous cycles. Endocrinology *97*:985.
25. Fraser, A. F., and Laing, A. H. (1969): Oestrus induction in ewes with standard treatments of reduced natural light. Vet. Rec. *84*:427.
26. Garnier, D.-H., Cotta, Y., and Terqui, M. (1978): Androgen radioimmunoassay in the ram: results of direct plasma testosterone and dehydroepiandrosterone measurement and physiological evaluation. Ann. Biol. Anim. Biochim. Biophys. *18*:265.
27. George, J. M. (1973): Post parturient oestrus in Merino and Dorset horn sheep. Aust. Vet. J. *49*:242.
28. Gerneke, W. H. (1965): Chromosomal evidence of the freemartin condition in sheep. J. S. Afr. Vet. Med. Assoc. *36*:99.
29. Ghannam, S. A. M., Bosc, M. J., and Du Mesnil-Du Buisson, F. (1972): Examination of vaginal epithelium of the sheep and its use in pregnancy diagnosis. Am. J. Vet. Res. *33*:1175.
30. Ginther, O. J., and Bisgard, G. E. (1972): Role of main uterine vein in local action of an intrauterine

device on the corpus luteum in sheep. Am. J. Vet. Res. *33*:1583.

31. Ginther, O.J., and Del Campo, C. H. (1973): Vascular anatomy of the uterus and ovaries and the unilateral luteolytic effect of the uterus: Areas of close apposition between the ovarian artery and vessels which contain uterine venous blood in sheep. Am. J. Vet. Res. *34*:1387.

32. Ginther, O. J., Del Campo, C. H., and Rawlings, C. A. (1973): Vascular anatomy of the uterus and ovaries and the unilateral luteolytic effect of the uterus. A local venoarterial pathway between uterus and ovaries in sheep. Am. J. Vet. Res. *34*:723.

33. Gunn, R. G., and Doney, J. M. (1979): Ewe management for control of reproductive performance. ADAS Quat. Rev. *35*:231.

34. Harding, C. F. (1981): Social modulation of circulating hormone levels in the male. Am. Zool. *21*:223.

35. Hauger, R. L., Karsch, F. J., and Foster, D. L. (1977): A new concept for control of the estrous cycle of the ewe based on the temporal relationships between luteinizing hormones, estradiol and progesterone in peripheral serum and evidence that progesterone inhibits tonic LH secretion. Endocrinology *101*:807.

36. Hidiroglou, M. (1979): Trace element deficiencies and fertility in ruminants: A review. J. Dairy Sci. *62*:1195.

37. Hoagland, T. A. and Bolt, D. J. (1986): Serum follicle stimulating hormone, luteinizing hormone, and testosterone in sexually stimulated intact and unilaterally castrated rams. Theriogenology *26*:671.

38. Hochereau–de Reviers, M.-T., and Courot, M. (1978): Sertoli cells and development of seminiferous epithelium. Ann. Biol. Anim. Biochim. Biophys. *18*:573.

39. Hogg, J. T. (1984): Mating in bighorn sheep: Multiple creative male strategies. Science *225*:526.

40. Hollis, D. E., Frith, P. A., Vaughan, J. D., et al. (1984): Ultrastructural changes in the oviductal epithelium of merino ewes during the estrous cycle. Am. J. Anat. *171*:441.

41. Hunter, R. H. F., and Nichol, R. (1983): Transport of spermatozoa in the sheep oviduct: Preovulatory sequestering of cells in the caudal isthmus. J. Exp. Zool. *228*:121.

42. Hunter, R. H. F., Barbwise, L., and King, R. (1982): Sperm transport, storage and release in the sheep oviduct in relation to the time of ovulation. Br. Vet. J. *138*:225.

43. Hunter, R. H. F., Nichol, R., and Crabtree, S. M., (1980): Transport of spermatozoa in the ewe: timing of the establishment of a functional population in the oviduct. Reprod. Nutr. Develop. *20*:1869.

44. Jenkins, G., Heap, R. B., and Symons, D. B. A. (1977): Pituitary responsiveness to synthetic LH-RH and pituitary LH content at various reproductive stages in the sheep. J. Reprod. Fertil. *49*:207.

45. Karsch, F. J., Foster, D. L., Legan, S. J., et al. (1979): Control of the preovulatory endocrine events in the ewe: Interrelationship of estradiol, progesterone, and luteinizing hormone. Endocrinology *105*:421.

46. Keverne, E. B., Levy, F., Poindron, P., et al. (1983): Vaginal stimulation: An important determinant of maternal bonding in sheep. Science *219*:81.

47. King, G. J., Atkinson, B. A., and Robertson, H. A. (1982): Implantation and early placentation in domestic ungulates. J. Reprod. Fertil., Suppl., *31*:17.

48. Kittok, R. J., and Britt, J. H. (1977): Corpus luteum function in ewes given estradiol during the estrous cycle or early pregnancy. J. Anim. Sci. *45*:336.

49. Knight, T. W. (1977): Methods for the indirect estimation of testes weight and sperm numbers in merino and romney rams. N. Z. J. Agric. Res. *20*:291.

50. Knight, T. W., and Lynch, P. R. (1980): Source of ram pheromones that stimulate ovulation in the ewe. Anim. Reprod. Sci. *3*:133.

51. Knight, T. W., Peterson, A. J., and Payne, E. (1978): The ovarian and hormonal response of the ewe to stimulation by the ram early in the breeding season. Theriogenology *10*:34.

52. Lacroix, M. C., and Kann, G. (1986): Aspects of the antiluteolytic activity of the conceptus during early pregnancy in ewes. J. Anim. Sci. *63*:1449.

53. Lamond, D. R., Hill, J. R., Godley, W. C., et al. (1973): Influence of nutrition on ovulation and fertilization in the Rambouillet ewe. J. Anim. Sci. *36*:363.

54. Lees, J. L. (1978). Functional infertility in sheep. Vet. Rec. *102*:232.

55. Legan, S. J., and Karsch, F. J. (1983): Importance of retinal photoreceptors to photoperiodic control of seasonal breeding in the ewe. Biol. Reprod. *29*:316.

56. Legan, S. J., Karsch, F. J., and Foster, D. L. (1977): The endocrine control of seasonal reproductive function in the ewe: A marked change in response to the negative feedback action of estradiol on luteinizing hormone secretion. Endocrinology *101*:818.

57. Lewis, P. E., and Warren, J. E., Jr. (1977): Effect of indomethacin on luteal function in ewes and heifers. J. Anim. Sci. *46*:763.

58. Lincoln, G. A. (1976): Seasonal variation in the episodic secretion of luteinizing hormone and testosterone in the ram. J. Endocrinol. *60*:213.

59. Lindsay, D. R., Pelletier, J., Pisselet, C., et al. (1984): Changes in photoperiod and nutrition and their affect on testicular growth of rams. J. Reprod. Fertil. *71*:351.

60. Lunstra, D. D., and Christenson, R. K. (1981): Fertilization and embryonic survival in ewes synchronized with exogenous hormones during the anestrous and estrous seasons. J. Anim. Sci. *53*:458.

61. Mallampati, R. S., Pope, A. L., and Casida, L. E. (1971): Effect of suckling on postpartum anestrus in ewes lambing in different seasons of the year. J. Anim. Sci. *32*:673.

62. Mapletoft, R. J., and Ginther, O. J. (1975): Adequacy of main uterine vein and the ovarian artery in the local venoarterial pathway for uterine-induced luteolysis in ewes. Am. J. Vet. Res. *36*:957.

63. Mapletoft, R. J., Lapin, D. R., and Ginther, O. J. (1976): The ovarian artery as the final component of the local luteotropic pathway between a gravid uterine horn and ovary in ewes. Biol. Reprod. *15*:414.

64. Mattner, E., and Voglmayr, J. K. (1962): A comparison of ram semen collected by the artificial vagina and by electroejaculation. Aust. J. Exp. Agr. Anim. Husb. *2*:78.

65. McNatty, K. P., Revfeim, K. J. A., and Young, A. (1973): Peripheral plasma progesterone concentrations in sheep during the oestrous cycle. J. Endo-

crinol. *58*:219.

66. McNatty, K. P., Gibb, M., Dobson, C., et al. (1981): Changes in the concentration of gonadotrophic and steroidal hormones in the antral fluid of ovarian follicles throughout the oestrous cycle of the sheep. Aust. J. Biol. Sci. *34*:67.

67. McNatty, K. P., Henderson, K. M., Lun, S., et al. (1985): Ovarian activity in booroola x romney ewes which have a major gene influencing their ovulation rate. J. Reprod. Fertil. *73*:109.

68. Mellin, T. N., and Bush, R. D. (1976): Corpus luteum function in the ewe: Effect of $PGF_{2\alpha}$ and prostaglandin synthetase inhibitors. Theriogenology *12*:303.

69. Murdoch, W. J. (1985): Follicular determinants of ovulation in the ewe. Domest. Anim. Endocrinol. *2*: 105.

70. Nayak, R. K., Albert, E. N., and Kassira, W. N. (1976): Cyclic ultrastructural changes in ewe uterine tube (oviduct) infundibular epithelium. Am. J. Vet. Res. *37*:923.

71. Noordhuizen-Stassen, E. N., Charbon, G. A., de Jong, F. H., et al. (1985): Functional arterio-venous anastomoses between the testicular artery and the pampiniform plexus in the spermatic cord of rams. J. Reprod. Fertil. *75*:193.

72. Osborne, H. G. (1970): The duration and intensity of oestrus in Finnsheep. Aust. Vet. J. *46*:605.

73. O'Shea, J. D., and Wright, P. J. (1985): Regression of the corpus luteum of pregnancy following parturition in the ewe. Acta Anat. *122*:69.

74. Pant, H. C., Hopkinson, C. R. N., and Fitzpatrick, R. J. (1977): Concentration of estradiol, progesterone, luteinizing hormone and follicle-stimulating hormone in the jugular venous plasma of ewes during the oestrous cycle. J. Endocrinol. *73*:247.

75. Pelletier, J. (1986): Contribution of increasing and decreasing daylength to the photoperiodic control of LH secretion in the Ile-de-France ram. J. Reprod. Fertil. *77*:505.

76. Pineda, M. H., Dooley, M. P., Hembrough, F. B., et al. (1987): Retrograde flow of spermatozoa into the urinary bladder of rams. Am. J. Vet. Res. *48*:562.

77. Ricketts, A. P., Sheldrick, E. L., Lindsay, K. S., et al. (1980): Induction of labour in sheep after fetal hypophysectomy: An investigation of the possible involvement of a fetal pituitary secretion in the activation of placental enzymes by fetal cortisol. Placenta *1*:287.

78. Rippel, R. H., Moyer, R. H., Johnson, E. S., et al. (1974): Response of the ewe to synthetic gonadotropin releasing hormone. J. Anim. Sci. *38*:605.

79. Robertson, H. A., Dwyer, R. J., and King, G. J. (1985): Oestrogens in fetal and maternal fluids throughout pregnancy in the pig and comparisons with the ewe and cow. J. Endocrinol. *106*:355.

80. Robertson, H. A., Chan, J. S. D., Hackett, A. J., et al. (1980): Diagnosis of pregnancy in the ewe at midgestation. Anim. Reprod. Sci. *3*:69.

81. Sanford, L. M., Winter, J. S. D., Palmer, W. M., et al. (1974): The profile of LH and testosterone secretion in the ram. Endocrinology *96*:627.

82. Scaramuzzi, R. J., Davidson, W. G., and Van Look, P. F. A. (1977): Increasing ovulation rate in sheep by active immunization against an ovarian steroid androstenedione. Nature *269*:817.

83. Segerson, E. C., Jr., Ulberg, L. C., Martin, J. E., et al. (1974): Fertility in ewes treated with luteinizing hormone-releasing factor. Proc. Soc. Exp. Biol. Med. *146*:518.

84. Thwaites, C. J. (1982): Semen quality after vasectomy in the ram. Livestock Prod. Sci. *8*:529.

85. Thorburn, G. D., Challis, J. R. C., and Currie, W. B. (1977): Control of parturition in domestic animals. Biol. Reprod. *16*:18.

86. Tilbrook, A. J., and Pearce, D. T. (1986): Time required for spermatozoa to remain in the vagina of the ewe to ensure conception. Aust. J. Biol. Sci. *39*: 305.

87. Trapp, M. J., and Slyter, A. L. (1983): Pregnancy diagnosis in the ewe. J. Anim. Sci. *57*:1.

88. Trounson, A. O., Willadsen, S. M., and Moor, R. M. (1977): Reproductive function in prepubertal lambs: Ovulation, embryo development and ovarian steroidogenesis. J. Reprod. Fertil. *49*:69.

89. Tryphonas, L., Hidiroglou, M., and Collins, B. (1979): Reversal by testosterone of atrophy of accessory genital glands of castrated male sheep. Vet. Pathol. *16*:710.

90. Turnbull, K. E., Braden, A. W. H., and Mattner, P. E. (1977): The pattern of follicular growth and atresia in the ovine ovary. Aust. J. Biol. Sci. *30*:229.

91. Tyrrell, R. N., and Plant, J. W. (1979): Rectal damage in ewes following pregnancy diagnosis by rectal-abdominal palpation. J. Anim. Sci. *48*:348.

92. Van Wyk, L. C., Van Niekerk, C., and Belonje, P. C. (1972): Involution of the post-partum uterus of the ewe. J. S. Afr. Vet. Assoc. *43*:19.

93. Walkley, J. R. W., and Smith, C. (1980): The use of physiological traits in genetic selection for litter size in sheep. J. Reprod. Fertil. *59*:83.

94. Wallace, J. M., McNeilly, A. S., and Baird, D. T. (1986): Induction of ovulation during anoestrous in two breeds of sheep with multiple injections of LH alone or in combination with FSH. J. Endocrinol. *111*:181.

95. Wheeler, A. G. (1978): Comparisons of the ovulatory and steroidogenic activities of the left and right ovaries of the ewe. J. Reprod. Fertil. *53*:27.

96. Willadsen, S. M., (1986): Nuclear transplantation in sheep embryos. Nature *320*:63.

97. Willingham, T., Shelton, M., and Thompson, P. (1986): An assessment of reproductive wastage in sheep. Theriogenology *26*:179.

98. Wooding, F. B. P., Flint, A. P. F., Heap, R. B., et al. (1981): Autoradiographic evidence for migration and fusion of cells in the sheep placenta: Resolution of a problem in placental classification. Cell Biol. *5*:821.

Goats

1. Ali, B. H., and Mustafa, A. I. (1986): Semen characteristics of nubian goats in the Sudan. Anim. Reprod. Sc. *12*:63.

2. Armstrong, D. T., and Evans, G. (1983): Factors influencing success of embryo transfer in sheep and goats. Theriogenology *19*:31.

3. Armstrong, D. T., and Evans, G. (1984): Hormonal regulation of reproduction: Induction of ovulation in sheep and goats with FSH preparations. Proc. 10th.

Int. Congr. Anim. Reprod. Art. Insem., Vol. VII. Univ. Illinois, Champaign/Urbana, June 10–14, 1984, p. 8.

4. Basrur, P. K. (1986): Goat-sheep hybrids. *In*: Current Therapy in Theriogenology 2, D. A. Morrow, ed., Philadelphia, W. B. Saunders Co., p. 613.

5. Basrur, P. K., and McKinnon, A. O. (1986): Caprine intersexes and freemartins. *In*: Current Therapy in Theriogenology 2, D. A. Morrow, ed., Philadelphia, W. B. Saunders Co., p. 596.

6. Beckett, S. D., Reynolds, T. M., and Bartels, J. E. (1978): Angiography of the crus penis in the ram and buck during erection. Am. J. Vet. Res. *39*:1950.

7. Bon Durant, R. H. (1981): Reproductive physiology in the goat. Mod. Vet. Pract. *62*:525.

8. Bon Durant, R. H., Darien, B. J., Munro, C. J., et al. (1981): Photoperiod induction of fertile oestrus and changes in LH and progesterone concentrations in yearling dairy goats (Capra hircus). J. Reprod. Fertil. *63*:1.

9. Bretzlaff, K. N., Hill, A., and Ott, R. S. (1983): Induction of luteolysis in goats with prostaglandin $F_{2\alpha}$. Am. J. Vet. Res. *44*:1162.

10. Bretzlaff, K. N., Ott, R. S., Weston, P. G., et al. (1981): Dose of prostaglandin $F_2\alpha$ effective for induction of estrus in goats. Theriogenology *16*:587.

11. Buttle, H. L. (1978): The maintenance of pregnancy in hypophysectomized goats. J. Reprod. Fertil. *52*:255.

12. Chemineau, P. (1983): Effect on oestrus and ovulation of exposing creole goats to the male at three times of the year. J. Reprod. Fertil. *67*:65.

13. Chemineau, P. (1986): Sexual behaviour and gonadal activity during the year in the tropical creole meat goat. I. Female oestrous behaviour and ovarian activity. Reprod. Nutr. Develop. *26*:441.

14. Chemineau, P. (1986): Sexual behaviour and gonadal activity during the year in the tropical creole meat goat. II. Male mating behaviour, testis diameter, ejaculate characteristics and fertility. Reprod. Nutr. Develop. *26*:453.

15. Chemineau, P., and Xande, A. (1982): Reproductive efficiency of creole meat goats permanently kept with males. Relationship to a tropical environment. Trop. Anim. Prod. *7*:98.

16. Cooke, R. G., and Homeida, A. M. (1983): Prevention of the luteolytic action of oxytocin in the goat by inhibition of prostaglandin synthesis. Theriogenology *20*:363.

17. Cooke, R. G., and Homeida, A. M. (1985): Suppression of prostaglandin $F_{2\alpha}$ release and delay of luteolysis after active immunization against oxytocin in the goat. J. Reprod. Fertil. *75*:63.

18. Cooke, R. G., and Knifton, A. (1980): Removal of corpora lutea in pregnant goats: Effects of intrauterine indomethacin. Res. Vet. Sci. *29*:77.

19. Currie, W. B. (1974): Regression of the corpus luteum of pregnancy and initiation of labour in goats. J. Reprod. Fertil. *36*:481.

20. Currie, W. B., and Thorburn, G. D. (1974): Luteal function in hysterectomized goats. J. Reprod. Fertil. *41*:501.

21. Currie, W. B., Cox, R. I., and Thorburn, G. D. (1976): Release of prostaglandin F, regression of corpora lutea and induction of premature parturition in goats treated with estradiol-17β. Prostaglandins *12*:1093.

22. Daudu, C. S. (1984): Spermatozoa output, testicular sperm reserve and epididymal storage capacity of the red sokoto goats indigenous to Northern Nigeria. Theriogenology *21*:317.

23. Day, A. M., and Southwell, S. R. G. (1979): Termination of pregnancy in goats using cloprostenol. N. Z. Vet. J. *27*:207.

24. Dhingra, L. D. (1979): Angioarchitecture of the arteries of the testis of goat (Capra aegagrus). Zbl. Vet. Med. *8*:193.

25. Erasmus, J. A., Fourie, A. J., and Venter, J. J. (1985): Influence of age on reproductive performance of the improved Boer goat doe. So. Afr. J. Anim. Sci. *15*:5.

26. Fielden, E. D. (1984): Reproductive diseases of sheep and goats. Proc. 10th. Int. Congr. Anim. Reprod. Art. Insem. Vol. VII. Univ. Illinois, Champaign/Urbana, June 10–14, 1984, p. 39.

27. Forsyth, I. A., Byatt, J. C., and Iley, S. (1985): Hormone concentrations, mammary development and milk yield in goats given long-term bromocriptine treatment in pregnancy. J. Endocrinol. *104*:77.

28. Gadgil, B. A., Zala, P. M., Shukla, K. P., et al. (1969): Effect of intrauterine spirals on reproduction in goats. Ind. J. Exp. Biol. *7*:82.

29. Hayden, T. J., Thomas, C. R., Smith, S. V., et al. (1980): Placental lactogen in the goat in relation to stage of gestation, number of fetuses, metabolites, progesterone and time of day. J. Endocrinol. *86*:279.

30. Hinkle, R. F., Howard, J. L., and Stowater, J. L. (1978): An anatomic barrier to urethral catheterization in the male goat. J. Am. Vet. Med. Assoc. *173*:1584.

31. Linzell, J. L., and Heap, R. B. (1966): A comparison of progesterone metabolism in the pregnant sheep and goat, sources of production and estimation of uptake by some target organs. J. Endocrinol. *41*:433.

32. Lyngset, O. (1968): Studies on reproduction in the goat. III. Functional activity of the ovaries of the goat. Acta Vet. Scand. *9*:268.

33. Meites, J., Webster, H. D., Young, F. W., et al. (1951): Effects of the corpora lutea removal and replacement with progesterone on pregancy in goats. J. Anim. Sci. *10*:411.

34. Memon, M. A., Bretzlaff, K. N., and Ott, R. S. (1986): Comparison of semen collection techniques in goats. Theriogenology *26*:823.

35. Mohammad, W. A., Grossman, M., and Vatthauer, J. L. (1984): Seasonal breeding in United States dairy goats. J. Dairy Sci. *67*:1813.

36. Mori, Y., Kano, Y., and Sawasaki, T. (1983): An application of culdoscopy to goats for serial observation of periovulatory ovary in the goats (sic). Jap. J. Vet. Sci. *45*:667.

37. Muduuli, D. S., Sanford, L. M., Plamer, W. M., et al. (1979): Secretory patterns and circadian and seasonal changes in luteinizing hormone, follicle stimulating hormone, prolactin, and testosterone in the male pygmy goat. J. Anim. Sci. *49*:543.

38. Ogunbiyi, P. O., Molokwu, E. C. I., and Sooriyamoorthy, T. (1980): Estrus synchronization and controlled breeding in goats using prostaglandin $F_{2\alpha}$. Theriogenology *13*:257.

39. Ott, R. S., Nelson, D. R., and Hixon, J. E. (1980): The effect of presence of the male on initiation of

estrous cycle activity of goats. Theriogenology *13*:183.

40. Ott, R. S., Nelson, D. R., and Hixon, J. E. (1980): Fertility of goats following synchronization of estrus with prostaglandin F$_{2\alpha}$. Theriogenology *13*:341.

41. Ott, R. S., Nelson, D. R., and Hixon, J. E. (1980): Peripheral serum progesterone and luteinizing hormone concentrations of goats during synchronization of estrus and ovulation with prostaglandin F$_{2\alpha}$. Am. J. Vet. Res. *41*:1432.

42. Price, E. O., and Smith, V. M. (1984/85): The relationship of male-male mounting to mate choice and sexual performance in male dairy goats. Appl. Anim. Behav. Sci. *13*:71.

43. Refsal, K. R. (1986): Collection and evaluation of caprine semen. *In*: Current Therapy in Theriogenology 2, D. A. Morrow, ed. Philadelphia, W. B. Saunders Co., p. 619.

44. Riera, G. S. (1984): Some similarities and differences in female sheep and goat reproduction. Proc. 10th. Int. Congr. Anim. Reprod. Art. Insem., Vol. VII, Univ. Illinois, Champaign/Urbana, June 10–14, p. 1.

45. Ritar, A. J., and Salamon, S. (1983): Fertility of fresh and frozen-thawed semen of the angora goat. Aust. J. Biol. Sci. *36*:49.

46. Salamon, S., and Ritar, A. J. (1982): Deep freezing of angora goat semen: Effects of diluent composition, method and rate of dilution on survival of spermatozoa. Aust. J. Biol. Sci. *35*:295.

47. Shelton, M. (1978): Reproduction and breeding of goats. J. Dairy Sci. *61*:994.

48. Sheldrick, E. L., Ricketts, A. P., and Flint, A. P. F. (1980): Placental production of progesterone in ovariectomized goats treated with a synthetic progestagen to maintain pregnancy. J. Reprod. Fertil. *60*:339.

49. Staples, L. D., Fleet, I. R., and Heap, R. B. (1982): Anatomy of the utero-ovarian lymphatic network and the composition of afferent lymph in relation to the establishment of pregnancy in the sheep and goat. J. Reprod. Fertil. *64*:409.

50. Thibier, M., Pothelet, D., Jeanguyot, N., et al. (1981): Estrous behavior, progesterone in peripheral plasma and milk in dairy goats at onset of breeding season. J. Dairy Sci. *64*:513.

51. Thompson, F. N., Abrams, E., and Miller, D. M. (1983): Reproductive traits in Nubian dairy goats. Anim. Reprod. Sci., *6*:59.

52. Tokashiki, S., and Kawashima, Y. (1976): Histochemical changes in the endometrium of the goats during the course of estrous cycle and pregnancy. Jap. J. Vet. Sci. *38*:639.

53. Wathes, D. C., Swann, R. W., Porter, D. G., et al. (1986): Oxytocin as an ovarian hormone. Current Topics Neuroendocrinol. *6*:129.

54. Williams, H. LL. (1984): The effects of the physical and social environments on reproduction in adult sheep and goats. Proc. 10th. Int. Congr. Anim. Reprod. Art. Insem. Vol. IV, Univ. Illinois, Champaign/Urbana, June 10–14, p. 31.

Reproductive Patterns of Swine*

L. E. EVANS

15

THE domestic female pig is polytocous and nonseasonally polyestrous with estrus occurring at intervals of about 21 days. Proestrus lasts about 2 days, estrus 2 to 3 days, and metestrus for 1 or 2 days. The remainder of the cycle is diestrus. The corpora lutea are functional for about 16 days after ovulation. Ovulation occurs spontaneously, 36 to 44 hours after the onset of estrus or shortly beyond mid-estrus.

Pregnancy lasts 112 to 116 days, common-ly resulting in litters of 8 to 10 pigs for gilts and 10 to 16 pigs for sows. During lactation the sow may have an abbreviated psychic estrus shortly after parturition but does not normally cycle and breed until after the pigs are weaned.

SEXUAL MATURITY (PUBERTY)

Several factors influence the onset of puberty in the gilt and continuance of regular estrous cycles. The most important of these include: (1) breed, (2) season of the year during sexual development, (3) boar exposure, (4) housing and degree of confinement, (5) nutrition and (6) general health. Under good management, puberty occurs in the young female, which is called a gilt, at approximately 6 to 7 months of age when the gilt reaches a body weight of 100 to 110 kg.

The age of puberty is influenced by the breed and selection within the breed. Generally, Landrace and the Large White breeds followed by Hampshires have earlier first estrus than other common breeds in the United States. Within breeds, some genetic lines cycle earlier than others.

The percentage of gilts showing normal estrous cycles by 9 months of age is lower for those gilts reaching breeding age during the summer than for gilts reaching breeding age during the other seasons. This effect is observed in both confinement and non-con-

---

* Additional information concerning reproduction in swine has been covered in Chapter 8 (Male Reproduction), Chapter 9 (Female Reproduction) and Chapter 10 (Artificial Insemination)

finement gilts. Confinement will reduce the number of gilts showing estrus at 7 to 9 months of age by 10 to 15% when compared to non-confinement housed gilts. Housing gilts individually, in small groups of 2 to 3 per pen, or in large groups of 50 or more, delays the first estrus. Other environmental factors such as lighting appear to have little effect on days to first estrus.

As the gilts are approaching pubertal age, exposure of gilts to a mature boar will shorten the interval to estrus and results in some synchronization of estrus. Puberty is often delayed if boar exposure is initiated when the gilts are only 3 to 4 months of age.

Under normal conditions of feeding and management, nutrition will have a minimal effect on puberty. A low protein diet will delay growth and puberty and a low energy diet may depress ovulation rates. Likewise unthriftiness due to disease can delay the first estrus.

The age at onset of puberty in the boar is similar to that in the gilt. Primary spermatocytes first appear in the seminiferous tubules by 3 months of age; secondary spermatocytes at 4 to 5 months and mature spermatozoa are present in the ejaculate at 5 to 6 months of age. At this age the boar has limited fertility and should not be used on a regular basis for breeding until 8 months of age. Young boars should be selected for early sexual maturity, since this characteristic is one of the more heritable reproductive traits and may be reflected in age of puberty in his offspring. Boars raised without interaction with the opposite sex often have delayed behavioral development. A castrated male is called a barrow.

BREEDING SEASON

A well-fed postpuberal non-pregnant sow or a gilt under ordinary environmental conditions is a non-seasonal polyestrous animal although fertility and cyclicity may be depressed in the late summer and early fall months. The sow will show estrus approximately every 21 days until the age of 10 to 12 years when senility begins to affect ovarian function. Most sows are culled from the breeding herd for other reasons long before senility sets in.

After parturition there is a period of anestrus when the ovaries are quiescent. This quiescence generally lasts throughout lactation. Soon after weaning, which occurs at 2 to 5 weeks postpartum under present husbandry conditions, there is a rapid growth of ovarian follicles, followed by estrus and ovulation within 3 to 7 days. It is desirable to breed the sow at this time since uterine involution is completed by 21 days postpartum and the sow's fertility is good. Weaning is often used as a means of achieving synchrony of estrus in a group of sows.

Most producers maximize sow productivity by rebreeding the sow as soon as possible. With a gestation period of 114 days and a lactational period of 21 days, sows which are bred 5 to 10 days after weaning can be expected to produce a litter every 5 months or an average of 2.4 litters per year. However, due to other factors which reduce fertility, the average sow herd falls considerably short of this potential production level.

THE ESTROUS CYCLE

The estrous cycle of the sow can be divided into events associated with the growth of the follicles and events associated with the growth and survival of the corpora lutea (Figs. 15-1 and 15-2). The histologic and secretory changes occurring in the tubular genital tract under the influence of rising estrogen levels at the time of proestrus and estrus or rising progesterone levels during metestrus and diestrus are similar to those of other species (Fig. 15-3). The vaginal smear is a poor indicator of the stage of estrous cycle in the sow.

Following ovulation at mid-estrus, follicular remnants luteinize resulting in the formation of progesterone-producing corpora lutea (CL). Plasma progesterone levels rise to a peak of 25 to 30 ng/ml at 12 to 14 days and are followed by a rapid decline, coincidental with luteolysis, 15 to 18 days after estrus. Prostaglandin $T_{2\alpha}$ is believed to be the natural luteolysin, however, porcine corpora lutea are not responsive to rising levels of $PGF_{2\alpha}$ until after day 12 of the estrous cycle.

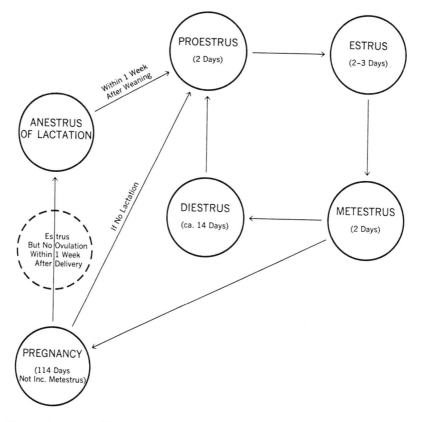

Fig. 15-1. The ovarian cycle of the sow with alternates.

As progesterone levels decline, the hypothalamo-hypophyseal axis responds by increasing the frequency of episodic release of LH. Ultimately there is increased binding of gonadotropins by the developing follicles and maturation of the follicles. An increase in circulating levels of estrogens, primarily 17β-estradiol, occurs between days 15 and 20 of the estrous cycle. Circulating estrogens peak about 24 hours before the onset of behavioral estrus. LH levels peak at the beginning of estrus and ovulation occurs 36 to 44 hours after the LH peak. The ova are shed from both ovaries over a range of 6 to 8 hours.

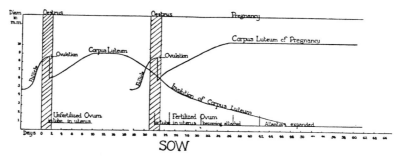

Fig. 15-2. The ovarian cycle in the sow. (Slightly modified from Corner. Dukes: The Physiology of Domestic Animals. Courtesy Comstock Pub. Assoc.)

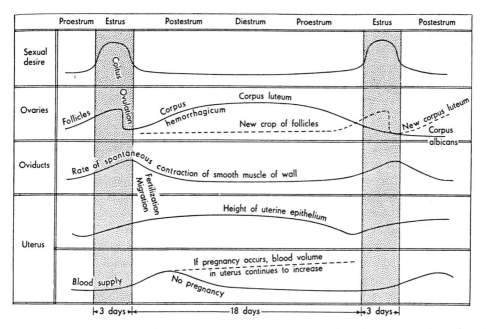

Fig. 15-3. Graph showing correlation of changes during the estrous cycle in the sow. (Compiled from the work of Corner, Seckinger, and Keye.) Note the coincidence of the important events leading toward pregnancy (coitus, ovulation, fertilization, and the migration of the ovum through the oviduct to the uterus, and finally its attachment to the uterine mucosa) with the height of local activity as indicated by the curves. (From Patten: Foundations of Embryology. Courtesy McGraw-Hill Book Co.)

Estrus and Sexual Behavior

Estrus in the sow lasts from 40 to 70 hours. Usually the sow seeks out the male when he is within sight, sound or vocal response. There may be nuzzling actions and attempts at mounting both sows and the boar, but more commonly the female assumes a characteristic immobile stance with elevation of the ears in response to the boar's vocal response, nuzzling, and attempts to mount.

The boar will test sows for estrus by vocalizing, urinating, nuzzling, and attempting to mount and randomly seeks the female with this pattern of courtship. Nasal-genital testing is common in the boar, but boars do not show the Flehman reaction. Erection occurs after mounting. The boar has a corkscrew glans penis that penetrates the female's cervix during ejaculation. Ejaculation lasts from 5 to 8 minutes. Ejaculate volumes of 150 to 200 ml are common and the ejaculate is deposited into the cervix and uterus.

Under pasture conditions, copulation may occur several times during estrus. With limited matings (hand mating), it is recommended that copulation be permitted once daily during estrus. Detection of estrus for hand mating or artificial insemination generally requires a teaser boar. The standing response of the sow in estrus to back pressure is often used by the herdsman. The swollen and red appearance of the vulva provides a clue to approaching estrus especially in gilts.

Within 2 to 3 days after parturition, approximately one-fourth of the sows will show a psychic estrus in response to the elevated estrogen levels at farrowing. However, there is not a concomitant ovarian response and normally ovulation does not occur.

Fertilization Time

The fertilization rate is usually low for single breeding occurring either on the first day of estrus or after ovulation. Breeding 6 to 12 hours before ovulation results in the highest rate of fertilization. Since estrus detection is not always accurate and ovulation time is even less predictable, it is a good practice to have the female bred on both the first and second days of estrus. Daily breeding during estrus is optimal and results in fertilization of nearly all of the oocytes shed.

EMBRYONIC MORTALITY

Under optimal breeding conditions, capacitated spermatozoa fertilize nearly 100% of the oocytes. The pig embryos enter the uterus at the four-celled stage, approximately 48 hours after fertilization. About 6 days after ovulation, the embryos hatch at the blastocyst stage from their zona pellucida. These embryos undergo intrauterine distribution into both horns especially during the 9th to 11th days. By day 13, the embryos are evenly distributed within the horns as implantation begins. If the embryos are not distributed into both horns of the uterus at this time or if less than four embryos are present, the pregnancy will fail. Maternal recognition of pregnancy is completed primarily by day 14 after ovulation.

Embryonic loss within any one pregnancy eventually may represent 25 to 40% of the oocytes ovulated. Nearly two-thirds of this loss occurs before the pregnancy recognition by the female. The remaining losses occur before day 40 of pregnancy. If embryo death occurs before day 40 of gestation, resorption of the tissue will take place. If death occurs after bone calcification, then fetal mummification, abortion or maceration will follow. The cause of this enormous loss of embryos during early pregnancy in the sow remains unknown and this loss cannot be fully compensated for by selecting for increased ovulation rates or by superovulation procedures. Thus, an innate limitation of litter size resides within the uterine functions of the sow.

LITTER SIZE

Fecundity or prolificacy (litter size) of the sow is dependent upon breed, age, days postpartum when bred, state of nutrition and, to a lesser extent, the environment and boar management at breeding.

Some breeds are more prolific than others. In general the white breeds, Landrace, Large White and bacon-type Yorkshires, have a modest advantage in litter size. However, there is as much variation between genetic lines within a breed as there is between breeds. In addition, attempts to improve litter size through genetic selection have not been successful. The heritability of reproductive traits is apparently low, thus, improvement of litter size in a given herd centers on selection of breeding stock from prolific herds, on maximizing heterosis within the breed, or in utilizing a cross-breeding system.

Ovulation rate and litter size increase with advancing age or parity, stabilizing after 6 or 7 litters (Table 15-1). The rate of stillbirth increases slowly after the fourth parity so the advantage of keeping older sows is gradually lost. The size of the first litter increases with the number of estrous cycles prior to mating. However, early-bred females perform as well as later-bred females when later parities are considered.

Early weaning, resulting in a shorter interval from farrowing to the next breeding, will generally result in smaller litter sizes through all parities. Breeding sows within 21 days after farrowing will significantly reduce litter size, while litter size will generally increase as the interval from farrowing increases up to about 35 days.

The nutritional status of the breeding herd may influence litter size, although these effects are minimal if adequate rations are fed. Nutritional deficits usually affect estrual cyclicity. Increasing feed intake (flushing) for 10 to 14 days before the expected time of breeding will increase ovulation rates by one or two oocytes in gilts. First and second parity sows are particularly vulnerable to energy deficits and weight loss during lactation. These sows will benefit from full feeding during lactation and after weaning; this results in better cyclicity and larger litters.

A high environmental temperature may adversely affect the ovulation rate and increase embryonic mortality. Likewise, boar fertility may be depressed by extremely low

Table 15-1   Relation Between Parity and Prolificacy in Pigs

No. of litters	1	2	3	4	5	6	7	8	9
Excess of young over first litter	0.0	0.68	1.36	1.58	1.90	1.92	1.89	1.71	1.45

Data from Lush and Molln. USDA Tech. Bul. 836, 1942.

or high environmental temperatures. Litter size and conception rate are also adversely affected by poor timing of the mating. Multiple matings help avoid this problem. Overuse of a boar results in a reduced impregnating dose of spermatozoa and can adversely affect litter size and conception rates.

PARTURITION

Parturition normally commences approximately 114 days after breeding. Filling of the mammary glands and vulvar swelling occur 2 to 3 days prior to delivery. Within a few hours of delivery, milk secretions may be expressed from the mammary glands. The sow shows restlessness, an increased temperature and respiration rate, and nesting during the hours preceding labor. Blood stained fluids and small amounts of meconium are usually released within 30 minutes of birth of the first pig.

Farrowing occurs with the sow in lateral recumbency and normally is completed within 2 to 4 hours, although this interval may be greatly extended if the sow is disturbed or dystocia occurs. The interval between pigs may range from a few minutes to 1 or 2 hours, but averages about 15 minutes. In most instances, the pig is born with the umbilical cord attached. Pigs born with broken cords are usually in the last one-third of the farrowed litter and have a higher incidence of stillbirths. Pigs may be born head first with the forelegs along the chest or rear feet first with the ventral part of the pig passing over the pubis of the sow. The fetal membranes are usually passed after the delivery of the litter, but some placenta may be passed between pigs. Retained fetal membranes are generally not a problem in the sow and usually indicate retained pigs in the reproductive tract.

The neonatal pig is particularly susceptible to hazards of the environment and up to one-fourth of the litter is often lost within the first 2 weeks. Newborn pigs require an environmental temperature of 28° to 30°C, which is normally supplied by supplemental heat. Pigs which get adequate milk (colostrum) early after birth have the best chance for survival. The newborn pigs receive maternal antibodies via the colostrum. Colostrum also supplies the pig with a high energy source, a critical need, since the pig is born with very little energy reserves. Early success in obtaining this energy source often determines which pigs survive particularly if the sow has more pigs than serviceable nipples. Cross fostering is the process of moving newborn pigs between sows to balance the number of available functional nipples among the litters. Once established, individual pigs return to the same nipple. Cross fostering or milk supplementation is necessary to save smaller, weaker pigs, which are in excess of available nipples.

Large birth weight is the most important factor favoring survival of the neonate. Good nutrition during late gestation, providing a favorable neonatal environment, and cross fostering of piglets are major factors for improving neonatal survival.

POSTPARTUM RETURN TO ESTRUS

In order to maximize reproductive performance, it is important to minimize the weaning-to-breeding interval in the sow. Under optimum performance, estrus should occur 4 to 10 days after weaning in 85 to 90% of the sows. Return to estrus may be influenced by season, sow parity, nutritional status of the sow, boar exposure, litter size at weaning, duration of lactation, and stressful conditions following weaning.

The most common cause of a delay in the return to estrus after weaning (anestrus) is insufficient dietary energy provided during lactation. This is particularly evident in sows weaning their first litters. Excessive weight loss during lactation or insufficient weight gain during late pregnancy often results in a post-weaning anestrus. Depressed feed consumption during the summer months may result in excessive weight loss during lactation. This may be minimized by increasing the percent of fat in the diet to improve energy levels.

The stress of grouping sows or withholding feed after weaning will generally lengthen the return to estrus interval. Housing sows in small groups and maintaining them on a high energy intake for the first 7 to 10 days after weaning is beneficial. Exposure to a mature boar will also hasten the return to estrus in the weaned sow. Periods of reduced cyclicity in the sow during the summer and fall months may prolong the return to estrus in weaned sows. Providing adequate energy during lactation and post-weaning boar exposure will help to reduce this problem.

The length of lactation also influences the return to estrus interval. Sows with short lactations, less than 21 days, usually require a slightly longer time to resume cyclicity. Weaning a portion of the litter, generally the largest pigs, at least 48 hours before the remaining pigs are weaned may improve cycling performance if delayed return to estrus is a problem in the herd.

OVARY

Since the sow is nonseasonal and polyestrous, the ovaries are cyclically active after puberty. During the luteal and early follicular phases, there are up to 30 small follicles (less than 5 mm) per ovary. About half of these ovulate during estrus, and the others regress to be followed in a few days by a new wave of follicles, even though there are functional corpora lutea present on the ovary. Senility eventually interrupts this pattern but, under practical farm conditions, the animal is usually slaughtered before senility is reached. Following ovulation, the follicle collapses, there is slight hemorrhaging into the central cavity and the granulosa cells begin to proliferate. The development of the corpus

luteum is progressive and requires about 1 week for full development. Progesterone production begins to rise soon after ovulation. The corpora lutea are elevated above the surface of the ovary, giving an appearance of a cluster of grapes (Fig. 15-4). If the sow becomes pregnant, the corpora lutea are maintained throughout pregnancy. If the animal does not become pregnant, luteolysis begins on the 14th to the 16th day of the estrous cycle. The physiologic factors regulating the maintenance or regression of the corpus luteum are discussed in Chapter 9 (Female Reproduction). The exterior of the newly formed corpora lutea are pink due to the high vascularity and the ovulation point remains visible on the corpus luteum until approximately day 12. By the end of diestrus, when the degenerative changes begin, the corpora lutea become yellowish-brown in color, especially on the cut surface.

The left ovary is more functional in the sow. Most studies indicate that about 55% of the oocytes are from the left ovary. Intrauterine migration of the embryos before implantation is common. If one ovary of the sow is removed, there will still be a relatively equal distribution of embryos in both horns of the uterus before implantation. Thus, even though the left ovary is more functional than the right, an equal number of embryos usually locate within each uterine horn. Bilateral ovariectomy causes abortion at any stage of pregnancy because of the ensuing drop in progesterone levels.

A detailed description of morphologic changes throughout the estrous cycle of the sow ovary is provided in Figure 9-24.

Estrous synchronization and embryo transfer are discussed in Chapter 19.

OVIDUCTS

The oviduct has a columnar epithelium which reaches its peak height (25 μm) during estrus and then declines to approximately 10 μm near the end of diestrus. The uterotubal junction does not have a true sphincter, but the surrounding mucosa projects in finger-like folds. These folds become edematous at the end of estrus and restrict the movement of fluids and ova through the junction to the

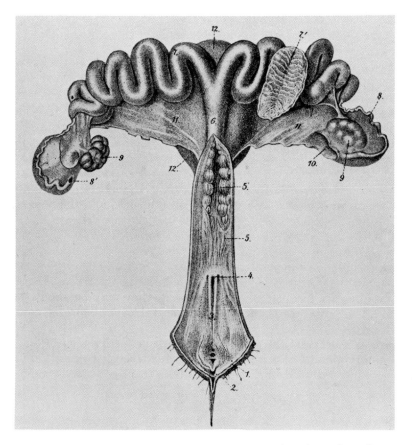

Fig. 15-4. Genital organs of sow; dorsal view. The vulva, vagina, and cervix uteri are slit open. *1*, Labium vulvae; *2*, glans clitoridis; *3*, vulva; *4*, external urethral orifice; *5*, vagina; *5'*, cervix uteri; *6*, corpus uteri; *7*, cornua uteri, one of which is opened at *7'* to show folds of mucous membrane; *8*, uterine tube; *8'*, abdominal opening of tube; *9*, ovaries; *10*, ovarian bursa; *11*, broad ligament of uterus; *12*, urinary bladder. (From Leisering's Atlas and Sisson and Grossman: The Anatomy of the Domestic Animals. Courtesy W. B. Saunders Co.)

uterus. The edema is thought to be caused by high levels of estrogen during estrus; the embryos are retained within the oviduct for 2 to 3 days, reaching the four-cell stage in the oviduct before entering the uterus. It has been suggested, but not confirmed, that the sow's multiple corpora lutea produce progesterone in sufficient amounts to override the estrogenic activity to reduce the edema, and hasten the movement of the oocytes or embryos to the uterus.

UTERUS

Figure 15-4 depicts the macroscopic appearance of the genital organs of the sow. Cyclic changes in the histology and glandular secretions of the uterus of the sow are similar to those in other species. Hemorrhage from the uterus during the cycle, as it occurs in the cow or in the bitch, does not occur in the sow or gilt. The development of the uterine mucosa is more conservative than in those species. As in other species, there is secretion of uterine milk by the endometrial glands for the nutrition of the developing preimplantation embryos. Since implantation of pig embryos does not occur until 15 to 18 days after conception, there is considerable need for nutrition during the preimplantation period. During early pregnancy myometrial activity is responsible for the spacing of embryos within the uterine horns.

Table 15-2 Classification of Swine Ovarian Cysts

| Type of Cyst | Avg. No. Cysts per Ovary | Histology | | | | Diagnosis and Treatment |
		Size	Effect on Cycle	Cyst Wall	Endometrium	
Single or retention cyst (1–2 follicles fail to ovulate)	1–2	Slightly larger than follicle (actually unruptured follicles)	None: cycle continues normally	Granulosa normal	Depends on stage of estrous cycle	Incidence low Relatively unimportant *Does not cause infertility*
Multiple large cysts (see Fig. 15-5)	5.6	Up to 10 cm (unruptured follicles)	Infrequent and irregular intense heats Prolonged anestrus Can be confused with pregnancy Ovary contains less estrogen than normal	Granulosa heavily luteinized, thick Secretes progesterone	Progestational type	Irregular cycle *Enlarged clitoris* (Fig. 15-5) (do not confuse with enlarged clitoris of pregnancy) Few recover Treatment useless Cannot distinguish from multiple small cyst cases, clinically Common cause of sterility
Multiple small cysts (see Fig. 15-5)	22.5	Only slightly larger than normal follicles but more numerous	Infrequent and irregular heats	Granulosa normal Secretes more estrogen than normal	Estrogen type	May recover spontaneously Usually no clitoris enlargement No known treatment Cannot distinguish from multiple large cyst cases, clinically

VAGINA AND VULVA

The vagina of the sow responds to rising levels of estrogens by a thickening of the epithelial cell layers, hyperemia, congestion, and edema. There is an increase in the amount of vaginal mucus during late estrus and an increase in leukocytes.

During estrus the internal portion of the vulva is congested and moistened by secretions from the vagina and other segments of the tract. Swelling of the vulva is intense and helps to identify those sows which are in estrus.

ANATOMIC ABNORMALITIES

A study of noninfectious infertility in swine[23] found that nearly half of the sterility of sows and gilts was due to ovarian cysts. The remaining infertility in this survey was primarily due to anatomic defects of the tubular genital tract of the female, especially hydrosalpinx. Unfortunately, little can be done to correct either condition. Therefore, early diagnosis is important so that affected females can be removed from the breeding herd.

A classification of ovarian cysts in swine is

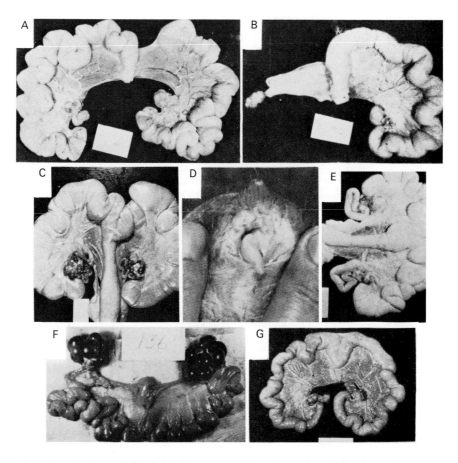

Fig. 15-5. A, Left uterine horn "blind," right horn patent. Note distension of blind horn due to accumulation of fluid. B, Right uterine horn missing but both ovaries are present. C, "Small" ovarian cysts. Compare with F. D, Greatly enlarged clitoris is frequently found in nonpregnant females with cystic ovaries. E, Bilateral hydrosalpinx, most common anatomic cause of sterility. F, "Large" ovarian cysts, most common cause of sterility. Compare with C. G, Cervix and vagina down to the vestibule are missing. Ovaries, uterine body, and horns are normal. (From Nalbandov, A. V.: Fertil. Steril. *3*(2):100, 1952.)

provided in Table 15-2. Figure 15-5 shows anatomic defects, hydrosalpinx, multiple small ovarian cysts, multiple large ovarian cysts, and other abnormalities of the reproductive organs of the sow or gilt.

THE MALE

The boar is a nonseasonal breeder. Photoperiod or artificial lighting apparently have little effect on production of semen or age of puberty. Adversely high or low environmental temperatures can result in reduced seminal quality.

Boars reach puberty as early as 5½ to 6 months of age but puberty may be delayed until 7 months of age. Limited use of the boar may begin soon after puberty, but use of the boar should be restricted until maturity. Boars approaching 1 year of age should not be used for breeding more than once daily or 5 times per week. Mature boars, 18 months or older, can be used more than once daily if the breedings are spaced. Mature boars will produce 5 to 15 billion spermatozoa per day. An inseminating dose for the sow should have at least 2 billion spermatozoa.

The ejaculate may vary from 70 to 500 ml. Most of the spermatozoa are released in the second fraction of the ejaculate. The gel fraction is produced by the Cowper's (bulbourethral) glands, while the gel free fluid is derived primarily from the seminal vesicles and the prostate gland. The seminal vesicles provide most of the protein and fructose in the ejaculate, while the prostatic secretions are high in electrolytes. These secretions enhance spermatozoal motility.

When exposed to a group of females, the boar randomly tests those females which are in close proximity. Sows in proestrus or estrus will actively seek the boar. Females in estrus will respond by standing to the boar's pheromones and smell, vocalization, nuzzling and attempted mounting. Copulation normally lasts from 3 to 6 minutes. During ejaculation, the tip of the boar's penis is fixed in the cervix enabling the ejaculate to be forcibly deposited into the uterus of the sow.

A few spermatozoa are present in the oviducts within 30 minutes after copulation, but the majority of the spermatozoa remain in the uterus and undergo capacitation. A small percentage of the capacitated spermatozoa are transported through the utero-tubal junction and reach the ampulla of the oviduct, where they serve as a spermatozoal reservoir for about 24 hours. If capacitated spermatozoa are present in the oviduct, fertilization occurs within minutes of arrival of the oocytes.

REFERENCES

1. Baldwin, D. M., and Stabenfeldt, G. H. (1975): Endocrine changes in the pig during later pregnancy, parturition and lactation. Biol. Reprod. *12:*508.
2. Bichard, M., and David, P. J. (1986): Producing more pigs per sow per year—genetic contributions. J. Anim. Sci. *63:*1275.
3. Britt, J. H. (1986): Improving sow productivity through management during gestation, lactation and after weaning. J. Anim. Sci. *63:*1288.
4. Britt, J. H., Szarek, V. E., and Levis, D. G. (1983): Characterization of summer infertility of sows in large confinement units. Theriogenology *20:*133.
5. Burger, K. F. (1952): Sex physiology of pigs. Onderstepoort J. Vet. Res., Suppl. No. 2,1.
6. Caton, J. S., Jesse, G. W., Day, B. N., et al. (1986): The effect of duration of boar exposure on the frequency of gilts reaching first estrus. J. Anim. Sci. *62:*1210.
7. Christenson, R. K. (1981): Influence of confinement and season of the year on puberty and estrous activity of gilts. J. Anim. Sci. *52:*821.
8. Christenson, R. K. (1986): Swine management to increase gilt reproductive efficiency. J. Anim. Sci. *63:* 1280.
9. Cronin, G. M., Hemsworth, P. H., and Winfield, C. G. (1982): Oestrous behaviour in relation to fertility and fecundity of gilts. Anim. Reprod. Sci. *5:*117.
10. Dutt, R. H., and Barnhart, C. E. (1959): Effect of plane of nutrition upon reproductive performance of boars. J. Anim. Sci. *18:*3.
11. Dziuk, P., Polge, J. C., and Rowson, L. E. (1964): Intrauterine migration and mixing of embryos in swine following egg transfer. J. Anim. Sci. *23:*37.
12. England, D. C. (1986): Improving sow efficiency by management to enhance opportunity for nutritional intake by neonatal piglets. J. Anim. Sci. *63:*1297.
13. Esbenshade, K. L., Britt, J. H., Armstrong, J. D., et al. (1986): Body condition of sows across parities and relationship to reproductive performance. J. Anim. Sci. *62:*1187.
14. Fenton, F. R., Bazer, F. W., Robinson, O. W., et al. (1970): Effect of quantity of uterus on uterine capacity of gilts. J. Anim. Sci. *31:*104.
15. Gleeson, A. R., Thorburn, G. D., and Cox, R. I. (1974): Prostaglandin F concentrations in the utero-ovarian venous plasma of the sow during the late luteal phase of the oestrous cycle. Prostaglandins *5:* 521.

16. Henricks, D. M., Guthrie, H. D., and Handlin, D. L. (1972): Plasma estrogen, progesterone and luteinizing hormone levels during the estrous cycle in pigs. Biol. Reprod. *6:*210.

17. Hunter, R. H. F., Hall, J. P., Cook, B., et al. (1972): Oestrogens and progesterone in porcine peripheral plasma before and after induced ovulation. J. Reprod. Fertil. *31:*499.

18. Hunter, R. H. F. (1977): Physiological factors influencing ovulation, fertilization, early embryonic development and establishment of pregnancy in pigs. Br. Vet. J. *133:*461.

19. Hurtgen, J. P., Leman, A. D. and Crabo, B. (1980): Seasonal influence on estrous activity in sows and gilts. J. Am. Vet. Med. Assoc. *176:*119.

20. Liptrap, R. M., and Raeside, J. I. (1978): A relationship between plasma concentrations of testosterone and corticosteroids during sexual and aggressive behavior in the boar. J. Endocrinol. *76:*75.

21. McKenzie, F. F. (1962): The normal estrous cycle in the sow. Mo. Agric. Expt. Sta. Res. Bull. No. 86.

22. Mavrogenis, A. P., and Robison, O. W. (1976): Factors affecting puberty in swine. J. Anim. Sci. *42:* 1251.

23. Molokwu, E. C. I., and Wagner, W. C. (1973): Endocrine physiology of the puerperal sow. J. Anim. Sci. *36:*1158.

24. Nalbandov, A. V. (1952): Anatomic and endocrinologic causes of sterility in female swine. Fertil. Steril. *3:*100.

25. Niswender, G. D., Dziuk, P. J., Kaltenbach, C. C., et al. (1970): Local effects of embryos and the uterus on corpora lutea in gilts. J. Anim. Sci. *31:*225.

26. Polge, C. (1978): Fertilization in the pig and horse. J. Reprod. Fertil. *54:*461.

27. Polge, C., Rowson, L. E. A., and Chang, M. C. (1966): The effect of reducing the number of embryos during early stages of pregnancy in the pig. J. Reprod. Fertil. *12:*395.

28. Reese, D. F., Moser, D. B., Peo E. R. Jr., et al. (1982): Influence of energy intake during lactation on the interval from weaning to first estrus in sows. J. Anim. Sci. *55:*590.

29. Robertson, H. A., and King, G. J. (1974): Plasma concentrations of progesterone, oestrone, oestradiol-17-β and oestrone sulphate in the pig at implantation during pregnancy and at parturition. J. Reprod. Fertil. *40:*133.

30. Stabenfeldt, G. H. Edqvist, L.-E., Kindahl, H., et al., (1978): Practical implications of recent physiologic findings for reproductive efficiency in cows, mares, sows, and ewes. J. Am. Vet. Med. Assoc. *172:*667.

31. Stevenson, J. S., Cox, N. M., and Britt, J. H. (1981): Role of the ovary in controlling luteinizing hormone, follicle stimulating hormone, and prolactin secretion during and after lactation in pigs. Biol. Reprod. *24:* 341.

32. Stevenson, J. S., Pollmann, D. S., Davis, D. L., et al. (1983): Influence of supplemental light on sow performance during and after lactation. J. Anim. Sci. *56:*1282.

33. Thompson, L. H., and Savage, J. S. (1978): Age at puberty and ovulation rate in gilts in confinement as influenced by exposure to a boar. J. Anim. Sci. *47:*1141.

34. Walton, J. S. (1986): Effect of boar presence before and after weaning on estrus and ovulation in sows. J. Anim. Sci. *62:*9.

35. Webel, S. K., and Dziuk, P. J. (1971): Pig fetal loss due to uterine space and fetal age. J. Anim. Sci. *33:*1165.

36. Wildt, D. E., Culver, A. A., Morcom, C. B., et al. (1976): Effect of administration of progesterone and oestrogen on litter size in pigs. J. Reprod. Fertil. *48:*209.

Reproductive Patterns of Dogs*

M. H. PINEDA

16

Puberty
Breeding Season
Litter Size
The Estrous Cycle
Oogenesis, Ovulation, and Fertilization
Endocrinology of the Reproductive Cycle
Corpora Lutea of the Bitch
Vaginal Cytology
Ovary, Oviducts, Uterus, and Vagina
Pseudopregnancy
Pregnancy and Parturition
The Dog
Response of Dogs and Bitches to Exogenous
    Hormones
Contraceptive Steroids for the Bitch

THE pattern of reproduction of the domestic male and female dog is remarkably different in several aspects from those of the farm animal species. The female dog, the bitch, is monoestric because in each breeding season she has only one estrus which is followed by a prolonged period of anestrus. During each estrous cycle, the bitch has prolonged follicular and luteal phases, compared to those of the cycling species of

* Much information concerned with reproduction in dogs has been covered in Chapter 9 (Female Reproduction), Chapter 8 (Male Reproduction), Chapter 10 (Artificial Insemination), and Chapter 2 (Pituitary Gland). The reader is encouraged to refer to these chapters in order to permit conciseness.

farm animals. Contrary to the norm in the farm animal species, the bitch ovulates at the beginning of estrus and releases primary oocytes. Oogenesis extends for about 2 months after birth, whereas in farm animals oogenesis is completed by the time of birth. The lifespan of the bitch's corpora lutea is about the same in the pregnant as in the nonpregnant bitch and the uterus of the bitch does not seem to exert a discernible role in the regression of the corpora lutea of the cycle. Lastly, the vagina of the bitch has a dorsal median postcervical fold, which together with the vaginal wall, contributes to the formation of a pseudocervix.

The male dog, called a dog, releases large volumes of ejaculates with a relatively low concentration of spermatozoa. About 97% of the volume of an ejaculate is contributed by the prostate gland,[94] the only accessory sex gland present in this species. The dog initiates copulation while the penis is only partially erected. Intromission of the dog's penis into the vagina of the bitch is facilitated by the os penis. Full erection is achieved after intromission has been completed and ejaculation has begun. The dog's penis remains "locked" in the bitch's vagina during ejaculation.

PUBERTY

Puberty, defined as the age at which the dog releases spermatozoa in his ejaculate or the bitch displays her first heat, occurs at 6 to 9 months of age for the male and between 9 to 16 months of age for the bitch. Puberty tends to occur earlier in smaller breeds than in larger breeds and kenneled dogs tend to reach puberty later than free-roaming animals. Age of puberty is less predictable in the female than in the male dog and is probably influenced more in the bitch than in the dog by nutritional and environmental factors, including social interactions with other dogs. Pubertal and maiden bitches often refuse mating, even though in heat, when exposed to young, sexually inexperienced dogs.

Prepubertal dogs respond with erection and coital movements when their penes are stimulated. These dogs may ejaculate small volumes of seminal fluid, devoid of spermatozoa, weeks in advance of puberty. The response to penile stimulation is faster and the volume of seminal fluid produced increases as the dog approaches puberty. Some prepubertal dogs, which produce azoospermic seminal fluid, have significant numbers of spermatozoa in their urine collected by cystocentesis from the bladder after penile stimulation. This suggests that young dogs may have the capability to release spermatozoa into the urethra, prior to or at the time of penile stimulation, at an earlier age than previously anticipated. Once in the urethra, these spermatozoa retrograde into the bladder probably following the path of least resistance.[73] As the dog approaches the age of puberty, it apparently acquires a more efficient ejaculatory mechanism to propel the spermatozoa through the penile urethra.

BREEDING SEASON

Although many dog breeders believe that there are two breeding seasons per year in the bitch, examination of available records does not substantiate this claim. Instead it appears that, under the controlled environmental conditions to which most dogs are now subjected, many of the seasonal breeding characteristics have been lost. Available records from dog colonies indicate that in the bitch estrus occurs year-round with a slight con-

centration of estruses occurring in late winter or early spring. Table 16-1 shows the number of estruses per year for some breeds of dogs.

American Kennel Club records for cockers, setters, great danes, and pekingese indicate that an even distribution of heat periods occurred throughout the year. Kenneled airedales and beagles show estrus throughout the year with a concentration in late summer and the fewest periods occurring in the fall. The basenjii has only one estrus each year, usually in the fall. The tendency for a single breeding season each year in the basenjii is due to a single recessive gene, because crossing the basenjii with other breeds gives a variable response in the offspring, some with one season, others with two breeding seasons. Environmentally protected, kenneled dogs show little or no seasonality, whereas a free-roaming dog may retain some seasonality. The household pet that roams may fall between these two extremes. Furthermore, there may be effects of latitude and climate similar to those in other species.

LITTER SIZE

Litter size is extremely variable, especially between breeds. Some toy or miniature breeds have litters of 1 to 3 puppies, whereas larger bitches, such as the setters, may have litters of 10 to 15 puppies. Considering all breeds, a litter of 5 to 8 puppies would probably be average.

Table 16-1 Number of Estruses per Year in Some Breeds of Dogs*

Breed	Mean pear Year
Basenjii	1.0
Basset hound	2.0
Beagle	1.5
Boston terrier	1.5
Cocker spaniel	2.0
German shepherd	2.4
Pekingese	1.5
Toy poodle	1.5

* Colony dogs. Compiled from information in: J. H. Sokolowski et al., J. Am. Vet. Med. Assoc. *171*:271, 1977.

THE ESTROUS CYCLE

The bitch has only one estrous period in each reproductive cycle, whether she is mated to fertile or infertile dogs, or not mated at all. The interestrous interval is highly variable between breeds (Table 16-2) and among bitches of the same breed, and probably is influenced by environmental conditions and social interactions. After puberty, bitches cycle every 4 to 12 months. The average interestrous interval is about 7 months. The timing of estrus and onset of heat is determined from the first day of standing for the male and acceptance to mating. The bitch is in estrus as long as she accepts the male for mating.

Determination of the stages of the estrous cycle is facilitated by the use of vasectomized, teaser dogs (Tables 16-3 and 16-4). When teaser dogs are not available, determination of the stages of the cycle, and particularly the timing of estrus, is more difficult. Observation of the external signs and behavioral responses of the bitch, as well as the examination of vaginal smears, is an acceptable and useful substitute.

The stages of the estrual cycle of the bitch are associated with recognizable, external signs. Figure 16-1 shows the stages and duration of the reproductive cycle of the bitch. The values indicated in Figure 16-1 are for the beagle bitch, but are reasonably valid for other breeds.

For the bitch, *proestrus* is the beginning of the period of sexual activity. The onset of proestrus is gradually established in a series of sequential anatomic and behavioral changes induced by gonadotropic stimulation, and subsequent follicular development and estro-

Table 16-2 Interestrous Intervals for Some Breeds of Dogs

Breed	Interval in Months
Basset hound	5.8
Beagle	7.4
Boston terrier	8.1
Boxer	8.0
Chihuahua	7.2
Cocker spaniel	6.0
Dachshund	7.0
German Shepherd	5.0
Pekingese	7.7
Scottish Terrier	6.5
Toy Poodle	8.0

Compiled from different sources.

genic influences exerted during late anestrus. For practical purposes, however, proestrus is considered to begin when the bitch discharges blood from the vulva. The first day of bloody discharge is generally agreed to represent the first day of proestrus. The blood discharged from the vulva at the time of proestrus is probably of uterine origin, and together with secretion from the uterine glands is usually first detected and reported as "spotting" by the bitch's owner. As the bitch progresses through proestrus and approaches estrus, the vulva becomes distinctly swollen. During proestrus, the bitch tends to be excitable, restless, and may lose her appetite; water intake is usually increased and the bitch tends to urinate frequently.

Bitches become attractive to males during proestrus. Pheromones released in the vaginal secretions and urine stimulate and attract males. Bitches in proestrus are inclined to roam and usually are followed by a pack of dogs. During proestrus, the bitch will not accept the male for mating and may even be ag-

Table 16-3 Criteria to Determine the Length of Proestrus and Estrus in the Bitch with Teaser Dogs

	Stage of the Cycle
First day of blood discharge from the vulva	Day 1 of Proestrus
First day of acceptance of the male for mating	Day 1 of Estrus
First day of refusal of the male for mating	Day 1 of Diestrus

Table 16-4 Patterns of Sexual Behavior in the Dog and Bitch

Dog Response	Bitch Response	Stage of the Cycle
Little or no interest for the bitch	Refuses advances of the male, barks or tries to bite	Anestrus
Shows interest and attempts to mount	Refuses male by retreating or hiding (no bloody discharge from vulva)	Late anestrus
Attempts to mount or sustained mounting with pelvic thrusting	Retreats or stands passively. Bloody discharge from the vulva	Proestrus
Sustained thrusting, intromission, and "locking" of the penis	Stands, displays vulva, and deviates tail	Estrus

gressive to the male. As the bitch approaches estrus, she becomes more receptive, and sexually experienced bitches may even allow mounting by the male.

Proestrus extends from the first day of bloody discharge from the vulva to the first day of acceptance of the male for mating, and lasts on the average 9 days, but may range from 2 to 15 days.

Estrus, the period of sexual receptivity, is reliably determined by the bitch's acceptance of the male for mating. The bitch is considered to be in estrus while she accepts, stands, and successfully forms a copulatory tie with the male. Estrus lasts an average of 10 days, but may range from 3 to 12 days. The estrous

bitch adopts a definite stance for mating, deviates and holds the tail to one side, and exposes the vulva by arching her back. Bitches in estrus actively seek males for mating. Since pheromonal release at this time is maximal, it is not unusual to observe dogs, attracted from blocks away, in the yard waiting for the bitch. This attractiveness of the bitch for the dogs during late proestrus and estrus is undesirable to pet owners and the public in general because of damage to property and public hazards. Roaming bitches are often followed by a pack of dogs, usually barking, polluting the environment, and fighting. As estrus progresses, the edema of the vulva becomes less noticeable and the bloody discharge becomes watery and reddish or yellowish in color.

Wild canides (coyotes and wolves) have only one estrus every year. The estrous cycle is characterized, particularly in the coyote, by an extended proestrus lasting for 2 to 3 months.

Methyl p-hydroxybenzoate, which stimulates the mounting reaction in the male dog, was proposed as a pheromone released from the vagina of the bitch. Recent evidences, however, question the pheromonal role of this compound.

Olfaction is the main determinant in communication between the canine sexes. Most of the courtship consists of the male seeking the female. Due to the lengthy proestrus and estrus, the period during which the male is attracted is prolonged.

Interaction between male and female dur-

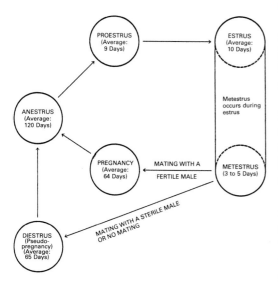

Fig. 16-1. The ovarian cycle of the bitch.

ing proestrus consists of frequent urination by both and attention shown toward each other. The male investigates and often licks the anogenital area of the female. The female may exhibit a bowing posture but does not allow mounting. Mounting may be discouraged by moving or by growling.

With the onset of estrus, the female lordoses for the male and allows mounting and intromission. Little courtship is involved during full estrus, but during late estrus, receptiveness declines.

Since the bitch ovulates while in estrus, *metestrus*, defined as the period of formation and beginning of secretion of progesterone by the newly formed corpora lutea, occurs in its entirety during the period of estrus. Based on blood levels of progesterone, metestrus lasts from 3 to 5 days and is only of academic interest in the bitch. However, some authors use the term metestrus to designate the stage of the cycle of the bitch that follows estrus and ovulation. In this chapter, metestrus is restricted to the short postovulatory period as indicated previously. The term diestrus is used to indicate that period which follows estrus, as applied to the other domestic species.

Diestrus begins with the bitch's refusal to mate and is the stage of the cycle in which the corpora lutea are fully functional. Toward the end of estrus, some bitches may refuse the male for mating on one day yet accept the male the following day. This is frequently observed in young bitches, particularly when the male is persistent and aggressive. Because of this dichotomous behavior, it is advisable to consider the bitch in diestrus when she refuses to mate on 2 consecutive days. Based on levels of progesterone greater than 1.0 ng/ml in the blood, diestrus lasts an average of 65 days but may range from 55 to 90 days or more. Figures for the length of diestrus given in the literature vary considerably depending on the criteria used to define the end of diestrus. During the initial stages of diestrus, vulvar swelling and vaginal discharge decrease rapidly and the bitch becomes more relaxed, as she progresses into diestrus.

If a fertile mating has occurred, pregnancy occupies most of diestrus. Bitches that are not mated, or bitches that are mated with sterile males may occasionally develop a false pregnancy (pseudopregnancy or pseudocyesis). Pseudopregnancy is characterized in some bitches by abdominal swelling, development of the mammary glands with light to full lactation, and profound behavioral changes.

Anestrus follows diestrus. This stage of the cycle is characterized as a period of sexual quiescence and used to be defined as the period of ovarian inactivity. This definition is no longer tenable since recent findings indicate that the ovaries of the bitch are quite active and responsive to endogenous gonadotropic stimulation, weeks in advance of the next proestrus. Anestrus lasts an average of 120 days, but may vary from 40 to 270 days. The duration of anestrus determines to a great extent the interestrous interval and the time elapsed from one cycle to the next varies considerably within an individual bitch or between bitches of the same breed.

OOGENESIS, OVULATION, AND FERTILIZATION

Oogenesis continues into the postnatal life of the bitch. At birth, the ovary of the pup does not contain primordial follicles, but oogonia are present and "pregranulosa" cells, forming irregularly shaped cords and lobules, are seen in apposition to or around oogonia. Oocytes entering the first meiotic prophase can be seen in the cortical area of the ovary by 5 days after birth, but oogonia continue mitotic divisions up to 14 days after birth. A few primordial follicles appear in the pup's ovary around days 17 to 22 after birth and continue to become more numerous until 54 to 56 days after birth, when oogenesis appears to be completed in the bitch (see Ref. No. 7 for further details). Polyovular follicles are frequent in the bitch. Individual follicles containing up to 9 oocytes have been reported. Spontaneous ovulation usually occurs within 5 days after the onset of estrus; 40% of the bitches ovulate within 2 days and 70% within 3 days (Fig. 16-2). The bitch is peculiar with respect to farm animals in that

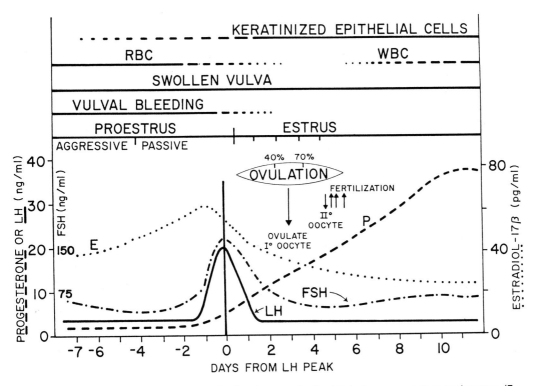

Fig. 16-2. Endocrine, cytological, and behavioral events in the bitch during proestrus and estrus. (E = estradiol; P = progesterone; RBC = red blood cells; WBC = white blood cells.)

she continues to accept the male for mating for several days after ovulation has occurred. Ovulation occurs 40 to 48 hours after the ovulatory surge of LH and all oocytes are discharged within 24 hours of the first ovulation. Variations reported in day of ovulation in the bitch appear to be caused by the method used to determine the stage of the cycle. When teaser dogs are used to detect onset and length of estrus, ovulation is remarkably constant and occurs within the first 3 days of standing estrus (Fig. 16-2).

In the bitch, each oocyte is released from the follicle before the completion of meiosis, at the stage of primary oocyte. Extrusion of the first polar body and completion of meiosis occurs during oviductal transport. In most species the fertilizability of ova decreases rapidly after ovulation. This is not the case in the bitch where oocytes are viable for several days and do not become fertilizable until 2 or 3 days after ovulation. In the bitch, concep-

tion is possible whether breeding has occurred on the first day of standing estrus or on the last day of estrus. Pregnancy and conception rates are not different when bitches are mated only once, either on the first or on the 7th day of estrus.

Oviductal transport of unfertilized or fertilized oocytes is prolonged in the bitch. It has been estimated that more than 7 days are needed for the oocytes or embryos to enter the uterus and thus complete oviductal transport.

The exact timing of pregnancy is difficult in the dog because dog spermatozoa retain their viability and probably their fertilizing capability for 11 days within the genital tract of the bitch. The bitch's oocytes appear to require a period of maturation in the oviduct before fertilization can actually occur. Thus, variable intervals from breeding to fertilization may contribute much of the variation observed in the length of gestation for the bitch.

ENDOCRINOLOGY OF THE REPRODUCTIVE CYCLE

Figure 16-2 depicts the changes in the blood levels of hormones and the associated changes in the reproductive organs during the follicular and the beginning of the luteal phases of the cycle in the bitch. Table 16-5 provides values for concentration of hormones during the reproductive cycle of the beagle bitch. These values were compiled from different sources and obtained using different radioimmunoassay systems. It is important to keep in mind that values for concentrations of hormones in the blood or tissues are greatly dependent on the assay system, the rate of secretion, and metabolic clearance rates for a given hormone, as well as other variables. Therefore, the values provided in Table 16-5 are intended to serve only as reference or guidelines and should not be used to determine normality or abnormality.

Proestrus and the first days of estrus, prior to ovulation, form the follicular phase of the cycle. Concurrent with the growth and secretory activity of the follicles, levels of estrogens progressively increase from basal to peak levels during the last 2 days of proestrus. FSH and LH levels also increase progressively, in a relative synchrony, to reach peak values by the end of proestrus (Fig. 16-2). The changes in concentration of LH in the blood are more pronounced than those of FSH. FSH levels tend to be suppressed during proestrus, as compared to the FSH levels during late anestrus. Recent evidences indicate that LH is released in a pulsatile fashion from the adenohypophysis of the bitch, whereas FSH release seems to be tonic. During proestrus, LH pulses in synergy with FSH stimulate the final maturation of the follicles. Estrogen secretion by the follicles probably stimulates secretion of inhibin, and then both inhibin and the elevated blood levels of estrogens would feed back to inhibit FSH release by the adenohypophysis. The ovulatory surge of LH occurs in most bitches during the last 2 days

Table 16-5 Hormonal Levels in the Blood of the Beagle Bitch

Reproductive Stage	LH (ng/ml)	FSH (ng/ml)	Prolactin (ng/ml)	Progesterone (ng/ml)	Estradiol (pg/ml)
Proestrus	2.8 ± 0.1	59 ± 9	27	1.7 ± 0.3	58 ± 7
Estrus	36.0 ± 10	168 ± 37 297*	32	< 2.0	69 ± 11
Metestrus	—	69 ± 15	20	24 ± 3*	18 ± 3
Diestrus	4.2 ± 1.1	108 ± 19	20 to 35	18 ± 6	23 ± 7
Pregnancy	3.0 ± 0.2	197 ± 21 255 ± 28**	57 ± 14**	15 ± 10 3.8 ± 2.4** 1.2 ± 0.4†	19 ± 2
Anestrus	2.8 ± 0.3	—	—	0.6 ± 0.1	33 ± 15
Late anestrus	21 to 156	240 to 294	1.95 to 33.15	<1.0	20 to 46

Mean ± standard deviation
* Peak values
** Days 55–58 of pregnancy
† At parturition
Compiled from different sources, including:
  Concannon et al., Biol. Reprod. *19:*1113, 1978.
  Nett et al., Proc. Soc. Exptl. Biol. Med., *148:*134, 1975.
  Olson et al., Biol. Reprod. *27:*1196, 1982.
  Reimers et al., Biol. Reprod., *19:*673, 1978.

of proestrus or first 2 days of standing estrus. However, there can be asynchrony between the behavioral responses of the bitch, corresponding with the stages of proestrus and standing estrus, and the ovulatory surge of LH. In some bitches, the ovulatory surge of LH may occur earlier in proestrus or even later in estrus. Most bitches ovulate within 48 hours after the ovulatory surge of LH, and LH levels rapidly decline to basal levels after the ovulatory surge.

As the blood levels of estrogens increase, the bitch develops those external signs and responses of the reproductive organs and of the nervous system associated with estrogenic stimulation. These include edema of the vulva, bloody discharge, and increased receptivity to the male and attraction of the male toward the bitch (Fig. 16-2). Toward the end of proestrus, increasing levels of LH promote follicular luteinization and as a result, there is a progressive increase in blood levels of progesterone. As the levels of progesterone produced by the luteinized follicles increase, blood levels of estrogens decline. The ovulatory surge of LH and ovulation bring about a further increase in progesterone secretion from the developing corpora lutea (Fig. 16-3). The

behavioral transition of the bitch from the proestrual rejection to mating, to standing and acceptance of the mating advances of the male is a relatively fast event. This often occurs within a 12- to 24-hour period, although in some bitches the transition may be more gradual.

As compared to farm animal species, the bitch is also peculiar in that behavioral estrus occurs when the blood levels of progesterone are rapidly increasing, while the levels of estrogens are rapidly declining. In ovariectomized bitches, estrogens alone do not induce a full behavioral estrus. The ovariectomized bitch will respond to treatment with estrogens with edema and vulvar discharge of blood and she will become attractive to males, but will not display standing estrus, even when estrogens are given in high doses. To induce standing estrus, ovariectomized bitches must be treated with progesterone after treatment with estrogens.

After ovulation, corpora lutea are formed and induced to secrete progesterone under the luteotropic stimulus of LH. The corpora lutea continue to secrete progesterone for 50 to 70 days from ovulation, regardless of whether the bitch is pregnant (Figs. 16-3 and

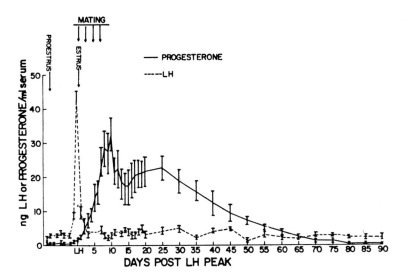

Fig. 16-3. LH and progesterone concentrations in sterile-mated beagles throughout the periods of proestrus, estrus, and diestrus. Vertical bars represent the standard error of the mean. Mating indicates the period of acceptance of the male. (From Smith, M. S. and McDonald, L. E.: Endocrinol. *94*(2):408, 1974.)

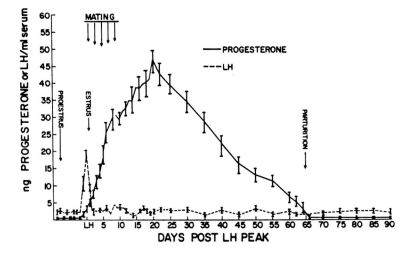

Fig. 16-4. LH and progesterone concentrations during pregnancy in beagles. Vertical bars represent the standard error of the mean. (From Smith, M. S. and McDonald, L. E.: Endocrinol. *94*(2):404, 1974.)

16-4). This peculiarity of the corpora lutea of the bitch will be discussed later in this chapter.

The luteal phase of the cycle includes the postovulatory, metestrual formative stage of the corpora lutea, and the diestrual stage of the cycle. Based on the blood levels of progesterone, the duration of the luteal phase of the cycle in the nonpregnant bitch is variable. Progesterone declines to basal levels of 1.0 ng/ml or less by 70 to 80 days (Fig. 16-3) or even longer after the ovulatory LH surge, particularly if the bitch has undergone an intense pseudopregnant reaction, including mammary gland development and secretion. In the pregnant bitch, however, progesterone levels decrease rapidly at parturition and become undetectable by the day after parturition (Fig. 16-4).

Prolactin levels in the bitch remain relatively constant throughout the follicular and luteal phases of the cycle. The major role of prolactin is probably expressed during pregnancy or pseudopregnancy, as a hormonal factor forming with LH the luteotropic complex. The severity of several of the undesirable and overt manifestations of pseudopregnancy of the bitch, such as mammary gland secretion, can be controlled with bromocriptine (2-bromo-α-ergocryptine), a dopamine ago-

nist, which selectively reduces prolactin secretion.

The endocrinology of anestrus in the bitch remained unexplored until recently. Researchers from Colorado State University[127] have demonstrated that neither the canine ovary, nor the pituitary gland are quiescent during the last 2 months of anestrus (Table 16-5). Mean concentrations of FSH were higher during the last month of anestrus than during proestrus. During this period, there were sporadic but significant increases in mean serum concentrations of LH. The mean concentration of prolactin also was elevated and variable during late anestrus, but no specific pattern could be detected. Estradiol-17β reached levels up to 46 ng/ml during late anestrus (Table 16-5), indicating that ovarian follicles developed and responded to gonadotropic stimulation. Progesterone levels, however, remained below 1.0 ng/ml of serum (Table 16-5). Even though it has not been determined whether similar adenohypophysial ovarian responses occur throughout the duration of anestrus in the bitch, the long-held view that the ovary of the bitch is inactive during anestrus is no longer tenable. However, despite gonadotropic activity and estradiol secretion by the ovarian follicles during late anestrus, the bitch remains in a quiescent reproductive stage during this period. The external signs and vaginal smears are those typical for anestrus and thus were thought to represent an inactive ovary. The mechanisms by which the reproductive organs and the nervous system of the bitch fail to respond to the estrogenic stimulation and the bitch fails to show behavioral responses have not been determined. During late anestrus the blood progesterone remains below basal levels. Therefore, it is possible that these follicles, which develop during late anestrus, are unable to luteinize and secrete progesterone, as they do during estrus. Since progesterone is needed for full expression of estrous behavior in the bitch, the low levels of progesterone may explain the absence of behavioral signs during anestrus.

The bitch has relatively high levels of testosterone in serum collected during late anestrus, proestrus, or early estrus. Blood levels of testosterone increase significantly during proestrus and decrease rapidly after the ovulatory surge of LH (Table 16-6). During diestrus, levels of testosterone remain at basal levels. The physiologic significance of these relatively high blood levels of testosterone in the bitch has not been determined. However, since levels of testosterone are highest at the onset of estrus, testosterone may contribute to the behavioral responses of the estrous bitch.

CORPORA LUTEA OF THE BITCH

The corpora lutea of the bitch, as those of most of the farm animal species, are chroni-

cally dependent on a pituitary luteotropic complex for maintenance and secretion. Of this luteotropic complex, LH seems to play the major role, probably in synergy with prolactin. In bitches hypophysectomized on days 10 through 50 of the luteal phase of the cycle, progesterone secretion is rapidly impaired and ceases 3 to 17 days following hypophysectomy. Similarly, administration of antiserum containing antibodies to LH severely impairs progesterone secretion by the bitch's corpora lutea. Prolactin also appears to be part of the luteotropic complex and necessary for luteal maintenance and secretion. Treatment of diestrual bitches with bromocriptine or other dopamine agonists selectively reduces prolactin levels in the blood and causes a rapid decline in blood levels of progesterone.

The nonpregnant uterus does not appear to play any significant luteolytic role in the bitch. Either the nonpregnant uterus of the bitch does not produce luteolytic factors or the transfer of these factors from the uterus to the ovary does not occur in the bitch. This could be due to the anatomic independence between the vein draining the bitch's uterus and the artery supplying the ovary. Recent studies on the effects of hysterectomy during diestrus in bitches indicate that neither the pregnant nor the nonpregnant uterus is an essential component of the regulatory mechanisms participating in luteal maintenance, secretion, or demise. During diestrus, blood levels of progesterone are not significantly different between nonpregnant and pregnant bitches. Blood levels of progesterone decline rapidly at parturition, whereas in the nonpregnant bitch they persist at basal levels for extended periods. This suggests that the corpora lutea of the nonpregnant bitch are either resistant to luteolytic factors or simply that luteolytic factors are lacking and the corpora lutea undergo retrogressive changes caused by their aging.

Exogenous prostaglandin $F_{2\alpha}$ or synthetic prostaglandin analogs can induce irreversible luteal regression during certain periods of diestrus or pregnancy in the bitch when given in a single, high dose or in lower, but repeat-

Table 16-6 Concentration of Testosterone (pg/ml) in the Serum of Bitches

Stage of the Cycle		
Anestrus	Proestrus	At the time of the preovulatory surge of LH
<150	239 ± 113*	56 ± 225*

* Mean ± SEM
Adapted From: P. N. Olson et al., Am. J. Vet. Res. *45:*145, 1984.

Table 16-7   *Clinical, Vaginal, and Hormonal Signs of the Estrous Cycle of the Bitch*

Observation	Proestrus (Mean = 9 days; Range = 2–15 days)	Estrus (Mean = 10 days; Range = 3–12 days)	Diestrus (Mean = 65 days; Range = 55–90 days)	Anestrus (Mean = 120 days; Range = 40–270 days)
Clinical Signs	Enlargement of the vulva and bloody discharge; male is attracted to the bitch in late proestrus but not accepted for mating.	Vulva is enlarged and swollen; reduced vaginal discharge; male is accepted for mating.	Refusal to mate; pregnancy or pseudopregnancy.	Sexual quiescence.
Vaginal Cytology	Number of cornified cells increases; numerous red blood cells but few leukocytes.	Mostly cornified cells.	Abrupt change from superficial to basal cells; number of leukocytes increases.	Foam cells; number of leukocytes is variable.
Hormonal Levels in Blood	Estrogens rise and peak; LH and FSH rise and may peak; slight rise in progesterone; testosterone increases to peak levels.	Estrogens decrease; progesterone rises; LH and FSH peak and decrease rapidly; testosterone decreases.	Progesterone peaks and decreases by the end of diestrus; LH declines to basal levels; FSH declines in nonpregnant bitches and increases in pregnant bitches. Testosterone remains at basal levels.	Late anestrus: LH, FSH, estrogens, and testosterone increase. Progesterone remains below basal levels.

ed doses. The effective single dose of prostaglandin to cause irreversible luteolysis in the bitch approaches toxic levels. A lower single dose causes only a transient decline in the blood levels of progesterone. In addition, the corpora lutea of nonpregnant bitches are more sensitive to the luteolytic activity of exogenous prostaglandin $F_{2\alpha}$ after day 30 of diestrus than earlier in diestrus. Similarly, the corpora lutea of the pregnant bitch are more sensitive to exogenous prostaglandin $F_{2\alpha}$ in the second half of pregnancy. Treatment with $PGF_{2\alpha}$ after day 30 of pregnancy causes a dramatic decrease in blood levels of progesterone and abortion usually occurs 4 to 5 days after treatment.

VAGINAL CYTOLOGY

The vaginal smear can be a fairly good indicator of the stage of the estrous cycle in the bitch, particularly if a series of daily smears are obtained. The smear represents secretions and cells from the uterus, cervix, and vagina. A smear that is quickly air dried and stained by the Giemsa technique is usually satisfactory for examination. Table 16-7 summarizes the clinical, hormonal, and changes in the vaginal smear of the bitch associated with the different stages of the cycle. Figure 16-5 shows the cellular changes observable in vaginal smears obtained during the phases of anestrus, proestrus, estrus, and diestrus. The

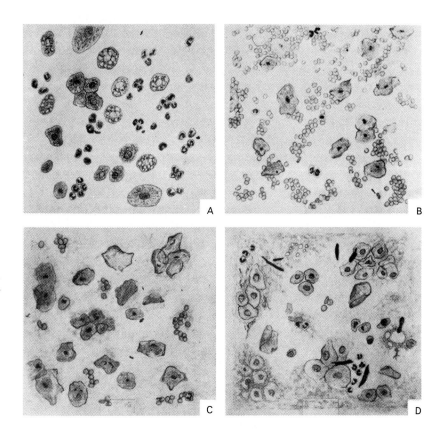

Fig. 16-5. Vaginal smears. A, Anestrus. Epithelial cells with cytoplasmic granules or vacuoles ("foam-cells"). Varying numbers of polymorphonuclear leukocytes. B, Proestrus. Erythrocytes numerous. Cornified epithelial cells with pyknotic nuclei. Leukocytes sparse. C, Estrus. Large numbers of cornified epithelial cells ("flakes"). Moderate number of erythrocytes. D, Diestrus. Epithelial elements varying in both size and staining characteristics, "boat-cells," leukocytes and detritus. (From Cole, H. H., and Cupps, P. T.: Reproduction in Domestic Animals. New York, Academic Press, 1959.)

anestrous smear consists mainly of exfoliate epithelial cells and leukocytes (Fig. 16-5A). Red blood cells and cornified epithelial cells appear in vaginal smears early in proestrus. By the end of proestrus, large cornified epithelial cells are present (Fig. 16-5B), and most of the bleeding has ceased. During estrus the smear consists almost completely of keratinized superficial cells with pyknotic nuclei or anuclear cells. There are few erythrocytes (Fig. 16-5C). Toward the end of estrus a few leukocytes begin to appear in the smear, and they are numerous 2 or 3 days after the end of estrus (Fig. 16-5D).

The epithelial lining of the vagina during anestrus is only 2 or 3 layers thick (Fig. 16-6), but by the beginning of proestrus it becomes stratified and increases to 6 to 8 layers (Fig. 16-7). During proestrus, growth of the vaginal epithelium continues, and by the time estrus occurs, the epithelial lining may contain 12 to 20 cell layers. Desquamation of the epithelium begins by late estrus.

OVARY, OVIDUCTS, UTERUS, AND VAGINA

The ovary of the bitch is encapsulated by the bursa ovarica, which has a ventrally located bursal slit through which the ovary can be visualized during estrus, using an endoscope. During anestrus, the bursal slit becomes

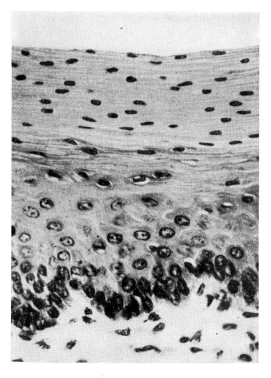

Fig. 16-7. The vaginal epithelium of the bitch at the beginning of proestrus shows the thickening and cornification of the surface layers. (Reproduced by permission, from Evans and Cole: The Oestrous Cycle in the Dog. Memoirs of the University of California, 9, no. 2.)

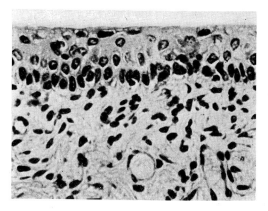

Fig. 16-6. The vaginal epithelium of the bitch at anestrus. The epithelium is low, tending toward a simple columnar type. (Reproduced by permission, from Evans and Cole: The Oestrous Cycle in the Dog. Memoirs of the University of California, 9, no. 2.)

closed. The ovaries of the newborn bitch contain an estimated 700,000 oocytes which decline to 250,000 at puberty, 33,000 at 5 years of age, and only 500 remain by 10 years of age. Obviously, most of these follicles undergo atresia at different stages of follicular development and the oocytes degenerate. After puberty a wave of follicles develops with each estrus. Many follicles reach about 6 mm in diameter, but not all are destined to ovulate.

Canine oocytes are 90 to 110 μm in diameter. They are released from the follicle at ovulation as primary oocytes, while the oocyte is at the dictyate stage of meiosis. The cytoplasm of the canine oocyte is rich in lipids and the oocytes are opaque in appearance. Studies on the *in vitro* fertilization of canine oocytes suggest that dog spermatozoa require capacitation to penetrate the zona pellucida.

After ovulation the granulosa luteal cells develop rapidly, and corpora lutea become functional before the end of estrus. Progesterone secretion by the corpora lutea throughout pregnancy is necessary for pregnancy maintenance in the bitch. Bilateral ovariectomy prior to day 56 of gestation is followed by abortion, indicating that the ovaries are the sole source of progesterone during most of pregnancy in the bitch. Pregnancy can be maintained in bilaterally ovariectomized bitches by daily administrations of progesterone.

The ovaries and uterus are attached to the dorsal abdominal wall by the broad ligaments, and the ovaries are attached to the dorsal aspects of the diaphragm by suspensory ligaments. The ovaries are attached to the anterior portion of the uterine horns by the proper ligament of the ovary. These attachments make it difficult to exteriorize the ovaries, oviducts, and anterior portion of the uterine horns at laparotomy. The infundibulum of the oviduct is attached to the bursa ovarica and the oviduct follows a convoluted course and encircles the ovary before reaching the uterine horn. The bicornuate uterus of the bitch is long and highly responsive to estrogenic and progestational stimulation. The cervix of the bitch is pendulous and the cervical canal is oblique in a dorsoventral direction, with the external os in close apposition to the ventral area of the vaginal fornix. The vagina of the bitch is bottle-shaped with the narrow end or neck directed rostrally and has numerous folds or rugae in its mucosa. The vagina of the bitch contains a dorsal-medial postcervical fold, which together with the vaginal wall forms a pseudocervix (Fig. 16-8). This pseudocervix is often mistaken as the cervix and cannulated as if it were the true cervix. In fact, the cervix of the bitch is difficult to visualize and generally is very difficult to cannulate, even when special endoscopic equipment is used. When palpated transabdominally, or observed during laparotomy, the anterior vagina, cervix, and pseudocervix of the bitch form a firm, long cord-like, cylindrical structure, which is also often mistaken to represent, as a unit, the

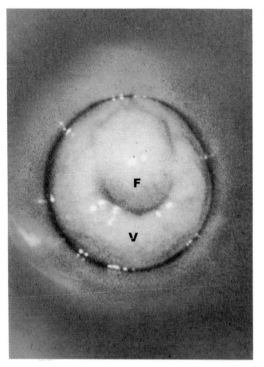

Fig. 16-8. Endoscopic view of the canine anterior vagina showing the pseudocervix[139] (also called paracervix[115]) of the bitch, which simulates the external os of the cervix. F = dorsal medial cervical fold; V = vaginal wall.

external correspondent to the cervix of the bitch.

During anestrus and early proestrus, the adult bitch has low cuboidal epithelium and no cilia in the oviducts. The basal cells of the oviductal epithelium undergo differentiation into ciliated and secretory cells during proestrus, under the influence of progressively increasing levels of estrogens. The response to estrogenic stimulation is rapid; within 3 days ciliogenesis and secretory cell differentiation can be observed in puppies treated with exogenous estrogens. With the onset of proestrus, the endometrium responds rapidly to the rising levels of estrogen by becoming edematous, hyperemic, and hyperplastic. Consequently, the rapid development of the vascular system leads to the loss of blood into the uterine lumen by diapedesis. The uterine glands continue to develop and serous secretion continues. As estrogen declines and progesterone rises, vaginal cornification decreases, noncornified cells reappear, and neutrophils are able to cross the epithelial lining.

The uterine response to progesterone during pregnancy or pseudopregnancy is similar to that of other species, but is prolonged and exaggerated. The uterus of the bitch is particularly susceptible to both, progestagens and estrogens. Many steroids that have powerful progestagenic activity in the bitch are found to be weak progestagens in other species, and several estrogens that have relatively weak estrogenic activities in other species are powerful bone marrow depressors in the bitch. Exogenous progestagens in general, particularly when given for extended periods, induce hyperplasia of the endometrium in the bitch. This endometrial response of the bitch is frequently conducive to a pathologic condition termed cystic hyperplasia or cystic hyperplastic complex of the endometrium. This complex is characterized by intense endometrial gland development and mucus secretion, which may develop into mucometra or pyometra. The incidence of hyperplastic reaction increases and tends to become the cystic hyperplastic complex when the bitch has been primed with estrogens prior to the administration of progestagens. In addition to this undesirable endometrial reaction, progestagens stimulate mammary gland development which, in time, tend to become nodular and often malignant.

Prolonged treatment with progestagens can induce electrolyte disturbances, affect water retention, and alter carbohydrate metabolism, promoting diabetogenic responses in bitches due to increased pituitary secretion and release of growth hormone.

Myometrial reaction is also pronounced and a characteristic dose-dependent response, termed "corkscrew," develops in bitches upon treatment with progestagens. The uterus normally enlarges (Fig. 16-9) and folds under the influence of progesterone. The reaction is more exaggerated when large doses of progesterone or progestagens are given and the uterine horns coil along their longitudinal axis giving the "cork screw" appearance.

In addition to the myelotoxic, bone marrow depressant activity of estrogens in dogs, which frequently leads to a severe and often fatal aplastic anemia, exogenous estrogens induce proestrual signs in the bitch, including hyperemia of the genital tract, and bloody discharge from the vulva. Large doses and extended treatments with estrogens are associated with mammary gland hyperplasia in the bitch, which can result in benign or malignant tumors.

PSEUDOPREGNANCY

Pseudopregnancy, false pregnancy, or pseudocyesis can be defined as an exaggerated diestrual response of the bitch. Pseudopregnancy is a condition of considerable clinical importance and likely is related to the extreme sensitivity of the canine endometrium and mammary gland to progesterone, in synergy with other hormonal factors, including prolactin. As previously discussed, the corpora lutea of the nonpregnant bitch remain functional for an extended period after ovulation. Development of the uterus is similar to that in early pregnancy, in spite of the fact that no embryos are present in the uterus (Fig. 16-9). The uterus enlarges, and the abdomen may actually become relaxed. In most cases, diestrual bitches do not display external signs of pregnancy and the progesterone-related enlargement of the uterus goes undetected. On occasions, however, the nonmated or sterile-mated bitch develops a series of behavioral responses and external signs of pregnancy, which has been termed "overt pseudopregnancy."

In overt pseudopregnancy, the mammary glands begin to develop in preparation for lactation. In addition, there is a relaxation of the pelvis and external genitalia similar to that during pregnancy. A maternal attitude develops toward her environment and associates. Pseudopregnancy often lasts as long as or longer than a normal pregnancy. With time, the psychological manifestations become intense and the bitch may attempt to build a

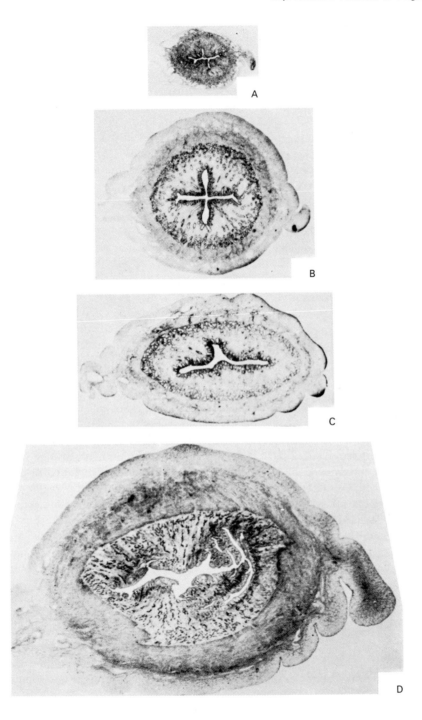

Fig. 16-9. Cross sections of uterus. A, Anestrus. B, Proestrus. Note increase in size and tubular appearance resulting largely from congestion and edema. C, Estrus. Note further enlargement due principally to hypertrophy of both myo- and endometrium. D, Diestrus. The increase in diameter is accompanied by a marked decrease in length of the cornu. (Bouin's, nitrocellulose, hematoxylin and eosin; section 12 microns thick. ×10.) (From Cole, H. H., and Cupps, P. T.: Reproduction in Domestic Animals. New York, Academic Press, 1959.)

whelping nest in preparation for parturition. Occasionally the bitch may experience labor, although this is rare. The mammary glands may even develop to such an extent that lactation begins. Some pseudopregnant bitches can adopt and effectively nurse puppies from other bitches.

In most cases, pseudopregnancy is so subtle in outward appearance that the owner is unaware of the condition. However, it is important for the veterinarian to understand and explain to the owner the known physiological processes involved. Administration of bromocriptine has proven to be effective to ameliorate the nesting behavior and other signs of overt pseudopregnancy, suggesting that increased pituitary prolactin secretion might contribute to these external manifestations of pseudopregnancy.

PREGNANCY AND PARTURITION

Even though conception is possible in the bitch, whether the breeding occurs once on the first day, subsequent days, or even on the last day of estrus without any apparent decrease in the pregnancy rate or the size of the litter, breeding on the first and either third or fourth days of estrus is recommended to increase the chances for pregnancy. Pregnancy lasts an average of 64 days, when the length of pregnancy is calculated from the first day of estrus for those bitches bred on the first day of standing estrus. Pregnancy may range between 56 to 68 days for bitches in dog colonies with controlled breeding programs. If the length of pregnancy is calculated from the first day that the bitch refuses to mate, that is the first day of diestrus, the length of pregnancy is remarkably constant and lasts an average of 57 days. Most of the variation in the length of pregnancy reported in the literature for the bitch, in which extreme values such as 72 days have been reported, is likely due to the methods used to determine estrus and diestrus, particularly those based on the vaginal smear. Other contributing factors may include variations due to breed and time of ovulation, effects of single versus multiple matings, and

false mounts of the male without actual genital lock and ejaculation. When teaser dogs are used to establish the onset of diestrus, variations in the length of gestation are reduced considerably.

Preimplantation embryonic development begins in the oviduct and the embryo enters the uterus of the bitch at the late morula or early blastocyst stage, 8 to 10 days after ovulation. Implantation sites are distinguishable by day 10 of diestrus. By day 16 of diestrus (approximately 23 days after the onset of estrus) the expansion of these implantation sites occurs and the deep endometrial penetration of the trophoblast is completed by day 18 of diestrus. Table 16-8 displays the stages and time of appearance of prenatal development for the beagle dog.

The uterine swellings at the implantation sites can be palpated transabdominally as early as day 20 to 22 and as late as day 30 to 31 of gestation. The detection of these swellings is not difficult in young, thin bitches, but becomes difficult or even impossible in obese bitches. Radiologic diagnosis of pregnancy is possible 42 to 46 days from the onset of estrus, when the bones of the fetus become radiopaque. Caution is imperative when performing radiologic examination of presumptively pregnant bitches. Excessive or prolonged exposure of the bitch and fetuses to the x rays may permanently alter the future reproductive function of both the mother and offspring, since the ionizing radiation is detrimental to gametogenesis. Ultrasonographic diagnosis of pregnancy is another technique being studied. Even though embryos can be detected in the uterus using ultrasound by day 10 after breeding, it is recommended that another scan be performed 4 to 10 days later. By day 28 or 29 of gestation, the heartbeat can be detected in the developing fetus, and the number of fetuses can be determined between days 28 and 35 of gestation.

The placenta of the bitch is endotheliochorial and zonary because it attaches to the endometrium only at a central zone of the placenta. The yolk sac persists in the bitch for most of the length of gestation and this organ

Table 16-8 States of Canine Prenatal Development
for the Beagle

Stage of Development	Days Post Breeding	Size (Diameter* or Length†)
Fertilized oocyte to blastocyst (in oviduct)	<8	230 to 250 μm*
Spherical blastocyst (in uterus)	12	250 to 1250 μm*
Oval blastocyst (spaced in uterus)	16	1250 to 2500 μm*
Implantation, no primitive streak	17	>2500 μm*
Primitive streak	18	1 to 2 mm
Neural groove, 1 to 4 somites	19	2 to 3 mm†
Cranial enlargement of neural groove, 5 to 9 somites	20	3 to 5 mm†
First limb buds, branchial arches	23	5 to 6 mm†
First appearance of eye, hindlimb buds	24	6 to 14 mm†
Abdomen closes to umbilicus	25	10 to 15 mm†
Eyelids, facial vibrissae	27	12 to 15 mm†
Sexual differentiation	32	23 to 27 mm†
Closed eyelids, claws	35	28 to 41 mm†
Fully formed fetus	42	40 to 90 mm†
Appearance of hair	49	90 to 100 mm†

Adapted From: P. A. Holst, and R. D. Phemister. Prenatal Canine Development. Description of Normal Development Stages. Annual Report. Collaborative Radiological Health Laboratory, Colorado State University, 1969.

may function as a supplementary liver during part of gestation.

An abrupt decline in progesterone levels 1 to 2 days before parturition is required for normal parturition in the bitch. This decline is probably in association with maturation of the pituitary-adrenal axis of the fetus. Exogenous progesterone delays parturition in the bitch. Androgens also decline at parturition time, but the role of androgens in the parturition of the bitch has not been determined. The elevation of maternal corticoid levels 1 to 4 days before parturition, at the time of maximal decline of blood levels of progesterone, may be due to fetal adrenal involvement in the parturition process.

Rectal temperature drops 1 to 1.5°F two days before parturition, a reflection of the disappearance of the thermogenic effect of progesterone. Rectal temperatures return to normal or slightly higher within 12 to 24 hours after parturition.

Bitches usually show increased restlessness and panting followed by nesting behavior, 24 hours before parturition. Delivery or whelping is usually completed within a period of 8 to 10 hours, but may take longer. Whelping time is influenced by the number of puppies to be born and varies among bitches. During whelping, there is an alternate expulsion of the puppies. The birth of the first pup, in relation to the left or right uterine horn, seems to be of random occurrence, but in most cases (78%) the second pup is born from the horn opposite to the one from which the first pup was born.

Lactation lasts from 6 to 9 weeks in the bitch, and during lactation, the levels of prolactin are elevated. The mean interestrus interval does not seem to be different between pregnant and nonpregnant bitches, suggesting that lactational anestrus does not contribute to or lengthen anestrus or the interval between consecutive estruses.

THE DOG

The testes of the dog pass through the inguinal canal on the third or fourth day after birth and reach their final scrotal location by 35 days after birth.

The average length of the cycle of the seminiferous epithelium (see Chapter 7) is estimated to be 13.6 days for the dog and coyote and the duration of spermatogenesis lasts an average of 54.4 days. Each spermatogonium of the dog is thought to have the potential of producing 64 to 96 spermatozoa. The epididymal transit time is estimated to last 10 to 11 days.

After puberty, dogs are capable of mating and producing fertile ejaculates year round. Mating in dogs is characterized by a genital lock between the male and the female (Fig. 8-19). Dogs attempting to mate mount the estrous bitch from the rear and perform several pelvic thrusts, releasing short bursts of pre-sperm secretion while the penis is only partially erected. When the tip of the penis enters the bitch's vagina, the dog performs a deep thrust to introduce the penis, followed by a short series of rapid thrusts, until the penis becomes fully erected and anchored in the vagina. After the genital lock has been established, the dog dismounts and either turns away from the bitch or remains by her side facing in the same direction. When the dog dismounts the bitch, the root of the penis is twisted 180 degrees, as the penis is reflected backwards between the hind legs of the dog, without any apparent rotation of the glans penis and bulbus glandis within the vagina. This backward reflection and twisting at the base of the penis, which truly constitutes a "paradox of flexible rigidity,"[81] compress the veins of the penis ensuring an extended erection and the genital lock that is essential, due to the large volume of the dog's ejaculate and prolonged ejaculation. At mating, some bitches fall to the ground after the genital lock or even twist and turn vigorously, while trying to bite the male. The genital lock of the penis within the vagina is firm enough to withstand those movements. Occasionally, dislodging of the penis from the vagina may occur when the male is unable to achieve or to keep a full erection, or when the mating partners are frightened or disturbed by un-

familiar surroundings. In this case, some dogs will continue to ejaculate discharging the ejaculate on the ground. Pressure from the prepuce on the erected penis appears to be a sufficient stimulus to maintain this ongoing ejaculation.

The dog's ejaculate is delivered in three fractions (Table 16-9). The first, the presperm fraction, is small in volume, clear, and usually contains only a few spermatozoa. The second, sperm rich fraction is small in volume, milky in appearance, and contains most of the spermatozoa to be released during ejaculation. The first two fractions are delivered within the first 2 or 3 minutes of ejaculation. The third, postsperm fraction is the most voluminous, may contain a few spermatozoa, and requires 3 to 40 minutes to be delivered. Most of the postsperm fraction is contributed by the prostate gland, thus the collection of samples of postsperm fraction can be very useful for studies on prostatic secretions and evaluation of prostatic diseases. After the completion of ejaculation, penile erection subsides and the dog separates from the bitch, by withdrawing the penis.

Samples of semen can be collected from dogs with an artificial vagina or by digital manipulation using a rubber directing cone (Fig. 16-10). The method of digital manipulation is effective, easy to perform, and suitable for clinical practice, since little or no previous training of the dog is required (see Chapter 10). Semen can also be collected from the dog by electrical stimulation when dogs do not respond to the digital stimulation

Table 16-9 Fractions of the Dog's Ejaculate

Fraction	Volume (ml)	
	Mean	Range
Presperm	0.8	0.25–2.8
Sperm rich	0.6	0.40–2.0
Postsperm	4.0	1.10–16.3
Total ejaculate	5.4	1.75–21.1

Adapted From: Boucher, J. H. et al., Cornell Vet. *48:* 72, 1958.

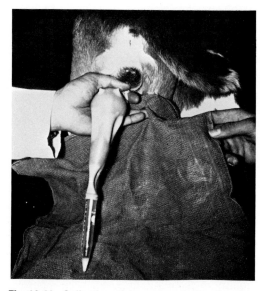

Fig. 16-10. Collection of dog semen by the directing cone method.

4 or 5 days. More frequent collections, especially for extended periods, result in a decreased output of spermatozoa per ejaculate. Depletion of spermatozoal reserves occurs when 5 or more ejaculates are obtained within 5 days.

RESPONSE OF DOGS AND BITCHES TO EXOGENOUS HORMONES

The pituitary of dogs and anestrous or cycling bitches responds within minutes to the intravenous injection of GnRH by releasing both LH and FSH. Similarly, both prolactin and thyroid stimulating hormone are released from the dog's pituitary gland following the injection of thyrotropin releasing hormone. Dopamine agonists effectively suppress levels of prolactin in the blood.

Natural or synthetic estrogens, androgens, and progestagens effectively inhibit the release of gonadotropins from the pituitary of dogs and bitches. The influence of these reproductive steroids on gonadotropin release makes them useful as contraceptive steroids for the management and control of reproduction of dogs.

Although the pituitary of dogs and bitches is responsive to the stimulatory activity of releasing factors, or to the inhibitory activity of steroids, the ovaries of anestrous bitches respond poorly and erratically to exogenous gonadotropic stimulation. Treatment of anestrous bitches with PMSG or with FSH preparations to induce estrus often fails, or results in only a small percentage of bitches respond-

of the penis. The process of inducing seminal emission by electrical stimulation is called electroejaculation and the resulting product, an electroejaculate. Electroejaculation is particularly useful to collect semen from wild canidae such as coyotes, dingoes, and foxes. Dogs and wild canidae should be anesthetized prior to electroejaculation.

Table 16-10 displays some of the physical characteristics of ejaculates from beagle dogs and Table 16-11 shows the daily sperm production, output, and extragonadal sperm reserves for the beagle dog. Seminal collections should not be performed more than once every

Table 16-10   Physical Characteristics of Beagle Ejaculates (Artificial Vagina)

Parameter	Mean	SD*	Range
Volume, ml	3.1	0.3	2.8–3.4
Motility (0 to 5)	3.0	0.3	2.2–3.9
Density (0 to 5)	1.5	1.1	0.0–4.2
Sperm concentration (10^6/ml)	111	22	57–164
Total sperm per ejaculate (10^6)	301	60	154–449
Percent sperm alive	90	2	84–95
Percent abnormal sperm	7	1	3–10

* SD = Standard deviation
Adapted From: R. W. James and R. Heywood, Vet. Rec. *104:*480, 1979.

Table 16-11 Daily Sperm Production (DSP), Daily Sperm
Output (DSO), and Extra Gonadal Sperm
Reserves (EGR) in the Beagle Dog

DSP (10^6)*	DSO (10^6)*	EGR (10^6)*
594 ± 102	464 ± 16	479 ± 175

* Mean ± standard error of the mean. Semen collected by the digital manipulation method using a teaser bitch.
Adapted From: T. T. Olar, et al., Biol. Reprod., *29:*1114, 1983.

ing with follicular development, standing estrous behavior, and ovulation. The ovulatory response to exogenous gonadotropins, particularly PMSG, is highly variable, and the treatment of those bitches that respond to the treatment with FSH or FSH-like gonadotropins with hCG, seems to improve their ovulatory response (Table 16-12). It is possible that the ovary of the bitch is similar to the ovary of the mare, which responds more reliably to homologous equine pituitary gonadotropins than to heterologous gonadotropins. Canine gonadotropins might allow for the reliable induction of estrus and ovulation in anestrous bitches. Unfortunately, canine pituitary gonadotropins are not commercially available and they have not been used to induce estrus in anestrous bitches.

Studies to determine the effectiveness of GnRH to induce estrous and ovulatory responses in anestrous bitches have not been reported.

Treatment of the dog with GnRH significantly increases the levels of testosterone in the blood and hCG increases testosterone secretion in perfused testes, but the effectiveness of GnRH, or of FSH, LH, and FSH- or LH-like hormones on reproductive problems of dogs, including their effects on libido, spermatogenesis, ejaculatory responses, and on the quality of ejaculate, have not been reported.

CONTRACEPTIVE STEROIDS FOR THE BITCH

The major aim of contraception is to prevent pregnancy by blocking or preventing estrus, ovulation, or any other appropriate interference in the reproductive processes. As stated previously, several natural or synthetic steroids effectively prevent estrus or inhibit the behavioral manifestations of estrus, thus preventing the bitch to accept the male for mating. Unfortunately, most steroids also produce objectionable or undesirable side effects in the bitch. Progestagens promote excessive

Table 16-12 Response of Anestrous Bitches to Daily
Injections of PMSG*
Followed by a Single Treatment with HCG**

Response	Ratio	%
Estrous behavior[†]	5/8	63
Vulval bleeding	3/8	38
Vulval swelling	7/8	88
Bitches in standing estrus that ovulated	5/8	63

* PMSG, 250 IU/day, subcutaneous injections for 14 to 20 days, until the bitch showed estrous vaginal smears.
** HCG, 500 IU, subcutaneous injection the first day of estrus after PMSG treatment was discontinued.
† Standing estrus, mating.
Adapted From: P. J. Wright, Aust. Vet. J. *59:*123, 1982.

endometrial and uterine growth; androgens tend to masculinize the bitch and the fetus when given to pregnant bitches, and estrogens may induce irreversible aplastic anemia in dogs and bitches. The demands created by the increasing population of pet animals prompted the search for safe and suitable steroids for use as contraceptives in dogs and cats. Of these, only two steroids have been approved by the U.S. Food and Drug Administration and are commercially available for canine contraception. These are: megestrol acetate, a synthetic progestational compound and mibolerone, a synthetic androgen derivative. Megestrol acetate, sold under the commercial name of Ovaban, is orally active and effective to block the progression of proestrus to estrus, when given early in proestrus. Ovaban is also effective to postpone estrus when given during anestrus. Ovaban will not block behavioral estrus and should not be given to bitches in estrus because of the increased endometrial responses and abnormal uterine growth, which is caused when this synthetic progestagen acts on an estrogen-primed uterus. Mibolerone, sold under the commercial name of Cheque is an effective and apparently safe oral contraceptive for bitches. Mibolerone blocks the appearance of estrus when given daily to anestrous bitches. The drug is effective to postpone estrus, while is being given to the bitch. Daily administration of Mibolerone for periods as long as 2 years does not appear to cause detrimental effects to the bitch.

Estrogens are and have been used in the veterinary clinical practice for years as a replacement therapy in spayed bitches with urinary incontinence, to treat prostatic hypertrophy and perianal edema in dogs, and to prevent pregnancies after mismatings or to terminate pregnancies. Recent evidences provided by carefully controlled studies indicate that the effectiveness of estrogen treatment to prevent or to terminate pregnancy needs to be re-evaluated. Particularly in view of the inefficacy of some of the more widely used estrogens and the detrimental and myelotoxic effects of estrogens in dogs and bitches.

REFERENCES

1. Abel, J. H., Jr., McClellan, M. C., Verhage. H. G., et al. (1975): Subcellular compartmentalization of the luteal cell in the ovary of the dog. Cell Tissue Res. *158:*461.
2. Abel, J. H., Jr., Verhage, H. G., McClellan, M. C., et al. (1975): Ultrastructural analysis of the granulosa-luteal cell transition in the ovary of the dog. Cell Tissue Res. *160:*155.
3. Al-Kafawi, A. A., Hopwood, M. L., Pineda M. H., et al. (1974): Immunization of dogs against human chorionic gonadotropin. Am. J. Vet. Res. *35:*261.
4. Allen, W. E. (1986): Pseudopregnancy in the bitch: the current view on aetiology and treatment. J. Small Anim. Pract. *27:*419.
5. Allen, W. E., and Meredith, M. J. (1981): Detection of pregnancy in the bitch: A study of abdominal palpation, A-mode ultrasound and doppler ultrasound techniques. J. Small Anim. Pract. *22:*609.
6. Allen, W. E., Daker, M. G. and Hancock, J. L. (1981): Three intersexual dogs. Vet. Rec. *109:*468.
7. Anderson, A. C., and Simpson, M. E. (1973): The ovary and reproductive cycle of the dog (Beagle). Los Altos, California, Geron-X, Inc.
8. Anderson, J. W. (1969): Ultrastructure of the placenta and fetal membranes of the dog. I. Placental labyrinth. Am. J. Anat. *165:*15.
9. Anderson, R. K., Gilmore, C. E., and Schnelle, G. B. (1965): Utero-ovarian disorders associated with use of medroxyprogesterone in dogs. J. Am. Vet. Med. Assoc. *146:*1311.
10. Aumuller, G., Stofft, E., and Tunn, U. (1980): Fine structure of the canine prostatic complex. Anat. Embryol. *160:*327.
11. Austad, R., Lunde, A., and Sjaastad, O. V. (1976): Peripheral plasma levels of estradiol-17β and progesterone in the bitch during the estrous cycle, in normal pregnancy and after dexamethasone treatment. J. Reprod. Fertil. *46:*129.
12. Awoniyi, C., Hasson, T., Chandrashekar, V., et al. (1986): Regulation of gonadotropin secretion in the male: effect of an aromatization inhibitor in estradiol-implanted, orchidectomized dogs. J. Androl. *7:*234.
13. Barrau, M. D., Abel, J. H., Jr., Verhage, H. G., et al. (1975): Development of the endometrium during the estrous cycle in the bitch. Am. J. Anat. *142:*47.
14. Barrau, M. D., Abel, J. H., Jr., Torbit, C. A., et al. (1975): Development of the implantation chamber in the pregnant bitch. Am. J. Anat. *143:*115.
15. Baumans, V., Dijkstra, G., and Wensing, C. J. G. (1981): Testicular descent in the dog. Zbl. Vet. Med. *10:*97.
16. Baumans, V., Dijkstra, G., and Wensing, C. J. G. (1983): The role of a non-androgenic testicular factor in the process of testicular descent in the dog. Int. J. Androl. *6:*541.
17. Baumans, V., Dieleman, S. J., Wouterse, H. S., et al. (1983): Testosterone secretion during gubernacular development and testicular descent in the dog. J. Reprod. Fertil. *73:*21.
18. Beach, F. A. (1970): Coital behavior in dogs. IX. Sequelae to "coitus interruptus" in males and fe-

males. Physiol. and Behav. *5:*263.

19. Bell, E. T., and Christie, D. W. (1971): The evaluation of cellular indices in canine vaginal cytology. Br. Vet. J. *127:*63.

20. Bell, E. T., and Christie, D. W. (1971): Duration of proestrus, oestrus and vulval bleeding in the beagle bitch. Br. Vet. J. *127:*25.

21. Bondestam, S., Alitalo, I., and Karkkainen, M. (1983): Real-time ultrasound pregnancy diagnosis in the bitch. J. Small Anim. Pract. *24:*145.

22. Boucher, J. H., Foote, R. H., and Kirk, R. W. (1958): The evaluation of semen quality in the dog and the effects of frequency of ejaculation upon semen quality, libido, and depletion of sperm reserves. Cornell Vet. *48:*67.

23. Boulanger, P., Desaulniers, M., Bleau, G., et al. (1983): Sex steroid concentrations in plasma from the canine deferential vein. J. Endocrinol. *96:*223.

24. Bowen, R. A., Olson, P. N., Behrendt, M. D., et al. (1985): Efficacy and toxicity of estrogens commonly used to terminate canine pregnancy. J. Am. Vet. Med. Assoc. *186:*783.

25. Boyden, T. W., Pamenter, R. W., and Silvert, M. A. (1980): Testosterone secretion by the isolated canine testis after controlled infusions of hCG. J. Reprod. Fertil. *59:*25.

26. Briggs, M. (1977): The beagle dog and contraceptive steroids. Life Sci. *21:*275.

27. Briggs, M. H. (1980): Progestogens and mammary tumours in the beagle bitch. Res. Vet. Sci. *28:*199.

28. Brodey, R. S., Fidler, I. J., and Howson, A. E. (1966): The relationship of estrous irregularity, pseudopregnancy, and pregnancy to the development of canine mammary neoplasms. J. Am. Vet. Med. Assoc. *149:*1047.

29. Capel-Edwards, K., Hall, D. E., Fellowes, K. P., et al. (1973): Long-term administration of progesterone to the female Beagle dog. Toxicol. Appl. Pharmacol. *24:*474.

30. Cartee, R. E., and Rowles, T. (1984): Preliminary study of the ultrasonographic diagnosis of pregnancy and fetal development in the dog. Am. J. Vet. Res. *45:*1259.

31. Catling, P. C. (1979): Seasonal variation in plasma testosterone and the testis in captive male dingoes, *Canis familiaris dingo.* Aust. J. Zool. *27:*939.

32. Chakraborty, P. K., and Fletcher, W. S. (1977): Responsiveness of anestrous labrador bitches to GnRH. Proc. Soc. Exp. Biol. Med. *154:*125.

33. Christiansen, Ib. J. (1984): Reproduction in the Dog and Cat. London, Bailliere Tindall.

34. Christie, D. W., Bailey, J. B., and Bell, E. T. (1972): Classification of cell types in vaginal smears during the canine oestrous cycle. Br. Vet. J. *128:*301.

35. Christie, D. W., and Bell, E. T. (1971): Some observations on the seasonal incidence and frequency of oestrus in breeding bitches in Britain. J. Small Anim. Pract. *12:*159.

36. Concannon, P. W. (1980): Effects of hypophysectomy and of LH administration on luteal phase plasma progesterone levels in the beagle bitch. J. Reprod. Fertil. *58:*407.

37. Concannon, P. W. (1983): Reproductive physiology and endocrine patterns of the bitch. *In:* Current Veterinary Therapy, Vol. VIII, Small Animal Prac-

tice, Philadelphia, W. B. Saunders Co., p. 886.

38. Concannon, P. W. (1983): Fertility regulation in the bitch: contraception, sterilization, and pregnancy termination. *In:* Current Veterinary Therapy, Vol. VIII, Small Animal Practice, Philadelphia, W. B. Saunders Co., p. 901.

39. Concannon, P. W., and Castracane, V. D. (1985): Serum androstenedione and testosterone concentrations during pregnancy and nonpregnant cycles in dogs. Biol. Reprod. *33:*1078.

40. Concannon, P. W., and Hansel, W. (1977): Prostaglandin $F_{2\alpha}$ induced luteolysis, hypothermia and abortion in beagle bitches. Prostaglandins *13:*543.

41. Concannon, P., and Rendano, V. (1983): Radiographic diagnosis of canine pregnancy: onset of fetal skeletal radiopacity in relation to times of breeding, preovulatory luteinizing hormone release, and parturition. Am. J. Vet. Res. *44:*1506.

42. Concannon, P., Cowan, R., and Hansel, W. (1979): LH release in ovariectomized dogs in response to estrogen withdrawal and its facilitation by progesterone. Biol. Reprod. *20:*523.

43. Concannon, P., Hansel, W., and McEntee, K. (1977): Changes in LH, progesterone and sexual behavior associated with preovulatory luteinization in the bitch. Biol. Reprod. *17:*604.

44. Concannon, P. W., Hansel, W., and Visek, W. J. (1975): The ovarian cycle of the bitch: plasma estrogen, LH and progesterone. Biol. Reprod. *13:*112.

45. Concannon, P. W., Powers, M. E., Holder, W., et al. (1977): Pregnancy and parturition in the bitch. Biol. Reprod. *16:*517.

46. Concannon, P. W., Spraker, T. R., Casey, H. W., et al. (1981): Gross and histopathologic effects of medroxyprogesterone acetate and progesterone on the mammary gland of adult beagle bitches. Fert. Steril. *36:*373.

47. Concannon, P. W., Weigand, N., Wilson, S., et al. (1979): Sexual behavior in ovariectomized bitches in response to estrogen and progesterone treatments. Biol. Reprod. *20:*799.

48. Concannon, P. W., Altszuler, N., Hampshire, J., et al. (1980): Growth hormone, prolactin and cortisol in dogs developing mammary nodules and an acromegaly-like appearance during treatment with medroxyprogesterone acetate. Endocrinology *106:*1173.

49. Concannon, P. W., Butler, W. R., Hansel, W., et al. (1978): Parturition and lactation in the bitch: Serum progesterone, cortisol and prolactin. Biol. Reprod. *19:*1113.

50. Connell, C. J. (1980): Blood-testis barrier formation and the initiation of meiosis in the dog. *In:* Testicular Development, Structure, and Function. Steinberger A. and Steinberger E. (eds.). New York, Raven Press, p. 71.

51. Connell, C. J., and Donjacour, A. (1985): A morphological study of the epididymides of control and estradiol-treated prepubertal dogs. Biol. Reprod. *33:*951.

52. Crafts, R. C. (1948): The effects of estrogens on the bone marrow of adult female dogs. Blood *3:*276.

53. Daniels, T. J. (1983): The social organization of free-ranging urban dogs. I. Non-estrous social behavior. Appl. Anim. Ethol. *10:*341.

54. Daniels, T. J. (1983): The social organization of free-ranging urban dogs. II. Estrous groups and the mating system. Appl. Anim. Ethol. *10:*365.
55. De Coster, R., Beckers, J.-F., Beerens, D. et al. (1983): A homologous radioimmunoassay for canine prolactin: plasma levels during the reproductive cycle. Acta Endocrinol. *103:*473.
56. Del Campo, C. H., and Ginther, O. J. (1974): Arteries and veins of uterus and ovaries in dogs and cats. Am. J. Vet. Res. *35:*409.
57. DePalatis, L., Moore, J., and Falvo, R. E. (1978): Plasma concentrations of testosterone and LH in male dog. J. Reprod. Fertil. *52:*201.
58. Doak, R. L., Hall, A., and Dale, H. E. (1967): Longevity of spermatozoa in the reproductive tract of the bitch. J. Reprod. Fertil. *13:*51.
59. Doty, R. L., and Dunbar, I. (1974): Attraction of Beagles to conspecific urine, vaginal and anal sac secretion odors. Physiol. and Behav. *12:*825.
60. Doty, R. L. and Mare, C. J. (1974): Color, odor, consistency and secretion rate of anal sac secretions from male, female, and early-androgenized female Beagles. Am. J. Vet. Res. *35:*669.
61. Drill, V. A. (1974): Some metabolic actions and possible toxic effects of hormonal contraceptives in animals and man. Acta Endocrinol. *75:*169.
62. Eigenmann, J. E., and Eigenmann, R. Y. (1981): Influence of medroxyprogesterone acetate (Provera) on plasma growth hormone levels and on carbohydrate metabolism. II. Studies in the ovariohysterectomized, oestradiol-primed bitch. Acta Endocrinol. *98:*603.
63. Eigenmann, J. E., and Rijnberk, A. (1981): Influence of medroxyprogesterone acetate (Provera) on plasma growth hormone levels and on carbohydrate metabolism. I. Studies on the ovariectomized bitch. Acta Endocrinol. *98:*599.
64. Ewing, L. L., Berry, S. J., and Higginbottom, E. G. (1983): Dihydrotestosterone concentration of beagle prostatic tissue: effect of age and hyperplasia. Endocrinology *113:*2004.
65. Ewing, L. L., Zirkin, B. R., Cochran, R. C., et al. (1979): Testosterone secretion by rat, rabbit, guinea pig, dog, and hamster testes perfused in vitro: correlation with Leydig cell mass. Endocrinology *105:*1135.
66. Falvo, R. E., and Vincent, D. L. (1980): Testosterone regulation of follicle-stimulating hormone secretion in the male dog. J. Androl. *1:*197.
67. Falvo, R. E., Vincent, D. L., Lathrop, J., et al. (1979): Effects of testosterone and testosterone propionate administration on luteinizing hormone secretion in the male mongrel dog. Biol. Reprod. *21:*807.
68. Falvo, R. E., Gerrit, M., Pirmann, J., et al. (1982): Testosterone pretreatment and the response of pituitary LH to gonadotropin-releasing hormone (GnRH) in the male dog. J. Androl. *3:*193.
69. Faulkner, L. C., Pineda, M. H., and Reimers, T. J. (1975): Immunization against gonadotropins in dogs. *In:* Immunization with Hormones in Reproduction Research, Nieschlag E. (ed.), Amsterdam, North-Holland Publishing Co., p. 199.
70. Foote, R. H., Swierstra, E. E., and Hunt, W. L. (1972): Spermatogenesis in the dog. Anat. Rec.
*173:*341.
71. Fowler, E. H., Feldman, M. K., and Loeb, W. F. (1971): Comparison of histologic features of ovarian and uterine tissues with vaginal smears of the bitch. Am. J. Vet. Res. *32:*327.
72. Frank, D. W., Kirton, K. T., Murchison, T. E., et al. (1979): Mammary tumors and serum hormones in the bitch treated with medroxyprogesterone acetate or progesterone for four years. Fertil. Steril. *31:*340.
73. Frenette, M. D., Dooley, M. P., and Pineda, M. H. (1986): Effect of flushing the vasa deferentia at the time of vasectomy on the rate of clearance of spermatozoa from the ejaculates of dogs and cats. Am. J. Vet. Res. *47:*463.
74. Froman, D. P., and Amann, R. P. (1983): Inhibition of motility of bovine, canine and equine spermatozoa by artificial vagina lubricants. Theriogenology *20:*357.
75. Gerber, J. G., Hubbard, W. C., and Nies, A. S. (1976): Uterine vein prostaglandin levels in late pregnant dogs. Prostaglandins *17:*623.
76. Gill, H. P., Kaufman, C. F., Foote, R. H., et al. (1970): Artificial insemination of beagle bitches with freshly collected, liquid-stored, and frozen-stored semen. Am. J. Vet. Res. *31:*1807.
77. Ginther, O. J. (1976): Comparative anatomy of uteroovarian vasculature. Vet. Scope *20:*2.
78. Goodwin, M., Gooding, K. M., and Regnier, F. (1979): Sex pheromone in the dog. Science *203:*559.
79. Graf, K.-J. (1978): Serum oestrogen, progesterone and prolactin concentrations in cyclic, pregnant and lactating beagle dogs. J. Reprod. Fertil. *52:*9.
80. Graf, K.-J., and El Etreby, M. F. (1979): Endocrinology of reproduction in the female beagle dog and its significance in mammary gland tumorogenesis. Acta Endocrinol. *90*, Suppl. 222:1.
81. Grandage, J. (1972): The erect dog penis: a paradox of flexible rigidity. Vet. Rec. *91:*141.
82. Hadley, J. C. (1975): Total unconjugated oestrogen and progesterone concentrations in peripheral blood during the oestrous cycle of the dog. J. Reprod. Fertil. *44:*445.
83. Hadley, J. C. (1975): Total unconjugated oestrogen and progesterone concentrations in peripheral blood during pregnancy in the dog. J. Reprod. Fertil. *44:*453.
84. Hadley, J. C. (1975): Unconjugated oestrogen and progesterone concentrations in the blood of bitches with false pregnancy and pyometra. Vet. Rec. *96:*545.
85. Hart, B. L. (1974): Gonadal androgen and sociosexual behavior of male mammals: a comparative analysis. Physiol. Bull. *81:*383.
86. Hart, B. L., and Kitchell, R. L. (1966): Penile erection and contraction of penile muscles in the spinal and intact dog. Am. J. Physiol. *210:*257.
87. Hart, B. L., and Ladewig, J. (1979): Serum testosterone of neonatal male and female dogs. Biol. Reprod. *21:*289.
88. Hinton, M., and Jones, D. R. E. (1977): Anaemia in the dog: an analysis of laboratory data. J. Small Anim. Pract. *18:*701.
89. Holst, P. A., and Phemister, R. D. (1971): The prenatal development of the dog: Preimplantation

events. Biol. Reprod. *5:*194.

90. Holst, P. A., and Phemister, R. D. (1974): Onset of diestrus in the Beagle bitch: Definition and significance. Am. J. Vet. Res. *35:*401.

91. Holst, P. A., and Phemister, R. D. (1975): Temporal sequence of events in the estrous cycle of the bitch. Am. J. Vet. Res. *36:*705.

92. Holt, P. E., and Sayle, B. (1981): Congenital vestibulo-vaginal stenosis in the bitch. J. Small Anim. Pract. *22:*67.

93. Hopkins, S. G., Schubert, T. A., and Hart, B. L. (1976): Castration of adult male dogs: Effects on roaming, aggression, urine marking, and mounting. J. Am. Vet. Med. Assoc. *168:*1108.

94. Huggins, C., Masina, M. H., Eichelberger, L. E., et al. (1939): Quantitative studies of prostatic secretion. 1. Characteristics of normal secretion, the influence of thyroid, suprarenal and testis extirpation and androgen substitution on the prostatic output. J. Exp. Med. *70:*543.

95. Ibach, B., Weissbach, L., and Hilscher, B. (1976): Stages of the cycle of the seminiferous epithelium in the dog. Andrologia *8:*297.

96. Ibach, B., Passia, D., Weissbach, L., et al. (1978): The effect of low-dose HCG on the testis of prepuberal dogs. Int. J. Androl. *6:*509.

97. James, R. W., Crook, D., and Heywood, R. (1979): Canine pituitary-testicular function in relation to toxicity testing. Toxicology *13:*237.

98. James, R. W., Heywood, R., and Street, A. E. (1979): Biochemical observations on beagle dog semen. Vet. Rec. *104:*480.

99. Joby, R., Jemmett, J. E., and Miller, A. S. H. (1984): The control of undesirable behaviour in male dogs using megestrol acetate. J. Small Anim. Pract. *25:* 567.

100. Jochle, W. (1975): Hormones in canine gynecology: A review. Theriogenology *3:*152.

101. Jochle, W., and Andersen, A. C. (1977): The estrus cycle in the dog: A review. Theriogenology *7:*113.

102. Jochle, W., Tomlinson, R. V., and Andersen, A. C. (1972): Prostaglandin effects on plasma progesterone levels in the pregnant and cycling dog (Beagle). Prostaglandins *3:*209.

103. Johnston, S. D., Buoen, L. C., Weber, A. F., et al. (1985): X-trisomy in an airedale bitch with ovarian dysplasia and primary anestrus. Theriogenology *24:*597.

104. Johnston, S. D., Kiang, D. T., Seguin, B. E., et al. (1985): Cytoplasmic estrogen and progesterone receptors in canine endometrium during the estrous cycle. Am. J. Vet. Res. *46:*1653.

105. Kennelly, J. J. (1969): The effect of mestranol on canine reproduction. Biol. Reprod. *1:*282.

106. Kennelly, J. J. (1972): Coyote reproduction. I. The duration of the spermatogenic cycle and epididymal sperm transport. J. Reprod. Fertil. *31:*163.

107. Kennelly, J. J., and Johns, B. E. (1976): The estrous cycle of coyotes. J. Wildlife Mngmt. *40:* 272.

108. Kirdani, R. Y., and Sandberg, A. A. (1974): The fate of estriol in dogs. Steroids *23:*667.

109. Kruse, S. M., and Howard, W. E. (1983): Canid sex attractant studies. J. Chem. Ecol. *9:*1503.

110. Kwan, P. W. L., Merk, F. B., Leav, I., et al. (1982): Estrogen mediated exocytosis in the glandular epithelium of prostates in castrated and hypophysectomized dogs. Cell Tissue Res. *226:*689.

111. Lee, S. Y., Anderson, J. W., Scott, G. L., et al. (1983): Ultrastructure of the placenta and fetal membranes of the dog. II. The yolk sac. Am. J. Anat. *166:*313.

112. Lein, D. H. (1983): Examination of the bitch for breeding soundness. *In*: Current Veterinary Therapy, Vol. VIII, Small Animal Practice, Philadelphia, W. B. Saunders Co., p. 909.

113. Lessey, B. A., Wahawisan, R., and Gorell, T. A. (1981): Hormonal regulation of cytoplasmic estrogen and progesterone receptors in the beagle uterus and oviduct, Mol. Cell. Endocrinol. *21:*171.

114. Levine, B. N. (1984): Small animal pet population trends and demands for veterinary service. *In*: Proc. 8th Kal Kan Symp. for the Treatment of Small Animal Diseases, edited by van Marthens E., Vernon, California, Kal Kan, p. 49.

115. Lindsay, F. E. F. (1983): The normal endoscopic appearance of the caudal reproductive tract of the cyclic and non-cyclic bitch: post-uterine endoscopy. J. Small Anim. Pract. *24:*1.

116. Lindsay, F. E. F. (1983): Endoscopy of the reproductive tract in the bitch. *In*: Current Veterinary Therapy, Vol. VIII, Small Animal Practice, Philadelphia, W. B. Saunders Co., p. 912.

117. Lunnen, J. E., Faulkner, L. C., Hopwood, M. L., et al. (1974): Immunization of dogs with bovine luteinizing hormone. Biol. Reprod. *10:*453.

118. Mahi, C. A., and Yanagimachi, R. (1976): Maturation and sperm penetration of canine ovarian oocytes in vitro. J. Exp. Zool. *196:*189.

119. Mahi, C. A., and Yanagimachi, R. (1978): Capacitation, acrosome reaction, and egg penetration by canine spermatozoa in a simple defined medium. Gamete Res. *1:*101.

120. Machi, C. A., and Yanagimachi, R. (1979): Prevention of in vitro fertilization of canine oocytes by antiovary antisera: a potential approach to fertility control in the bitch. J. Exp. Zool. *210:*129.

121. Mahi-Brown, C. A., Yanagimachi, R., Hoffman, J. C., et al. (1985): Fertility control in the bitch by active immunization with porcine zonae pellucidae: use of different adjuvants and patterns of estradiol and progesterone levels in estrous cycles. Biol. Reprod. *32:*761.

122. McRae, G. I., Roberts, B. B., Worden, A. C., et al. (1985): Long-term reversible suppression of oestrus in bitches with nafarelin acetate, a potent LHRH agonist. J. Reprod. Fertil. *74:*389.

123. Myers, R. K., Cook, J. E., and Mosier, J. E. (1984): Comparative aging changes in canine uterine tubes (oviducts): electron microscopy. Am. J. Vet. Res. *45:*2008.

124. Okkens, A. C., Dieleman, S. J., Bevers, M. M., et al. (1985): Evidence for the non-involvement of the uterus in the lifespan of the corpus luteum in the cyclic dog. Vet. Quart. *7:*169.

125. Okkens, A. C., Dieleman, S. J., Bevers, M. M., et al. (1986): Influence of hypophysectomy on the lifespan of the corpus luteum in the cyclic dog. J. Reprod. Fertil. *77:*187.

126. Olar, T. T., Amann, R. P., and Pickett, B. W.

(1983): Relationships among testicular size, daily production and output of spermatozoa, and extragonadal spermatozoal reserves of the dog. Biol. Reprod. *29:*1114.

127. Olson, P. N., Bowen, R. A., Behrendt, M. D., et al. (1982): Concentrations of reproductive hormones in canine serum throughout late anestrus, proestrus, and estrus. Biol. Reprod. *27:*1196.

128. Olson, P. N., Bowen, R. A., Behrendt, M. D., et al. (1984): Validation of radioimmunoassays to measure prostaglandins $F_{2\alpha}$ and E_2 in canine endometrium and plasma. Am. J. Vet. Res. *45:*119.

129. Olson, P. N., Bowen, R. A., Behrendt, B. S., et al. (1984): Concentrations of testosterone in canine serum during late anestrus, proestrus, and early diestrus. Am. J. Vet. Res. *45:*145.

130. Olson, P. N., Bowen, R. A., Behrendt, M. D., et al. (1984): Concentrations of progesterone and luteinizing hormone in the serum of diestrous bitches before and after hysterectomy. Am. J. Vet. Res. *45:*149.

131. O'Shea, J. D., and Jabara, A. G. (1967): The histogenesis of canine ovarian tumours induced by stilboestrol administration. Path. Vet. *4:*137.

132. Paisley, L. G., and Fahning, M. L. (1977): Effects of exogenous follicle-stimulating hormone and luteinizing hormone in bitches. J. Am. Vet. Med. Assoc. *171:*181.

133. Paradis, M., Post, K., and Mapletoft, R. J. (1983): Effects of prostaglandin $F_{2\alpha}$ on corpora lutea formation and function in mated bitches. Canad. Vet. J. *24:*239.

134. Phemister, R. D., Holst, P. A., Spano, J. S., et al. (1973): Time of ovulation in the Beagle bitch. Biol. Reprod. *8:*74.

135. Picon, R., Picon, L., Chaffaux, S., et al. (1978): Effects of canine fetal testes and testicular tumors on Mullerian ducts. Biol. Reprod. *18:*459.

136. Pineda, M. H. (1977): A simple method for collection of semen from dogs. Canine Pract. *4:*14.

137. Pineda, M. H. (1986): Contraceptive procedures for the male dog. *In:* Current Therapy in Theriogenology, Morrow D. A. (ed.), Philadelphia, W. B. Saunders Co., p. 563.

138. Pineda, M. H., and Hepler, D. I. (1981): Chemical vasectomy in dogs. Long-term study. Theriogenology *16:*1.

139. Pineda, M. H., Kainer, R. A., and Faulkner, L. C. (1973): Dorsal median postcervical fold in the canine vagina. Am. J. Vet. Res. *34:*1487.

140. Pineda, M. H., Reimers, T. J., and Faulkner, L. C. (1976): Disappearance of spermatozoa from the ejaculates of vasectomized dogs. J. Am. Vet. Med. Assoc. *168:*502.

141. Pineda, M. H., Reimers, T. J., Faulkner, L. C., et al. (1977): Azoospermia in dogs induced by injection of sclerosing agents into the caudae of the epididymides. Am. J. Vet. Res. *38:*831.

142. Reimers, T. J., Phemister, R. D., and Niswender, G. D. (1978): Radio-immunological measurement of follicle stimulating hormone and prolactin in the dog. Biol. Reprod. *19:*673.

143. Roszel, J. F. (1975): Genital cytology of the bitch. Vet. Scope. *19:*3.

144. Schardein, J. L., Reutner, T. F. Fitzgerald, J. E.,

et al. (1973): Canine teratogenesis with an estrogen antagonist. Teratology *7:*199.

145. Schutte, A. P. (1967): Canine vaginal cytology. J. Small Anim. Pract. *8:*301.

146. Schwartz, E., Tornaben, J. A., and Boxill, G. C. (1969): Effects of chronic oral administration of a long-acting estrogen, quinestrol, to dogs. Toxicol. Appl. Pharmacol. *14:*487.

147. Shille, V. M., Dorsey, D., and Thatcher, M.-J. (1984): Induction of abortion in the bitch with a synthetic prostaglandin analog. Am. J. Vet. Res. *45:*1295.

148. Shille, V. M., Thatcher, M. J., and Simmons, K. J. (1984): Efforts to induce estrus in the bitch, using pituitary gonadotropins. J. Am. Vet. Med. Assoc. *184:*1469.

149. Smith, M. S., and McDonald, L. E. (1974): Serum levels of luteinizing hormone and progesterone during the estrous cycle, pseudopregnancy and pregnancy in the dog. Endocrinology *94:*404.

150. Sokolowski, J. H. (1971): The effects of ovariectomy on pregnancy maintenance in the bitch. Lab. Anim. Sci. *21:*696.

151. Sokolowski, J. H. (1973): Reproductive features and patterns in the bitch. J. Am. Anim. Hosp. Assoc. *9:*71.

152. Sokolowski, J. H. (1977): Reproductive patterns in the bitch. Vet. Clin. North Am. *7:*653.

153. Sokolowski, J. H., and Geng, S. (1977): Effect of prostaglandin $F_{2\alpha}$-Tham in the bitch. J. Am. Vet. Med. Assoc. *170:*536.

154. Sokolowski, J. H., and Kasson, C. W. (1978): Effects of mibolerone on conception, pregnancy, parturition, and offspring in the Beagle. Am. J. Vet. Res. *39:*837.

155. Sokolowski, J. H., and van Ravenswaay, F. (1978): Summary of studies evaluating the efficacy of mibolerone in the mature female Beagle. Canine Pract. *5:*53.

156. Sokolowski, J. H., and Zimbelman, R. G. (1974): Canine reproduction: Effects of multiple treatments of medroxyprogesterone acetate on reproductive organs of the bitch. Am. J. Vet. Res. *35:*1285.

157. Sokolowski, J. H., and Zimbelman, R. G. (1976): Evaluation of selected compounds for estrus control in the bitch. Am. J. Vet. Res. *37:*939.

158. Sokolowski, J. H., Stover, D. G., and van Ravenswaay, F. (1977): Seasonal incidence of estrus and interestrous interval for bitches of seven breeds. J. Am. Vet. Med. Assoc. *171:*271.

159. Sokolowski, J. H., Zimbelman, R. G., and Goyings, L. S. (1973): Canine reproduction: Reproductive organs and related structures of the nonparous, parous, and postpartum bitch. Am. J. Vet. Res. *34:*1001.

160. Taha, M. B., and Noakes, D. E. (1982): The effect of age and season of the year on testicular function in the dog, as determined by histological examination of the seminiferous tubules and the estimation of peripheral plasma testosterone concentrations. J. Small Anim. Pract. *23:*351.

161. Taha, M. B., Noakes, D. E., and Allen, W. E. (1982): Hemicastration and castration in the beagle dog; the effects on libido, peripheral plasma testosterone concentrations, seminal characteristics and

testicular function. J. Small Anim. Pract. *23:*279.

162. Teunissen, G. H. B. (1952): The development of endometritis in the dog and the effect of estradiol and progesterone on the uterus. Acta Endocrinol. *9:*407.

163. Thompson, D. L., Jr., Ewing, L. L., and Lasley, B. L. (1983): Oestrogen secretion by in vitro perfused testes: species comparison and factors affecting short-term secretion. J. Endocrinol. *96:*97.

164. Thornton, D. A. K. (1967): Uterine cystic hyperplasia in a Siamese cat following treatment with medroxyprogesterone. Vet. Rec. *80:*380.

165. Thun, R., Watson, P., and Jackson, G. L. (1977): Induction of estrus and ovulation in the bitch, using exogenous gonadotropins. Am. J. Vet. Res. *38:*483.

166. Tsutsui, T. (1981): Process of development of uterus, fetus, and fetal appendices during pregnancy in the dog. Bull. Nippon Vet. Zootech. Coll., No. *29:*175.

167. Tsutsui, T., Takatani, H., Hirose, O., et al. (1982): Effects of prostaglandin $F_{2\alpha}$ on implantation and maintenance of pregnancy in the dog. Jap. J. Vet. Sci. *44:*403.

168. Tyslowitz, R., and Dingemanse, E. (1941): Effect of large doses of estrogens on the blood picture of dogs. Endocrinology *29:*817.

169. Van der Weyden, G. C., Taverne, M. A. M., Okkens, A. C., et al. (1981): The intrauterine position of canine foetuses and their sequence of expulsion at birth. J. Small Anim. Pract. *22:*503.

170. Varga, B., and Folly, G. (1977): Effects of prostaglandins on ovarian blood flow in the bitch. J. Reprod. Fertil. *51:*315.

171. Verhage, H. G., Abel, J. H., Jr., Tietz, W. J., Jr., et al. (1973): Development and maintenance of the oviductal epithelium during the estrous cycle in the bitch. Biol. Reprod. *9:*460.

172. Verhage, H. G., Abel, J. H., Jr., Tietz, W. J., Jr., et al. (1973): Estrogen-induced differentiation of the oviductal epithelium in prepubertal dogs. Biol. Reprod. *9:*475.

173. Vickery, B., and McRae, G. (1980): Effect of a synthetic prostaglandin analogue on pregnancy in beagle bitches. Biol. Reprod. *22:*438.

174. Vincent, D. L., Kepic, T. A., Lathrop, J. C., et al.

(1979): Testosterone regulation of luteinizing hormone secretion in the male dog. Int. J. Androl. *2:*241.

175. Wales, R. G., and White, I. G. (1965): Some observations on the chemistry of dog semen. J. Reprod. Fertil. *9:*69.

176. Weikel, J. H., Jr., and Nelson, L. W. (1977): Problems in evaluating chronic toxicity of contraceptive steroids in dogs. J. Toxicol. and Env. Health *3:*167.

177. Weissbach, L., and Ibach, B. (1976): Quantitative parameters for light microscopic assessment of the tubuli seminiferi. Fertil. Steril. *27:*836.

178. Wildt, D. E., and Lawler, D. F. (1985): Laparoscopic sterilization of the bitch and queen by uterine horn occlusion. Am. J. Vet. Res. *46:*864.

179. Wildt, D. E., Levinson, C. J., and Seager, S. W. J. (1977): Laparoscopic exposure and sequential observation of the ovary of the cycling bitch. Anat. Rec. *189:*443.

180. Wildt, D. E., Chakraborty, P. K., Panko, W. B., et al. (1978): Relationship of reproductive behavior, serum luteinizing hormone and time of ovulation in the bitch. Biol. Reprod. *18:*561.

181. Wildt, D. E., Panko, W. B., Chakraborty, P. K., et al. (1979): Relationship of serum estrone, estradiol-17β and progesterone to LH, sexual behavior and time of ovulation in the bitch. Biol. Reprod. *20:*648.

182. Winter, M., Falvo, R. E., Schanbacker, B. D., et al. (1983): Regulation of gonadotropin secretion in the male dog. J. Androl. *4:*319.

183. Winter, M., Pirmann, J., Falvo, R. E., et al. (1982): Steroidal control of gonadotrophin secretion in the orchiectomized dog. J. Reprod. Fertil. *64:*449.

184. Wright, P. J. (1980): The induction of oestrus and ovulation in the bitch using pregnant mare serum gonadotrophin and human chorionic gonadotrophin. Aust. Vet. J. *56:*137.

185. Wright, P. J. (1982): The induction of oestrus in the bitch using daily injections of pregnant mare serum gonadotrophin. Aust. Vet. J. *59:*123.

186. Zirkin, B. R., and Strandberg, J. D. (1984): Quantitative changes in the morphology of the aging canine prostate. Anat. Rec. *208:*207.

Reproductive Patterns of Domestic Cats*

M. H. PINEDA

17

Little is known about the reproductive biology of the domestic cat. In this regard, the domestic cat is a neglected species. In the last few years, considerable attention has been paid to the endocrinology of the reproductive cycle and to the mechanisms involved in the ovulatory process of the queen, the female domestic cat. The male cat, called a tom, has not received the same level of attention. Consequently, little is known about the reproductive physiology of the tom.

The queen will undergo a series of non-ovulatory estruses in each breeding season. Although follicles will develop and secrete estrogens during each of these estruses, ovulation does not occur unless the queen is mated. The glans penis of the tom is covered with corneal spines and, during mating, these penile spines appear to be essential to elicit the ovulatory surge of LH in the queen. Toms mate frequently with the estrous queen. The number of matings determine the magnitude of the ovulatory surge of LH and the number of oocytes released by the queen.

PUBERTY AND SEXUAL MATURITY

The queen reaches puberty at 8 to 13 months of age (Table 17-1), but there is considerable variation between breeds. Puberty may be reached as early as 5 months or as late as 18 months of age. Toms are thought to reach puberty at about the same age as the queen; however, the age of puberty of the tom cat has not been accurately determined, probably because of the difficulties in collecting semen with an artificial vagina from untrained, pubertal toms. The recent development of electroejaculation protocols for the collection of semen from the domestic cat may promote and facilitate studies in this regard. Environmental factors may also influence the age of puberty in domestic cats and it is thought that free-roaming cats reach puberty earlier than animals confined in breeding colonies.

*Much information concerned with reproduction in domestic cats has been covered in Chapter 9 (Female Reproduction), Chapter 8 (Male Reproduction), Chapter 10 (Artificial Insemination), and Chapter 2 (Pituitary Gland). The reader is encouraged to refer to these chapters in order to permit conciseness.

Table 17-1   Onset* of Puberty in the Queen

Breed	Average age in months
Abyssinian	11.3
Birman	11.3
Burmese	7.7
Colourpoint	13.0
Persian	10.4
Siamese	8.9
Long-haired domestic	11.0
Short-haired domestic	9.4

*Survey data.
Adapted From: J. E. Jemmett and J. M. Evans, J. Small Anim. Pract. *18:*31, *1977.*

BREEDING SEASON

In the northern hemisphere, domestic cats have two main breeding seasons per year, one in the spring (January to March) and the other in late summer and early fall (August to October). Environmental factors, particularly the amount of light, influence the length of the breeding season. The greatest incidence of estruses occurs in February and March in the northern hemisphere, while in temperate climates, matings may occur throughout the year. Cats maintained in colonies under controlled light schedules (12 hours of light: 12 hours of darkness or 14 hours of light: 10 hours of darkness) cycle throughout the year, yet exhibit peak periods of estruses in March, July, and October.

Female cats tend to have a definite nonbreeding season beginning in late October and extending through December. Household cats, depending upon the amount of supplemental artificial lighting, are more likely to behave, with regard to their breeding season, as cats kept within a colony.

After puberty, tom cats are capable of mating and will ejaculate throughout the year, without any discernible seasonal effect on the number of spermatozoa or fertility of the ejaculate.

THE ESTROUS CYCLE

The queen is seasonally polyestrus and an induced ovulator. As a consequence, the characteristics of the reproductive cycle of the

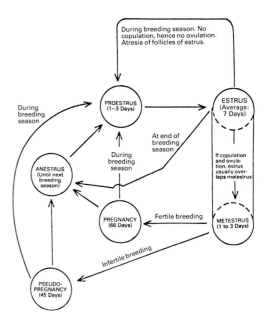

Fig. 17-1. The ovarian cycle of the queen.

queen are greatly influenced by mating (Fig. 17-1). The *nonmated queen* displays a series of nonovulatory estruses, each lasting an average of 7 days, with a range of 3 to 20 days. Each of these nonmated estruses is followed by an interestrous period of nonsexual receptivity, lasting an average of 10 days, with a range of 8 to 30 days (Table 17-2, Fig. 17-1). Values reported for the length of the nonmated estrus and interestrous intervals vary considerably, probably because it is difficult to accurately assess the onset and end of estrus solely by behavioral signs in the absence of a tom (see queen responses in Table 17-3). The length of the *nonmated* estrus and the interestrous interval are also influenced by breed, environmental conditions, and social interactions with other queens. Nonmated queens, in colonies maintained under controlled light and temperature, display an average of 13 estruses per year, with a range of 4 to 25 estruses. The average time elapsed from the onset of one nonovulatory estrus to the next is 17 days.

The proestrual, follicular growth occurs rather rapidly in the queen. Proestrus lasts from 1 to 3 days, before the onset of behav-

Table 17-2   Length of the Reproductive Cycle of the Queen

Stage	Average, days	Range, days
Estrous	7	3 to 20
Interestrus		
Nonmated	10	8 to 30
Sterile-mated (pseudopregnancy)	45	30 to 70
Anestrus	90	30 to 210

ioral estrus, and is associated with increased secretion of estradiol 17-β and elevated blood levels of estrogens, which may reach peak values as high as 100 pg of estradiol 17-β ml. Due to the short period of follicular growth, the phase of proestrus is difficult to detect clinically.

Blood levels of estrogens decline during the first 5 days of estrus as the follicles reach a mature stage. The follicles appear to retain their capability to respond to the ovulatory surges of LH, should mating occur during the period of sexual receptivity. The follicles that have reached the mature stage during a given estrus undergo atresia if the queen is not mated in that estrus, and the blood levels of estrogens, as well as the intensity of the associated behavioral signs, decline rapidly. The process is repeated several times during the breeding season if mating does not occur. A new wave of follicles will develop at each proestrus and the beginning of the subsequent estrus. Blood levels of progesterone remain at basal levels, less than 0.5 ng/ml of blood, during these nonovulatory estruses.

Mating Behavior

The behavioral responses of estrous queens are recognized with ease when the queen is exposed to the tom. The tom also displays a characteristic behavioral pattern when confronted with an estrous queen (Table 17-3, Fig. 17-2 A and B). During the breeding season, the behavior of the male changes drastically. The male becomes aggressive and roams great distances, particularly at night,

Table 17-3   Patterns of Sexual Behavior of the Queen and Tom

Stage of the Cycle	Queen Response	Tom Response
Onset of Proestrus (lasts for 1 to 3 days)	Rubbing of head and neck against objects; rolling on the floor. Refuses advances of the male; does not stand and does not allow intromission.	Shows interest, sniffs or attempts to sniff the female body, and in particular the anogenital region. Mounting is attempted.
Estrus	Responds by treading and crouching with her forequarters pressed to the ground. May vocalize for prolonged periods. When approached by the male or when stroked on the back shows lordosis, lateral deviation of the tail, and presentation of the perineal region with exposure of the vulva. Minor vulvar discharge may be observed, but in general there are not conspicuous changes in the size or appearance of the external genitalia. Allows grasping of the neck and mounting by the male.	Intensely attracted to the queen; sniffing, scratching, and grooming. Grips the neck of the queen and mounts with vigorous pelvic thrusts leading to intromission. Licks the female's anogenital region.
Anestrus or interestrus	Ignores the male or shows defensive spitting, hisses, and fights the male with paw-swipes.	Little or no interest in the queen.

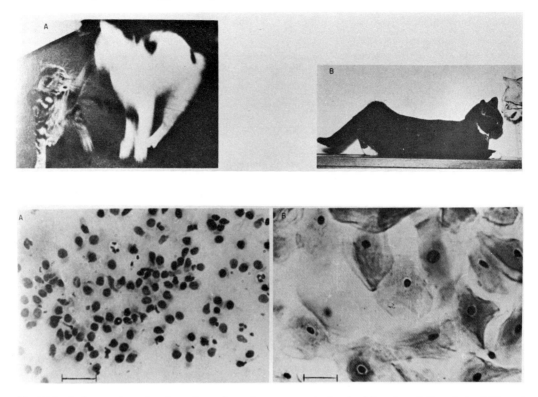

Fig. 17-2. A, Aggressive refusal reaction of anestrous or ovariectomized female cat. Female is striking at the male, which is leaping away. Typical anestrous vaginal smear for the reaction: only basal cells and leukocytes are seen. B, Receptive reaction by the female when in estrus or when treated with estrogen. Estrual crouch and lordosis posture are adopted in presence of a male. Estrous vaginal smear corresponding to reaction: large cornified cells with pyknotic nuclei and perinuclear halos are seen. Scale 100 μ. (From Michael, R. P.: *In* Handbook of Physiology, Sec. 7, Endocrinology, vol. 2, Female Reproduction, Part I, p. 189. Edited by R. O. Greep and E. B. Astwood. The American Physiological Society. Baltimore, Williams & Wilkins, 1973.)

since cats are nocturnal. If a female in the neighborhood is in proestrus or estrus, males can detect this, probably by an olfactory mechanism (pheromones). A male may guard a female for days or weeks, or sometimes several males are in intense competition for the affections of the female. This may lead to destructive attacks by the males on each other. The owners of cats should be warned of this hazard, and if a female is to be bred, she should be housed with the male of choice and not allowed to run at will. If the male and female are to be housed together during the breeding period, the female should be brought to the male after he has had several days to become accustomed to his surroundings. Unfamiliar surroundings often prevent the mating response even in sexually active males.

The estrous queen readily stands and accepts mounting, neck biting by the male, and intromission. During intromission, particularly during thrusting by the male or during withdrawal of the penis from the vagina, the queen emits a loud, piercing cry, sometimes referred to as the "mating cry." Coitus is relatively brief and may last up to half a minute. Experienced and vigorous males may intromit several times during a single copulation. If left unrestricted, as in free-mating situations, toms may attempt to copulate within minutes after penile withdrawal. Queens have been observed to allow multiple matings, 10 times or more in a few hours. It is not yet clear, however, whether the tom ejaculates each time that he copulates with the queen.

Copulation with either fertile or sterile

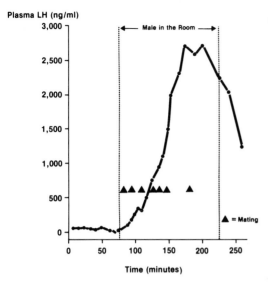

Plasma LH (ng/ml)

Fig. 17-3. Plasma levels of LH in two estrous queens permitted self-paced matings. (Drawn from data in: L. M. Johnson and V. L. Gay, Endocrinology *109*:247, 1981.)

males induces the release of the ovulatory surge of LH in the queen. The magnitude of the surge and subsequent levels of LH in the blood are greatly influenced by the number of matings (Fig. 17-3, Table 17-4). In self-paced matings, maximal levels of LH are reached within 2 hours after 6 to 8 matings. The corneal spines of the tom appear to play an important role in eliciting the vaginal and pos-

sibly the cervical stimulation, which results in the release of LH from the pituitary gland. The corneal spines of the penis of the tom are prominent and directed caudally toward the base of the penis. The penile spines may also play a role in preventing the premature withdrawal of the penis from the vagina of queens that attempt to separate from the copulating male.

Ovulation occurs 24 to 50 hours after mating. The number of follicles that ovulate and number of oocytes released are dependent upon the number of matings and may be related to the day of estrus, since ovulation is more likely to occur after the second day of estrus. Mounting by the male, without intromission, is not a sufficient stimulus to induce the ovulatory surge of LH (Table 17-4). A single mating induces ovulation in only 50% of the queens, yet increasing the number of copulations beyond 4 copulations within a 4-hour period does not improve the ovulatory response of the queen (Table 17-4).

Ovulation can also be induced in the queen by repeated mechanical stimulation of the cervix via the vagina, but the ovulatory response is erratic. The administration of hCG in doses of 250 IU on the first and second days of estrus reportedly induces ovulation in more than 85% of the queens. Ovulatory responses can

Table 17-4   *Incidence of Ovulation and Serum LH Peak in Cats Following Single or Multiple Copulations on Day 3 of Estrus.*

Treatment	Ratio of Queens Ovulating (%)	LH Peak ng/ml
Unmounted	0/2 (0)	1.0 ± 0.8
Mounted without intromission	0/4 (0)	4.1 ± 1.1
One copulation	9/18 (50)	23.9 ± 5.8
Four copulations in a 4-hr period	23/23 (100)	88.9 ± 14.8
Eight to twelve copulations in a 4-hr period	13/13 (100)	120.5 ± 23.8

Adapted From: P. W. Concannon et al., Biol. Reprod. *23*:111, 1980.

Table 17-5   *Ovulatory Response of Anestrous and Estrous Queens after a Single Intramuscular Injection of GnRH*

Dose of GnRH (μg)	Number of Queens Ovulating (%)	
	Anestrous	Estrous
5	0/4 (0)	1/4 (25%)
10	0/4 (0)	2/4 (50%)
25	0/4 (0)	4/4 (100%)

Adapted From: P. K. Chakraborty et al., Lab. Anim. Sci. *29*:338, 1979.

also be induced in estrous queens by exogenous GnRH (Table 17-5).

Blood levels of estradiol-17β decline rapidly from about 50 pg/ml of serum at the time of the ovulatory surge of LH to less than 20 pg/ml by 96 hours after coitus (Fig. 17-4). Corpora lutea form within 1 to 3 days (metestrus) after coitus and progesterone levels in the blood rise rapidly from baseline levels reaching 2 to 3 ng/ml by 96 hours after coitus (Fig. 17-4). Blood levels of progesterone reach peak levels of 15 to 90 ng/ml 15 to 25 days after coitus. The period of metestrus, only of academic

significance in the cat, is included within the period of estrus.

Pseudopregnancy

Queens that are induced to ovulate by mechanical stimulation of the vagina, exogenous hormones, or by matings with sterile males become pseudopregnant. Pseudopregnancy lasts an average of 45 days, with a range of 30 to 70 days. Up to about day 30, levels of progesterone in the blood of pseudopregnant queens are similar to that of pregnancy. Progesterone levels then decline in the pseudo-

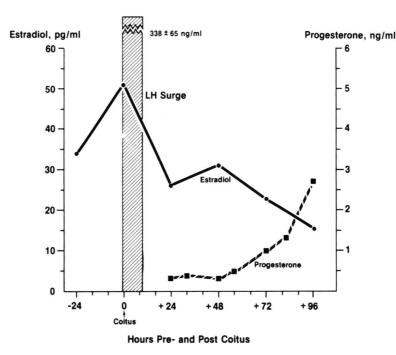

Fig. 17-4. Pre- and postcoital changes in estradiol-17β and postovulatory changes in progesterone in the blood of the queen. (Adapted from: D. H. Banks, and G. Stabenfeldt, Biol. Reprod. *26*:603, 1982.)

pregnant queen and become significantly lower than those found in the pregnant queen. Progesterone levels return to baseline levels of less than 1.0 ng/ml of blood by about day 40 of pseudopregnancy. If pseudopregnancy is induced early in the breeding season, the queen may display one or more estruses during that breeding season. If the pseudopregnancy is induced late in the breeding season, the queen enters into a period of anestrus lasting until the next breeding season.

The corpora lutea of pseudopregnancy, as those of pregnancy, are resistant to the luteolytic actions of prostaglandins. Repeated treatments with prostaglandin $F_{2\alpha}$ cause a transient decline in blood levels of progesterone and do not induce abortion or shorten the length of pseudopregnancy. It is not known whether the uterus exerts any control on the function of the corpus luteum of the queen. The anatomic features of the ovarian and uterine vasculature of the queen would not appear to favor the transfer of luteolytic substances, if any, from the uterus to the arteries supplying the ovary. Furthermore, corpora lutea of pseudopregnant queens produce progesterone in comparable amounts to that of pregnant queens, up to about day 30 of pseudopregnancy. Therefore, it is doubtful that the non-pregnant uterus influences luteal function in the pseudopregnant queen. It is possible that the ovulatory surge of LH provides enough luteotropic support for the corpus luteum to remain functional for extended periods after ovulation. The luteotropic stimulus from developing embryos may provide additional support for luteal maintenance beyond day 30 or 40 of pregnancy, since the corpora lutea of the pseudopregnant queen undergo gradual retrogressive changes at that time.

Pseudopregnancy in the queen is not associated with the profound organic and behavioral changes observed in the bitch (Chapter 16) and seldom leads to lactation and nesting behavior. However, pseudopregnant queens undergo vaginal, uterine, and oviductal changes induced by the progesterone secreted by the corpora lutea.

The tubular genitalia of the queen respond to the gonadal hormones, estradiol and progesterone, in a manner similar to that described for the bitch. During anestrus, the oviductal and uterine epithelium are low. The uterine glands are straight and barely extend into the mucosa. At proestrus and estrus, rising levels of estrogens stimulate the development of the oviductal and uterine epithelium which increase in both height and mitotic activity. The oviductal secretory and ciliated cells also differentiate under estrogenic stimulation. After ovulation, the endometrial glands increase in diameter and coil under the influence of progesterone secreted by the developing corpora lutea. As progesterone levels increase, endometrial glandular development continues, leading to the secretion of "uterine milk" to nourish the preimplantation embryos.

VAGINAL CYTOLOGY

The vaginal smear of the queen is less distinct and defined than in the bitch. During anestrus, the vaginal epithelium consists only of a few layers of cells. The anestrous smear contains nucleated, basal epithelial cells and leukocytes. Cornified cells are absent or only present in small numbers (Fig. 17-2A). Under the influence of estrogens, the vaginal epithelium thickens, and becomes cornified in its superficial layers. During the follicular phase, prior to ovulation, the vaginal smear consists mainly of anuclear, cornified cells, and intermediate and superficial, partially cornified cells (Fig. 17-2B, Table 17-6). After ovulation, during the luteal phase, the superficial and intermediate cells become predominant although a few parabasal cells may be found (Table 17-6).

The mechanical stimulation provided during the collection of vaginal samples for smears may induce ovulation in some queens. This possibility must be considered when repeated vaginal smears are to be taken from a queen.

OOGENESIS

Sexual differentiation occurs in the fetus around day 30 of pregnancy and continues in the newborn kitten, until day 37 of age.[49]

Table 17-6   Vaginal Smear of the Queen-Cytological Changes*

FOLLICULAR PHASE (Proestrus and estrus, prior to ovulation)	LUTEAL PHASE AND INTERESTRUS (Estrus after ovulation, pregnancy, pseudopregnancy)
Absence of noncellular debris (clearing of the vaginal smear) is the earliest sign of follicular activity.	A few anuclear cells may be found.
Increased proportion of *anuclear, cornified cells* (from 5 to 40% of total cell population), remaining around 40% through the first day of the luteal phase.	Superficial and intermediate cells are the dominant type (> 80% of the total cell population).
Intermediate cells, partially cornified with intact nucleus, progressively decrease from 45 to 6 % from the first to the fourth day of the follicular phase.	Parabasal cells are present, their relative percentage varying between 1 to 6%.
Superficial cells, partially cornified with signs of nuclear degeneration, remain about 50% throughout estrus.	
Parabasal, noncornified cells are not found.	
Erythrocytes are rarely seen.	

*Cotton swabs moistened with saline solution were used to obtain material for the smears. Smears fixed with 90% ethanol, air-dried, and stained with Giemsa.
Adapted from: V. M. Shille et al., Biol. Reprod. *21*:953, 1979.

Oocytes in meiotic prophase can be observed in the fetal queen from day 50 of pregnancy until up to about day 40 of the postnatal period, when it appears that all of the oocytes have reached the dictyate stage of meiosis.[49]

FERTILIZATION AND OVIDUCTAL TRANSPORT

The oocytes of the queen are ovulated as secondary oocytes. As in the other domestic species, fertilization occurs in the ampullary region of the oviduct. The embryos or the unfertilized oocytes migrate toward the uterus over a 4- to 5-day period, reaching the uterus by day 6 after ovulation. Since ovulation in the queen is induced by mating, spermatozoa are usually in the oviducts by the time the oocytes are shed from follicles. Thus, infertility due to aging of the gametes in asynchronous matings is seldom a problem in the queen. The ejaculated spermatozoa of the tom must be capacitated to fertilize the oocytes. Capacitation requires a 1 to 2 hour exposure to the fluids secreted by the genital tract of the queen. Epididymal spermatozoa are capable of fertilizing the queen's oocytes in vitro, suggesting that the accessory sex glands of the tom contribute a decapacitation factor or factors to the semen at the time of ejaculation.

PREGNANCY

Counting from the first mating of the queen, the length of pregnancy in cat colonies is 66 days on the average, with a range of 62 to 70 days (Table 17-7). Mean litter size in cat colonies is 4.3 and an average of 84% of the kittens are successfully reared. In breeding colonies, under controlled environmental conditions, the average number of litters per cat per year is 2.2 and the mean interval between litters is 5.2 months (Table 17-7). The average litter size varies over the reproductive life of the queen (Fig. 17-5).

Placentation is zonary in the cat and implantation is believed to occur between 13 to 14 days after the first fertile mating. The low aromatase activity in the trophoblasts of the cat embryo suggests that estrogens do not play a role in implantation. The levels of estradiol-17β and progesterone in the

Table 17-7   Reproductive Performance in a Cat* Colony

Mean gestation length, days	66
Range, days	62–70
Mean litter size	4.3
Mean percentage of kittens reared	84.0
Mean interval between litters, months	5.2
Average number of litters/cat per year	2.2
Average age of replacement of brood queens, years	6.0

*Controlled light (12-hour light/darkness, 150 Lux), humidity (55 ± 10%), and temperature (23 ± 2°C).
Adapted from: H. Hurni, Z. Versuchstierk. *23*:102, 1981.

blood of pregnant queens are not different from those of pseudopregnant queens up to about day 20 of pregnancy. After day 30 of pregnancy, levels of progesterone in the blood are higher in pregnant than in pseudopregnant queens. Levels of progesterone in the blood of pregnant queens begin to decline gradually, returning to a baseline of less than 1.0 ng of progesterone per ml of blood at the time of parturition. Prolactin levels remain relatively constant during pregnancy, increase severalfold 2 to 3 days before parturition, and remain elevated during the first 4 weeks after parturition. Lactation and kitten's suckling appear to be powerful inhibitors of

ovarian follicular development and of estrus in the queen. The interestrus interval for lactating queens is usually 120 days (66 days of gestation plus 54 days of lactation). Weaning of the kittens is followed by estrus, on the average, 18 days after weaning. However, there is considerable variation in the time of return to estrus after weaning between queens, particularly for those not in breeding colonies and exposed to variable environmental conditions.

Luteal progesterone secretion is needed for normal gestation for the major part of pregnancy in the queen. Bilateral ovariectomy causes abortion when performed before day 49 of gestation. After day 50 of pregnancy, abortion does not occur following bilateral ovariectomy. Gestation continues to term, apparently without harmful effects to the kittens. Exogenous progesterone can maintain pregnancy in queens bilaterally ovariectomized prior to day 49 of pregnancy.

Relaxin has been detected in the blood of pregnant queens approximately by day 25 of pregnancy. Relaxin levels plateau by day 30 to 35 of pregnancy, remain high during most of the gestation and decline gradually beginning 10 days before parturition. Relaxin is undetectable in the blood within 24 hours after parturition.

Pregnancy Diagnosis

Abdominal palpation allows the detection of fetuses from day 20 to 30 of pregnancy. Pregnancy can also be diagnosed in the queen by ultrasound or by x-ray examination. The same considerations described in Chapter 16

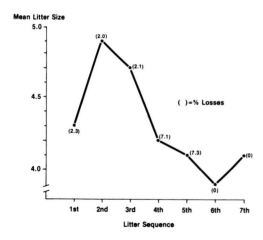

Fig. 17-5. Breeding performance of cats in a breeding colony. Queens were approximately 10 months old (n = 61 queens) when first introduced to the colony and the total length of the observation period was 2.6 years. (Drawn from data in: H. Hurni, Z. Versuchstierk. *23*:102, 1981.)

for the x-ray examination of the pregnant bitch are applicable to the pregnant queen.

THE TOM

There is no published information concerning the duration of the cycle of the seminiferous epithelium and of spermatogenesis, daily sperm production, epididymal transport, spermatozoal reserves, or daily spermatozoal output for the domestic tom. The male kitten is born with the testicles already descended and located in the external inguinal ring or in the scrotum. After puberty, the tom is capable of mating and releasing fertile ejaculates year round. Toms usually approach the queen cautiously, assessing her reactions. When the queen is receptive, the tom will approach her from the rear and grasp the skin of the neck of the female with his teeth, positioning himself for mounting and intromission. Ejaculation appears to be fast, lasting only a few seconds, and is nearly simultaneous with intromission. Toms tend to intromit the penis in the vagina several times during mating, but it is not clear whether or not they ejaculate during each intromission. Similar responses are observed in some toms when semen is collected with an artificial vagina. Frequency of intromission during mating and the number of copulations of the tom with the estrous queen may be an evolutionary trait. The small volume and relatively low numbers of spermatozoa in the tom's ejaculate may have evolved to prevent depletion of the spermatozoal reserves in view of the frequent matings needed for the ovulatory response of the queen. Multiple matings may ensure the release of sufficient amounts of GnRH, conducive to an adequate ovulatory surge of LH in the queen.

The deposition of cat odor by urine spraying is a form of territorial marking pronounced in wild felids, but also present in the domestic tom. Tomcat odor is androgen dependent and can be suppressed by castration. Urine spraying by the domestic tom may also have an estrus synchronizing effect on the queen. Pheromones produced by the convoluted tubules of the kidneys and possibly by the anal glands of the tom, which appear to be added to the urine during spraying, facilitate the expression of behavioral estrus in the queen. Valeric acid in the vaginal secretions from estrous queens has been suggested as a candidate pheromone which would synchronize estrus between queens. Valeric acid may also attract and stimulate mating behavior in the tom.

Toms and queens, when exposed to the smell of bruised leaves of catnip or cat mint (Nepeta cataria L), develop a characteristic behavioral response, which includes sniffing, licking, and cheek and body rubbing. An active compound, nepetalactone, has been isolated from catnip. This compound induces hallucinogenic effects in cats, which mimic the estrous-like responses induced by pheromones. Cat owners buy the catnip as dry leaves or as an extract in spray cans in supermarkets and pet shops, and they often provide the catnip as a treat to their pets. However, it is doubtful that catnip has any estrous-facilitating effects.

Little is known about the reproductive endocrinology and blood levels of reproductive hormones in the tomcat. Table 17-8 shows the concentration of testosterone and androstenedione in the blood of the domestic tom. Both, testosterone and androstenedione decrease rapidly after castration.

Semen Collection

Semen can be collected from tom cats with an artificial vagina (AV) or by electroejaculation. Although an AV can be easily assembled from inexpensive components (Fig. 10-10 and Fig. 17-6 A and B), the AV method is not practical for clinical use in veterinary medicine, because the toms are not easily trained to ejaculate in the AV and often require a prolonged period of training. Only 10 to 20% of toms can be trained to ejaculate in the AV. Furthermore, estrous queens, either naturally cycling or hormonally induced, are needed to stimulate the mating behavior needed for training the toms to ejaculate in the AV (Fig 17-6 A and B).

A regimen of electrical stimulation has been developed[21] to collect semen from the anesthe-

Table 17-8   Testosterone and Androstenedione
Concentrations in the Blood of the Domestic
Cat

	Testosterone (ng/ml)	Androstenedione (ng/ml)
Intact*	6.33 ± 1.81	7.10 ± 2.98
castrated[+]		
24 hours after castration	0.03 ± 0.19	1.16 ± 0.51
96 hours after castration	0.08 ± 0.11	0.29 ± 0.43

*Hourly samples over 24 hours during two seasons of the year from 4 intact males. Mean ± SD.
[+]From 2 castrated males.
Adapted from data in: I. P. Johnstone et al., Anim. Reprod Sci., 7:363, 1984.

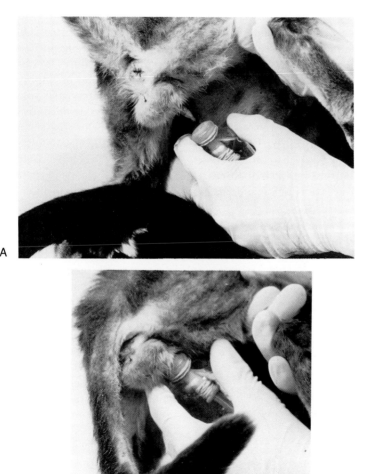

A

B

Fig. 17-6. Collection of semen from the tom with an AV. Notice that the AV was constructed using a glass vial so that the semen could be visualized in the AV. The right leg of the tom is raised to facilitate the photography of the process. A. After the tom mounts and grips the queen's neck, the AV is placed over the erect penis. B. The tom is allowed to thrust and ejaculate in the AV.

tized tom. Even though general anesthesia must be given prior to electrical stimulation, electroejaculation appears to be the method of choice for the routine collection of semen from tomcats. Semen can be collected consistently and reliably from any tom without previous training and estrous queens are not needed to successfully complete the seminal collection. These characteristics make the method of electroejaculation to be suited for most clinical settings. Figure 17-7 shows semen collection by electroejaculation in an anesthetized tomcat. Table 17-9 displays the seminal characteristics of ejaculates obtained with an AV and by electroejaculation from the same toms. The method of electroejaculation is safe and can be used repeatedly, without apparent harmful effects to the tom.[58]

Seminal samples obtained with an AV have lower volume and pH and tend to have more spermatozoa per ejaculate than semen collected by electroejaculation (Table 17-9). The larger volume of semen collected by electroejaculation is apparently due to the secretions contributed by the prostate and bulbourethral glands, the only accessory sex glands in the tomcat.

Through use of an appropriate regimen of electrical stimulation,[21] electroejaculation produces semen that is comparable to seminal samples obtained with an AV. An assay to evaluate spermatozoal viability, based on the

exclusion of a micromolar concentration of eosin B, has been developed[21] for cat semen, but critical studies to correlate seminal parameters with the fertility of an ejaculate have not been done for the cat. Thus, there are no reliable guidelines for the clinician to assess the potential fertility of an ejaculate and the breeding soundness of a given tom.

Insemination of queens, which have been induced to ovulate with exogenous gonadotropins, using freshly collected and diluted semen has produced litters. Ejaculates collected from toms with an AV appear to have enough spermatozoa to inseminate several queens, and artificial insemination with frozen-stored semen has been reported. The rate of conception and litter size obtained with frozen semen is low and procedures for cryopreservation of cat semen need to be improved.

After vasectomy, the volume of ejaculate does not change significantly from the volume of ejaculate before vasectomy,[56] indicating that most of the ejaculate volume is contributed by the secretion of the prostate and bulbourethral glands in the tom. Most of the spermatozoa present in a tom's ejaculate originate from the epididymides. Vasectomized toms become azoospermic 56 to 63 days after bilateral vasectomy, but intact spermatozoa are cleared from the ejaculate by day 49 post-vasectomy. If pregnancies are to be prevented, a period of restraint of at least 49 days post-vasectomy should be observed. Flushing the vasa deferentia at the time of vasectomy will dramatically decrease the time from vasectomy to the potentially safe utilization of cats as teasers, from 63 days to 7 days.[26]

Variable but significant numbers of spermatozoa flow into the urinary bladder at the time of ejaculation in the tomcat. Retrograde flow into the urinary bladder occurs during natural mating, when semen is collected with an AV, or during electroejaculation, when seminal emission is induced by electrical stimulation in the anesthetized cat. The total number of spermatozoa displaced from the sites of storage in the epididymides and vasa deferentia during ejaculation or electroejaculation can be estimated by adding the total

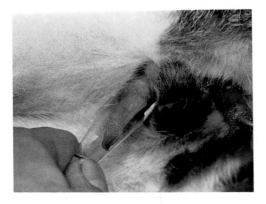

Fig. 17-7. Electroejaculation in an anesthetized tom cat. Notice the penile spines and the seminal fluid in the collecting tube.

Table 17-9   Effect of Method of Collection on the Seminal Characteristics of the Domestic Cat

Seminal Characteristic	Method of Collection					
	Artificial Vagina			Electroejaculation*		
	Mean[+]	SD	Range	Mean[+]	SD	Range
Volume (ml)	0.06[†]	0.02	0.03–0.09	0.26	0.13	0.11–0.49
Number of spermatozoa (10^6)	60.97	31.05	21.50–117.00	42.70	20.51	11.10–65.96
Spermatozoal:						
Motility (%)	58	27	4–87	65	14	44–85
Viability (%)[‡]	67	28	5–95	73	14	49–93
pH	8.32[†]	0.15	8.15–8.57	8.61	0.09	8.45–8.77
Osmolality (mOsm/kg)	324	31	274–368	339	22	317–390

*Spermatozoa and seminal fluid obtained during the application of 240 stimuli (4 series of 60 stimuli) at 6 V.
[+] Means for each method of collection were obtained from 4 cats with replication, n = 8 (see ref. 21 for details).
[†]Significantly different (P < 0.005) from the corresponding mean in the same row.
[‡]Percentage of spermatozoa that were unstained after incubation for 15 minutes in a micromolar solution of eosin B.
Adapted from: M. P. Dooley, and M. H. Pineda, Am. J. Vet. Res. 47:286, 1986.

number of spermatozoa in the ejaculate or electroejaculate to the total number of spermatozoa in the urine obtained from the bladder by cystocentesis after ejaculation. The percentage of the total number of spermatozoa displaced, which is found in the urine, is considered to represent the percentage of retrograde flow of spermatozoa. Table 17-10 displays the volume and concentration of spermatozoa in the urine obtained by cystocentesis before electroejaculation, the volume and total number of spermatozoa in the urine, also obtained by cystocentesis, after electroejaculation, the volume of the electroejaculate, the total number of spermatozoa in the electroejaculate, and the calculated per-

Table 17-10   Total Number of Spermatozoa (10^6) in the Ejaculate and in the Urine Obtained by Cystocentesis Before and After Electroejaculation (EE) of the Domestic Cat

Cat	Urine				Ejaculate		Retrograde Flow (%)*
	Pre-EE		Post-EE				
	Volume (ml)	Spermatozoal Concentration (10^6/ml)	Volume (ml)	Total No. Spermatozoa (10^6)	Volume (ml)	Total No. Spermatozoa (10^6)	
1	2.0	0	6.5	0.20	0.10	0.05	80.0
2	1.6	0.015	6.4	17.28	0.29	5.22	76.8
3	2.1	0	1.6	3.92	0.25	4.00	49.5
4	1.5	0	10.5	74.03	0.39	27.30	73.1
5	1.0	0	6.4	21.76	0.22	27.50	44.2
6	0.8	0.005	6.9	69.28	0.15	8.25	89.4
7	0.7	0.050	17.0	31.96	0.26	49.40	39.3
8	0.6	0.005	2.7	31.62	0.24	1.92	94.3

*The percentage of the total number of spermatozoa displaced during EE that were recovered in the urine.
Adapted from: M. P. Dooley, et al. Proc. 10th Internat. Congr. Anim. Reprod. and Art. Insem, Univ. Illinois, Urbana-Champaign, 1984, Vol. III, Brief Comm. No. 363.

centage of retrograde flow for each of 8 cats. Notice that retrograde flow accounted for 39.3 to 94.3% of the estimated total number of spermatozoa displaced. These results indicate that urinary losses of spermatozoa, because of the retrograde flow of spermatozoa into the bladder of the tom cat during electroejaculation, are considerable and should not be ignored when performing breeding soundness examinations in cats. Retrograde flow of spermatozoa into the bladder during periods of sexual rest, has not been reported for the cat, but may also occur. The finding that the fluid used to flush the vasa deferentia of toms at the time of vasectomy retrograded into the bladder, instead of being eliminated through the penile urethra,[26] suggests that the passage of fluid from the urethra into the bladder follows the pathway of least resistance.

Male tortoiseshell cats are rare (1:3000). The male tortoiseshell cat is infertile because of a genetic defect. The genes for orange or black hair are allelic on the X chromosome; consequently if the phenotype includes both colors, he would have two X and one Y chromosomes, which usually results in infertility due to aspermatogenesis. In the presence of white spotting ("piebald") (an autosomal dominant) the phenotype is often described as tortoiseshell and white, tortie and white, "tricolor," or "calico."

RESPONSE OF CATS TO EXOGENOUS HORMONES

The pituitary gland of the cat responds to intravenous injections of GnRH by releasing LH. It is likely that FSH is also released, but to date there are no published data in this regard.

The ovary of the queen is responsive to exogenous gonadotropins, such as PMSG, FSH, LH, and hCG. These hormones are used to induce estrus in anestrous queens, as well as superovulatory responses (see Chapter 19).

There is no published information regarding the effects of GnRH, pituitary or placental gonadotropins on male libido, spermatogenesis, ejaculatory responses, or quality of ejaculates.

CONTRACEPTIVES FOR THE QUEEN

To date, there is no approved contraceptive for the queen in the U.S. In other countries synthetic progestagens, such as medroxyprogesterone acetate and megestrol acetate (Ovaban), are used to control estrus in queens. The queen seems to be less susceptible to the hyperplastic reactions of the endometrium and the nodular development of tumors of the mammary gland, which are associated with exogenous progestagens in the bitch. Nevertheless, treatment of queens with progestagens must be approached with caution, particularly when uterine infections are suspected.

Synthetic progestagens, such as megestrol acetate, appear to control urine spraying in queens and toms.

Mibolerone, the orally effective, synthetic androgenic compound sold in the U.S. under the commerical name of Cheque for blocking estrus in bitches, appears to be effective and safe to control estrus, when given to anestrous queens. Mibolerone has not yet been cleared for use in queens in the U.S.

Estrogens are reportedly effective to prevent pregnancies after mismatings in the queen, particularly when given about 40 hours after coitus. Exogenous estrogens appear to retard oviductal transport and delay passage of the developing embryos to the uterus. Estrogens may be toxic to cats and, therefore, must be used with caution.

REFERENCES

1. Banks, D. H., and Stabenfeldt, G. (1982): Luteinizing hormone release in the cat in response to coitus on consecutive days of estrus. Biol. Reprod. *26*:603.
2. Banks, D. R., Paape, S. R., and Stabenfeldt, G. H. (1983): Prolactin in the cat: I. Pseudopregnancy and lactation. Biol. Reprod. *28*:923.
3. Bareither, M. L., and Verhage, H. G. (1981): Control of the secretory cell cycle in cat oviduct by estradiol and progesterone. Am J. Anat. *162*:107.
4. Beaver, B. V. (1977): Mating behavior in the cat. Vet. Clin. North Am. *7*:729.
5. Bland, K. P. (1979): Tom-cat odour and other pheromones in feline reproduction. Vet. Sci. Comm. *3*:125.
6. Boomsa, R. A., and Verhage, H. G. (1982): The

uterine progestational response in cats: ultrastructural changes during chronic administration of progesterone to estradiol-primed and nonprimed animals. Am. J. Anat. *164*:243.

7. Bowen, R. A. (1977): Fertilization in vitro of feline ova by spermatozoa from the ductus deferens. Biol. Reprod. *17*:144.

8. Burke, T. J., Reynolds, H. A., and Sokolowski, J. H. (1977): A 180-day tolerance-efficacy study with mibolerone for suppression of estrus in the cat. Am. J. Vet. Res. *38*:469.

9. Chakraborty, P. K., Wildt, D. E., and Seager, S. W. J. (1979): Serum luteinizing hormone and ovulatory response to luteinizing hormone-releasing hormone in the estrous and anestrous domestic cat. Lab. Anim. Sci. *29*:338.

10. Chan, S. Y. W., Chakraborty, P. K., Bass, E. J., et al. (1982): Ovarian-endocrine-behavioural function in the domestic cat treated with exogenous gonadotrophins during mid-gestation. J. Reprod. Fertil. *65*:395.

11. Cline, E. M., Jennings, L. L., and Sojka, N. J. (1980): Analysis of the feline vaginal epithelial cycle. Feline Reprod. *10*:47.

12. Cline, E. M., Jennings, L. L., and Sojka, N. J. (1980): Breeding laboratory cats during artificially induced estrus. Lab. Anim. Sci. *30*:1003.

13. Colby, E. D. (1970): Induced estrus and timed pregnancies in cats. Lab. Anim. Care *20*:1075.

14. Concannon, P. W., and Lein, D. H. (1983): Feline reproduction. *In*: Current Veterinary Therapy. VIII. Small Animal Practice, Philadelphia, W. B. Saunders Co., p. 932.

15. Concannon, P., Hodgson, B., and Lein, D. (1980): Reflex LH release in estrous cats following single and multiple copulations. Biol. Reprod. *23*:111.

16. Concannon, P., Lein, D., and Hodgson, B. (1982): Sexual behavior and self-limiting reflex LH release during extended periods of ad libitum copulatory activity in domestic cats. J. Anim. Sci. *55*(Suppl.1):344.

17. Christiansen, Ib. J. (1984): Reproduction in the Dog and Cat. London, Bailliere Tindall.

18. Courrier, R., and Gros, G. (1932): Remarques sur la nidation de l'oeuf chez la chatte. C. R. Soc. Biol. (Paris): *111*:787.

19. Dawson, A. B. (1981): The development and morphology of the corpus luteum of the cat. Anat. Rec. *79*:155.

20. Del Campo, C. H., and Ginther, O. J. (1974): Arteries and veins of uterus and ovaries in dogs and cats. Am J. Vet. Res. *35*:409.

21. Dooley, M. P., and Pineda, M. H. (1986): Effect of method of collection on seminal characteristics of the domestic cat. Am. J. Vet. Res. *47*:286.

22. Dooley, M. P., Murase, K., and Pineda, M. H. (1983): An electroejaculator for the collection of semen from the domestic cat. Theriogenology *20*:297.

23. Dooley, M. P., Pineda, M. H., Hopper, J. G., et al. Retrograde flow of semen caused by electroejaculation in the domestic cat. Proc. 10th Int. Congr. Anim. Reprod. and AI., Univ. Illinois, Champaign/Urbana, June 10–14, 1984, Vol. III, Brief Comm. No. 363.

24. Elcock, L. H., and Schoning, P. (1984): Age-related changes in the cat testis and epididymis. Am. J. Vet. Res. *45*:2380.

25. Foster, M. A., and Hisaw, F. L. (1935): Experimental ovulation and the resulting pseudopregnancy in anestrous cats. Anat. Rec. *62*:75.

26. Frenette, M. D., Dooley, M. P., and Pineda, M. H. (1986): Effect of flushing the vasa deferentia at the time of vasectomy on the rate of clearance of spermatozoa from the ejaculates of dogs and cats. Am. J. Vet. Res. *47*:463.

27. Gadsby, J. E., Heap, R. B., and Burton, R. D. (1980): Oestrogen production by blastocyst and early embryonic tissue of various species. J. Reprod. Fertil. *60*:409.

28. Glover, T. E., and Watson, P. F. (1985): Cold shock and its prevention by egg yolk in spermatozoa of the cat (Felis catus): Cryo-letters *6*:239.

29. Glover, T. E., and Watson, P. F. (1985): The effect of buffer osmolality on the survival of cat (Felis catus) spermatozoa at 5°C. Theriogenology *24*:449.

30. Glover, T. E., Watson, P. F., and Bonney, R. C. (1985): Observations on variability in LH release and fertility during oestrus in the domestic cat (Felis catus): J. Reprod. Fertil. *75*:145.

31. Hammer, C. E., Jenning, L. L. and Sojka, N. J. (1970): Cat (Felis catus, L.) spermatozoa require capacitation. J. Reprod. Fertil. *23*:477.

32. Hart, B. L. (1980): Objectionable urine spraying and urine marking in cats: evaluation of progestin treatment in gonadectomized males and females. J. Am. Vet. Med. Assoc. *177*:529.

33. Hart, B. L., and Cooper, L. (1984): Factors relating to urine spraying and fighting in prepubertally gonadectomized cats. J. Am. Vet. Med. Assoc. *184*:1255.

34. Henderson, R. T. (1984): Prostaglandin therapeutics in the bitch and queen. Aust. Vet. J. *61*:317.

35. Hughes, B. J., Bowen, J. M., Campion, D. R., et al. (1983): Effect of denervation or castration on ultrastructural and histochemical properties of feline bulbocavernosus muscle. Acta Anat. *115*:97.

36. Hurni, H. (1981): Daylength and breeding in the domestic cat. Lab Anim. *15*:229.

37. Hurni, H. (1981): SPF-cat breeding. Z. Versucht. *23*:102.

38. Jemmett, J. E., and Evans, J. M. (1977): A survey of sexual behaviour and reproduction of female cats. J. Small Anim. Pract. *18*:31.

39. Johnson, L. M., and Gay, V. L. (1981): Luteinizing hormone in the cat. I. Tonic secretion. Endocrinology *109*:240.

40. Johnson, L. M., and Gay, V. L. (1981): Luteinizing hormone in the cat. II. Mating-induced secretion. Endocrinology *109*:247.

41. Johnston, S. D., Hayden, D. W., Kiang, D. T., et al. (1984): Progesterone receptors in feline mammary adenocarcinomas. Am. J. Vet. Res. *45*:379.

42. Johnstone, I. P., Bancroft, B. J., and McFarlane, J. R. (1984): Testosterone and androstenedione profiles in the blood of domestic tomcats. Anim. Reprod. Sci. *7*:363.

43. Jones, T. C. (1969): Sex chromosome anomaly, Klinefelter's syndrome. Comp. Pathol. Bull. *1*:1.

44. Kelly, R. E., and Verhage, H. G. (1981): Hormonal effects on the contractile apparatus of the myometrium. Am. J. Anat. *161*:375.

45. Legay, J.-M., and Pontier, D. (1985): Relation age-Fecondite dans les populations de chats domestiques,

Felis catus. Mammalia *49*:395.

46. Lein, D. H., and Concannon, P. W. (1983): Infertility and fertility treatments and management in the queen and tom cat. *In*: Current Veterinary Therapy. VIII. Small Animal Practice, Philadelphia, W. B. Saunders Co., p. 936.

47. Levine, B. N. (1984): Small animal population trends and demands for veterinary service. *In*: Proc. 8th Kal Kan Symp. for the Treatment of Small Animal Disease, edited by E. Van Marthens, Vernon, California, Kal Kan, p. 49.

48. Manwell, E. J., and Wickens, P. G. (1928): The mechanisms of ovulation and implantation in the domestic cat. Anat. Rec. *38*:54.

49. Mauleon, P. (1967): Cinetique de l'ovogenese chez les mammiferes. Arch d'Anat. Microsc. Morphol. Exp. *56*:125.

50. Michael, R. P. (1961): Observations upon the sexual behavior of the domestic cat (*Felis catus L.*) under laboratory conditions. Behavior *18*:1.

51. Michael, R. P. (1973): The effects of hormones on sexual behavior in female cat and rhesus monkey. *In* Handbook of Physiology, Section 7: Vol. II. edited by R. O. Creep and E. B. Astwood. Washington. D. C., American Physiology Society, pp. 187–221.

52. Motta, P., and Van Blerkom, J. (1979): Morphodynamic aspects of the ovarian superficial epithelium as revealed by transmission, scanning and high voltage electron microscopy. Ann. Biol. Anim. Bioch. Biophys. *19*:1559.

53. Neville, P. F., and Remfry, J. (1984): Effect of neutering on two groups of feral cats. Vet. Rec. *114*:447.

54. Niwa, K., Ohara, K., Hosoi, Y., et al. (1985): Early events of in vitro fertilization of cat eggs by epididymal spermatozoa. J. Reprod. Fertil. *74*:657.

55. Paape, S. R., Shille, V. M., Seto, H., et al. (1975): Luteal activity in the pseudopregnant cat. Biol. Reprod. *13*:470.

56. Pineda, M. H., and Dooley, M. P. (1984): Surgical and chemical vasectomy in the cat. Am. J. Vet. Res. *45*:291.

57. Pineda, M. H., and Dooley, M. P. (1984): Effects of voltage and order of voltage application on seminal characteristics of electroejaculates of the domestic cat. Am. J. Vet. Res. *45*:1520.

58. Pineda, M. H., Dooley, M. P., and Martin, P. A. (1984): Long-term study on the effects of electro-ejaculation on seminal characteristics of the domestic cat. Am. J. Vet. Res. *45*:1038.

59. Rees, H. D., Swite, G. M., and Michael, R. P. (1980): The estrogen-sensitive neural system in the brain of female cats. J. Comp. Neurol. *193*:789.

60. Remfry, J. (1978): Control of feral cat populations by long-term administration of megestrol acetate. Vet. Rec. *103*:403.

61. Robinson, R., and Cox, H. W. (1970): Reproductive performance in a cat colony over a 10-year period. Lab. Anim. *4*:99.

62. Schmidt, P. M., Chakraborty, P. K., and Wildt, D.E. (1983): Ovarian activity, circulatory hormones and

sexual behavior in the cat. II. Relationships during pregnancy, parturition, lactation and the postpartum estrus. Biol. Reprod. *28*:657.

63. Shille, V. M., and Stabenfeldt, G. H. (1979): Luteal function in the domestic cat during pseudopregnancy and after treatment with prostaglandin $F_{2\alpha}$. Biol. Reprod. *21*:1217.

64. Shille, V. M., Kerstin, E., Lundstrom, E., et al., (1979): Follicular function in domestic cats as determined by estradiol-17β concentrations in plasma: Relation to estrous behavior and cornification of exfoliated vaginal epithelium. Biol. Reprod. *21*:953.

65. Shille, V. M., Munro, C., Farmer, S. W., et al. (1983): Ovarian and endocrine responses in the cat after coitus. J. Reprod. Fertil. *68*:29.

66. Sojka, N. J., Jennings, L. L., and Hamner, C.E. (1970): Artificial insemination in the cat, (*Felis catus L.*): Lab. Anim. Care *20*:198.

67. Stabenfeldt, G. H. (1974): Physiologic, pathologic and therapeutic roles of progestins in domestic animals. J. Am. Vet. Med. Assoc. *164*:311.

68. Stewart, D. R., and Stabenfeldt, G. H. (1985): Relaxin activity in the pregnant cat. Biol. Reprod. *32*: 848.

69. Stover, D. G., and Sokolowski, J. H. (1978): Estrous behavior of the domestic cat. Feline Pract. *8*:54.

70. Strasser, H., Brunk, R., and Baeder, C. (1971): Studies in the sexual cycle of the cat. Berl. Munch. Tieraerztl. Wochenschr. *84*:253.

71. Thuline, H. C., and Norby, D. E. (1961): Spontaneous occurrence of chromosome abnormality in cats. Science *134*:554.

72. Van der Stricht, R. (1911): Vitellogenese dans l'ovule de chatte. Arch. de Biol. *26*:365.

73. Verhage, H. G., Beamer, N. B., and Brenner, R. M. (1976): Plasma levels of estradiol and progesterone in the cat during polyestrus, pregnancy and pseudopregnancy. Biol. Reprod. *14*:579.

74. West, N. B., Verhage, H. G., and Brenner, R. M. (1976): Suppression of the estradiol receptor system by progesterone in the oviduct and uterus of the cat. Endocrinology *99*:1010.

75. Whalen, R. E. (1963): Sexual behavior of cats. Behavior *20*:321.

76. Wildt, D. E., and Lawler, D. F. (1985): Laparoscopic sterilization of the bitch and queen by uterine horn occlusion. Am. J. Vet. Res. *46*:864.

77. Wildt, D. E., Seager, S. W. J., and Chakraborty, P. K. (1980): Effect of copulatory stimuli on incidence of ovulation and on serum luteinizing hormone in the cat. Endocrinology *107*:1212.

78. Wildt, D. W., Chan, S. Y. W., Seager, S. W. J., et al. (1981): Ovarian activity, circulating hormones, and sexual behavior in the cat. I. Relationships during the coitus-induced luteal phase and the estrous period without mating. Biol. Reprod. *25*:15.

79. Younglai, E. V., Belbeck, L. W., Dimond, P., et al. (1976): Testosterone production by ovarian follicles of the domestic cat (Felis catus): Hormone Res. *7*:91.

Pregnancy and Parturition

L. E. McDonald

18

A consideration of the physiology of pregnancy rests heavily on a careful understanding of embryology. Since veterinary students have had a detailed course in embryology, the discussion is based on an assumption of such knowledge. The student is encouraged to review embryology.

PREGNANCY

Pregnancy or gestation in mammals is the result of millions of years of evolutionary changes which led to the development of a new organ, the placenta. For viviparity to be developed, many processes had to be coordinated to bring about a successful pregnancy. Foremost of course, was a coordination of the endocrine system which is directly concerned with a successful pregnancy. In late pregnancy, the placenta assumes the role of an endocrine organ. The general metabolism of the maternal organism must also change to accommodate the stress of pregnancy.

Preparation of the Uterus For Pregnancy

Since the uterus is to serve as an incubator, preparation must begin even before pregnancy. Most incubators are warm, moist, dark, and sterile and contain a nutrient medium. Such is the case in the uterus.

The gonadal hormone levels have important effects on the uterus, a prime *target organ* of these hormones. Even during proestrus the rising level of estrogen acts on the endometrium to cause a proliferation of the epithelium and straight duct growth of the glands. Also the myometrium responds to the rising estrogen level. Soon after ovulation, the rising level of progesterone enhances and acts synergistically with the existing estrogen level to bring about additional endometrial and myometrial changes. The uterine glands become branched and coiled and secrete a thick mucous material which can serve as the nutrient medium for the zygote until implantation occurs. After ovulation and development of the corpus luteum, the progesterone output is sufficient to cause a quietening of the myometrium and a more favorable physical environment for the zygote. The "uterine milk," consisting of uterine gland secretions, uterine tubal fluid, and cellular debris, provides an ideal nutritional medium for the zygote.

The Three Periods of Pregnancy

Winters et al. suggested that prenatal life be subdivided into three periods: (1) *The period of the ovum* is the period during which the developing zygote sheds its zona pellucida and becomes a blastocyst and lasts until it makes its first loose attachment to the endometrium. This is a free living stage when the zygote is subsisting on uterine tubal or uterine fluids (milk). (2) *The period of the embryo* consists of the time from blastocyst development until there is differentiation of the organ systems in the embryo and more complete placenta formation. (3) *The period of the fetus* is the time during which most of the growth of the placenta and fetus occurs and lasts until parturition.[64].

Of the three periods of gestation the longest is the third period, but perhaps the most critical in the life of the new organism is the second period. It is during the period of the embryo when most embryonic deaths occur.

Period of the Ovum

The period of the ovum begins with ovulation and is soon followed by union of the male and female gametes which results in a zygote. (Fertilization has been covered in Chapters 7, 8, and 9.) Strictly speaking, as soon as fertilization occurs, the fertilized ovum should be referred to as the *zygote*.

With the union of the two gametes the diploid number of chromosomes is restored, and cell division can continue. The first cell division results in two cells, these two cells divide into four, the four into eight cells, and the eight-cell stage divides into the sixteen-cell stage. This cell division occurs at the rate of about one division each day. So within 4 days a sixteen-cell zygote has developed. In most domestic animals, movement of zygote through the uterine tube takes 4 to 5 days. In the bitch, however, 5 to 10 days and in the sow only 2 days are required for the zygotes to move through the uterine tube. During this time the free-living zygote is nourished by a small amount of nutrients carried by the gametes, but more importantly by the uterine tube secretion.

While the zygote is in the uterine tube, it is subject to heat stress. Ewes kept at 90°F (32.2°C) during the 3 days following estrus have lowered fertility because of morphologically abnormal zygotes rather than fertilization failure. Zygotes are less susceptible to heat stress after leaving the uterine tube.[3,17] There is evidence that similar deleterious effects occur in some other species (sows;[62] cows[37]).

At the end of 4 or 5 days, the zygote reaches the tubouterine junction and passes into the uterus. The uterus is a receptive incubator and has sufficient uterine milk to provide nutrients for additional cell division. By about the eighth postovulation day in the cow, cell division is sufficient to cause the zona pellucida to rupture (hatch) and the growing cell mass to extend outward. Cavitation, which leads to formation of the blastula or hollow sphere, has begun. On one side of the sphere a mass of cells that is to become the embryo proper begins to accumulate. The thin single layer extending around the rest of the sphere becomes a trophoblast which finally develops into the extraembryonic membranes or the fetal placenta. For the next several days (until the third week in the cow and sow and days 35 to 60 in the mare) the blastocyst moves freely in the uterus, while the developing membranes become elongated to conform to the inner dimensions of the uterus.

The free floating blastocyst may move up or down the uterine horn or into the body of the other horn if the uterine anatomy permits. This is possible in all domestic animals, but the rabbit has separate cervices which prohibit such transuterine migration. In litter-bearing animals, the blastocysts move from horn to horn with considerable ease, and during the first 2 to 3 weeks an *even spacing* occurs. The mechanisms regulating spacing are not clearly understood, but it must be due in part to random location because of regular uterine contractions and abdominal movement. In the sow there is a very even spacing. As the fetal membranes begin to grow during the second and third week of pregnancy, there appears to be some force preventing the membranes of one fetus from overlapping another.

Transuterine migration through the body of the uterus appears to be common in litter-bearing animals, but less common in mono-tocous animals. Pregnancy in a monotocous animal usually is in the uterine horn adjacent to the ovary with the corpus luteum. In rare cases there is external migration—an ovum from one ovary is captured by the uterine tube on the opposite side. Scanlon found no trans-uterine migration in 643 single ovulating cows, but 2 of 10 cows with two ovulations on the same ovary had transuterine migration of one of the embyros.[45] Ewes experienced more transuterine migration: 8% of 834 ewes with one ovulation and 87.5% of 120 ewes with two ovulations on the same ovary. Even though a single fetus may migrate to the opposite horn, some of the placenta will extend into the horn on the side of ovulation, thereby preventing PG formation and early luteolysis.

As the delicate fetal membranes develop, there is a weak adherence of these membranes to the uterine wall. The attachment is not firm and consists more of an apposition of tissues. But these developing membranes provide a large surface area for *absorption of nutrient materials* from the uterine surface and permit the *excretion of waste substances* from the zygote.

Period of the Embryo

The period of the embryo lasts from about the 15th to the 45th days in cattle and is correspondingly shorter or longer in other species, depending on the length of gestation. This period is characterized by the formation of the organ systems of the body, development of the embryonic membranes, and implantation or attachment to the uterus (nidation).

During the early part of the period of the embryo, zygote nutrition continues to be from the uterine fluids. By the end of the period, the embryo is firmly attached to the uterus through formation of the placenta which provides a more specialized means of gaining nutritive substances and losing waste products. By the end of the period of the embryo, the organism has developed the appendages and organ systems. One can observe a particular conformation and determine the species of the embryo. Some authors use this as the criterion for distinguishing between an embryo and a fetus.

Period of the Fetus

The period of the fetus is the longest period in all species and in the cow begins about the 46th day of pregnancy and lasts until parturition. Tremendous gross changes must occur in the uterus, placenta, and fetus. The nutritive requirements of the fetus are high. Once development has progressed to this stage, fetal death is uncommon.

Fetal Membranes and Placentation Types

Placentation is a complex subject that has been carefully reviewed by Amoroso.[5] The placenta represents a means for two organisms to communicate but to a restricted degree. The attachment is intimate enough that nutritive materials can cross with considerable ease from the dam to the fetus and waste substances can pass from the fetus to the dam. During pregnancy, the dam not only serves as a host providing nourishment, but also shares respiratory and urinary systems with the fetus.

Classifications of placentas have been made by many authors. The classification by Grosser is based on the number of layers of tissue separating the maternal blood from the fetal blood (Table 18-1). The epitheliochorial attachment seen in the sow and mare consists

Table 18-1 Tissues Separating the Maternal Blood from the Fetal Blood in the Various Species

Placental Class (Grosser)	Shape of Attachment	Species	Layers	(Uterus Mucous Membrane) Maternal Tissues			(Allantochorion) Fetal Tissues		
				Endothelium of Blood Vessels	Connective Tissue	Epithelium of Uterus	Trophoblast (Chorion)	Connective Tissue	Endothelium of Blood Vessels
Epithelio-chorial	Diffuse	Pig, horse, donkey	6	+	+	+	+	+	+
Syndesmo-chorial*	Cotyledonary	Cattle, sheep, goat	5	+	+	−*	+	+	+
Endothelio-chorial	Zonary or discoid	Cat, dog, ferret	4	+	−	−	+	+	+
Hemochorial	Discoid or zonary	Primates	3	−	−	−	+	+	+
Hemoendo-thelial	Discoid or spheroidal	Guinea pig, rat, rabbit	1	−	−	−	−	−	+

*Bjorkman found a syncytium between the trophoblast and the maternal connective tissue of the sheep which could cause the syndesmochorial class to be considered as epitheliochorial.

of six intervening layers. This is the simplest form of placentation and consists merely of an apposition of the tissues of the placentas of the two organisms. The syndesmochorial type in the ruminant involves the loss of one of the layers—the epithelial lining of the uterus. Bjorkman found a syncytium between the trophoblast and the maternal connective tissue of the sheep which could cause the syndesmochorial class to be considered as epitheliochorial.[11]

If two layers are lost, then four layers separate the blood of the two organisms, and this is termed an endotheliochorial type of placenta. It is seen in the queen and the bitch. The two layers lost are the uterine epithelium and the connective tissues surrounding the uterine capillaries. If further tissue layers are lost, then only three would be left. This is termed a hemochorial attachment and is seen in primates. In these animals the chorion is bathed by the blood of the dam because it has eroded the endothelium of the uterine blood supply. No domestic species has two layers separating the two blood systems, but the rat, rabbit, and guinea pig have the hemoendothelial type of placenta. Only one tissue layer, the endothelium of the fetal capillary, separates the two blood systems.

All animals start the placentation process with six layers of tissue in the maternal and fetal placentas, but as implantation becomes more highly developed, fewer tissue layers remain. Many look upon the comparative nature of placentation just described as being a progressive process in which the fetuses of certain species are more successful in invading the uterus. This aggressive process on the part of the fetus appears to be most highly developed in the rabbit and rat and least developed in the pig or horse. During the early part of the implantation process a full complement of tissue layers separates the blood supplies in the rabbit, but with time, successively more layers are eroded until finally only a single layer separates the two blood supplies.

The classification of placentation according to Grosser is too simplified to explain intricate cellular interactions that develop between the trophoblast and the uterine epithelium. First, the epithelial layers come into apposition; then microvilli from the chorion slowly begin interdigitating with maternal epithelium. There may be an actual invasive process in dogs and cats that may be facilitated by lytic enzymes, since there is a decidual reaction followed by the trophoblast eroding or penetrating the maternal tissue. In pigs, mares, ewes, and cows there are no decidual reactions and no invasion of maternal tissue, since the apposition of fetal and maternal placenta is passive, except for microvilli attachments and adhesiveness. Nonetheless, the apposition in the latter group is sufficient to signal pregnancy and consequently to prevent the production and release of PG which, if released, would kill the corpus luteum.

The matter of the possible immunological rejection of the "foreign" fetus by the dam requires conjecture. Since the fetus contains antigens from the sire as well as the dam, the fetus represents "non-self" tissue to the dam and could be rejected. The fetus is a homograph which usually succeeds, but the exact mechanism is not known. One theory is that progesterone is the "immunosuppressant" hormone for the uterus much as glucocorticoids are elsewhere. Possibly the fetus is immunologically immature. Perhaps a barrier exists against the transfer of antigens from fetus to dam.

In animals with mamy tissue layers separating the blood supplies, there is seldom hemorrhage following parturition and the attendant separation of the fetal from the maternal placenta. In such species, the maternal blood supply is well protected. Therefore, postpartum uterine hemorrhage is seldom seen in the mare, ewe, or cow. But in primates this is a serious problem because there are few if any tissues left to protect the continuity of the vessel walls in the dam after the placenta is separated. The size of the fetus also affects the tendency toward hemorrhage; consequently, postpartum hemorrhage in the rat and rabbit is seldom severe because the uterus is so small that a blood clot would soon develop and fill the uterine cavity.

The time of implantation is difficult to determine in domestic species. It varies from about 12 to 24 days postovulation in the sow and cow to 35 to 60 days in the mare. These times must be regarded as estimates, since the first attachment is very tenuous and it is difficult to define exactly what constitutes attachment and to pinpoint when it occurs. It is unusual, though, that implantation in the mare waits so long to occur when compared to the times for other domestic animals. Also the queen and the bitch do not have implantation until up to 21 days which is one third of pregnancy. Certain marsupials have delayed implantation of the blastocyst until lactation ceases. The roe deer may carry a free floating blastocyt for up to 5 months, thereby causing a variable gestation period.

Prenatal Nutrition

A consideration of prenatal nutrition could be divided in accordance with the three periods of pregnancy, i.e., the *period of the ovum*, the *period of the embryo*, and the *period of the fetus*. Another breakdown could include nutrition during the *preplacentation period* and during the *postplacentation period*. The preplacentation period includes all of the period of the ovum and that part of the period of the embryo while placentation is occurring. After attachment, the consideration of prenatal nutrition falls in the postplacentation period. However, the means of nutrition does not change sharply between the two periods but instead involves a gradual change.

During the preplacentation period the ovum or early blastocyst absorbs foodstuffs from the surrounding fluids in either the uterine tube or the uterus. Uterine milk is available in most species and provides a good nutritional medium. As the blastocyst grows, its outer layer becomes an absorbing layer and is called a trophoblast. Finally, there is fusion of the ectodermal trophoblast with the mesodermal allantois and together these are called the chorion. Even before attachment to the uterine wall, the trophoblast or chorion utilizes its external surface as an absorptive surface. In the pig, early attachment consists merely of the trophoblastic cells lying in close contact with the uterus. In other species, such as the ewe or cat, degeneration and disappearance of the epithelium of the uterus allow the trophoblast or chorion to "attach" more intimately.

During the preplacentation period in the pig, the chorion lies close to the uterine epithelium facilitating absorption of the uterine gland secretion. There is no erosion of either the maternal or fetal placental tissue layers so the full six layers separate the two blood systems in the sow and mare (see Table 18-1). In the epitheliochorial type of attachment, the uterine glands serve as an important source of nutrition throughout intrauterine life. Obviously, there must be a good blood supply to the uterine glands in order to provide the nutrients which form the glandular secretions.

In the syndesmochorial type of placenta as seen in the cow and ewe, the uterine epithelium eventually erodes, and a more intimate attachment forms at the sites of the cotyledons-caruncles. In these species, nutrition of the fetus consists of two components: (1) the usual uterine gland secretion, the residue from the damaged epithelium, the blood cells, and tissue fluids that escape at the placentation site and (2) the regular exchange of nutrients at the cotyledon-caruncle.

In the queen and bitch with the endotheliochorial type of placenta, erosion of the uterus has proceeded a step further (two layers have been eroded). With such loss of maternal tissue layers, loss of blood from the maternal vessels leads to stagnant pools of blood at the placentation sites. This blood undergoes autolysis, and the liberated hemoglobin forms a green pigment called *uteroverdin*. This pigment is iron-free but remains at the placentation site and gives a brilliant green coloration to the placenta at parturition. This harmless discoloration is poorly understood by the layman. The role of the uterine gland is minor after nidation in the queen and bitch. Direct exchange of substances from one blood supply to the other is the important route.

In rodents, all layers have been destroyed

except one, and the two blood systems are barely separated. Nutrition of the rodent fetus occurs with considerable ease, since nutritive substances need pass only one layer of tissue. This is in contrast with the transfer of nutritive substances across the six layers in ungulates. Consequently, ungulate nutrition of the fetus depends considerably on uterine gland secretions.

As the period of the embryo progresses in any species and placentation becomes more intimate and successful, there is a shift from the embryo living by absorbing uterine milk or histotroph to a situation in which the embryo lives from transfer of nutrients across the placenta (hemotroph). As pointed out previously, this varies among the species and becomes more intimate later in pregnancy in any given species. Even in the pig in which the six tissue layers persist, nutrient substances are transferred from the maternal blood to the fetal blood.

Small molecules like CO_2, O_2, water, or electrolytes move across the placental membranes by *simple diffusion*, the mere movement of the molecule from an area of high concentration to an area of low concentration. Some larger molecules, such as certain hormones or drugs, also diffuse. *Active transport* (biological pumping) moves many important substances, such as amino acids, sugar, and some minerals, across the placental membrane against a gradient.

Prenatal Excretion

In domestic animals there is functional development of the mesonephros; this occurs by the 18th day in the lamb. Function apparently begins at this time, since there is a gradual expansion of the allantois, and fluid (urine) begins to accumulate within it. Carbon dioxide tension in fetal blood is considerably higher than in maternal blood. Barcoft concluded that the transfer of carbon dioxide to the maternal organism is by diffusion. Apparently the placenta of most domestic animals is sufficiently permeable to nitrogenous waste products that these are passed to the maternal organism by diffusion.

Relative Growth of Uterus and Contents During Pregnancy

The fetus and the fetal membranes grow at different rates (Fig. 18-1). The fetal membranes grow faster early in pregnancy while the fetus remains stable in size. There is an exaggerated accumulation of fluids relative to the other two components during the first half of pregnancy. The accumulation of fluids and the growth of the fetal membranes require less energy than growth of the fetus. This is reflected in the nutritional needs of the dam, since the *energy requirements during the first half of pregnancy are low*. During the second half of pregnancy the energy requirements increase tremendously because this is the stage in which the fetus makes its greatest growth (see Fig. 11-2).

The uterine wall makes a slow but constant gain in weight throughout pregnancy. The delay in the growth rate of the fetus is probably because it must await placentation before a sufficient transfer of nutrients can occur. The fetus will often double its weight in the last one fifth of pregnancy. Needham has pointed out that the *absolute growth* of the fetus is greater each succeeding week. On the other hand, the *relative growth* rate becomes progressively slower during fetal life. This is calculated by taking the growth increment in any week and dividing by the mean weight in that week.

Nutrition of the Pregnant Dam

Desired Weight Gain

The pregnant animal should have a well-balanced diet throughout pregnancy. It should include the proper amounts of minerals, vitamins, protein, and total energy. Total energy is particularly important. Experimental results have shown that overfeeding sows during the first half of pregnancy increases the incidence of embryonic deaths. In fact, the sow should not be allowed to gain much body weight during the first half of pregnancy or there will be small litter size. During the last half of pregnancy in the sow

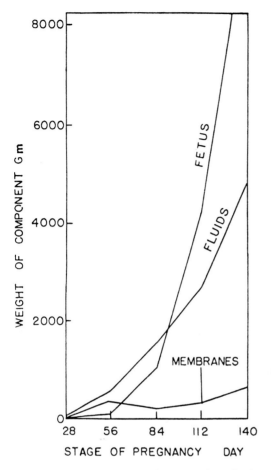

Fig. 18-1. Weight changes of fetuses, fetal fluids, and membranes during pregnancy in ditocous ewes. (From Wallace: J. Agric. Sci., 38, 93, 1948.)

the energy supply can be increased until she gains at a moderate rate. Obesity should be aovided (see Fig. 11-2).

In cows, overfeeding during pregnancy often results in the birth of weak calves. Owners often wish to give the pregnant animal additional feed and care. Extra energy intake should be discouraged during the first half of pregnancy in all species, with only moderate weight gains permitted during the last half of pregnancy. The weight of the pregnant animal should increase enough to offset the weight of the fetus, fetal fluids, and placenta with a moderate additional increase in body weight of animals in average condition. In cows, over-feeding until obesity occurs dur-

ing pregnancy causes fat deposits to replace the lactiferous tissue in the mammary gland. This damage is permanent, and the mammary gland is incapable of normal lactation. Obese cows often suffer from dystocia because of fat deposits impinging on the birth canal.

An excellent review of the effect of nutrition on reproduction is given by van Tienhoven.[57]

Priority of the Fetus for Nutrients

The fetus has priority over the dam for nearly all nutritive materials. The dam, if deprived of sufficient total energy to make a normal body weight gain during late pregnancy, will usually sacrifice her own body in order that the fetus can make most of its expected body growth.

There are a few elements for which the dam is reluctant to sacrifice her own body. For example, the sow on an iodine-deficient diet is often unable to spare enough iodine for the fetus; consequently a hairless pig is born. A cow on a prolonged vitamin A-deficient diet may be unable to spare enough vitamin A to prevent the fetus from being born blind.

Hormones of Pregnancy

In all species the production of estrogens and progesterone continues to rise throughout most of pregnancy. Implantation is especially dependent on critical levels of and balance between progesterone and estrogen. Progesterone is needed first and then estrogen to cause the reaction leading to implantation. High levels of estrogen from injections can prevent nidation. Corpus luteum production of these hormones is augmented, perhaps even replaced, by hormone production by the placenta after it develops in mid- or late pregnancy in some species. There is usually a drop in the production of these hormones, especially progesterone, just before parturition (this is discussed under parturition). Gonadotropin production by the pituitary usually falls during pregnancy because of gonadal steroid inhibition. There is placental production of some gonadotropin-like hormones, particularly in the mare (PMSG) and the woman (HCG).

Relaxin is produced during late pregnancy in several species. This water-soluble hormone apparently is produced by the corpus luteum or possibly the placenta and will be covered in the consideration of parturition. Oxytocin production and release during pregnancy are highest during the second stage of parturition and will be considered later. During pregnancy, there can be a release of oxytocin to cause milk letdown or in response to genital tract stimulation. The level is low, but there may be some stimulation of myometrial contraction.

Duration of Gestation

The duration of gestation varies considerably. Breed differences occur: the mean gestation length of Holstein-Friesian cattle is about 278 days but that for Brown-Swiss cattle is about 292 days. Even within a breed there can be differences due to the genotype of the fetus. Male calves and foals are usually carried a day or two longer, but the sex of the fetus does not affect the length of pregnancy in sheep. In polytocous species, larger litter sizes are usually delivered earlier.

Removal of the corpus luteum of pregnancy in the cow invariably causes parturition to occur earlier. The administration of progesterone lengthens gestation in the rabbit but not in the intact cow.

Sheep that ingest skunk's cabbage during the first two weeks of gestation experience abnormalities in the development of the fetus, such as cyclops-like malformation and pituitary absence. These fetuses are usually delivered late and may require a cesarean section.[10]

An autosomal recessive gene in the fetuses of certain strains of Holstein-Friesian cattle prevents delivery at the normal time. These cows do not show pelvic outlet relaxation. The blood progesterone concentration remains high when it should drop several days before the expected time of parturition. Some of these fetuses are carried for several months beyond term and may die in the uterus unless cesarean section is performed. These calves seldom survive. In Guernsey cattle, a similar failure to deliver has been found, but the calf has a homozygously recessive gene; the fetus lacks a pituitary, and fetal growth stops at the seventh month of pregnancy. The uteri of both breeds fail to respond to oxytocin. See Table 11-5 for gestation data.

Diagnosis of Pregnancy

Diagnosis of pregnancy in domestic animals has considerable practical value. A number of animals show estrus even though pregnant. In domestic animals, diagnosis may depend on either a physical examination or a test of body fluids. In the larger domestic animals a physical or clinical examination of the animal is the preferred method. In the mare and the cow this can be accomplished by manual examination of the uterus through the rectal wall. Experienced practitioners can sometimes detect the presence of an embryo as early as 25 to 35 days after conception.

The milk progesterone test in the cow is being used for pregnancy diagnosis, especially in England. The principle is based on the cycling level of progesterone in the nonpregnant cow and the stable level in the pregnant cow. Milk progesterone levels reflect plasma levels. A decline in progesterone about days 17 to 21 after estrus and breeding indicates nonpregnancy; a stable or rising level indicates pregnancy. The obtaining of an appropriate milk sample is relatively simple and the laboratory procedure has been simplified. The test is about 80% accurate for a positive pregnancy diagnosis and nearly 100% accurate as a nonpregnancy test. The difference is due to the fact that the corpus luteum may continue functioning during 17 to 21 days postestrus period for reasons other than pregnancy. For details of the test see Hoffman et al.[26] This test should aid manual palpation and even give earlier information.

The MIP test for pregnancy in the mare depends on an immunologic reaction to PMSG in blood as early as days 35 to 45 postbreeding.

In the bitch and queen, palpation of the fetus through the abdominal wall can be useful in the last half of pregnancy, but this should be discouraged because of possible damage to the developing embryo. In small species, such as the bitch or the cat, x-ray examination will often detect pregnancy if the fetuses are sufficiently developed (last quarter).

In the sow and ewe many attempts have been made to develop tests of the urine or blood for hormone changes during pregnancy but so far none has proved reliable. Of course, in farm species (not bitch and queen), the prolonged blood progesterone rise is present only during pregnancy or persistent corpus luteal function of nonpregnancy. Pseudopregnancy in the bitch or queen or persistent corpus luteal function of the farm species would give a false positive test.

Ultrasound has been used to determine pregnancy in several species, especially smaller ones such as the sow, ewe, and bitch. The principle is based on the fact that the pregnant uterus and its contents have different conductivity and reflectivity of the sound waves compared to those of other viscera. The instrument is usually placed on the abdominal wall near the uterus. Several commercial instruments are available. Accuracy and satisfaction are improving and use of the instruments is increasing.

PARTURITION

Parturition is the climax of the great drama of pregnancy. Few physiological processes can rival parturition in complexity or lack of understanding on the part of scientists. We need only to reflect on the writings of Foster in 1891:

> We may be said to be in the dark as to why the uterus, after remaining for months subject only to futile contractions, is suddenly thrown into powerful and efficient action, and within it may in a few hours, or even less, gets rid of the burden which it has borne with such tolerance for so long a time. None of the various hypotheses which have been put forward can be considered as satisfactory. We can only say that labour is the culminating point of a series of events, and must come sooner or later, though its immediate advent may sometimes be decided by accident.[19]

Although we now have a better understanding of the processes associated with parturition than Foster had in 1891, we still lack a full understanding of the causes of parturition.

Since that time the roles of oxytocin, adrenal corticoids, estrogen, and progesterone have been partially elucidated but much remains to be learned.

Laymen, herdsmen, and stockmen often use unique terms for the act of parturition, i.e., bitches "whelp," cows "calve," mares "foal," sows "farrow" or "pig," ewes "lamb."

Relaxation of the Symphysis Pubis, Cervix, Pelvic Tissues, and Ligaments

This relaxation occurs throughout the later part of pregnancy but with greater intensity in the last days before parturition. These changes are most noticeable in the cow, in part because of its size and the size of the fetus that must pass through the birth canal. *Relaxin* is a water-soluble hormone (polypeptide, MW 5,500) produced in the granulosa lutein cells of the ovary, whose effect on the relaxation of the pelvic structures is somewhat disputed. Like insulin, porcine relaxin is composed of an A chain of 22 amino acids and a B chain of 26 amino acids connected by 2 disulfide bridges. This hormone is probably important in some domestic animals, especially the cow and sow, and acts with the rising level of estrogen of late pregnancy to bring about a relaxation of the structures surrounding the birth canal. The symphysis pubis of the young female undergoes sufficient demineralization or dissolution of connective tissue to allow some separation at the time of parturition. This may not occur in the older female in which ossification of the symphysis pubis is more complete. With each approaching parturition, though, the cervix must dilate to allow passage of the fetus. Estrogen and relaxin apparently facilitate this process. The changes occurring in the pelvic tissues and ligaments are dramatic in large animals such as the cow and are one sign of impending delivery. There are some elevation of the tailhead, a relaxation of the muscles surrounding the pelvis, and a relaxation of the sacrosciatic and sacroiliac ligaments, all of which cause the pelvic bones to become more prominent as parturition approaches. The soft tissues of the perineal region, the vulva, and vagina become relaxed, enlarged, and flabby. Relaxin increases distensibility of the uterus and favors fetal accommodation.

Signs of Approaching Parturition

Signs for approaching parturition vary from species to species, but it is important for a veterinarian or animal husbandryman to know and recognize them. Maternal behavior begins to appear even before parturition, and the female usually seeks solitude from the herd for parturition. For several days before delivery the sow will build a nest or bed in some isolated place. The bitch likewise tries to prepare a nest or bed for the puppies to be delivered. The mare and the cow begin leaving the herd for increasing periods in the days preceding parturition. As the time of parturition draws closer, the female of all species begins to show inappetence, distress, and anxiety and withdraws from her usual environment as much as possible. Withdrawal is a natural process and should be encouraged and enhanced if possible.

By this time, the mammary glands have developed in preparation for lactation and there may be considerable secretion in the udder. In some species distention of the udder may be so great that there may be some dripping of secretion from the teats, especially in the dairy cow. The mare may have enough dripping from the teats that the drying of secretion on the teats forms a "waxy seal." This usually indicates impending parturition.

As the time of parturition nears, the beginning uterine contraction may bring distress to the animal. The dam may pace about, often in circles, and kick toward her flank. In monotocous animals, the movements of the fetus often can be seen through the abdominal wall. During this latter stage the dam should not be encouraged to eat but should be provided with adequate water and solitude.

Body temperature changes are a signal of impending parturition in several species. Body temperature rises approximately 1°C about 12 to 15 hours before the birth of the first pig in sows or gilts regardless of the ambient temperature.[18] This is in contrast to the prepar-

turient *drop* in body temperature in the cow, bitch, ewe, and rat. The drop is in response to the decline in circulating progesterone levels in the latter group, since it is known that progesterone is thermogenic in most species. The temperature *rise* in the sow is contrary to the expected change, since the sow also has a preparturient decline in progesterone. Another important aspect of the sow is that the elevated temperature persists throughout lactation and must not be confused with the fever response seen in disease states.

Theories of Causes of Parturition

Parturition is an important but poorly understood process involving an interplay of maternal hormones, fetal hormones, and several physical or mechanical factors. The role of the fetus in initiating parturition has been given increased emphasis as the function of the fetal adrenal cortex has been elucidated in the last two decades. Some of the evidence for each of the theories will be presented with a summary suggesting how these may affect parturition in domestic animals. It is quite likely that each species differs somewhat in its fine control of the process of parturition.

MATERNAL HORMONES. *Progesterone* has long been recognized as a hormone which discourages uterine contraction by adversely affecting the repolarization process. In most domestic animals there is a rising level of progesterone throughout pregnancy which comes from either the corpus luteum or the placenta. In most species (woman excepted) progesterone declines a few hours or days before parturition. The withdrawal of the progesterone block would allow the myometrial stimulatory effects of estrogen and PGF to be more manifest. Possibly progesterone production is stopped by the interaction of prostaglandin with fetal glucocorticoids acting as a stimulus for PG synthesis.

Estrone and estradiol increase during pregnancy in domestic animals and reach a peak a few days before parturition. This rising level of estrogen during pregnancy causes growth of the myometrium, synthesis of actomyosin, and consequently an increase in the contractile capacity of the uterus. Estrogen increases spontaneous myometrial activity and favors rapid repolarization of the membrane potential. During the last hours or days of pregnancy, the declining influence of progesterone and the increasing influence of estrogen favor myometrial contractility. Estrogen also causes a relaxation (along with relaxin) of the birth canal, especially the cervix and vagina.

Adrenal corticoids rise immediately before parturition in the maternal plasma, but the total effect on the process may be negligible. This is in contrast to the important role of the fetal adrenal cortex which will be considered presently.

Prostaglandins of the F group appear to be of considerable importance in parturition in the sheep and goat. Liggins et al. found an increase of PGF in uterine vein blood within the 24 hours before parturition (Fig. 18-2).[32] The source may be the placenta or the endo-

metrium. Stimulus for PGF synthesis may come from the fetal adrenal level of corticoids. PGF is luteolytic and a strong myometrial stimulant.

Oxytocin levels rise sharply during the second stage of parturition. The uterine response to oxytocin increases throughout pregnancy. It is somewhat difficult to say whether this is entirely associated with the rising sensitization of the uterus by estrogen or whether it is due to a disappearance of the progesterone block. Nonetheless, most authorities agree that the uterus becomes critically sensitive to low physiologic concentrations of oxytocin near parturition. Work in several species indicates there is a sudden release of oxytocin just before the final expulsion of the fetus. This is particularly defined in the cow (Fig. 18-3). Debackere and Peeters found that vaginal distension in the cow causes an increased release of oxytocin.[15] Perhaps this is the final signal

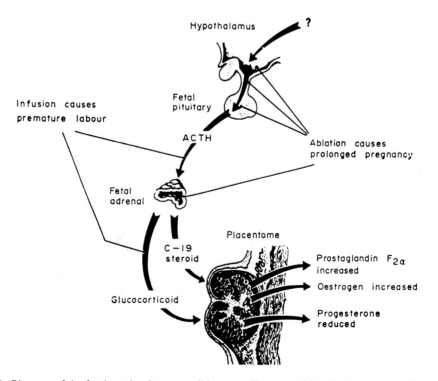

Fig. 18-2. Diagram of the fetal mechanisms possibly controlling parturition in the ewe. The fetal hypothalamus invokes the fetal pituitary-adrenal axis to increase glucocorticoid output in most mammals. The placentome then releases estrogen and PGF, but progesterone declines. (From Liggins et al: J. Reprod. Fertil., Suppl. *16*:85, 1972.)

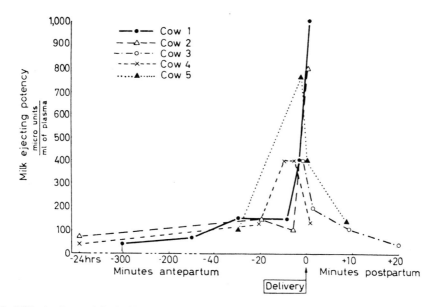

Fig. 18-3. Milk-ejecting activity in blood plasma, estimated as oxytocin, is shown in relation to progress of labor in 5 cows. Potency increases dramatically during the last few minutes before delivery and declines rapidly in the first few minutes postpartum. (From Fitzpatrick, R. J.: The posterior pituitary gland and the female reproductive tract. *In* The Pituitary Gland, edited by G. W. Harris and B. T. Donovan. London, Butterworth, 1966.)

to cause a sudden release of oxytocin needed for complete expulsion of the fetus. Its importance in the initiation of labor is minimal, but it is important in the expedition of parturition.

FETAL HORMONES. The output of adrenal cortical hormones by the fetus is important in parturition. Prolonged gestation in Holstein and Guernsey cows is due to hypoplastic or aplastic pituitaries in the fetuses. These cows with prolonged gestation maintain high plasma progesterone levels, the uterus is insensitive to oxytocin, and if the fetuses are surgically delivered, they are weak and usually die in a hypoglycemic state. Prolonged gestation has also been found in sheep that have ingested a weed, *Veratrum californicum*. The lambs have facial anomalies (cyclopean) and an absence of the pituitary. In South Africa there is a prolonged gestation disease of sheep known as Grootlamsiekte, apparently due to ingestion of the shrub *Salsola tuberculate*. Likewise, there is fetal hypophyseal and adrenal atrophy.

Experimental destruction of the fetal lamb's

pituitary-adrenal axis results in prolonged gestation. From the foregoing it is seen that failure of the fetal adrenal cortex to secrete normal levels of the adrenal corticoids leads to prolonged gestation. In the normal fetus there is a rise in fetal plasma corticoids as parturition approaches. In fact, hyperplasia of the fetal adrenal has been found in a group of habitually aborting Angora goats.

In the normal fetus high levels of fetal corticoids appear the last few hours before parturition. From the work of Liggins (Fig. 18-2) and others the rising level of fetal glucocorticoids is temporarily associated with an increased prostaglandin $F_{2\alpha}$ and estrogen output from the placentome of the sheep and the goat (Fig. 18-4). Furthermore, progesterone production is reduced. The rising levels of estradiol and PGF precede declining progesterone, thereby setting the stage for myometrial contractions.

Experimentally, small amounts of a potent glucocorticoid such as dexamethasone, when infused into the fetal circulation, will induce the above hormone changes and parturition. Likewise giving dexamethasone in massive

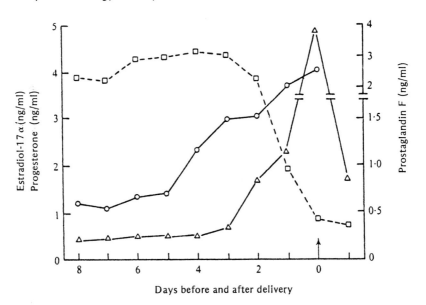

Fig. 18-4. Changes in the uterine venous plasma of Østradiol-17α (○), progesterone (□), prostaglandin F(△), before and after delivery (arrow). The values are the means of 5 to 6 daily observations in 4 goats (*n* = 20 or 24). (From Umo et al.: J. Endocrinol. *68*:385, 1976.)

amounts to the maternal organism will initiate parturition in cows, ewes, goats, and mares.

An interesting additional effect of the prepartum rise in fetal glucocorticoids is their stimulation of *surfactant* production. The surfactant decreases alveoli surface tension thereby allowing lung expansion and easier breathing in preparation for extrauterine life.

PHYSICAL OR MECHANICAL FACTORS. The *size* and *weight of the fetus* increase during pregnancy causing distension of the uterus, increased irritability of the myometrium, and uterine contractions. Evidence for this is that twin pregnancies in usually monotocous animals often experience a shortened gestation period. In fact, the length of gestation in all monotocous or polytocous species is inversely related to the number of fetuses. Increased movement of the large fetus has been suggested as a stimulus to myometrial contractions which could lead to parturition.

Central nervous system control has been studied fairly well. Parturition cannot be prevented by uterine denervation, or by other methods of negating the influence of the nervous system. Parturition in such a preparation lacks some

of the normal aspects. Probably the intact nervous system enhances the normal processes but it is not entirely necessary.

In *conclusion*, parturition is probably caused by a combination of many factors, with some factors being more dominant in one species than in another. In domestic animals, attention should be focused on the role of fetal corticoids acting on the uterus and placenta and causing increased estrogen which probably increases PGF output (Fig. 18-2). The PGF would then cause progesterone output to drop. The estrogen-dominated but progesterone-deprived myometrium would respond to PGF, and labor would begin (Fig. 18-4). The final spurt of oxytocin which culminates in parturition could come from a neuroendocrine reflex originating from genital tract stimulation by the fetus (Fig. 18-2) and involves the hypothalamoneurohypophyseal system. *But* we cannot consider oxytocin essential because, in the absence of the hypophysis, parturition can occur—probably because of the compensating effects of the other mechanisms. In the normal animal all these forces work together in an integrated fashion to cause parturition (see Wagner et al.[59] and Thorburn et al.[54] for excellent reviews of parturition in domestic animals).

Induction of Parturition

The control of the time of parturition in farm animals, particularly those on the range such as beef cattle or sheep, would be an important management technique. The control of parturition within a few hours' period would permit veterinary care and husbandry to be concentrated and lead to the efficient use of facilities and personnel (providing no adverse effects were induced in the dam or the newborn). Control of the time of parturition would be an advantage in all species provided the above conditions could be met.

Oxytocin, PGF, and parasympathomimetic drugs have been used to induce myometrial contractions and labor in many species for several years. Oxytocin-induced labor is similar to spontaneous labor, but the success of such parturition is dependent upon a dilated cervix. If the cervix is not dilated, then uterine rupture is possible in the large domestic animals. Once the cervix is dilated, it is practical in most large domestic animals to effect delivery by physical means. In valuable mares, oxytocin-facilitated delivery can be effected with 120 units, intramuscularly provided the cervix is dilated, the fetus is properly positioned, and term has been reached as evidenced by milk formation. Slow intravenous drip is preferred and less dosage is required. In small animals in which physical intervention is difficult or impossible such treatment might be considered. Cross induced delivery in the rabbit by a single intravenous injection of 100 to 200 mμ of oxytocin.[13] Obviously even in small animals the cervix must be dilated, or the induced contractions may cause fetal death or uterine damage.

After the report by Adams in 1969 that the synthetic glucocorticoids in large doses induce parturition in cattle, sheep, and goats, many trials have been conducted.[1] Parturition can be induced in a large percentage of the dams at or even preceding the expected date of parturition. An adverse side effect has been the frequent retention of the placenta in cattle. The administration of 10 to 30 mg of dexamethasone intramuscularly in the cow within 2 weeks of the expected date of parturition usually causes delivery within 72 hours. The calves are somewhat weak, although survival is good, with the stronger calves being those delivered nearer the expected time of delivery. Retained placenta occurs in up to 90% of the treated cows, and follow-up therapy for this pathological condition is necessary. The onset of milk production is somewhat slower than normal and the return of the uterus to the normal state is somewhat delayed compared to normal parturition, but the procedure has potential.

Estrogens, particularly DES, have been used during the first trimester of pregnancy to cause abortion, particularly in feedlot heifers. During the second and third trimesters, though, the efficacy of DES declines.

The mechanism of action of the corticosteroids in inducing parturition in the cow is likely due to its luteolytic effect which causes a sharp drop in the progesterone level. Also there is a short but dramatic rise in estrogen. These events indicate that the administered corticosteroid acts much as would a signal from the fetal adrenal to induce parturition (Fig. 18-2). The ewe does not appear to be responsive to corticosteroids before day 130 of gestation. During days 130 to 150, parturition can be induced by the corticosteroids, and placenta retention does not occur in the ewe. The mechanism of action in the ewe is probably not mediated through the corpus luteum, since it is not essential in the final days of pregnancy. Instead, the corticosteroids probably mimic the effect of the fetal adrenal to induce the chain of events shown in Figure 18-2.

In the mare induction of parturition with dexamethasone has been reported, although repeated administration of an extremely high dosage was necessary.

PGE or PGF given intravenously induces premature parturition in the cow. PG has successfully terminated prolonged gestation in the cow, although retained placenta occurs as in corticoid-induced parturition. PG has induced parturition in swine without adverse effects other than restlessness and defecation. Fifteen mg of $PGF_{2\alpha}$ (Prostin, Upjohn) intramuscularly on day 111 induced delivery in 32 ($\pm$ 14) hours (Elmore et al.). Further work is needed to determine the ultimate value of PG for parturition induction in cows and sows. $PGF_{2\alpha}$ is an effective abortifacient in cats only after 40 days of gestation, but preliminary studies in the dog have not been encouraging, except with repeated high doses.

Stages of Parturition

The events occurring during parturition could be considered more appropriately in obstetrics, but a brief discussion will be given of the three stages of parturition in domestic animals. Parturition in all species of domestic animals usually occurs with the dam in lateral recumbency.

The *first stage* of parturition is the preparatory one and consists of dilation of the cervix caused by beginning myometrial contractions forcing the fetus and the fluid-filled membranes against and through the cervix. The fluid-filled membranes act as a wedge seeking out the cervical canal and expanding it with each uterine contraction until finally the cervix can accommodate the forefeet of the fetus. This stage may last for a day, but usually is limited to only several hours. The reactions of the dam to this first stage of labor include evidence of discomfort and distress. Sometimes rupture of the fetal membranes at this stage allows some allantoic fluid to escape. During the preparatory stage, the fetus of the monotocous species rotates from a position of lying on its side or back to a dorsal position with the forelimbs and head forced against the cervix. In polytocous animals, the posterior fetus from one uterine horn is forced into the uterine body and against the cervix. In polytocous animals the first contractions are concentrated in the cervical end of the uterus. Otherwise, fetuses from the ovarian end of the uterine horn would be dislodged and jammed against one another. The dam usually

lies down a while, then rises, and paces about during this stage.

The *second stage* of parturition, the expulsive stage, consists of complete dilation of the cervix and delivery of the fetus. The uterine contractions increase in intensity and frequency, and their action is reinforced by the abdominal press which provides the additional force necessary for parturition. The time involved in the second stage depends on the species and is considered in the following section.

The *third stage* of parturition consists of expulsion of the placenta. This varies with the species, occurring quickly in the mare, sometimes only a few minutes after delivery. In the cow, placenta expulsion up to 12 hours post-delivery is considered normal. In some polytocous species, the fetal membranes are expelled with or after each fetus and before the next fetus is delivered. In other species the placenta does not follow each fetus and may be expelled as a group after several fetuses are delivered (i.e., sow).

The period following parturition required for the reproductive tract to return to normal is called the puerperium. This varies with the species, but in the mare and cow usually requires 35 to 60 days. In smaller animals less time is required, since less uterine tissue is involved. The bitch appears to be an exception because her uterus is so sensitive to progesterone, the corpus luteum functions throughout pregnancy and pseudopregnancy, and her uterus requires 100 to 159 days to return to normal.

Parturition in Various Species

In the *cow* the fetus usually lies on its side during late pregnancy, but during the preparatory stage of parturition it rotates a quarter-turn, thereby presenting the forelimbs and head to the birth canal. In monotocous species such as the mare and cow, contractions begin at the anterior end of the uterine horn, whereas in polytocous species, contractions begin near the cervix in order to expel the fetus nearest the cervix. During parturition, the separation of the cotyledons occurs slowly, if at all; consequently the circulation exchange between maternal and fetal organisms continues until the calf is fully expelled. The umbilical cord is sufficiently long to allow the fetus to move through most of the birth canal before it is severed. This permits survival of the fetus during a lengthy parturition which in the cow may last 2 hours. As the calf leaves the vulva, the umbilical cord often breaks. Usually the calf has begun respiration by this time and is no longer dependent on oxygenation of its blood through the maternal organism. If a placenta is not expelled within 12 hours after parturition, the cow is usually considered to have a "retained placenta." This is a pathologic condition that follows approximately 10% of deliveries. This incidence is higher in cases of infectious uterine conditions, twinning, difficult parturition, or premature delivery. Removal of the corpus luteum of pregnancy is a way to induce experimentally retained placenta. If progesterone is given to these corpus luteum-deficient animals, then the retention can be prevented.[34] Likewise, induction of parturition in the cow with the corticosteroids causes a high incidence of placenta retention.

During the second stage of parturition in the *mare* the chorion separates completely from its uterine attachment. Therefore, once the expulsion of the fetus begins, parturition must be completed quickly or the foal will suffocate. Consequently, the second stage of parturition in the mare usually takes only 5 to 15 minutes. The fetal membranes leave the uterus along with the fetus. Once the head and forelegs pass through the vulva, the fetus usually ruptures the amnion to allow respiration to begin.

Mahaffey has cautioned against severance of the umbilical cord in the foal too quickly after delivery.[35] He has found that the foal is completely delivered during a normal unassisted birth except that portions of the hind legs remain in the vagina. After 5 to 15 minutes, either the foal or the mare begins to move, the legs are withdrawn and the umbilical cord breaks. But during this 5- to 15-minute period the fetus has been accumulating blood which was formerly in the fetal pla-

centa. This may amount to as much as 30% of the fetal blood. If the umbilical cord is cut immediately after delivery, there is a loss of 1,200 to 1,500 ml of blood or about 30% of the potential blood volume of the fetus. This amount of blood is critical to the life of the newborn foal, and Mahaffey cautions against early severance of the umbilical cord in assisted births. Since the fetal membranes become separated from the uterus during the second stage of parturition in the mare, the membranes are usually expelled shortly after the fetus. In some cases, several hours may pass after parturition before the uterus recovers sufficient contractility to expel the placenta.

Parturition in the *ewe* usually takes about 15 minutes for each lamb, and separation and expulsion of the placenta usually follow within 2 hours after delivery. Since the ewe has a firm placental attachment typical of a cotyledonary type of placentation, separation of the fetal placenta (cotyledon) from the uterus (caruncle) may be slow. The fetal membranes from the first delivered lamb are expelled before delivery of the second or third lambs in cases of twinning or tripleting.

Hindson et al. studied parturition in the ewe by implanting a pressure-sensitive radio transmitter in the uterus.[25] They found that uterine contractions did not begin until about 12 hours before parturition, and these contractions were responsible for dilation of the cervix. Once cervical dilation occurs, the myometrial contractions assume a lesser role, since abdominal contractions and straining constitute the effective means of expelling the fetus. The abdominal contractions are synchronized with the peak of uterine myometrial contraction waves. Postpartum myometrial contraction waves continue with equal intensity for several hours after delivery to effect the third stage of labor—expulsion of the placenta.

Parturition in the *sow* is different because of the many fetuses in the uterus. Perry recorded the gross intrauterine state after parturition had begun in two sows. Myometrial contraction waves apparently begin near the cervix. Several chorionic sacs may rupture near the cervix before the first delivery, but the umbilical cords remain intact. The umbilical cords are long enough to permit the piglets to be delivered before severing the cord. The ruptured chorionic sacs provide a slippery tunnel through which the piglets are forced. Fetuses are usually delivered randomly from both horns, beginning and continuing with those nearest the cervix. About 60% of the piglets are delivered headfirst, their orientation during pregnancy. Reversal seldom occurs during parturition.

The piglets may be delivered rapidly (one each 3 to 8 minutes) or there can be delays of an hour or more. Little information has been recorded on the time of expulsion of the placental membranes. Apparently several piglets can be followed by several placentas, or most piglets can be delivered before their placentas are expelled. Perry estimates that in 25% of the sows some placentas are shed before parturition is completed.

The long umbilical cords are the reason that so few piglets suffocate during a rather disorganized parturition process in the sow.

Parturition in the *bitch* and *queen* is similar to that in the sow, since a litter is involved. In most litter-bearing animals the dam may rise and walk around after delivery of one or several fetuses. Fetal membranes are shed with the fetus, and rupture is important in order that respiration can begin. The dam usually licks the newborn to remove the fetal membranes from the nose and stimulate respiration and circulation. The dam usually ingests the membranes soon after delivery of the puppy. The bitch may deliver a puppy each 10 to 30 minutes and there may be an interval of an hour or more between deliveries. The uterine horn that contains the most pupies usually expels the first pup (Gunther). The parturition process is usually completed within 3 to 6 hours from the onset of labor.

Ingestion of the fetal membranes by the dam occurs in nearly all species, and carnivorous animals can digest the membranes satisfactorily. In herbivorous animals there is some danger that the ingested membranes may obstruct the gastrointestinal tract and lead to digestive upsets. Therefore, access to the membranes should be prevented, if possible, in the cow, ewe, or mare. Ingestion of fetal membranes is probably an innate protective characteristic by which the dam is attempting to destroy evidence of a recent delivery and thereby discourage predators.

Parturition occurs during the night at a greater frequency in most species. Rossdale and Short reported data on 501 thoroughbred mares and found that 86% of the parturitions occurred between 7 P.M. and 7 A.M.[43] The peak delivery was from 10 to 11 P.M. This circadian rhythm in the time of birth is also reported in women and pigs. *Sheep* favor the daytime hours, but there is even distribution of parturition throughout the 24 hours in cattle. The causes of circadian rhythm in parturition time are unknown. The fetus influences the day of delivery, but the dam must exert some influence on the hour. Koch also reported a circadian rhythm in equine parturition.[30]

Maternal Behavior

Ethology is the study of animal behavior. A segment of ethology includes maternal behavior, which is the response of the dam from preparturition to weaning. Likewise, neonatal behavior is the response of the neonate from birth until weaning. Ethology has been a poorly studied science, but it is becoming more important in domestic species because abnormal maternal and neonatal behaviors are limiting reproduction in modern but artificial environments.

As parturition approaches, the dam of all species seeks seclusion. This is particularly true in herd animals in which the expectant dam leaves the herd in preparation for parturition. Seclusion and quiet should be encouraged and provided. The intrusion of man during this period should be minimal. The nesting reaction is strong in queens, bitches, and sows (young born immature—altricial), but is nearly absent in ewes, cows, and mares (young born mature—precocial). After delivery, the licking and grooming response of the newborn is strong in all domestic dams except the sow. The grooming response is important, since licking the nasal area often removes placental tissue and mucus which may obstruct respiration. Since the sow does not groom, piglets often suffocate from nasal obstruction. The nesting species nurse their litters while lying, whereas the cow, mare, and ewe nurse their young while standing.

Within the first few hours after delivery, a strong bond develops between dam and neonate which lasts until weaning. Experienced dams are quicker and more successful in developing this bond, whereas inexperienced dams sometimes will abandon their newborn. The imprinting of the bond depends primarily upon olfaction which depends on a pheromone. Vocalization is a means of communication and encourages dam-neonate recognition which is confirmed by olfaction. This bond lasts until weaning after which the dam usually shows an indifferent response toward her offspring. Sometimes the offspring will return and attempt to nurse during subsequent lactations and even compete with the next generation. Once the bond is broken, though, the relationship is usually as indifferent as those between unrelated animals in a herd. Immediately after delivery, a protective impulse develops, varying with the species. The sow and cow develop the strongest protective reaction, and the least protective reaction is shown by the bitch and queen. The ewe and the mare are intermediate in this response.

The role of the male following parturition in domestic animals is minor. Usually it consists of little more than curiosity, and in none of the domestic species does the male exert a protective role often seen in birds and some wild animals. In fact, the tomcat will often destroy a litter of kittens which, of course, shortens lactation but hastens the onset of the next estrus.

The *ewe* rises within a matter of minutes after delivery, turns, thereby breaking the umbilical cord, and begins the grooming and licking response. This is desirable for the newborn, since it dries the coat as a protection against adverse weather and stimulates the cardiovascular and respiratory systems. The ewe has difficulty in caring for twin or triplet births, since she may become imprinted with a bond to only one and ignore the other lambs. The best protection that management has against such a problem is to have the ewe penned separately from the flock so that she is exposed only to her own lambs in a relatively small pen. The lamb usually rises within 15 to 20 minutes after parturition and begins unsteady movements which eventually lead to searching for the teat. Newborn animals have an innate behavioral response which causes them to search the underside of the dam for the teat. Fortunately, this response is strong and usually successful. It is at this point that the owner can be of value to the well-being of dam and neonate by helping the newborn with the first suckling experience. Because wool tags often obscure the teats, the lamb seems to have more difficulty than other species. Once the first intake of colostrum has been accomplished, the suckling experience will usually follow on its own.

Cows usually rise soon after delivery and begin an intense grooming of the newborn. The dam may attempt to ingest the fetal membranes, a practice which should be discouraged. The calf does not rise for approximately one-half hour and within the next hour attempts to nurse. The cow is quite protective of her newborn and is best left alone at this stage. If the calf has not nursed within several hours, then help should be provided. Under pasture conditions the cow will often "hide" the calf in vegetation. The calf usually remains recumbent for several hours while the dam is away grazing. She returns several times daily for nursing. This is an unusual reaction not often seen in other species.

Mares usually do not arise immediately after delivery, and this delay is good because the placental blood needs time to enter the foal's circulation as previously discussed. Suffocation seldom occurs because the foal's forelimb pedaling ensures membrane rupture. Upon standing, the mare begins the licking reaction which is stimulatory to the fetus. The foal usually makes standing attempts within one-half hour to one hour, and once it arises, it is surprising how coordinated such a large neonate can be after having spent gestation in such a restricted space. The nursing reflex is strong in the foal, and suckling usually occurs within a few hours, but should be confirmed by the owner. Separation of mare and neonate from the herd is important for several days.

Sows have a lengthy duration of farrowing which may last several hours during which the dam alternately lies down and stands up. Since she does not have a nuzzling and licking reaction, the newborn may suffocate from respiratory obstruction. Although the sow has a strong protective reaction against other animals and man, she is unable to provide much maternal help to the piglets. Newborn pigs tend to seek the warmth of the underside of the belly which facilitates nursing. Suckling occurs soon after delivery and may occur before the entire litter is delivered. The maternal-neonate bond is less developed in swine than in most species probably due to the litter effect. Piglets from other litters may be accepted by a sow during their first 2 days of life; this acceptance of other newborn is greater than in any other domestic species. Pigs tend to follow only one sow in a herd. Pigs acquire teat preferences which usually last throughout lactation. The suckling response by the dam is highly developed in swine. The piglets may pester the dam for frequent nursing opportunities, but it is only when the sow decides to lie down on one side, thereby exposing the udders, that she releases oxytocin to cause milk letdown. This interesting neuroendocrine reflex is easily observed and the time involved for the reflex is easily pinpointed, since the letdown of milk stops the teat trading, squealing, and hyperactivity of the piglets. Sows have little discrimination toward physical harm to their newborn; consequently, under modern husbandry conditions, they are often housed with protective bars to keep them from lying on the litter.

The *bitch* and *queen* seek seclusion several hours to days before parturition and initiate a strong nest-building reaction. Even a domestic house pet should be afforded privacy unless parturition is difficult. Newborn puppies, and especially newborn kittens, are immature at birth and the nest is important for their well-being. Puppies and kittens are born blind and deaf and do not acquire these special senses for several days. The bitch and queen show strong retrieval responses if the young stray from the nest. A strong grooming response exists in both species; the dam usually licks the fetal membranes away quickly and may even ingest them. The dam may arise between individual deliveries and care for the newborn before again lying down to complete delivery. Sometimes the dam may remain recumbent, but move the newborn where she can groom it. The neonates have a strong nursing instinct and quickly find their way to the dam, probably attracted by the warmth of the dam. Suckling should occur within the first few hours and help might be provided at this point if there seems to be difficulty. Thereafter, the dam should be provided with seclusion and privacy for the next few days. Much distress can be inflicted on the dam and newborn by human interference.

TRANSMAMMARY AND TRANSPLACENTAL PASSAGE OF PARASITES

Transplacental passage of *Toxocara cati* has not been demonstrated from queens to kittens, but transmammary passage has been shown by Swerczek et al.[52] Evidence of transmammary passage of nematode larvae has been shown for *Strongyloides ransomi* in pigs, *Ancylostoma caninum* in dogs, *Toxocara canis* in dogs, *Strongyloides westeri* in horses, and *Neoascaris vitulorum* in cattle.

Krakowka summarized transplacentally acquired microbial and parasitic diseases of dogs (Table 18-2).

TRANSPLACENTAL TRANSFER OF IMMUNOGLOBULINS (Ig)

Transplacental passage of immunoglobulins is of tremendous importance in domestic animals, since the newborn is immediately subjected to an environment containing infectious

Table 18-2 Transplacentally Acquired Microbial and Parasitic Diseases of Dogs

Viral
  Canine herpesvirus
  Canine adenovirus 1 (infectious canine hepatitis)
  Canine distemper virus

Bacteria
  Brucella canis
  Streptococcus
  Leptospira canicola, icterohaemorrhagiae (?)

Rickettsial
  Haemobartonella canis

Protozoan
  Toxoplasma gondii

Metazoan
  Toxocara canis
  Ancylostoma caninum
  Dirofilaria immitis

From Krakowka, S.: Transplacentally acquired microbial and parasitic diseases of dogs. J. Am. Vet. Med. Assoc. *171*:750, 1977.

microorganisms. When the maternal and fetal blood supplies are separated by only a few layers of tissue, such as in primates and rabbits (Table 18-1), there is considerable transfer of immune bodies from dam to fetus before delivery. In the endotheliochorial type of placentation (dog and cat), there is limited transfer across the placenta of maternal immunoglobulins. In farm animals, such as pigs, cattle, sheep, and particularly the mare (epitheliochorial placenta), there is little, if any, transplacental passage of molecules as large as immunoglobulins. In the mare, however, a good alternate system for transfer of immune bodies exists via colostrum. Mammary tissue is unable to synthesize immunoglobulins but is able to selectively secrete and concentrate serum immunoglobulin in the colostrum before delivery. Because of the need of the newborn foal for immunoglobulins, it is important that the foal suckle soon after delivery. The epithelium of the foal's small intestine is unique tissue, since it can absorb large molecules such as colostral immunoglobulin by an active process called pinocytosis or "cell drinking." Unfortunately, these intestinal epithelial cells have a short life and are replaced within 24 to 36 hours by mature cells which will not permit passage of immunoglobulin. Occasionally, a mare's milk may be low in immunoglobulin due to premature lactation several days or weeks before parturition. Since colostrum is secreted only once each pregnancy, a loss before parturition can result in a lowered level of immunoglobulin.[44]

In other domestic species, transplacental transfer is insufficient to ensure a high neonatal level of immunoglobulin; consequently the need for colostral immunoglobulin is important.

REFERENCES

1. Adams, W. M. (1969): The elective induction of labor and parturition in cattle. J. Am. Vet. Med. Assoc. *154*:261.
2. Allen, W. R. (1970): Endocrinology of early pregnancy in the mare. Equine Vet. J. *2*:64.
3. Alliston, C. W., and Ulberg, L. C. (1961): Early pregnancy loss in sheep at ambient temperatures of 70° and 90°F as determined by embryo transfer. J. Anim. Sci. *20*:608.
4. Alm, C. C., Sullivan, J. J., and First, N. L. (1974): Induction of premature parturition by parenteral administration of dexamethosone in the mare. J. Am. Vet. Med. Assoc. *168*(8):721.
5. Amoroso, E. C. (1952): Placentation. In: Marshall's Physiology of Reproduction, edited by A. S. Parkers. London, Longmans, Green & Co.
6. Barben, E. E. (1969): A practical laboratory test for diagnosing pregnancy in the mare. Vet. Med. Small Anim. Clin. *64*:231.
7. Barcroft, J. (1946): Researches on Pre-natal Life. Oxford, Oxford University Press.
8. Barnes, R. J., Comline, R. S., Jeffcott, L. B., et al. (1978): Foetal and maternal plasma concentrations of 13, 14-dihydro-15-oxo-prostaglandin F in the mare during late pregnancy and at parturition. J. Endocrinol. *78*:201.
9. Beaver, B. G. (1973): Supernumerary fetation in the cat. Feline Pract. *3*:24.
10. Binn, W., James, L. F., Shupe, J. L., et al. (1963): A congenital cyclopian-type malformation in lambs induced by maternal ingestion of *Veratrum californicum*. Am. J. Vet. Res. *24*:1164.
11. Bjorkman, N. (1965): Fine structure of the ovine placentome. J. Anat. *99*:283.
12. Cox, J. E. (1969): Rectal temperature as an indicator of approaching parturition in the mare. Equine Vet. J. *1*:174.
13. Cross, B. A. (1958): On the mechanism of labour in the rabbit. J. Endocrinol. *16*:261.
14. Csapo, A. (1956): Progesterone "block," Am. J. Anat. *98*:273.
15. Debackere, M., and Peeters, G. (1960): The influence

of vaginal distention on milk ejection and diuresis in the lactating cow. Arch. Int. Pharmacodyn. Ther. *123*:462.

16. Drost, M. (1972): Failure to induce parturition in pony mares with dexamethasone. J. Am. Vet. Med. Assoc. *160*:462.
17. Dutt, R. H., Ellington, E. F., and Carlton, W. W. (1971): Fertilization rate and early embryo survival in sheared and unsheared ewes exposed to high ambient temperatures. J. Anim.Sci. *18*:1308.
18. Elmore, R. G., Martin, C. E., Riley, J. L., et al. (1979): Body temperatures of farrowing swine. J. Am. Vet. Med. Assoc. *174*:620.
19. Foster, M. (1891): Textbook of Physiology. London.
20. Gee, C. D. (1971): A case of superfoetation in the cow. Aust. Vet. J. *47*:179.
21. Gunther, S. (1955): Die geburtsfunktion des uterus bicornis unter physiologischen verhaltnissen. Arch. Exp. Veterinaermed. *9*:93.
22. Hart, B. L. (1972): Feline behavior. Maternal behavior. I. Feline Pract. *2*:6.
23. Heap, R. B., Linzell, J. L., and Laing, J. A. (1974): Pregnancy diagnosis in cows: use of progestagen concentration in milk. Vet. Rec. *94*:160.
24. Helper, L. C. (1970): Diagnosis of pregnancy in the bitch with an ultrasonic Doppler instrument. J. Am. Vet. Med. Assoc. *156*:60.
25. Hindson, J. C., Schofield, B. M., Turner, C. B., et al. (1965): Parturition in sheep. J. Physiol. *181*:560.
26. Hoffman, B., Gunzler, O., Hamburger, R., et al. (1976): Milk progesterone as a parameter for fertility control in cattle. Br. Vet. J. *132*:469.
27. Hoffman, B., Wagner, W. C., Rattenberger, E., et al. (1977): Endocrine relationships during late gestation and parturition in the cow. *In* The Fetus and Birth. Ciba Foundation Symp. 47, p. 107. Amsterdam, Elsevier/Excerpta Medica/North Holland.
28. Inskeeps, E. K. (1973): Potential use of prostaglandins in control of reproductive cycles of domestic animals. J. Anim. Sci. *36*:1149.
29. Kilgour, R. (1972): Behavior of sheep at lambing. N.Z. J. Agric. *125*:24.
30. Koch, W. (1951): Psychogene beeinflussing des geburtstermins bei pferden. Z. Tierpsychol. *8*:441.
31. Legors, J. J., Peeters, G., Marcus, S., et al. (1977): Release of neurohysins I and II during and after parturition in cows. J. Endocrinol. *74*:487.
32. Liggins, G. C., Grieves, S. A., Kendall, S. F., et al. (1972): The physiological roles of progesterone, oestradiol-17 and prostaglandin 2 in the control of ovine parturition. J. Reprod. Fertil. *16*:85.
33. Maarten, D. (1972): Failure to induce parturition in pony mares with dexamethasone. J. Am. Vet. Med. Assoc. *160*:321.
34. McDonald, L. E., McNutt, S. H., and Nichols, R. E. (1954): Retained placenta—experimental production and prevention. Am. J. Vet. Res. *15*(54):22.
35. Mahaffey, L. W. (1961): *In* Ciba Foundation Symposium on Somatic Stability in the Newly Born, edited by G. E. W. Walstenholme and Maeve O'Connor. Boston, Little, Brown & Co.
36. Moller, K. (1970): A review of uterine involution and ovarian activity during the post parturient period in the cow. N.Z. Vet. J. *18*:83.
37. Monty, D. E., and Wolff, L. K. (1974): Summer heat

stress and reduced fertility in Holstein-Friesian cows in Arizona. Am. J. Vet. Res. *35*:1495.
38. Needham, J. (1931): Chemical Embryology. Cambridge, Cambridge University Press.
39. Omtvedt, I. T., Nelson, R. E., Edwards, R. L., et al. (1971): Influence of heat stress during early mid and late pregnancy of gilts. J. Anim. Sci. *32*:312.
40. Perry, J. S., and Rowlands, I. W. (1962): Early pregnancy in the pig. J. Reprod. Fertil. *4*:175.
41. Rawlings, N. C., and Ward, W. R. (1978): Correlations of maternal and fetal endocrine events with uterine presure changes around parturition in the ewe. J. Reprod. Fertil. *54*:1.
42. Reimers, T. J., Dziuk, P. J., Bahr, J., et al. (1973): Transuterine embryonal migration in sheep, anteroposterior orientation of pig and sheep fetuses and presentation of piglets at birth. J. Anim. Sci. *37*:1212.
43. Rossdale, P. D., and Short, R. V. (1967): The time of foaling of thoroughbred mares. J. Reprod. Fert. *13*:341.
44. Rumbaugh, G. E., Ardans, A. A., Ginno, D., et al. (1979): Identification and treatment of colostrum-deficient foals. J. Am. Vet. Med. Assoc. *174*:273.
45. Scanlon, P. F. (1972): Frequency of transuterine migration of embryos in ewes and cows. J. Anim. Sci. *34*:791.
46. Sharafeldin, M. A., Ragab, M. T., and Kandeel, A. A. (1971): Behavior of ewes during parturition. J. Agric. Sci. *76*:419.
47. Shemesh, M., Ayalon, N., and Lindner, H. R. (1973): Early pregnancy diagnois based upon plasma progesterone levels in the cow and ewe. J. Anim. Sci. *36*:726.
48. Sittmann, K. (1973): Intrauterine migration of pig embryos in litters without losses. Can. J. Anim. Sci. *53*:71.
49. Smith, V. G., Edgerton, L. A., Hafs, H. D., et al. (1973): Bovine serum estrogens, progestins and glucocorticoids during late pregnancy, parturition and early lactation. J. Anim. Sci. *36*:391.
50. Stabenfeldt, G. H., Edqvist, L.-E., Kindhal, et al. (1978): Practical implications of recent physiologic findings for reproductive efficiency in cows, mares, sows, and ewes. J. Am. Vet. Med. Assoc. *172*:667.
51. Stone, W. M., and Girardeau, M. H. (1967): Transmammary passage of infective-stage nematode larvae. Vet. Med. Small Anim. Clin. *62*:252.
52. Swercezek, T. W., Nielsen, S. W., and Helmboldt, C. F. (1971): Transmammary passage of *Toxocara cati* in the cat. Am. J. Vet. Res. *32*:89.
53. Tavern, M., Van Der Weyden, G., Fontijne, P., et al. (1977): Uterine position and presentation of minipig-fetuses and their order and presentation at birth. Am. J. Vet. Res. *38*:1761.
54. Thorburn, G. D., Challis, J. R. C., and Currie, W. B. (1977): Control of parturition in domestic aniamls. Biol. Reprod. *16*:18.
55. Umo, I., Fitzpatrick, R. J., and Ward, W. R. (1976): Parturition in the goat: Plasma concentrations of prostaglandin F and steroid hormones and uterine activity during late pregnancy and parturition. J. Endocrinol. *68*:383.
56. Van Rensberg, S. J. (1971): Reproductive physiology and endocrinology of normal and habitually aborting Angora goats. Onderstepoort J. Vet. Res. *38*:1.

57. van Tienhoven, A. (1968): Chapter 12. *In* Reproductive Physiology of Vertebrates. Philadelphia, W. B. Saunders Co.

58. Veznik, Z., Holub, A., Zraly, Z., et al. (1979): Regulation of bovine labor with a long-acting carba-analog of oxytocin: A preliminary report. Am. J. Vet. Res. *40*:425.

59. Wagner, W. C., Thompson, F. N., Evans, L. E., et al. (1974): Hormonal mechanisms controlling parturition. J. Anim. Sci. *38*:39.

60. Wagner, W. C., Willham, R. L., and Evans, L. E. (1974): Controlled parturition in cattle. J. Anim. Sci. *38*:485.

61. Walker, D. (1972): Pregnancy diagnosis in pigs. Vet. Rec. *90*:139.

62. Warnick, A. C., Wallace, H. D., Palmer, A. Z., et al. (1965): Effect of temperatures in early embryo survival in gilts. J. Anim. Sci. *24*:89.

63. Warren, E. G. (1969): Nematode larvae in milk. Austl. Vet. J. *45*:388.

64. Winters, L. M., Green, W. W., and Comstock, R. E. (1942): Prenatal development of the bovine. Minn. Agric. Exp. Sta. Tech. Bull. 151.

Embryo Transfer in Domestic Animals

R. A. BOWEN and M. H. PINEDA

19

EMBRYO transfer refers to the techniques by which fertilized oocytes are collected from a female called the *donor* and transferred, for development to term, to another female known as the *recipient*. The chain of events in the process of embryo transfer includes management of the donor for production of a suitable number of viable oocytes, mating or artificial insemination, collection, evaluation, and short-term storage of embryos from the donor, and finally, the transfer of these embryos to suitable recipients. Also associated with embryo transfer are a number of ancillary procedures, including maintenance of a rigorous health program for both donors and recipients and the keeping of a detailed series of records for every aspect of the program.

For simplicity and consistency in nomenclature, the term *embryo* will be used in this chapter to refer to any stage of embryonal development from the one-cell fertilized oocyte to the preattachment blastocyst.

The main objective of embryo transfer is the improvement of animal populations through increased utilization of superior females. Artificial insemination in several mammalian species, and especially in dairy cattle, has substantially contributed to the dissemination of superior genetic material from the male, allowing acceleration of genetic selection at a much greater rate than could be hoped for with natural matings. Theoretical arguments have been developed which imply that embryo transfer will never be a tool for genetic improvement as efficient as artificial insemination, primarily because of the comparatively small number of oocytes released even in superovulated animals. However, there is no doubt that embryo transfer allows expansion of desirable genetic pools for breed improvement.

The expansion of genetic pools provided by embryo transfer is especially important for monotocous species, such as the bovine and equine, which have long gestation periods and low rates of reproduction. In these species, the intensity of selection that can be applied and the natural rate of genetic improvement are limited by this relatively low reproductive efficiency. It has been estimated that the ovaries of a prepubertal heifer contain more than 100,000 oocytes. Even under ideal conditions of health and management, a highly productive cow may produce only 8 to 12 calves in her reproductive lifetime. Using current technology for superovulation and embryo transfer, it is feasible to obtain 30 to 40 calves from a single cow over a period of a year. The intensity of genetic selection of females is thus facilitated by embryo transfer, since it is possible to obtain several daughters, all of the same age, from a single mating of a superior dam, by using recipients of a lesser genetic value as foster mothers. Due to the enhancement of reproductive potential, careful selection of embryo donors is as important as the selection of the sire to avoid propagation of undesirable, heritable traits.

The transfer of embryos also offers other important, potential, or real contributions to the livestock industry. Reliable induction of twinning in cattle would be of great benefit, and embryo transfer appears as the most promising of the available methods to induce twinning. The generation interval from birth to reproductive age can be shortened by obtaining and transferring embryos from prepubertal animals. Control of sex ratio has been an extremely sought after technique for many years, and fulfillment of this ideal would revolutionize animal production. Separation of X-bearing from Y-bearing spermatozoa would represent the ultimate tool for control of the sex ratio, but to date, results in this area have been disappointing (see Chapter 7). The sexing of early embryos and the transfer of only those of the desired sex have been achieved experimentally in laboratory animals and cattle. The use of this technique, especially when coupled with low temperature preservation of sexed embryos, offers exciting possibilities for the livestock industry in the near future.

Infertility, especially in the older animal, is one of most wasteful and economically devastating problems of the livestock industry. In the majority of cases, infertile food-producing animals should be culled. There are, however, many genetically superior females which become infertile due to uterine or oviductal diseases or to old age, and in many instances embryo transfer techniques can be used to obtain additional progeny from such animals.

Embryo transfer also offers new opportunities for reproduction of other domestic and nondomestic animals. Embryo transfer may some day be used in companion animals as it is today in farm animals. There is also increasing interest in managing reproduction in endangered species and some zoo animals, and this has prompted the development of superovulation and embryo transfer techniques in a variety of wild animals.

Embryo transfer has expanded rapidly in the last few years. Only a few years ago, problems in development of technology for recovery, storage, and transfer of embryos, variability in results, and the high costs of performing embryo transfer precluded its extensive application to farm animals. As a result of stimulation for research in this field, prompted in large part by economic demand, embryo transfer is now utilized commercially throughout the world in cattle, sheep, and swine and to a lesser extent, in horses. Table 19-1 shows an example of the demand for and success achieved in transferring bovine embryos during the early years of its commercial application. In 1985, approximately 100,000 calves were born in North America alone from embryo transfer.

In addition to commercial applications, embryo transfer technology is being used at an ever-increasing rate in basic and applied research. Embryo transfer has been useful in investigations of spermatozoal capacitation, *in vitro* fertilization, and embryonic differentiation. Furthermore, investigations of viral infections of embryos and attempts to detect carriers of heritable diseases provide another application for embryo transfer techniques.

Table 19-1 Example of Increasing Demand and Success Achieved at Bovine Embryo Transfer in a Large Embryo Transfer Center

Year	1971	1973	1975*
Number of donors accepted	11	142	501
Number of successful donors	4	94	396
Average number of oocytes recovered (range)	8.1 (0–70)	7.9 (0–43)	10.4 (0–44)
Average number of embryos transferred (range)	11.4 (0–34)	5.6 (0–21)	8.2 (0–37)
Average number of successful pregnancies per donor (range)	2.1 (1–6)	3.4 (1–15)	4.4 (1–20)

Adapted from Church, R. B., and Shea, B. F.: Can. J. Anim. Sci. *57*:33, 1977.

* Includes first, second, third, and fourth superovulations of the same donor.

INCREASING THE AVAILABILITY OF EMBRYOS

The availability of embryos for transfer may be increased by inducing superovulation in adult and prepubertal animals or by using oocytes harvested directly from the ovarian follicles of prepubertal or adult animals. Induction of twinning in monotocous species by transfer of two embryos has been successful, but the higher abortion rate and other complications of twin pregnancy limit the routine use of this technique.

Superovulation in Adult Animals

Superovulation can be defined as the increased ovulatory response, above the number that would be expected to occur naturally, generated in an animal by the administration of exogenous gonadotropic hormones. The main objective of superovulatory treatment with gonadotropins is to increase the number of oocytes released by an animal, and thereby the potential number of embryos. The yield of viable embryos after superovulation is more important for a successful embryo transfer program than the number of ovulations induced in each individual animal. Superovula-

tory treatment in the cow, ewe, goat, sow, and queen can generally increase the number of ovulations 2- to 10-fold over the normal rate of ovulation. The mare can also be superovulated, but the increase in ovulations is usually modest. Limited work has been done with superovulation in the bitch, and the results have been disappointing.

Pregnant mare serum gonadotropin (PMSG), partially purified follicle-stimulating hormone (FSH), and crude pituitary extracts containing both FSH and luteinizing hormone (LH) are used to stimulate follicular growth and ovulation in domestic animals (Table 19-2). Of these gonadotropins, FSH is currently the most widely used in cattle.

Administration of superovulatory hormones is generally begun 3 to 5 days prior to the onset of estrus. Estrus and ovulation are then allowed to occur naturally. A much more reliable and commonly used method of timing superovulation is based on the discovery that prostaglandin $F_{2\alpha}$ ($PGF_{2\alpha}$) induces luteolysis in several species. $PGF_{2\alpha}$ and a series of synthetic analogues are now available to regulate the length of the estrous cycle when administered during the luteal phase of the cycle. The use of prostaglandins to synchronize the cycle in conjunction with superovulatory regimens allows for a more constant length of exposure to gonadotropins, and cows treated with $PGF_{2\alpha}$ during superovulation yield larger numbers of transferable embryos than cows superovulated without the use of $PGF_{2\alpha}$. Superovulatory treatments commonly used in cattle are shown in Table 19-2.

The greatest problem with superovulation is the large degree of variation in superovulatory response between individuals of the same species. At this time, there is no reliable way of predicting the number of oocytes that will be released from an animal in response to exogenous gonadotropins. Much of this variability may be due to genetic differences between animals, but differences in the potency, purity, and quality of commercially available gonadotropic preparations, and also in the species of origin of the preparation, may con-

Table 19-2   Superovulatory Treatments for Cattle

Gonadotropin Treatment	Prostaglandin Treatment	Days from Treatment to Estrus Interval
PMSG: 1500 IU as a single intramuscular injection on day* 15 or 16 of the estrous cycle	None	2–8 after PMSG
PMSG: 1500 IU as a single intramuscular injection, given on any day from 8–12 of the estrous cycle	$PGF_{2\alpha}$[†]: 25–30 mg as a single intramuscular injection 40–48 hours after PMSG	2–3 after $PGF_{2\alpha}$
PMSG: 5 IU/kg body weight as a single intramuscular injection on any day from 9–13 of the estrous cycle	$PGF_{2\alpha}$: 25 mg as a single intramuscular injection 48 hours after PMSG	2–3 after $PGF_{2\alpha}$
FSH[‡] mixed with LH[§] in a ratio of 5 : 1 and injected subcutaneously twice daily in doses of 5, 4, 3, 2, 2 mg FSH (5 days); total dose of 32 mg FSH	$PGF_{2\alpha}$: 30 mg split into two intramuscular injections 8 hours apart on the third or fourth day of FSH	2–3 after $PGF_{2\alpha}$
FSH: Mixed with LH in a ratio of 5 : 1 and injected subcutaneously twice daily, but given at a dose schedule of 7, 6, 4, 1 mg FSH (4 days); total dose of 36 mg FSH	Cloprostenol: 1 mg as a single intramuscular injection 48 hours after the first FSH treatment	2–3 after Cloprostenol

Data from Betteridge, K. J.: Embryo Transfer in Farm Animals. Canada Department of Agriculture, Monograph 16, 1977, p. 1; Elsden, R. P., et al.: Theriogenology *9*:17, 1978; Hasler, J. F.: Personal communication. 1979; Phillipo, M., and Rowson, L. E. A.: Ann. Biol. Anim. Biochem. Biophys. *15*:233, 1975; and Moore, N. W.: Aust. J. Agric. Res. *26*:295, 1975.

* First day of estrus = day 0.
† THAM salt of prostaglandin $F_{2\alpha}$.
‡ Porcine FSH (Armour); manufacturer's claim: 1.0 mg is equivalent to 9.4–13.2 IU.
§ Equine LH (Armour).

tribute to the variable response to superovulatory treatment. The general health, lactational status, and past reproductive performance of the donor certainly influence the response to superovulation. Cows that are "problem breeders" ovulate significantly lower numbers of oocytes in response to superovulatory treatments, and significantly fewer transferable embryos can be recovered from these cows than from reproductively healthy cows (Table 19-3). Older cows appear to be less responsive to superovulatory treatments with gonadotropins than heifers (Table 19-4). Other factors that may contribute to this variability include breed differences and seasonal effects.

PMSG and pituitary gonadotropins have been satisfactorily used to superovulate cycling ewes, or ewes synchronized with progestagens or prostaglandins (Table 19-5). The superovulatory response is poor in anestrous ewes during the nonbreeding season. Superovulation can be induced in the goat with a regimen similar to that used in ewes (Table 19-5).

The cycling sow responds well to superovulatory treatments with PMSG and does not require supplementary treatment to induce ovulation, although hCG can be administered to more precisely time ovulation. Most sows come into estrus 3 to 7 days after weaning and superovulating doses of PMSG can be administered to match that event. Also, superovulation can be initiated 24 hours prior to $PGF_{2\alpha}$-induced luteolysis in pregnant or pseudopregnant sows (Table 19-6). Suppression of estrus by administration of progestins, followed by their withdrawal has been used to synchronize estrus in donor sows, but is associated with a relatively high incidence of adverse effects.

Even though follicular growth can be induced, the ovaries of both the mare and the bitch appear to be resistant to ovulatory stimulation by exogenous gonadotropins. Pro-

Table 19-3   Superovulatory Response* in Reproductively "Healthy" and "Problem" Lactating Holstein Cows

	Reproductive Status	
	Healthy	Problem
Superovulation treatments	174	122
Number of cows superovulated	144	94
Age (years)	$7.8 \pm 3.2^{\dagger}$	10.1 ± 3.1
Months in lactation	5.2 ± 3.6	15.4 ± 7.9
Number of:		
corpora lutea	11.5 ± 7.6	8.2 ± 6.8
oocytes recovered	9.2 ± 8.2	5.9 ± 7.0
fertilized oocytes	6.4 ± 6.1	2.7 ± 5.2
transferable embryos	5.9 ± 5.9	2.1 ± 4.1
Number of cows with:		
at least one transferable embryo	139/174 (80%)	56/122 (46%)
three or more corpora lutea	160/174 (92%)	91/122 (75%)

From J. F. Hasler: Personal communication. 1979.
* Superovulation induced with Armour porcine FSH and LH; see Table 19-2.
† Mean $\pm$ standard deviation.

longed treatment with crude or with partially purified equine pituitary gonadotropins containing both FSH and LH activities produces a restricted superovulatory response in cycling or seasonally anovulatory pony mares (Table 19-7). Seasonally anovulatory mares require daily treatment for 14 days, and cycling mares for up to 6 days to induce a maxi-

mum of 4 ovulations per mare. Pregnancy rates after transfer of embryos from superovulated mares are generally lower than the pregnancy rates obtained after the transfer of embryos from normally ovulating mares. Thus, while some progress has been made in equine superovulation, it has not advanced to the point of routine use. Although some

Table 19-4   Response of Heifers and Cows to Superovulatory Treatments*

		Dose of PMSG, IU† or AP, mg‡	Number of Animals		Number of Oocytes		
	Treatment		Treated	In Estrus	Ovulated	Recovered	Fertilized
Heifers	Prog-PMSG§	1500–2700 IU	11	9 (82%)	82	48 (59%)	43 (90%)
Cows	Prog-PMSG§	1500–2700 IU	36	29 (81%)	74	53 (72%)	38 (72%)
Heifers	Prog-AP	60–107 mg	12	11 (92%)	74	60 (81%)	59 (98%)
Cows	Prog-AP	60–107 mg	33	21 (64%)	66	49 (74%)	39 (80%)
Heifers	PG-AP$^{\|}$	107 mg	4	3 (75%)	21	14 (67%)	14 (100%)
Cows	PG-AP.	60–107 mg	35	24 (69%)	88	59 (67%)	48 (81%)
	PG-PMSG	1500–2700 IU	36	24 (67%)	119	93 (78%)	76 (82%)

Adapted from Moore, N. W.: Tables 2, 3, and 5. Aust. J. Agric. Res. *26:*295, 1975.
* Heifers, 14 to 18 months of age; cows, $\geq$ 8 years of age.
† Pregnant mare serum gonadotropin given as a single subcutaneous injection on the day of the second-last injection of progesterone or the day before $PGF_{2\alpha}$.
‡ Equine anterior pituitary extracts given in three equal daily subcutaneous injections from the day before the last injection of progesterone or the day before the first injection of prostaglandin.
§ Prog = progesterone, 40 mg in daily intramuscular injections for 17 to 30 days, beginning on the 8th to 14th day after estrus.
$^{\|}$ PG = prostaglandin $F_{2\alpha}$, 500 μg/day, infused into the uterus for 2 consecutive days between the 8th and 14th day after estrus.

Table 19-5 Superovulatory Treatments for Ewes and Goats

Species	Gonadotropin Treatment	Estrus Synchronization Treatment	Treatment to Estrus Interval
Ewe	PMSG: 20–45 IU/kg body weight (maximum of 2000 IU) in a single intramuscular injection on day* 11, 12, or 13 of the estrous cycle	None	2–4 days after PMSG
	PMSG: 700–1300 IU in a single intramuscular injection on any day from 4 to 13 of the estrous cycle	Cloprostenol: intramuscular injection of 100 μg, 24 to 72 hrs after PMSG	36–40 hours after prostaglandin
	PMSG: as above; 24 hours before or at the time of progestogen withdrawal	Progesterone in oil: daily intramuscular injection of 10 mg	2–4 days after PMSG
Goat	PMSG: 1000–1500 IU in a single intramuscular injection on day 16, 17, or 18 of the estrous cycle; 1000 IU hCG at the onset of estrus	None	2–4 days after PMSG
	Equine pituitary extract:[†] 12–15 mg by daily intramuscular injection on three consecutive days, beginning on the day before the final injection of progesterone	Progesterone: 12 mg/day for 16 to 18 days	Within 2 days of progesterone withdrawal

Data from: Betteridge, K. J., and Moore, N. W.: Embryo Transfer in Farm Animals. Canada Department of Agriculture, Monograph 16, 1977, p. 37; Hancock, J. L., and Hovel, G. J. R.: J. Reprod. Fertil. *2*:295, 1961; Moore, N. W.: Proc. Aust. Soc. Anim. Prod. *10*:246, 1974, Nishikawa, Y., et al.: Proc. Jpn. Acad. *39*:610, 1963, cited by Betteridge, K. J., et al.; Trounson, A. O., et al.: J. Agri. Sci. *86*:609, 1976.
* First day of estrus = day 0.
[†] Prepared by the authors (Moore, N. W.).

degree of success has been achieved in stimulating follicular growth and ovulation in the anestrous bitch, the results have been disappointing.

Porcine or ovine FSH has been successfully used to induce estrus in anestrous cats, followed by hCG treatment to induce ovulation (Table 19-8). PMSG in single or in multiple injections induces follicular growth in cats, but the ovulatory response to hCG treat-

ment after PMSG seems more variable than the ovulatory response to hCG after FSH treatment.

It is desirable to superovulate valuable donors repeatedly to obtain as many embryos as possible. However, repeated treatment with gonadotropins may induce the formation of antibodies to the gonadotropins, resulting in a lower number of oocytes ovulated with each successive treatment. Heterologous gonado-

Table 19-6 Superovulatory Treatments for Sows and Postpubertal Gilts

Gonadotropin Treatment		Days from Treatment to Estrus
to Induce Follicular Growth	to Induce Ovulation	
PMSG: 1000–1500 IU in a single intramuscular injection on day* 15 of the estrous cycle	None	3–4 after PMSG
PMSG: 1500 IU in a single intramuscular injection 24 hours after PGF$_{2\alpha}$ in sows synchronized by being made pregnant or pseudopregnant	hCG: 500, IU 3 days after PMSG	3–4 after PMSG

Data from Betteridge, K. J.: Embryo Transfer in Farm Animals. Canada Department of Agriculture, Monograph 16, 1977, p. 41; Martin, P. A.; Embryo Transfer in Swine. In: Current Therapy in Theriogenology 2, 1986, p. 66.
* First day of estrus = day 0.

Table 19-7   Superovulatory Treatments for Mares

	Gonadotropin Treatment		Treatment to Estrus Interval
	to Induce Follicular Growth	to Induce Ovulation	
Seasonally anovulatory mares	Crude equine pituitary gonadotropins,* injected subcutaneously twice daily for 14 days for a total dose of 13.2 mg/kg body weight over the 14-day period	hCG:[†] 2000 IU given by intramuscular injection on day 14[‡]	Some mares were in estrus at the time of treatment; ovulation occurred on days 14 or 15
Cycling mares	Equine pituitary gonadotropin preparation,[§] 750 Fevold-Hisaw rat units, injected subcutaneously daily for 7 days from day 14 through day 20 postovulation	hCG: 4000 IU by subcutaneous injection on day 20 postovulation	Ovulation occurred in most mares on the day of hCG injection (day 20)

Data from Douglas, R. H.: Theriogenology *11*:33, 1979; Douglas, R. H., et al.: Theriogenology *2*:133, 1974.
   * The total dose of 13.2 mg of crude pituitary fraction (prepared by the authors, Douglas, et al.) was equivalent to 6.5 units NIH-FSH-S1 and 0.6 units NIH-LH-S1.
   [†] hCG was not necessary to induce ovulation after treatment with equine pituitary gonadotropins, but synchronized ovulation within 2 days after administration.
   [‡] day 1 = first day of treatment.
   [§] Pitropin, Biological Specialties, Middleton, Wisconsin.

tropins are more likely to induce antibodies than homologous gonadotropins. Experimentally, cattle and various laboratory animals produce antibodies to gonadotropins in response, to superovulatory treatments, but the clinical effects of this response has not been adequately investigated. Another possible consequence of the immunogenicity of gonadotropins is anaphylaxis upon repeated treatments. Clinically, however, this does not appear to be a common problem. When repeated superovulatory treatments are required, it is advisable to use purified, homologous gonadotropins whenever possible.

Superovulation in Prepubertal Animals

Follicular growth and ovulation can be induced in prepubertal animals of some species by treatment with exogenous gonadotropins. Although this technique has not advanced to the point of commercial or routine experimental use, induction of superovulation and transfer of embryos from prepubertal animals would allow early progeny testing and shortening of the generation interval. However, the genetic implications of transferring embryos from young animals, which have not been proven, need to be carefully evaluated. The

Table 19-8   Superovulatory Treatments for Anestrous Cats

Gonadotropin		Days from Treatment to Estrus
to Induce Follicular Growth	to Induce Ovulation	
FSH*: 2.0 mg daily; intramuscular injections until onset of estrus	hCG: 250 IU, intramuscular injections on days 1 and 2 of estrus	4 to 5 after first FSH treatment
PMSG: 200 or 400 IU; single injection	hCG: 200 IU on day 2 of estrus	3 to 6 after PMSG

Data from Wildt, D. E., et al.: Lab. Anim. Sci. *28*:301, 1978; Bowen, R. A.: Unpublished.
   * Porcine FSH, Armour-Baldwin Laboratories.

age of the prospective donor appears to be a limiting factor in the response to superovulation and in the quality of embryos recovered. Although there is species variation, sensitivity of the ovaries to stimulation with exogenous gonadotropins increases gradually from birth to puberty, and the closer the animal is to puberty, the better the response to superovulatory treatments.

Calves of one month of age or older can be superovulated with high doses of PMSG, followed by supplementary treatment with LH or hCG to induce ovulation. The rates of fertilization, embryo recovery, and embryonic viability are low and PMSG alone does not assure ovulation in young calves. The administration of progestagens with PMSG treatment apparently induces the release of endogenous LH, resulting in ovulation, but the quality of the embryos recovered is unsatisfactory for transfer.

Superovulation can be induced in lambs older than one month of age by priming the lambs with progesterone injections before PMSG treatment. Exogenous LH or hCG does not appear to be necessary for inducing ovulation in this situation.

Prepubertal gilts can be superovulated with PMSG followed in 48 hours by treatment with hCG or by combining PMSG and hCG in a single injection. The embryos recovered from superovulated prepubertal gilts appear to be suitable for transfer.

Induction of Twinning

The economical implications of a controlled increase in ovulation rate to obtain maximal numbers of offspring per pregnancy in meat-producing animals has prompted research to artificially induce twin pregnancies in cows and multiple pregnancies in the ewe. The economical advantage of producing two calves per pregnancy in the cow, even at the cost of an increased incidence of freemartins, and two or three lambs per pregnancy in the ewe are obvious for a world in urgent need of increased food production. Genetic selection, treatment with exogenous gonadotropins, and embryo transfer have been the major approaches used to induce twin pregnancies in cattle and sheep.

The natural frequency of twin births in cattle ranges between 1 and 5%. Genetic selection to increase the incidence of twinning in cattle has not been successful, due to the low heritability and repeatability of the trait for twinning. In the ewe, genetic selection programs carried out in Australia have been successful, over a number of generations, in establishing groups of Peppin Merino ewes with high and low reproductive rates. The difference in fecundity between these two groups appears to be due to an increased number of ovulations in the line of ewes selected for high reproductive rate.

Exogenous gonadotropins have been given to cows and ewes in attempts to induce twin pregnancies. These efforts have not been successful, chiefly because the superovulatory response to gonadotropins has not been reliable, and in a majority of animals, either the number of ovulations was not increased, or more than the desired number of ovulations was induced. Fetal death and abortion is a common consequence of pregnancies of more than two calves in the cow or three lambs in the ewe; the prenatal mortality and abortions are believed due to uterine crowding. Thus, it appears that only when a reliable superovulatory treatment has been developed to induce moderate superovulation can this method of twinning be used with success on a practical scale.

Currently, embryo transfer seems to be the most promising tool available for inducing twin pregnancies in cattle. Two methods have been investigated in this regard: transfer of two embryos to an unbred recipient or transfer of one embryo to a recipient that has been inseminated at the most recent estrus and is presumed to be pregnant.

In heifers and cows, surgical transfer of one embryo to each uterine horn of recipients in close synchrony with the donor has resulted in twin pregnancy rates of over 60%, whereas the transfer of two embryos to one uterine horn results in a considerably lower incidence of twin pregnancies. A high rate of embryonal death occurs when bovine embryos are transferred to the uterine horn contralateral to the corpus luteum (Table 19-9; see also Chapter 9, Fig. 9-28), indicating the need to take into account the local utero-ovarian relationship for maintenance of the corpus luteum, when transferring embryos in species that ovulate unilaterally. Therefore, it is advisable to transfer one embryo to each horn, or to transfer a single embryo to the horn contralateral to the corpus luteum in recipients which have been inseminated. Each of these approaches furnishes an embryo to the horn ipsilateral to the ovary bearing the corpus luteum to provide the initial luteotropic stimulus for luteal maintenance.

Management procedures, especially in regard to nutrition and supervision of parturition, must be adjusted if twinning is to be used successfully. Clinical problems such as dystocia and increased incidence of retained placentae have been associated with twin births.

RECOVERY OF EMBRYOS

Embryo transfer evolved around the use of surgical techniques for the recovery of embryos. After the initial demonstration of the commercial feasibility of embryo transfer in cattle, the development and improvement of the less costly and less traumatic methods of embryo collection became a major goal in

Table 19-9 *Embryo Survival in Single Pregnancies Relative to Site of Corpus Luteum Following Twin Egg Transfers in Cows*

	Ipsilateral To CL	Contralateral to CL
No. of eggs transferred	13	13
No. of embryos at slaughter	9	4
% Survival	69.2	30.8

From Sreenan, J. M., et al.: Egg transfer in the cow: factors affecting pregnancy and twinning rates following bilateral transfers. J. Reprod. Fertil. *44*:77, 1975.

embryo transfer programs. As a result of the combined research efforts of several groups, techniques have been improved, and the recovery of embryos from cattle and horses is today carried out almost exclusively by nonsurgical means. Routine embryo recovery from sheep and swine remains a surgical procedure. Experimentally, however, embryos can be recovered by nonsurgical methods from these two species.

Surgical Methods

Even though there are minor differences in the techniques applied to each species, the basic approach for surgical recovery of embryos is similar for all species. Several variations in technique and equipment have been developed by different groups for surgical recovery of embryos. This discussion is intended to serve only as a general guide.

The donor of embryos is bred at estrus by natural service or, more commonly, by artificial insemination. Since superovulated animals tend to ovulate over an extended period of time, they are commonly inseminated more than once to ensure a high fertilization rate. In cattle, the donor is usually inseminated twice at approximately 12 and 24 hours after the onset of estrus.

Several factors influence the decision as to when the embryos should be recovered for transfer. Since the transfer of embryos to the uterus rather than to the oviducts generally is easier to perform and results in higher pregnancy rates, the recovery of embryos should coincide with the time when the embryos would normally be in the uterus of the donor. The requirements of synchrony of the estrus cycle between the donor and recipient appear to be less critical for older embryos. The upper limit for recovery time is determined by the size and fragility of the developing embryos, and in some species by the implantation time. Large, elongating blastocysts, such as those found in the cow after day 13, are difficult to recover without damage. In general, embryos are recovered between the 8-cell and blastocyst stages while still within the zona pellucida.

Surgical recovery of embryos is best carried out with the donor under general anesthesia. Feed and water should be withheld for 24 to 36 hours before the operation. This period of preoperative starvation is especially critical in ruminants, since they tend to bloat quickly, making exposure of the reproductive tract difficult and traumatic. Anesthesia may be induced with a short-acting thio- or oxybarbiturate given as an intravenous bolus. After intubation, anesthesia is maintained with halothane or a similar agent. The ventral abdomen is clipped, disinfected, and draped for aseptic surgery. The ovaries and uterine horns are exteriorized for flushing through a midline incision. After recovery of the embryos, the reproductive tract is replaced into the abdominal cavity and the incision is closed in a standard fashion.

The surgical procedures for the recovery of embryos often reduce the fertility of the donor at subsequent inseminations by causing periovarian adhesions. The fimbriae, where even minor adhesions can greatly interfere with oocyte transport, are the most critical sites for such problems. Consequently, surgical procedures should be carried out aseptically and as carefully as possible, making every effort to minimize trauma to the tissues. The exposed reproductive tract should be kept moist with saline solution and handled as little as possible.

Several basic techniques have been used for the actual recovery of embryos. In all procedures, a warm medium is flushed through the lumen of the reproductive tract and collected at some distal site. A variety of balanced salt solutions or complete cell culture media such as medium 199 have been used for recovering embryos; one of the most widely used media is Dulbecco's phosphate buffered saline (Table 19-10). These media are usually supplemented with blood serum or serum components to provide a source of protein and reduce the problem of embryos sticking to the glassware.

A method for the recovery of embryos from the uterus and oviducts of cattle utilizes a glass or plastic cannula and a blunt hypodermic needle attached to a syringe containing the flushing medium. The cannula is inserted in the fimbrial opening of the oviduct and maintained in position by finger pressure or with a small atraumatic clamp. The uterine horn is punctured at a site close to the intercornual bifurcation, and the medium is forced through the uterine horn and oviduct and out through the cannula into a collection dish (Fig. 19-1A). The surgeon should keep pressure on the uterus around the needle to prevent loss of medium. Passage of the medium through the tract is aided by gently milking the uterus. The volume of fluid to be infused depends on the size of the uterus, but generally varies between 25 and 100 ml. This method cannot be used in the mare, sow, or queen due to valve-like papillae at the uterotubal junction, which prevents fluid from being milked from the uterus into the oviduct. In these species the medium is flushed from the uterine horn.

When embryos are expected to be located exclusively in the uterus, because of the elapsed time from ovulation, only the uterine horns need be flushed (Fig. 19-1B). An important advantage of this approach is that the oviducts are not handled and fimbrial adhesions are less likely to be induced.

Nonsurgical Methods

To recover embryos nonsurgically, the donor cow is restrained in a standing position in a chute, and the perineal area is clipped of hair and disinfected. Epidural anesthesia is usually administered to prevent straining

Table 19-10 Phosphate-buffered Saline for Recovery and Storage of Embryos*

Compound	Concentration (g/l)	mM
NaCl	8.00	136.9
$CaCl_2$	0.10	0.9
$MgCl_2 \cdot 6H_2O$	0.10	0.5
KCl	0.20	2.7
KH_2PO_4	0.20	1.5
$Na_2HPO_4 \cdot 7H_2O$	2.16	8.1

* Commonly supplemented with serum.

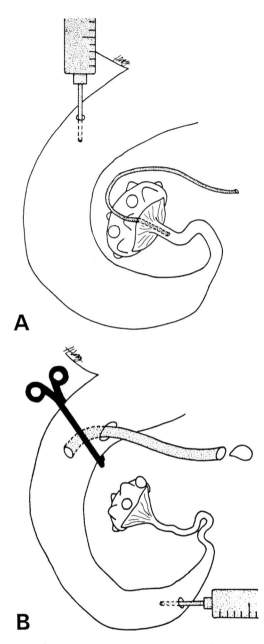

A

B

Fig. 19-1. Schematic representations of methods for surgical recovery of embryos. A, From the oviduct. B, From the uterus.

during the recovery. A variety of instruments have been used for nonsurgical recovery of embryos; one of the most successful of these is a soft rubber catheter such as the Foley catheter (Fig. 19-2C). This catheter is made of flexible latex and has three channels: one

to inflate a balloon near the tip of the catheter and two for the inflow and outflow of the flushing medium. The cervix is usually tightly closed at the time of embryo recovery, and a cervical dilator is required to dilate the cervical canal. Once the cervix is dilated, the catheter is maneuvered through the cervix with the aid of a stiff metal stylet. The balloon is inflated just proximal to the uterine bifurcation, and the uterine horns are flushed individually. After one horn is flushed, the balloon is deflated, the stylet is reinserted, and the catheter is placed in the other uterine horn. The medium used for flushing is fed through the inflow channel of the catheter by gravity flow from a suspended reservoir and the uterine horn is distended until it becomes turgid. The inflow is then interrupted, the out-flow channel is opened, and the accumulated fluid is allowed to drain into a collection cylinder. The whole procedure is monitored by palpation per rectum and aided by gentle massage of the uterine horns. The flushing and recovery procedure is repeated until approximately one liter of medium is flushed through each uterine horn. Few adverse effects of this type of nonsurgical recovery have been observed, and the fertility of the donor subsequent to several nonsurgical recoveries appears to be normal.

Excluding primates, the mare is the only other animal for which a routine procedure for nonsurgical recovery has been developed. The methods used for mares are basically modifications of those for cattle. Passage of the catheter through the cervix is much easier in the mare and the entire uterus is flushed at once.

The relative advantages and disadvantages of nonsurgical versus surgical methods for the recovery of embryos are compared in Table 19-11. The major disadvantage of surgical methods for the recovery of embryos is the virtually unavoidable induction of periovarian adhesions, which can reduce subsequent fertility. In addition, surgery under general anesthesia always carries the risks of anesthetic-related mortality, aspiration pneumonia from regurgitation, postoperative herniation,

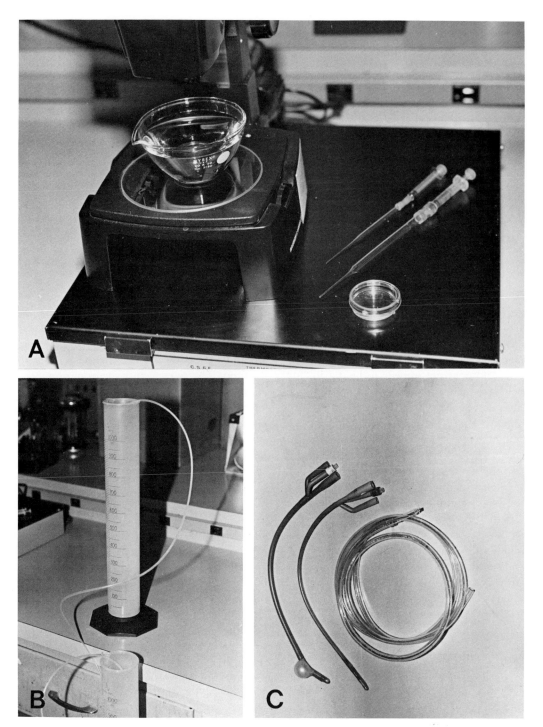

Fig. 19-2. Equipment used in bovine embryo transfer. A, Dissecting microscope, large glass dish used in searching for embryos, small Petri dish for short-term storage of embryos, glass pipets attached to syringes for manipulating embryos. B, Cylinders for collecting medium from nonsurgical embryo recoveries; C, Foley catheters and tubing used in nonsurgical recovery.

*Table 19-11 Comparison of Surgical and Nonsurgical
Methods for Recovery of Embryos*

	Method of Recovery	
End point	Surgical	Nonsurgical
Anesthesia	General	Epidural
Fasting	Required	Helpful, but not required
Ability to recover embryos at any stage	Excellent	Limited
Ability to accurately assess number of ovulations	Excellent	Poor
Risk of acute complications to donor	Definite possibility	Virtually nil
Risk to future reproductive performance of donor	Yes	Probably none
Embryo recovery rate	Excellent	Good
Ability to assess and give prognosis for reproductive tract pathology	Good	Poor
Can be performed on the farm	No	Yes

and other surgical complications. Even though these complications are actually rare, they do occur. Nonsurgical recovery, on the other hand, rarely results in any acute complications and does not appear to be detrimental to long-term fertility. Two major disadvantages of nonsurgical recovery are that 1) the embryos which are still in the oviduct at the time of recovery cannot be collected and 2) even a person skilled at rectal palpation can gain only a rough idea of the number of corpora lutea on superovulated ovaries as an indication of the number of ovulations. Finally, if a pathologic condition is present, such as oviductal obstruction or minor periovarian adhesions, rectal palpation of the genital tract while performing nonsurgical recovery cannot substitute for the direct visualization of such lesions, which is possible during surgical exposure of the reproductive tract.

HANDLING, EVALUATION, AND STORAGE OF EMBRYOS

After flushing the reproductive tract and collecting the flushing medium, the embryos must be located in the collection medium, recovered, and prepared for transfer or storage.

Location of Embryos after Recovery

The medium collected after flushing the reproductive tract is examined with a dissecting microscope to locate the embryos. A microscope is necessary due to the small size of the embryos and the presence of varying amounts of cellular debris in the recovered medium. The size of embryos from domestic animals changes little from fertilization to the onset of cavitation, the beginning of the blastocyst stage; the diameter across the zona pellucida in these embryos is approximately 150 microns. At later stages of embryonal development, the expanding blastocysts can be located without the aid of a microscope.

Finding the embryos, even in the large volume of fluid collected in a nonsurgical recovery, is greatly facilitated by the fact that embryos have a density greater than that of the collection medium and therefore sink to the bottom of the recovery vessel. Occasionally, however, embryos may be found floating near the surface of the medium. When the embryos are recovered in a large volume of fluid, a common practice is to collect the medium directly into a vessel with steep sides, such as a large graduated cylinder. Time is allowed for the embryos to settle to the bottom of the cylinder, and all but a small quantity of medium is gently siphoned from the top. The first quantity of medium to be siphoned should be collected in another cylinder, allowed to resettle, and then be resiphoned (Fig. 19-2B). The small quantity of medium left in the cylinders is then poured into a clear, glass or plastic dish for searching under the microscope. When only a small amount of medium is flushed from the donor, as with surgical collections, it may be collected directly into the searching dish. An alternative technique involves passing the recovered media directly from the donor animal through a nylon mesh filter that retains the embryos, but allows fluid and much of the cellular debris to pass through. The embryos retained on the surface of the filter are then washed into a small dish. Once located, embryos are transferred to another dish containing fresh, sterile medium. These and subsequent manipulations of the embryos are performed with small glass pipets or plastic catheters, which are attached to a syringe or operated by suction from a mouth-piece. The embryos are "washed" through several changes of fresh medium to remove contaminating debris and to dilute possible bacterial contamination. Mammalian embryos do not appear to be adversely affected by short-term exposure to room temperature, but the recovered medium and dishes containing the embryos are usually kept in an incubator at approximately 38°C. Exposure to cold drafts or especially to temperatures above body temperature should be avoided.

Short-term Storage of Embryos

A variety of media, ranging from simple balanced salt solutions supplemented with blood serum to complex cell culture media, have been used for maintenance of embryos between recovery and transfer. For short-term storage up to several hours, a simple medium such as described in Table 19-10 appears to be adequate. The pH of the storage medium should be in the range of 7.2 to 7.4. Media buffered with phosphate or one of the organic buffers such as HEPES (N-2-hydroxyethyl-piperazine-N'-2-ethanesulfonic acid) allow for the media to be kept in room atmosphere. Most standard cell culture media are based on a bicarbonate buffer system and these must be maintained in an atmosphere containing carbon dioxide (usually 5% CO_2 in air) to prevent a detrimental rise in pH. Another important variable in culture medium is osmolality. Media with an osmolality between 270 and 310 mOsm per kg are acceptable for embryo culture.

Transfer of embryos from cows, ewes, or sows to the oviduct of a rabbit has been used for short-term embryo storage. Such embryos continue to develop normally for a period of 2 to 3 days, after which they can be recovered and re-transferred to the original donor species. This technique has been used for long distance transport of embryos and for a variety of experimental purposes.

Evaluation of Embryos

A preliminary assessment of embryonic viability and differentiation between embryos and unfertilized oocytes can be made by examination under the dissecting microscope. A more definitive evaluation, especially with embryos of questionable quality, is done with a compound microscope (Fig. 19-3). An embryo is initially classified as being either transferable or nontransferable, according to whether it is judged to have a significant probability of establishing a pregnancy in the recipient. This can be a difficult judgment and is based primarily on how closely the recovered embryo corresponds with the expected stage of development normally found on that day of gestation (Table 19-12, Figs. 19-4 and 19-5). Unfertilized oocytes or an embryo whose development has been arrested early are generally easy to recognize as nontransferable (Fig. 19-6). However, cell fragmentation, which can give the false impression that a morula has been recovered, often occurs. Fragmented, nonviable embryos are often recognized because of large differences in the sizes of the various cellular fragments.

The next level of difficulty in classifying embryos occurs when the embryo is only moderately retarded in development. An example of this situation in cattle would be the recovery on day 7 of an early morula, generally seen on day 4 or 5, when one would expect an early blastocyst. Often, a mixture of embryos, some normal and some develop-

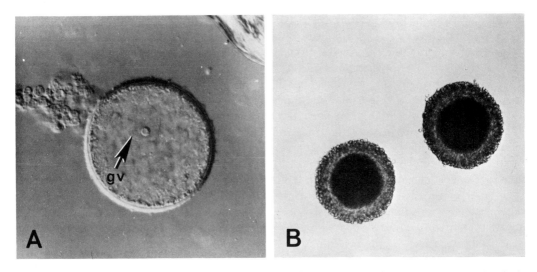

Fig. 19-3. Normal unfertilized oocytes. A, Follicular oocyte from a raccoon showing germinal vesicle (gv). B, Recently ovulated canine oocytes surrounded by cumulus cells.

mentally retarded, is recovered. The question that arises is whether the retarded embryo died at an earlier stage, or whether it is truly retarded in development, perhaps from being fertilized late, but still viable. Deciding whether an embryo is transferable rests primarily on economic considerations, and the probability of establishing a pregnancy from a retarded embryo must be weighed against the potential value of that offspring.

Table 19-12　Cleavage and Hatching of Embryos

Stage of Development	Species					
	Cow*	Ewe*	Sow*	Mare*	Bitch[†]	Cat*
1-cell	0–1	0–1	0–1	0–1	1–8	0–1
2-cell	1–2	0–1	0–1	0–1	—	1–2
4-cell	1–2	1–2	1–2	1–2	—	1–2
8-cell	2–3	2–3	2–3	2–3	—	2–3
Morula	3–6	3–6	3–5	2–5	5–12	4–6
Blastocyst	6–9	5–8	4–6	5–8	8–20	6–7
Hatching or hatched blastocyst	8–10	8–9	5–7	8–9	17–20	7–9

Data for Cow: Seidel, G. E., Bowen, R. A., and Elsden, R. P.: Colorado State University Embryo Transfer Program. Unpublished, 1979.

Ewe: Moore, N. W., and Shelton, J. N.: J. Reprod. Fertil. 7:145, 1964; Rowson, L. E. A., and Moore, R. M.: J. Anat. *100*:777, 1966.

Sow: Hunter, R. H. F.: Anat. Rec. *178*:169, 1974.

Mare: Betteridge, K. J.: Embryo Transfer in Farm Animals. Monograph No. 16, Canada Department of Agriculture, 1977.

Bitch: Holst, P. A., and Phemister, R. D.: Biol. Reprod., *5*: 194, 1971.

Cat: Bowen, R. A.: Unpublished, 1979.
* Days after ovulation.
[†] Days after onset of estrus.

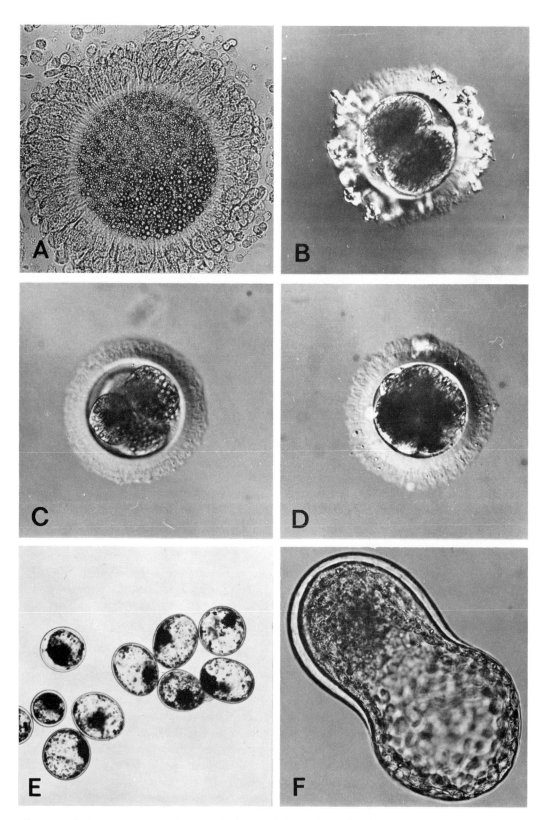

Fig. 19-4. Early embryonic development in the cat. A, Recently ovulated oocyte before fertilization, showing cumulus cells surrounding the zona pellucida. B, Two-cell embryo; C, Four-cell embryo. D, Early morula. E, Group of expanding blastocysts still within the zona pellucida. F, Hatching blastocyst.

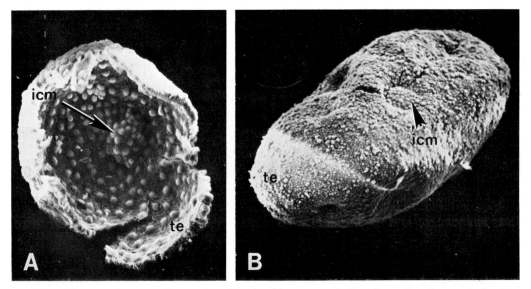

Fig. 19-5. Scanning electron micrographs of bovine blastocysts. A, Ten days after the onset of estrus (broken open to show blastocoel). B, Thirteen days after the onset of estrus. At this time the embryo is 3 to 4 mm long. Trophectoderm (te) and inner cell mass (icm).

Sexing Embryos before Transfer

In many cases, especially in cattle and horses, the offspring of one sex are much more valuable than those of the opposite sex. A demand for transfer of "presexed" embryos is thus created. Several approaches have been taken to fulfill this demand, but to date no technique has proven to be simple and reliable enough for routine use.

Direct examination of sex chromosomes from the embryonic cells can be used for sexing. The first step in such a procedure is to biopsy a group of cells from the embryo. Older embryos, such as day 13 or 14 blastocysts from cattle, tolerate the removal of small pieces of trophoblast relatively well. The biopsied embryo is then held in culture while the cells which have been removed are processed for cytogenetic analysis. Briefly, this procedure consists of a short-term culture for several hours of the fragment of trophoblast in the presence of an agent which arrests cells in metaphase and then staining the cells for determination of which sex chromosomes are present. If the embryo is of the desired sex, it is then taken from the culture medium and transferred; otherwise it is discarded. Using this technique, the sex of approximately two-thirds of the embryos examined can be determined. The preparations from the remaining one-third of the embryos are generally not of sufficient quality for accurate determination. An alternative method of sexing involves using specific antibodies to detect the presence of a male-specific antigen (H-Y antigen) on the surface of male embryos. After exposure of the embryo to H-Y antiserum and washing to remove unbound antibody, two general methods can be used to detect whether antibodies to H-Y antigen are bound to the embryos. One approach is to add complement to the culture medium, which results in membrane lysis and death of male embryos due to binding of the H-Y antibody. This technique has the obvious disadvantage that only female embryos survive the procedure. Alternatively, the antibody to the H-Y antigen can be fluorescently labeled so that only those embryos coated with antibody fluoresce during a brief exposure to ultraviolet light. Much of the developmental work with these immunologically-based sexing techniques is being conducted with rodent embryos and at the present time, must still be considered experimental. Improvements in accuracy and mod-

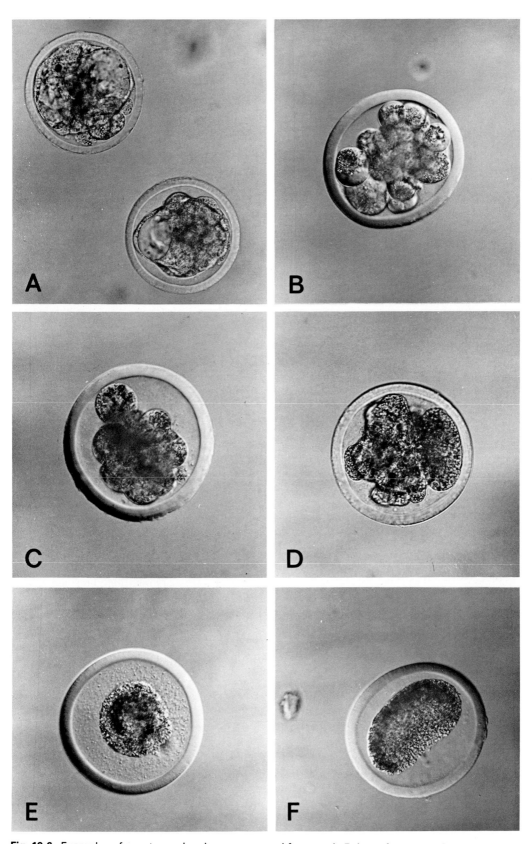

Fig. 19-6. Examples of oocytes and embryos recovered from cattle 7 days after onset of estrus. A, Early blastocysts. B, C, and D, Embryos with varying degrees of developmental retardation or fragmentation; classified as having a low probability of establishing a pregnancy if transferred. E and F, Degenerate, unfertilized oocytes.

ifications of the technique to ameliorate damage to the embryo will provide an extremely valuable addition to the technology of embryo transfer.

Long-term Storage of Embryos

Advances in the theory and practice of low temperature preservation of mammalian cells led to the report in 1972 of the birth of mammals (mice) which had been frozen as embryos. Within a short time, these cryobiological techniques had been successfully applied to embryos from cattle, sheep, mares and goats. Porcine embryos, on the other hand, are extremely sensitive to cooling and numerous attempts to freeze embryos from swine have been unsuccessful.

Frozen storage of embryos from farm animals offers several practical applications. The time for which embryos can be stored *in vitro* limits the distance over which embryos can be transported from donors in one area to recipients in another. These time limitations are abolished by low temperature preservation. The establishment of banks of frozen embryos has already begun with valuable laboratory animals and may be useful for livestock improvement programs. If large numbers of embryos are obtained from a donor, the excess embryos can be frozen and then transferred at some later time.

MANAGEMENT OF RECIPIENTS AND TRANSFER OF EMBRYOS

The methods for transferring embryos to recipient females have followed a similar developmental pattern as with recovery of embryos. Surgical transfer was developed first; nonsurgical transfer, later.

Surgical and Nonsurgical Transfer

Different techniques have been successfully applied for the actual process of transferring embryos surgically. The original method for embryo transfer in cattle, sheep, and goats required general anesthesia and a midline laparotomy to expose the reproductive tract of the recipient. More recently, many centers have begun transferring embryos using a para-

lumbar incision under local anesthesia, and there appears to be no significant difference in success rates between these two methods. In either case, the uterine horn ipsilateral to the corpus luteum is exteriorized through the abdominal incision, and a probe or the blunt end of a suture needle is used to puncture the uterine wall. A small quantity of medium containing the embryo or embryos to be transferred is taken up into a slender glass pipet, and after insertion of the pipet into the uterine lumen, the embryos are gently expelled. Before expulsion of the embryos, one must be certain that the tip of the pipet is indeed in the lumen, rather than in the subendometrial tissues.

Embryo transfer in the sow is carried out in a similar fashion, and several embryos are transferred to each recipient. Since transuterine migration of embryos readily occurs in the sow, all the embryos can be transferred to one uterine horn.

Surgical transfer of embryos in the mare has been performed basically as outlined for cattle. Work on embryo transfer in dogs and cats has been extremely limited and only a small number of offsprings have been obtained by embryo transfer in these species.

Perhaps more work has been done to develop a successful system for non-surgical transfer of embryos in cattle than was done for the development of nonsurgical recovery. Initially, success rates following nonsurgical transfer were disappointing. This lack of success was thought to be due to stimulation of uterine contractions as a consequence of invading the cervix. However, many groups have now reported a high pregnancy rate using transcervical transfer of embryos in the cow. Straws, such as those for freezing semen, are used to carry the embryos through the cervix to be deposited into the uterine lumen. A similar technique has been used successfully in mares, but the rate of success in this species is lower than with surgical transfer. Nonsurgical transfer also requires considerable skill and experience, but if done correctly, pregnancy rates are similar to those achieved with surgical transfer. Today, most commercial bovine embryo transfer centers utilize non-surgical transfer, because it entails fewer personnel, less time and expenses, and can be conducted on the farm.

Regardless of method of transfer, one of the primary factors affecting *success* in transferring embryos is the degree of *estrous cycle synchrony between donor and recipient.* In cattle and sheep, in which the bulk of the work with embryo transfer has been done, it has been clearly demonstrated that the highest degree of success is achieved when the donor and recipient are in estrus at the same time or within one-half day of each other. When normal embryos are transferred to synchronous recipients, 60 to 70% of the recipients usually become pregnant. Pregnancy rates decline, although not drastically, if the recipient is out of synchrony with the donor by one day. However, asynchrony of greater than one day results in a substantial reduction in pregnancy rates and virtually no pregnancies result from transfers made between animals out of synchrony by more than 2 days.

Synchronization and Induction of Estrus

Reliable methods for the artificial regulation of the estrous cycle have long been sought for the purpose of increasing productivity and decreasing costs in food-producing animals. The widespread application of artificial insemination to cattle, and more recently to other species, has prompted interest in developing methods for the artificial regulation of estrous cycles in order to inseminate maximal numbers of animals on a single day. Methods that were first developed often resulted in acceptable synchronization of estrus, but were associated with poor fertility at the first post-synchronization insemination. Techniques are now available to predictably alter the time of estrus within the breeding season (estrus synchronization) and to induce estrus during periods of anestrus (estrus induction), while maintaining a high level of fertility. Two basic approaches are used for synchronization of estrus: (1) administration of prostaglandins to cause regression of the corpus luteum, with a subsequent return to estrus; or (2) adminis-tration of progesterone, or more commonly synthetic progestins, to temporarily suppress ovarian activity while the animals are under treatment. Table 19-13 shows commonly used treatments for synchronization of estrus in domestic animals.

Prostaglandin-induced synchronization treatments were based on the finding that $PGF_{2\alpha}$ was luteolytic in several species. Several synthetic analogues of $PGF_{2\alpha}$ have been developed which have greater potency and in some cases fewer undesirable side effects than $PGF_{2\alpha}$. It is important to keep in mind that pregnant animals will often abort upon treatment with prostaglandins. Moreover, these agents are effective only in animals with a functional corpus luteum. Because of this requirement, prostaglandins are ineffective for estrous synchronization in animals that are not cycling due to age, poor nutrition, postpartum or lactational anestrus, or other causes.

In cattle, $PGF_{2\alpha}$ is effective in causing luteolysis only between days 5 and 16 of the estrous cycle. Synchronization of estrus can be induced by a single injection of $PGF_{2\alpha}$, but when a large group of cows is to be synchronized, a "double injection" schedule, with treatments 10 to 12 days apart, is often used. In this program, the first $PGF_{2\alpha}$ injection causes luteolysis and induces return to estrus in those cows that are in the stage of the cycle between days 5 and 16. At the time of the second injection, all cows should have a functional corpus luteum which can then be induced to regress. Synchronization treatments with $PGF_{2\alpha}$ in cattle are successful and are accompanied in most instances by good fertility. The luteolytic dose of $PGF_{2\alpha}$ in the cow is dramatically influenced by route of administration. Intrauterine instillation of only a small fraction of the dose required for subcutaneous or intramuscular injection will induce luteolysis. However, intrauterine treatment may be followed by uterine infection, if administration is not done aseptically. Synchronization of estrus with prostaglandins in sheep and goats during the breeding season is similar to that in cattle.

Table 19-13 Methods for Synchronization of Estrus in Farm Animals

Species	Treatments	Interval to Estrus
Cattle	20–30 mg $PGF_{2\alpha}$* by intramuscular injection on any day from 5 to 16 of the estrous cycle	2–4 days after $PGF_{2\alpha}$
	5 mg $PGF_{2\alpha}$ by intrauterine infusion on any day from 5 to 16 of the estrus cycle	2–3 days after $PGF_{2\alpha}$
	30 mg $PGF_{2\alpha}$ by intramuscular injection twice, 10 days apart, without regard to stage of the cycle	2–4 days after second injection of $PGF_{2\alpha}$
	Subcutaneous implant containing 6 mg SC2 1009[†] combined with an intramuscular injection of 3 mg SC21009 plus 5 mg estradiol valerate; implant removed in 9–14 days	24–52 hours after withdrawal of progestin
Sheep and Goats[§]	12.5 mg progesterone in oil daily for 16 days by intramuscular injection	1–3 days after last progesterone injection
	10–15 mg $PGF_{2\alpha}$ by intramuscular injection on any day from 5–14 of the estrous cycle	1–3 days after $PGF_{2\alpha}$
	Sponge containing 20 mg flurogestone acetate placed in the vagina for 16 to 20 days; intramuscular injection of 500 IU PMSG and 500 IU hCG at the time of sponge withdrawal	1–2 days after sponge removal
Swine	100 mg methallibure[‡] orally in feed daily for 20 days	2–4 days after cessation of feeding progestin
	100 mg methallibure[‡] orally in feed daily for 16 to 25 days; 1000–1500 IU PMSG on the day after last feeding of methallibure, followed in 96 hours by 500–1000 IU hCG	1–2 days after hCG

Data from Christenson, R. K., et al.: J. Anim. Sci. *36*:914, 1973; Cullen, R., et al.: Vet. Rec. *83*:10, 1968; Dhindsa, D. S., et al.: J. Anim. Sci. *32*:301, 1971; Gordon, I.: Proc. Br. Soc. Anim. Prod. *4*:79, 1975; Hafs, H. D., et al.: J. Anim. Sci. Suppl., 1, *30*:10, 1974; King, G. J., and Robertson, H. A.: Theriogenology *1*:123, 1974; Roche, J. F.: J. Reprod. Fertil, *37*:135, 1974; Webel, S. K., et al.: J. Anim. Sci. *30*:79, 1970; Wishart, D. F., and Young, I. M.: Vet. Rec. *95*:503, 1974.
* THAM salt of prostaglandin $F_{2\alpha}$.
† 17α-acetoxy-11β-methyl-19-nor-preg-4-ene-20, dione.
‡ 1α-methylallylthiocarbamoyl-2-methylthiocarbamoyl-hydrazine, ICI 33828.
§ Treatments for animals during the breeding season.

In the cycling sow, $PGF_{2\alpha}$ effectively induces luteolysis, but only on days 11 and 12 of the estrous cycle, which is very close to the time at which natural luteal regression takes place. Therefore, it is not practical to use prostaglandins to synchronize estrus in the normally cycling sow. However, the use of prostaglandins for estrous synchronization becomes practical and effective if the cycling sow is first treated with estrogens to prolong the lifespan of the corpora lutea or when gilts or sows are treated with gonadotropins to induce accessory corpora lutea. Estrus can also be synchronized in mated sows by inducing abortion with prostaglandins during early gestation, with good post-abortion rates of conception.

The corpus luteum of the mare is sensitive to $PGF_{2\alpha}$-mediated luteolysis after approximately day 5 of diestrus, and synchronization with normal fertility can be induced by administration of small doses of $PGF_{2\alpha}$. Groups of mares can be synchronized by a "double injection" schedule with $PGF_{2\alpha}$ treatments given 14 days apart. HCG is given 6 days after each treatment with $PGF_{2\alpha}$ to induce and synchronize ovulation in mares that returned to estrus after treatment with $PGF_{2\alpha}$. Prostaglandin treatment also appears to be of benefit in the treatment of anestrus in the nonpregnant mare due to a persistent corpus luteum. Horses are more susceptible to the side effects of $PGF_{2\alpha}$, such as sweating and colic; these are less of a problem with some of the prostaglandin analogues than with $PGF_{2\alpha}$ itself.

Synchronization of estrus by treatment with progestins is based on the finding that progestins suppress follicular activity by preventing release of gonadotropins from the pituitary. If treatment is continued for a period equal to or longer than the life span of the corpus luteum, all progestin-treated animals should have regressed corpora lutea at the end of treatment. Thus, follicular growth is reinitiated in a relatively synchronous manner upon withdrawal of the progestin treatment. Several routes of administration are available: oral administration in feed, daily injections, vaginal pessaries, and subcutaneous implants. Several of the schedules for synchronization of estrus with progestins also involve administration of estrogens at the termination of progestin treatment.

In cattle, the most successful programs for synchronization of estrus with progestins have utilized subcutaneous implants. Implants are also used in sheep, but pessaries are perhaps in more widespread use. Estrus and ovulation can be induced during the nonbreeding season in sheep and goats through treatment with gonadotropin, generally PMSG, in combination with progestin and withdrawal. In cycling sows, oral administration of progestins, such as Altrenogest, results in effective synchronization of estrus.

Relatively little research has been devoted to the induction or synchronization of estrus in dogs and cats. Attempts to induce estrus in anestrous bitches with exogenous gonadotropins frequently fail. At best, the results are erratic and unpredictable (see Chapter 16). Follicular growth can be induced in the queen by treatment with PMSG or FSH, and many of these queens come into a fertile estrus. As in naturally cycling queens, seasonal influences play a role in natural or artificial induction of estrus. Administration of estrogen and testosterone has also been reported to induce behavioral estrus in the queen, but fertility following these treatments has not been adequately investigated.

Treatments for synchronization of estrus are used in embryo transfer programs for the regulation of the estrous cycles of both the donors and recipients. An almost universal practice in programs for the transfer of bovine embryos is to combine superovulation induced by gonadotropins and estrous synchronization induced by prostaglandins. There are two major reasons for this practice. First, in programs in which embryos are recovered from a significant number of donors, it is advantageous to be able to reliably schedule when each donor will be collected, both for the sake of convenience and for optimal use of the recipient herd. Secondly, induced luteolysis allows more consistent superovulation and has been shown to result in the recovery of more transferable embryos than from gonadotropin treatment alone. As an example, a typical regimen for inducing superovulation without prostaglandin treatment is to inject FSH 4 to 5 days before the anticipated onset of estrus. Without artificial control of luteal regression, cows will return to estrus anytime between 1 and 10 days after FSH treatment. This results in either a short or an extended period of superovulation for many of the cows; as a consequence, the recovery of transferable embryos is reduced. Embryo recovery in sheep is also commonly carried out with donors that have been synchronized by either progestin or prostaglandin treatment. In mares, estrus is commonly synchronized either by feeding oral progestins or by parenteral administration of progesterone and estradiol. Superovulation and embryo recovery in wild ruminants, an area only recently explored, is an endeavor in which synchronization of estrus of the donor is mandatory because of the difficulty in detecting estrus in these animals.

Synchronization of estrus in the recipients of a large embryo transfer program is used to a lesser extent than the synchronization for donors. When dealing with large numbers of recipients, the costs of labor and drugs for repeated synchronization of estrus can become prohibitory. In addition, the high degree of variability in the number of embryos recovered causes many of the synchronized recipients to go unused, and when large numbers of embryos are recovered, not enough recipients may be synchronized. However, estrous synchronization of recipients can be a useful tool in small programs of embryo transfer when limited numbers of embryos are to be recovered or when the owner of the donor desires to use his own recipients.

OTHER APPLICATIONS OF TECHNOLOGY RELATED TO EMBRYO TRANSFER

In Vitro Fertilization

In vitro fertilization is the process by which mature oocytes are fertilized outside the female; the resulting embryos are then transferred back to the same or different females for development to term. Oocytes are collected by flushing the oviducts shortly after ovulation or by aspiration of preovulatory follicles. Follicular aspiration can be done by laparoscopy, which avoids some of the disadvantages of major abdominal surgery. Follicular oocytes are generally not yet mature at the time of aspiration, and must be cultured for a period of time prior to fertilization to allow nuclear maturation. Sperm must be capacitated before they are capable of fertilizing the oocyte, although this process appears to be less stringent in some species (cattle) compared to others (rabbits). Capacitation can be achieved either by recovering spermatozoa from another inseminated female or by incubation for several hours in the appropriate "capacitation medium." Fertilization occurs several hours after mixing cultured oocytes and capacitated spermatozoa, and the resulting embryos are generally cultured *in vitro* for a period of time before transfer back to the recipient. *In vitro* fertilization has resulted in offspring from cattle, sheep, and swine, but the rate of success in terms of live births is still quite low. As techniques for oocyte maturation and *in vitro* fertilization of gametes from domestic animals become more successful, there will be numerous applications for this technology. Many more offspring could be obtained from females with certain types of acquired infertility, such as periovarian adhesions. Frozen semen from valuable males, which may be long dead, could also be utilized much more efficiently. *In vitro* fertili-

zation may also become a commonly used technique for assessing the fertility of both male and female gametes. Finally, fertilization in vitro may be a valuable adjunct technology in efforts to apply genetic engineering techniques to domestic animals.

Control of Disease Transmission

Many genetically valuable animals are isolated and restricted from international trade because of the risk of transmitting infectious diseases. Also, a large number of animals, particularly swine, are maintained in specific pathogen-free, closed herds that eventually require the introduction of new genetic material. Today, livestock germ plasm can be dispersed by movement of live animals, semen, or embryos. Of these procedures, transfer of embryos appears to be the one that offers the least risk of transmitting agents causing infectious diseases. There are several arguments to support this contention: (1) Early embryos at the stages used for embryo transfer appear to be relatively resistant to viral infection because the zona pellucida that encases them has been shown to prevent contact with most, but not all classes of viruses. (2) If viruses were present in the maternal environment, the embryo and thus the medium used to recover them, would also be contaminated with the viruses. However, the standard procedure of washing the embryos several times in sterile medium prior to transfer would serve to greatly diminish the quantity of infectious agent present, probably to a level that would not establish an infection in the recipient. (3) Embryos can be frozen and the transfer postponed until sufficient time has elapsed to assure that the donor was not in the incubation stage of a particular disease at the time of embryo recovery. A limited number of studies have indicated that embryos can be recovered and transferred from animals infected with viruses such as those causing bovine leukemia, bluetongue, pseudorabies and bovine rhinotracheitis, without transmission of these agents to either the embryo or the recipient. Many more trials will have to be conducted to conclusively prove that embryo transfer is virtually free of the danger of transmitting a given disease.

Embryo Transfer in Exotic and Endangered Species

Many animal species are now endangered or extinct in their native habitats, with only small populations residing in zoos. Reproductive management in captivity is thus of critical importance in attempts either to prevent extinction or to return populations of the animals to the wild. Recently, embryo transfer techniques have successfully been applied to several species of exotic animals. As with embryo transfer in domestic animals, the goal of this work is to maximize the reproductive performance of a valuable female (the endangered animal) by superovulation and transfer of her embryos to less valuable recipients. The recipients, in this case, are from a different species that is not threatened or is less endangered. In most exotic species, there is a relative paucity of data concerning basic reproductive physiology, which makes successful embryo transfer particularly challenging.

Intergeneric transfer of embryos has been unsuccessful in a number of attempts. Often, as is seen with goat-sheep transfer, the transferred embryo develops normally for a time, but then, as the placenta begins to develop,

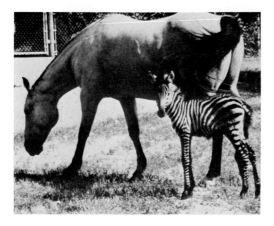

Fig. 19-7. Grant's zebra carried to term after transfer of the embryo to a domestic mare (courtesy of the Louisville Zoo, Louisville, KY).

the fetus is resorbed or aborted. In certain instances, a recipient from one genus can carry the fetus of another genus to term if the transferred embryo is chimeric (see below). Transfer between different species in the same genus has been much more successful. Thus, recipient elands have given birth to bongo antelopes, domestic mares to donkeys and zebras (Fig. 19-7), a domestic cow to a gaur and domestic ewes to mouflon sheep. Many other possibilities exist for interspecific embryo transfer of exotic animals and this technique will certainly be utilized more extensively in the future.

Production of Identical Multiplets and Chimeras

A recent advance in technology to manipulate embryos is the ability to reliably produce identical twins by splitting embryos. It has long been known that the cells of the early embryo are totipotent; that is, if one blastomere of a two-cell embryo is destroyed, the other blastomere can continue to develop to a normal adult. If, instead of destroying one blastomere, the two blastomeres are separated and allowed to develop independently, identical twins can result. Separation of blastomeres has resulted in the production of identical twin, triplet, and quadruplet lambs. A more common practice, and one that is used commercially, is to surgically divide a morula or early blastocyst into two parts, and then transfer both half-embryos (demi-embryos) to one or preferably two recipients. The microsurgical dissection of the embryo is conducted under the microscope with the aid of a micromanipulator, an instrument that translates relatively large movements of the operator's hands into small movements of the microsurgical tool. In cattle, this seemingly crude technique works remarkably well and, in many cases, 50 to 65% of the half-embryos develop into calves (Fig. 19-8). Embryo splitting is an extremely valuable tool for producing identical twins for research studies. Commercial interest in this technique occurs not only because it produces identical twins, but also because it allows pregnancy rates to exceed

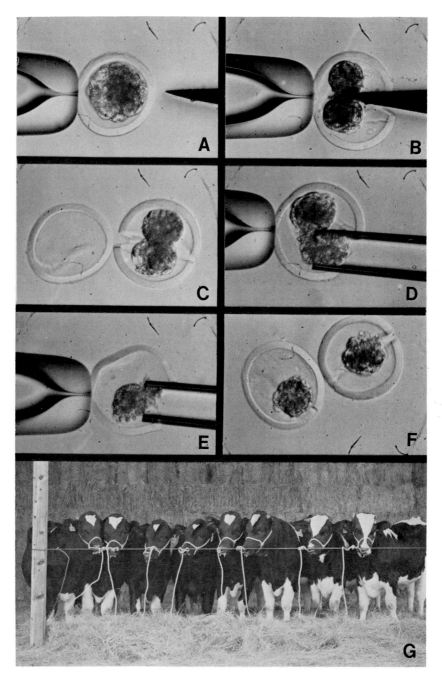

Fig. 19-8. Procedure for producing identical twin calves by bisecting embryos. A, Early blastocyst held by suction pipet; B, Bisection of embryo; C, Bisected embryo and empty surrogate zona pellucida; D, Removal of the demi-embryo from original zona pellucida; E, Placement of demi-embryo into surrogate zona pellucida; F, Two demi-embryos ready for transfer; G, four pairs of identical twin Holstein bulls produced by embryo splitting (courtesy of G. E. Seidel, Jr. and R. P. Amann, Colorado State University).

100%. If 60% of these half embryos develop into calves, then each original embryo will yield 1.2 calves, whereas with transfer of intact embryos, one can rarely expect more than a 75% pregnancy rate. A number of interesting applications exist with embryo splitting. For example, one-half of the split embryo can be frozen while the other is transferred, and then, if the transferred embryo has an outstanding phenotype as an adult, the twin can be thawed to double that genetic material.

If whole embryos or blastomeres from different embryos are combined instead of being split, a chimeric embryo is formed which can often develop into a viable offspring after transfer. Chimeras can be produced by combining blastomeres from two or more cleavage-stage embryos in a common zona pellucida or by microinjecting blastomeres or an inner cell mass from one embryo into the blastocoel of another embryo. If cells from each original embryo survive and populate the resulting fetus, the offspring is said to be a chimera. This technique has proven to be extremely valuable in a number of research settings. Because each chimeric animal is unique and not reproducible by breeding, production of chimeras has limited commercial potential. However, one possible application of the chimeras is to allow successful intergeneric embryo transfers. As mentioned above, when embryos from one genus are transferred to recipients of another genus, the embryos almost inevitably fail to develop to term. This incompatibility can be circumvented by making chimeras with embryos from the two different genera. If chimeric sheep-goat embryos are produced such that the placenta is derived exclusively from sheep cells and the fetus from goat cells, a recipient ewe can give birth to a normal goat kid.

Production of Transgenic Animals

One of the most exciting recent developments in embryo transfer technology and genetic engineering involves transferring a selected gene into embryos so that the resulting offspring carry and express that gene later in life. This procedure, like embryo splitting, is conducted with the aid of a micromanipulator. The solution containing the DNA sequence of interest is drawn into a fine pipet and a small volume is injected into one of the pronuclei of the recently fertilized oocyte. In some of these microinjected embryos, the introduced DNA will become integrated into the genome of the embryo, and because the DNA was introduced at the one-cell stage, the gene will be present in each of the cells of the resulting offspring. Animals that carry a copy of a foreign gene are referred to as transgenic. In a now classical demonstration of this technique, the gene for growth hormone was isolated from rats, linked to the regulatory sequences from another gene, and then was introduced into the pronuclei of mouse embryos. In some of those embryos, the rat gene was integrated into the mouse's genome and the transgene was expressed in large quantities after birth, leading to "giant mice" that displayed rapid growth and a large body size. The prospect of engineering strains of domestic livestock that display rapid growth, resistence to disease or other desirable characteristics is obviously of great interest. To date, growth hormone-transgenic pigs, sheep, and rabbits have been born, but accelerated growth has not been observed. The technology for producing transgenic animals, still in its infancy, has already contributed substantially to our understanding of gene expression. Much more work will be required before this technology has a practical impact on animal agriculture.

REFERENCES

1. Betteridge, K. J. (1981): A historical look at embryo transfer. J. Reprod. Fertil. *62:*1.
2. Bowen, R. A., Elsden, R. P., and Seidel, G. E., Jr. (1978): Embryo transfer for cows with reproductive problems. J. Am. Vet. Med. Assoc. *172:*1303.
3. Bradford, G. E., and Kennedy, B. W. (1980): Genetic aspects of embryo transfer. Theriogenology *13:* 13.
4. Brackett, B. G., Seidel, G. E., Jr., and Seidel, S. M. (Editors): (1981): New Technologies in Animal Breeding. New York, Academic Press.
5. Church, R. B., and Shea, B. F. (1977): The role of embryo transfer in cattle improvement programs. Can. J. Anim. Sci. *57:*33.
6. Cunningham, E. P. (1976): The use of egg transfer

techniques in genetic improvement. *In* Egg Transfer in Cattle, edited by L. E. A. Rowson. Luxembourg, EUR 5491, Commission of the European Communities, p. 345.

7. Land, R. B., and Hill, W. G. (1975): The possible use of superovulation and embryo transfer in cattle to increase response to selection. Anim. Prod. *21:*1.

8. Mapletoft, R. J., Johnson, W. H., and Miller, D. M. (1980): Embryo transfer techniques in repeat breeding cows. Theriogenology *13:*103.

9. Seidel, G. E. (1981): Superovulation and embryo transfer in cattle. Science *211:*351.

10. Van Vleck, L. D. (1981): Potential genetic impact of artificial insemination, sex selection, embryo transfer, cloning and selfing in dairy cattle. *In:* New Technologies in Animal Breeding, edited by B. G. Brackett, G. E. Seidel, Jr., and S. M. Seidel. New York, Academic Press, p. 221.

11. Whittingham, D. G. (1974): Embryo banks in the future of developmental genetics. Genetics *78:*395.

Superovulation in Adult Animals

12. Armstrong, D. T. and Evans, G. (1983): Factors influencing success of embryo transfer in sheep and goats. Theriogenology *19:*31.

13. Betteridge, K. J., Editor (1977): Embryo Transfer in Farm Animals. A Review of Techniques and Applications. Monograph 16, Canada Department of Agriculture, Station H, Ottawa K2H8P9, Canada, pp. 1, 37, 41.

14. Christenson, R. K., Pope, C. E., Zimmerman-Pope, V. A., et al. (1973): Synchronization of estrus and ovulation in superovulated gilts. J. Anim. Sci. *36:*914.

15. Donaldson, L. E. (1983): The effect of prostaglandin $F_{2\alpha}$ treatments in superovulated cattle on estrus response and embryo production. Theriogenology *20:*279.

16. Douglas, R. H. (1979): Review of induction of superovulation and embryo transfer in the equine. Theriogenology *11:*33.

17. Elsden, R. P., Nelson, L. D., and Seidel, G. E., Jr. (1978): Superovulating cows with follicle stimulating hormone and pregnant mare's serum gonadotrophin. Theriogenology *9:*17.

18. Greve, T. (1976): Egg transfer in the bovine: effect of injecting PMSG on different days. Theriogenology *5:*15.

19. Hasler, J. F., McCauley, A. D., Schermerhorn, E. C., et al. (1983): Superovulatory responses of Holstein cows. Theriogenology *19:*83.

20. Henricks, D. M., Hill, J. R., Jr., Dickey, J. F., et al. (1973): Plasma hormone levels in beef cows with induced multiple ovulations. J. Reprod. Fertil. *35:*225.

21. Hunter, R. H. F. (1966): Superovulation and fertility in the pig. Anim. Prod. *8:*457.

22. Imel, K. J., Squires, E. L., Elsden, R. P., et al. (1981): Collection and transfer of equine embryos. J. Am. Vet. Med. Assoc. *179:*987.

23. Killeen, I. D., and Moore, N. W. (1970): The effect of pregnant mare serum gonadotrophin and human chorionic gonadotrophin on ovulation and fertility in the ewe. Aust. J. Agric. Res. *21:*807.

24. Laster, D. B. (1973): Ovulation, fertility and prenatal mortality in heifers treated with PMSG or porcine FSH. J. Reprod. Fertil. *33:*275.

25. McIntosh, J. E. A., Moor, R. M., and Allen, W. R. (1975): Pregnant mare serum gonadotrophin: rate of clearance from the circulation of sheep. J. Reprod. Fertil. *44:*95.

26. Menino, A. R., Jr., and Wright, R. W., Jr. (1978): The influence of ovulation number and ovarian dimensions on embryo production in superovulated cattle. Theriogenology *9:*259.

27. Monniaux, D., Chupin, D., and Saumande, J. (1983): Superovulatory responses of cattle. Theriogenology *19:*55.

28. Moore, N. W. (1974): Multiple ovulation and ovum transfer in the goat. Proc. Aust. Soc. Anim. Prod. *10:*246.

29. Phillips, L. G., Simmons, L. G., Bush, M., et al. (1982): Gonadotropin regimen for inducing ovarian activity in captive wild felids. J. Am. Vet. Med. Assoc. *181:*1246.

30. Schneider, H. J., Jr., Castleberry, R. S., and Griffin, J. L. (1980): Commercial aspects of bovine embryo transfer. Theriogenology *13:*73.

31. Sreenan, J. M., and Beehan, D. (1976): Methods of induction of superovulation in the cow and transfer results. *In* Egg Transfer in Cattle, edited by L. E. A. Rowson. Luxembourg, EUR 5491, Commission of the European Communities, p. 19.

32. Wildt, D. E., Kinney, G. M., and Seager, S. W. J. (1978): Gonadotropin induced reproductive cyclicity in the domestic cat. Lab. Anim. Care *28:*301.

33. Willet, E. L., Buckner, P. J., and McShan, W. H. (1953): Refractoriness of cows repeatedly superovulated with gonadotrophins. J. Dairy Sci. *36:*1083.

34. Woods, G. L., and Ginther, O. J. (1983): Recent studies relating to the collection of multiple embryos in mares. Theriogenology *19:*101.

Superovulation in Prepubertal Animals

35. Woods, G. L., Scraba, S. T., and Ginther, O. J. (1982): Prospects for induction of multiple ovulations and collection of multiple embryos in the mare. Theriogenology *17:*61.

36. Baker, R. D., and Coggins, E. G. (1968): Control of ovulation rate and fertilization in prepuberal gilts. J. Anim. Sci. *27:*1607.

37. Baker, R. D., and Rajamahendran, R. (1973): Induction of estrus, ovulation, and fertilization in prepuberal gilts by a single injection of PMSG, HCG, and PMSG:HCG combination. Can. J. Anim. Sci. *53:*693.

38. Bedirian, K. N., and Baker, R. D. (1975): Follicular development, oocyte maturation and ovulation in gonadotrophin-treated prepuberal calves. Can. J. Anim. Sci. *55:*193.

39. Seidel, G. E., Jr., Larson, L. L., and Foote, R. H. (1971): Effects of age and gonadotropin treatment on superovulation in the calf. J. Anim. Sci. *33:*617.

40. Testart, J., and Arrau, J. (1973): Maturation ovocytaire apres stimulation folliculaire chez la genisse impubere. Ann. Biol. Anim. Biochim. Biophys. *13:*157.

41. Trounson, A. O., Willadsen, S. M., and Moor,

R. M. (1977): Reproductive function in prepubertal lambs: ovulation, embryo development and ovarian steroidogenesis. J. Reprod. Fertil. *49:*69.

Induction of Twinning

42. Anderson, G. B. (1978): Methods for producing twins in cattle. Theriogenology *9:*3.
43. Boland, M. P., Crosby, T. F., and Gordon, I. (1976): Birth of twin calves following a simple transcervical non-surgical egg transfer technique. Vet. Rec. *99:*274.
44. McCaughey, W. J., and Dow, C. (1977): Hormonal induction of twinning in cattle. Vet. Rec. *44:*29.
45. Pope, C. E., Christenson, R. K., Zimmerman-Pope, V. A., et al. (1972): Effect of number of embryos on embryonic survival in recipient gilts. J. Anim. Sci. *35:*805.
46. Rowson, L. E. A., Lawson, R. A. S., and Moor, R. M. (1971): Production of twins in cattle by egg transfer. J. Reprod. Fertil. *25:*261.
47. Sreenan, J. M., Beehan, D., and Mulvehill, P. (1975): Egg transfer in the cow: factors affecting pregnancy and twinning rates following bilateral transfers. J. Reprod. Fertil. *44:*77.

Recovery of Embryos

48. Brand, A., and Drost, M. (1977): Embryo collection by non-surgical methods. *In* Embryo Transfer in Farm Animals. A Review of Techniques and Applications, edited by K. J. Betteridge. Monograph 16, Canada Department of Agriculture, Station H, Ottawa K2H8P9, Canada, p. 16.
49. Day, B. N. (1979): Embryo transfer in swine. Theriogenology *11:*27.
50. Dziuk, P. J. (1971): Obtaining eggs and embryos from sheep and pigs. *In* Methods in Mammalian Embryology, edited by J. C. Daniel, Jr. San Francisco, W. H. Freeman and Co., p. 76.
51. Elsden, R. P., Hasler, J. F., and Seidel, G. E., Jr. (1976): Non-surgical recovery of bovine eggs. Theriogenology *6:*523.
52. Greve, T., Lehn-Jensen, H., and Rasbeck, N. O. (1977): Non-surgical recovery of bovine embryos. Theriogenology *7:*239.
53. Hunter, R. H. F., Polge, C., and Rowson, L. E. A. (1967): The recovery, transfer and survival of blastocysts in pigs. J. Reprod. Fertil. *14:*501.
54. Imel, K. J., Squires, E. L., Elsden, R. P., et al. (1981): Collection and transfer of equine embryos. J. Am. Vet. Med. Assoc. *179:*987.
55. Allen, W. R., Stewart, F., Trounson, A. O., et al. (1976): Viability of horse embryos after storage and long distance transport in the rabbit. J. Reprod. Fertil. *47:*387.
56. Anderson, G. B. (1978): Advances in large mammal embryo culture. *In:* Methods in Mammalian Reproduction, edited by J. C. Daniel, Jr. New York, Academic Press, p. 273.
57. Bilton, R. J., and Moore, N. W. (1976): *In vitro* culture, storage, and transfer of goat embryos. Aust. J. Biol. Sci. *29:*125.
58. Braden, A. W. H. (1964): The incidence of morphologically abnormal ova in sheep. Aust. J. Biol.

Sci. *17:*499.
59. Davis, D. L., and Day, B. N. (1978): Cleavage and blastocyst formation by pig eggs *in vitro.* J. Anim. Sci. *46:*1043.
60. Gardner, R. L., and Edwards, R. G. (1968): Control of the sex ratio at full term in the rabbit by transferring sexed blastocysts. Nature *218:*346.
61. Hare, W. C. D., and Betteridge, K. J. (1978): Relationship of embryo sexing to other methods of prenatal sex determination in farm animals: a review. Theriogenology *9:*27.
62. Holst, P. A., and Phemister, R. D. (1971): The prenatal development of the dog: preimplantation events. Biol. Reprod. *5:*194.
63. Hunter, R. H. F. (1974): Chronological and cytological details of fertilization and early embryonic development in the domestic pig, Sus scrofa. Anat. Rec. *178:*169.
64. Hunter, R. H. F. (1977): Physiological factors influencing ovulation, fertilization, early embryonic development and establishment of pregnancy in pigs. Br. Vet. J. *133:*461.
65. Lawson, R. A. S., Adams, C. E., and Rowson, L. E. A. (1972): The development of sheep eggs in the rabbit oviduct and their viability after retransfer to ewes. J. Reprod. Fertil. *29:*105.
66. Leibo, S. P. (1981): Preservation of ova and embryos by freezing. *In:* New Technologies in Animal Breeding, edited by B. G. Brackett, G. E. Seidel, Jr., and S. M. Seidel. New York, Academic Press, p. 127.
67. Lindner, G. M., and Wright, R. W., Jr. (1978): Morphological and quantitative aspects of the development of swine embryos *in vitro.* J. Anim. Sci. *46:*711.
68. Massip, A., Mulnard, J., Vanderzwalmen, P., et al. (1982): The behavior of cow blastocyst *in vitro.* Cinematographic and morphometric analysis. J. Anat. *134:*399.
69. Menino, A. R., Jr., and Wright, R. W., Jr. (1983): Effect of pronase treatment, microdissection, and zona pellucida removal on the development of porcine embryos and blastomeres in vitro. Biol. Reprod. *28:*433.
70. Moore, N. W., and Shelton, J. N. (1964): Egg transfer in the sheep. Effect of degree of synchronization between donor and recipient, age of egg, and site of transfer on the survival of transferred eggs. J. Reprod. Fertil. *7:*145.
71. Newcomb, R., and Rowson, L. E. A. (1975): Conception rate after uterine transfer of cow eggs in relation to synchronization of oestrus and age of eggs. J. Reprod. Fertil. *43:*539.
72. Renard, J. P., and Heyman, Y. (1979): Variable development of superovulated bovine embryos between day 6 and day 12. Ann. Biol. Anim. Biochim. Biophys. *19:*1589.
73. Shea, B. F. (1981): Evaluating the bovine embryo. Theriogenology *15:*31.
74. Tervit, H. R., Whittingham, D. G., and Rowson, L. E. A. (1972): Successful culture *in vitro* of sheep and cattle ova. J. Reprod. Fertil. *30:*493.
75. Trounson, A. O., Willadsen, S. M., Rowson, L. E. A., et al. (1976): The storage of cow eggs at room temperature and at low temperatures. J. Reprod. Fertil. *46:*173.

76. Wachtel, S. S. (1984): H-Y antigen in the study of sex determination and control of sex ratio. Theriogenology *21:*18.

77. White, K. L., Lindner, G. M., Anderson, G. B., et al. (1983): Cytolytic and fluorescent detection of H-Y antigen on preimplantation mouse embryos. Theriogenology *19:*701.

78. Whittingham, D. G., Leibo, S. P., and Mazur, P. (1972): Survival of mouse embryos frozen to −196° and −269°C. Science *178:*411.

79. Willadsen, S. M., Polge, C., Rowson, L. E. A., et al. (1976): Deep freezing of sheep embryos. J. Reprod. Fertil. *46:*151.

80. Willadsen, S. M., Polge, C., Rowson, L. E. A. (1978): The viability of deep frozen cow embryos. J. Reprod. Fertil. *52:*391.

81. Wilmut, I., and Rowson, L. E. A. (1973): Experiments on the low-temperature preservation of cow embryos. Vet. Rec. *92:*686.

82. Wright, J. M., (1985): Commercial freezing of bovine embryos in straws. Theriogenology *23:*17.

83. Wright, R. W., Jr., Anderson, G. B., Cupps, P. T., et al. (1976): Blastocyst expansion and hatching of bovine ova cultured *in vitro.* J. Anim. Sci. *43:*170.

Transfer of Embryos and Management of Recipients

84. Allen, W. R., and Rowson, L. E. A. (1973): Control of the mare's oestrous cycle by prostaglandins. J. Reprod. Fertil. *33:*539.

85. Allen, W. R., and Rowson, L. E. A. (1975): Surgical and non-surgical egg transfer in horses. J. Reprod. Fertil., Suppl. *23:*525.

86. Brand, A., Gunnink, J. W., Drost, M., et al. (1976): Non-surgical embryo transfer in cattle. II. Bacteriological aspects. *In* Egg Transfer in Cattle, edited by L. E. A. Rowson, Luxembourg, EUR 5491, Commission of the European Communities, p. 57.

87. Colby, E. D. (1970): Induced estrus and timed pregnancies in cats. Lab. Anim. Care *20:*1075.

88. Christenson, R. K., Pope, C. E., Zimmerman-Pope, V. A., et al. (1973): Synchronization of estrus and ovulation in superovulated gilts. J. Anim. Sci. *36:*914.

89. Cullen, R., Hovell, G. J. R., and Shearer, G. C. (1968): The control of oestrus and the effect on fertilization following progesterone treatment of ewes. Vet. Rec. *83:*10.

90. Del Campo, M. R., Rowe, R. F., Chaicharoen, D., et al. (1983): Effect of the relative locations of embryo and corpus luteum on embryo survival in cattle. Reprod. Nutr. Develop. *23:*303.

91. Dhindsa, D. S., Hoversland, A. S. and Metcalfe, J. (1971): Reproductive performance in goats treated with progestogen impregnated sponges and gonadotrophins. J. Anim. Sci. *32:*301.

92. Donaldson, L. E. (1977): Synchronization of oestrus in beef cattle artificial breeding programs using prostaglandin F$_{2\alpha}$. Aust. Vet. J. *53:*72.

93. Douglas, R. H. (1986): Equine embryo transfer. *In*: Current Therapy in Theriogenology 2, edited by D. A. Morrow. Philadelphia, W. B. Saunders Co., p. 70.

94. Gordon, I. (1975): Hormonal control of reproduction in sheep. Proc. Br. Soc. Anim. Prod. *4:*79.

95. Hafs, H. D., Louis, T. M., Noden, P. A., et al. (1974): Control of the estrous cycle with prostaglandin F$_{2\alpha}$ in cattle and horses. J. Anim. Sci. (Suppl.)1, *30:*10.

96. Hahn, J., and Hahn, R. (1976): Experiences with non-surgical embryo transfer techniques. *In* Egg Transfer in Cattle, edited by L. E. A. Rowson. Luxembourg, EUR 5491, Commission of the European Communities, p. 199.

97. Horton, M. B., Anderson, G. B., BonDurant, R. H., et al. (1986): Freemartins in beef cattle twins induced by embryo transfer. Theriogenology *14:*443.

98. Iuliano, M. F., Squires, E. L., and Cook, V. M. (1985): Effect of age of equine embryos and method of transfer on pregnancy rate. J. Anim. Sci. *60:*258.

99. King, G. J., and Robertson, H. A. (1974): A two injection schedule for the regulation of the ovulatory cycle in cattle. Theriogenology *1:*123.

100. Kraemer, D. C. (1983): Intra- and interspecific embryo transfer. J. Exp. Zool. *228:*363.

101. Kraemer, D. C., Flow, B. L., Schriver, M. D., et al. (1979): Embryo transfer in the non-human primate, feline and canine. Theriogenology *11:*51.

102. Lawson, R. A. S., Rowson, L. E. A., Moor, R. M., et al. (1975): Experiments on egg transfer in the cow and ewe: dependence of conception rate on the transfer procedure and stage of the oestrus cycle. J. Reprod. Fertil. *45:*101.

103. Loy, R. G., Pemstein, R., O'Canna, D., et al. (1981): Control of ovulation in cycling mares with ovarian steroids and prostaglandins. Theriogenology *15:*191.

104. Maurer, R. R., and Chenault, J. R. (1983): Fertilization failure and embryonic mortality in parous and nonparous beef cattle. J. Anim. Sci. *56:*1186.

105. Moore, N. W., Rowson, L. E. A., and Short, R. V. (1960): Egg transfer in sheep. Factors affecting the survival and development of transferred eggs. J. Reprod. Fertil. *1:*332.

106. Moore, N. W., and Shelton, J. N. (1964): Egg transfer in sheep. Effect of degree of synchronization between donor and recipient, age of egg, and site of transfer on the survival of transferred eggs. J. Reprod. Fertil. *7:*145.

107. Newcomb, R. (1979): Surgical and non-surgical transfer of bovine embryos. Vet. Rec. *105:*432.

108. Newcomb, R., and Rowson, L. E. A. (1980): Investigation of physiological factors affecting non-surgical transfer. Theriogenology *13:*41.

109. Newcomb, R., Christie, W. B., and Rowson, L. E. A. (1980): Fetal survival rate after the surgical transfer of two bovine embryos. J. Reprod. Fertil. *59:*31.

110. Oguri, N., and Tsutsumi, Y. (1974): Non-surgical egg transfer in mares. J. Reprod. Fertil. *41:*313.

111. Polge, C., and Day, B. N. (1968): Pregnancy following non-surgical egg transfer in pigs. Vet. Rec. *82:*712.

112. Pope, W. F., and First, N. L. (1985): Factors affecting the survival of pig embryos. Theriogenology *23:*91.

113. Pope, W. F., Maurer, R. R., and Stormshak, F.

(1982): Survival of porcine embryos after asynchronous transfer. Proc. Soc. Exp. Biol. Med. *171:* 179.

114. Roche, J. F. (1974): Synchronization of oestrus and fertility following artificial insemination in heifers given prostaglandin F$_{2\alpha}$. J. Reprod. Fertil. *37:*135.

115. Rowson, L. E. A., Lawson, R. A. S., Moor, R. M., et al. (1972): Egg transfer in the cow: synchronization requirements. J. Reprod. Fertil. *28:*427.

116. Schneider, H. J., Jr., Castleberry, R. S., and Griffin, J. L. (1980): Commercial aspects of bovine embryo transfer. Theriogenology *13:*73.

117. Squires, E. L., Stevens, W. B., McGlothlin, D. E., et al. (1979): Effect of an oral progestin on the estrous cycle and fertility of mares. J. Anim. Sci. *49:* 729.

118. Sreenan, J. M. (1975): Successful non-surgical transfer of fertilized cow eggs. Vet. Rec. *96:*490.

119. Thompson, C. K., and Fogwell, R. L. (1982): A paracervical method for non-surgical transfer of bovine embryos. Theriogenology *18:*629.

120. Tischner, M., and Bielanski, A. (1980): Non-surgical embryo collection in the mare and subsequent fertility of donor animals. J. Reprod. Fertil. *58:*357.

121. White, K. L., Lindner, G. M., Anderson, G. B., et al. (1982): Survival after transfer of "sexed" mouse embryos exposed to H-Y antisera. Theriogenology *18:*655.

122. Wilmut, I., Sales, D. I., and Ashworth, C. J. (1985): The influence of variation in embryo stage and maternal hormone profiles on embryo survival in farm animals. Theriogenology *23:*107.

Applications of Embryo Transfer

123. Allen, W. R. and Pasken, R. L. (1984): Production of monozygotic (identical) horse twins by embryo micromanipulation. J. Reprod. Fertil. *71:*607.

124. Ball, G. D., Leibfried, M. L., Lenz, R. W., et al. (1983): Factors affecting successful in vitro fertilization of bovine follicular oocytes. Biol. Reprod. *28:* 717.

125. Bowen, R. A., Howard, T. H., Elsden, R. P., et al. (1983): Embryo transfer from cattle infected with bluetongue virus. Am. J. Vet. Res. *44:*1625.

126. Brackett, B. G. (1983): A review of bovine fertilization in vitro. Theriogenology *19:*1.

127. Brackett, B. G., Bousquet, D., Boice, M. L., et al. (1982): Normal development following in vitro fertilization in the cow. Biol. Reprod. *27:*147.

128. Curnock, R. M., Day, B. N., and Dziuk, P. J. (1975): Embryo transfer in pigs: a method for introducing genetic material into primary specific-pathogen-free herds. Am. J. Vet. Res. *37:*97.

129. Dresser, B. L., Pope, C. E., Kramer, L., et al. (1985): Birth of Bongo antelope (Tragelaphus euryceros) to Eland antelope (Tragelaphus oryx) and cryopreservation of Bongo embryos. Theriogenology *23:*190.

130. Drost, M., Wright, J. M., and Elsden, R. P. (1986): Intergeneric embryo transfer between water buffalo and domestic cattle. Theriogenology *25:*13.

131. Durrant, B., and Benirschke, K. (1981): Embryo transfer in exotic animals. Theriogenology *15:*77.

132. Durrant, B. S., Oosterhuis, J. E., and Hoge, M. L. (1986): The application of artificial reproduction techniques to the propagation of selected endangered species. Theriogenology *25:*25.

133. Fehilly, C. B., Willadsen, S. M. and Tucker, E. M. (1984): Interspecific chimaerism between goat and sheep. Nature *307:*634.

134. Hammer, R. E., Pursel, V. G., Rexroad, C. E., et al. (1985): Production of transgenic rabbits, sheep and pigs by microinjection. Nature *315:*680.

135. Hare, W. C. D. (1984): Embryo transfer and disease transmission (An Overview): Proc. 10th Int. Cong. Anim. Reprod & AI. Univ. Illinois, Urbana-Champaign, Vol. IV, p. IX-1.

136. Kraemer, D. C. (1983): Intra- and interspecific embryo transfer. J. Exp. Zool. *228:*363.

137. Lambert, R. D., Sirard, M. A., Bernard, C., et al. (1986): In vitro fertilization of bovine oocytes matured in vivo and collected at laparoscopy. Theriogenology *25:*117.

138. Martin, P. A. (1983): Commercial embryo transfer in swine. Who is interested and why. Theriogenology *19:*43.

139. Meinecke-Tillmann, S., and Meinecke, B. (1984): Experimental chimaeras-removal of reproductive barrier between sheep and goats. Nature *307:*637.

140. Newcomb, R., Christie, W. B., and Rowson, L. E. A. (1978): Birth of calves after in vivo fertilization of oocytes removed from follicles and matured in vitro. Vet. Rec. *102:*461.

141. Seidel, G. E., Jr. (1982): Applications of microsurgery to mammalian embryos. Theriogenology *17:* 23.

142. Singh, E. L. and Hare, W. C. D. (1986): Embryo-pathogen interactions in relation to disease transmission. *In:* Current Therapy in Theriogenology 2, edited by D. A. Morrow. Philadelphia, W. B. Saunders Co., p. 84.

143. Wagner, T. E., Murray, F. A., Minhas, B., et al. (1984): The possibility of transgenic livestock. Theriogenology *21:*29.

144. Williams, T. J., Elsden, R. P., and Seidel, G. E. (1984): Pregnancy rates with bisected bovine embryos. Theriogenology *22:*521.

Index

Page numbers in italics indicate figures. Page numbers followed by a "t" refer to tables.